MEDICAL RADIOLOGY

Diagnostic Imaging

Springer
Berlin
Heidelberg
New York
Barcelona
Hong Kong
London
Milan
Paris
Tokyo

Armando Rossi · Giorgio Rossi

CT of the Peritoneum

Foreword by

A.E. Cardinale and A.L. Baert

With 425 Figures in 1418 Separate Illustrations, Some in Color

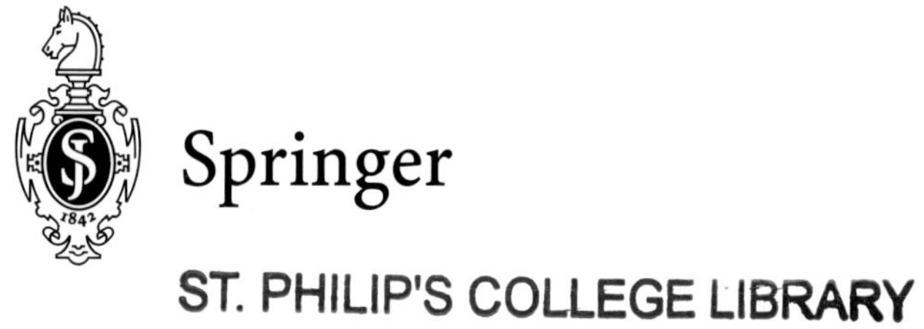

Springer

Armando Rossi, M.D.
Senior Researcher
Institute of Radiological Sciences
University of Parma
Via Gramsci 14
43100 Parma
Italy

Giorgio Rossi, M.D.
Supervisor of the Radiological Service
Local Health Unit (ASL)
Hospital of Fidenza
Via Borghesi 1
43036 Fidenza (Pr)
Italy

MEDICAL RADIOLOGY · Diagnostic Imaging and Radiation Oncology

Continuation of
Handbuch der medizinischen Radiologie
Encyclopedia of Medical Radiology

ISBN 3-540-41400-2 Springer-Verlag Berlin Heidelberg New York

Library of Congress Cataloging-in-Publication Data

Rossi, Armando, 1950–
[Tomografia computrizzaata del peritoneo. English]
CT of the peritoneum / Armando Rossi, Giorgio Rossi ; foreword by A.E. Cardinale and A.L. Baert.
p. ; cm. -- (Medical radiology)
Includes bibliographical references and index.
ISBN 3540414002 (alk. paper)
1. Peritoneum--Tomography. I. Rossi, Giorgio, 1952- II. Title. III. Series.
[DNLM: 1. Peritoneum--radiography. 2. Diagnostic Imaging. 3. Tomography, X-Ray Computed. WI575R831t2002a]
QM367.R6713 2002
617.5'5807572--dc21 2001020846

The Italian edition 'Tomografia compterizzata del peritoneo' was published by Athena Audiovisuals Publishing House, Modena, in 1999 (all rights reserved).

Drawings by Arch. M. L. Pusterla Cortesini

Springer-Verlag Berlin Heidelberg New York
a member of BertelsmannSpringer Science+Business Media GmbH

http://www.springer.de

Printed in Germany

Cover Design and Typesetting: Verlagsservice Teichmann, Mauer

SPIN: 107 908 27 21/3130 – 5 4 3 2 1 0 – Printed on acid-free paper

Foreword

I have not embarked on the foreword to this scientific monograph by Armando and Giorgio ROSSI in the expectation that it will be an easy task, because these two authors are the last remaining members of a family that has left its mark in the field of radiology in our country: therefore, the writer's enthusiasm and detachment could be jeopardized by memories of his own teachers and elders and the respect he still feels towards them.

The line stretches from Armando Rossi Sr., a pioneer in the field of radiology in Italy, a scientist and a versatile teacher, a student of Beclère and Busi, to Lucio Rossi, an eminent teacher, a learned man and a gentleman. An official biography of Armando Rossi shows that in his last years, his wide didactic interests were directed towards his own family, leading him to devote his attention to those of his grandchildren who were then getting ready to embrace the medical profession.

The passion and the pedagogic skills of this past master have left long-lasting signs, as is evident in the volume "Computed tomography of the peritoneum." This splendid book presents a complete and updated survey of diagnosis by means of CT of the peritoneum: this text is unique in the Italian radiology literature, because up to now this subject matter has been treated only patchily. This brilliant book is written with originality and with scrupulous accuracy, not without an organic and scholarly bent to synthesis in a field described up to now only in notes and not allocated more than small amounts of space.

A look through these pages immediately makes it obvious how profoundly the approach to diagnosis of the peritoneum has changed since the days of the traditional radiology taught to us by our teachers, and how CT has enriched our knowledge and extended the armamentarium at our disposal for dealing with diagnosis in this field.

The very rich graphic material and the large number of clinical cases on which this book is based are the fruits of long and patient work devoted to the collection, selection, and classification of clinical material and an in-depth analysis, all of which was certainly not done in a short time, also demonstrating the authors' profound competence. Indeed, it is this expertise that has permitted them to deal with difficult and sometimes complex arguments in a simple and comprehensible way.

The development of the text follows a logical and systematic scheme: the first part consists of four chapters that are essential for the understanding of what is presented later: "Normal Anatomy," "Physiology and Physiopathology of the peritoneum," "CT Study Techniques," and "CT Anatomy."

The second part comprises nine chapters dealing with a systematic discussion of primary and secondary pathology of the peritoneum. Particular emphasis is given to effusions and acute and chronic inflammatory processes. Then follows a careful, close examination of posttraumatic peritoneal and subperitoneal lesions in which CT, when associated with clinical and hemodynamic investigations, proves to be a technique of fundamental importance for selection of the treatment.

After an exhaustive examination of nonneoplastic pathologies, particular attention is given to the classification and evaluation of herniae; in these circumstances CT clarifies the nature and the characteristics of swellings in the abdominal wall and yields information that is valuable preoperatively. The book ends with an analysis of benign and malignant tumors of the peritoneum, which can originate from numerous embryonic structures.

Overall, the book is an up-to-date work with a very high cultural niveau, but nonetheless versatile and easy to read.

Particular care has been given to the selection and reproduction of the illustrations: these are unusual in their clarity, being presented with didactic insight and accompanied by informative legends.

Not only the clarity and the essential nature of the presentation but also the wealth of literature references – for use in any in-depth study – will recommend this volume selectively to specialists in the field. Such specialists will be able to adhere to balanced and specific indications in their use of CT and – while remaining within correct diagnostic protocols – will be able to complement CT with other methods to study the pathology of the peritoneum.

Older, and eminent students of Armando Rossi Sr. will recall his assertion that it is not possible to practice a profession well without loving it. This volume on CT of the peritoneum, a truly comprehensive treatise on this subject matter, demonstrates how a love of radiology has been transmitted "genetically" in this scientific family saga.

For all these reasons, I am pleased to record my appreciation of the authors, who have infused into this book the enthusiasm and expertise that have matured in the course of their daily work and research.

I hope the book will be well received by its readers and will be for them a source of satisfaction and of motivation towards increasingly earnestly desired and well-deserved scientific goals.

A. E. Cardinale

Foreword

The peritoneal cavity is an anatomical space involved in a large variety of medical and surgical conditions and has been the focus of much radiological research in the past.

The advent of cross-sectional imaging and more specifically of CT has, however, completely changed the approach of the radiologist to the different diagnosis and the management of many pathological conditions involving the peritoneum.

This volume presents the results of many years of innovative clinical research by the authors in the field of peritoneal pathology, which is covered in comprehensive fashion.

I sincerely hope that this book will meet the expectations of all those interested in updating their knowledge on the peritoneum. I am convinced it will be an excellent tool for the daily clinical work of the general and abdominal radiologist; in addition it merits the interest of abdominal surgeons, oncologists and gastroenterologists.

I wish this book the same success as the previous volumes in our series "Medical Radiology".

I welcome any constructive critism that might be offered.

Leuven

ALBERT L. BAERT

Preface

Even though many years have passed since the introduction of CT, few authors have dedicated themselves to the assessment of its systematic application in the study of the peritoneum.

Following both a family tradition and scholastic tradition, the almost life-long habit of interpreting radiological data on the basis of problems arising from clinical observations (with the collaboration of highly competent colleagues) has given us the incentive to systematically gather together the results of the observations we have made and of the teachings we have received in a single work.

It has been difficult, but extremely useful, to re-examine the numerous case studies and histories tested and monitored over so many years, to make a selection, to undertake an accurate evaluation of the results obtained in them and to compare our results with those published in the literature.

The data have been organized in two parts according to a general pre-established scheme: the first part is introductory, including information on the normal anatomy, physiology, physiopathology and CT anatomy of the peritoneum and of the subperitoneal spaces; the second part is dedicated to primary and secondary pathology of the peritoneum.

Agreat deal of attention was devoted to solutions to the wide range of problems that occur most frequently in daily practice or which sometimes overwhelm clinicians and radiologists because they are so difficult to solve and their solutions are so urgent: from the anatomical to the physiological study, from the functional to the inflammatory aspect, from the detection of the benign or malignant nature of tumoral forms and of their precise location and extension to the possibility of determining how they relate to organs and apparatuses before surgical operations and indicating what clinically silent complications may be encountered.

An accurate CT study of the abdominopelvic pathology, besides the pathology of the organ -- often already known from a simple echographic examination or through conventional radiological techniques -- should always assess the involvement of the peritoneum, the ligaments, the mesenteries, and the subperitoneal spaces; these elements often have a decisive role in the choice of the most suitable treatment.

The extensive bibliography contains reports from Anglo-Saxon, Asiatic and European authors.

Overall, we have tried to realize a simple, but thorough-going work, from which we hope practitioners will derive elements that will be useful and make for easier daily practice.

Parma

Armando Rossi · Giorgio Rossi

Contents

Abbreviations

Ligaments, Mesenteries and Fasciale

Supramesocolic

an retrohepatic bare area
ft transverse fascia
lco coronal ligament
led hepatoduodenal ligament
lf falciform ligament
lgc gastrocolic ligament
lge gastrohepatic ligament
lgs gastrosplenic ligament
lr round ligament
lt triangular ligament
mt transverse mesocolon

Submesocolic

flc lateroconal fascia
fov umbilicovesical fascia
fso supraumbilical fascia
o greater omentum
me mesentery
ma ascending mesocolon
md descending mesocolon
ms sigmoid mesocolon

Pelvic subperitoneal

ar ala recti
fp pelvic fascia
fpp prostatoperitoneal (Denonvilliers') fascia
lrc cardinal ligament
ll broad ligament
lov umbilicovesical ligament
lr round ligament
lsrgp sacro-recto-genito-pubic ligament
lus uterosacral ligament
lvr vesicorectal ligament
lvu vesicouterine ligament

Peritoneal Cavities

Supramesocolic

esr superior expansion of the lesser sac
re lesser sac
rgs gastrosplenic recess
rire inferior recess of the lesser sac
rM Morrison's recess
rps perisplenic recess
rses left subhepatic recess
rsp splenopancreatic recess
rsre superior recess of the lesser sac
rsves left suprahepatic recess
rvre vestibular recess of the lesser sac
ssed right subhepatic space
sses left subhepatic space
ssd right subphrenic space
sss left subphrenic space
W Winslow's foramen

Submesocolic

cmdc right inframesocolic cavity
cmcs left inframesocolic cavity
csme submesocolic cavity
dpd right paracolic gutter
dps left paracolic gutter

Pelvic

cpsd right parasigmoidal cavity
cpss left parasigmoidal cavity
cp pelvic cavity
fil lateral inguinal fossa
fim median inguinal fossa
rlv laterovesical recess
rpr pararectal recess
rrv retrovesical recess
rur uterorectal recess
rvr vesicouterine recess
ssv supravesical space

Abdominal Extraperitoneal Spaces

sov umbilicovesical space
spp preperitoneal space
srp suprapubic retromuscular space
sso supraumbilical space(umbilical canal)

Retroperitoneal Spaces

slc lateroconal space
spa anterior pararenal space
spp posterior pararenal space
sper perirenal space

Pelvic Subperitoneal Spaces

sper perirectal
spev perivesical
spr prerectal
spv prevesical
srl laterorectal
srr retrorectal
srv retrovesical

Arteries

A aorta
ACM middle colic
ACMA marginal colic
ACO left gastric or coronarostomachic
ACS left colic
AD duodenal
ADF inferior diaphragmatic
ADG jejunal
ADR Drummond's arcade
AE hepatic
AEP epiploic
AES superior hemorrhoidal
AGB short gastric
AGD gastroduodenal
AGE gastroepiploic
AI common iliac
AIC ileocolic
AIE external iliac
AII internal iliac
AMI inferior mesenteric
AMS superior mesenteric
APIDAI anteroinferior pancreatoduodenal
APDAS anterosuperior pancreatoduodenal
APDPI posteroinferior pancreatoduodenal
APDPS posterosuperior pancreatoduodenal
AR renal
ARIOL Riolan's arcade
AS splenic
ASI sigmoidal
TC celiac trunk
VaRe vasa recta

Pelvic arteries
AEI inferior epigastric
AES superior hemorrhoidal
AIC common iliac
AIE external iliac
AII internal iliac
AO obturator
AOV umbilicovesical
ASL lateral sacral
AUO utero-ovarian
AVD vesiculodeferential
AVI inferior vesical
AVS superior vesical

Veins

CI inferior cava
TP portal trunk
TVGC gastrocolic venous trunk
VCM middle colic
VCMA marginal colic
VCO left gastric
VCS left colic
VEP epiploic
VES superior hemorrhoidal
VGB short gastric
VGD gastroduodenal
VGE gastroepiploic
VIC ileocolic
VMI inferior mesenteric
VMS superior mesenteric
VO umbilical
VPCD paracolic or right marginal
VPCS paracolic or left marginal
VPDAI anteroinferior pancreatoduodenal
VPDAS anterosuperior pancreatoduodenal
VPDPI posteroinferior pancreatoduodenal
VPDPS posterosuperior pancreatoduodenal
VR renal
VS splenic
VSI sigmoidal

Pelvic veins
VEI inferior epigastric
VEM middle hemorrhoidal
VI common iliac
VIE external iliac
VII internal iliac
VSP spermatic
VSL lateral sacral
VUO utero-ovarian

Lymph Nodes

C	celiac
CD	right colic
CE	cecal
CI	cystic
CMA	marginal colic
CME	middle colic
CS	left gastric
CSI	left colic
D	duodenal
DI	jejunoileal
EMS	superior hemorrhoidal
EP	deep hepatic
ES	superficial hepatic
GED	right gastroepiploic
GES	left gastroepiploic
IC	ileocolic
IE	external iliac
II	internal iliac
ILC	common iliac
LA	lumboaortic
MC	mesocolic
MI	inferior mesenteric
MS	superior mesenteric
O	omental
P	pyloric
PA	pancreatic
PCA	anterior paracaval
PCP	posterior paracaval
PDA	anterior pancreatoduodenal
PDP	posterior pancreatoduodenal
R	renal
S	splenic
SC	supra- and subcardial
SI	sigmoidal
SP	splenopancreatic
UO	utero-ovarian
V	vesical
W	of the Winslow's foramen

Organs

C	colon
CA	ascending colon
CD	descending colon
CE	cecum
CO	gallbladder
CT	transverse colon
D	duodenum
DG	jejunum
F	liver
FDD	duodenojejunal flexure
FT	transverse fissure
I	ileum
LC	caudate lobe
M	spleen
O	ovary
P	pancreas
PL	pleura
PP	papilliferous process of the caudate lobe
R	rectum
RE	kidney
S	stomach
SI	sigmoid
T	small bowel
U	uterus
UR	ureter
V	urinary bladder (or vesica)
VE	seminal vesicles

Section 1

Introduction

1 Normal Anatomy

CONTENTS

1.1 Peritoneum, Ligaments and Peritoneal Cavity

1.1.1 Peritoneum

The peritoneum* is a thin continuous serous lamina that lines the wall of the abdominopelvic cavity; inside, it curves to surround the hollow viscera, the liver and the spleen and to give ligaments and mesenteries. All in all, the peritoneum limits and confines a wide and complex cavity: the *peritoneal cavity*.

The peritoneum is made up of two layers: a superficial stratum made of mesothelial cells and a deep connective stratum.

The *mesothelium* is characterized by a single layer of polygonal pavement epithelium (1–2 μm thick) lying on a thin and homogeneous limiting membrane. At the diaphragmatic and omental level, the continuity of the mesothelial layer is interrupted by microscopic fenestrations (Von Recklinghausen's stomata) 1–10 μm in diameter, which provide direct communications between the peritoneal cavity, the stromal framework and the diaphragmatic lymphatic structures.

The soft-fibrillated connective deep layer is made up of elastic collagen-reticular fibers; even though fibers are knotted and extend in all directions, their prevalent orientation is parallel to the surface. The deep layer is constituted of four strata: the tunica propria, the superficial elastic limiting stratum, the tela subserosa, and the deep elastic limiting stratum. The thickness of the parietal peritoneum is 100–150 μm, whereas the visceral peritoneum is 50–60 μm thick.

The peritoneum is composed of two parts: parietal and visceral.

The *parietal peritoneum* lines the walls of the abdominopelvic cavity; above, on the sides and anteriorly, it joins the transverse abdominal fascia, with the interposition of a connective, prevalently adipose, layer that is thin higher up and becomes thicker on the sides and anteriorly. At the lower levels it covers the urinary bladder, the seminal vesicles (in men), the uterus and the ovaries (in women) and the rectum. Posteriorly, it adheres to the anterior renal fascia, with the interposition of a thin adipose layer, reducing the pararenal space to a virtual compartment. However, at various levels the posterior parietal peritoneum moves away from the fascia to cover

From the Greek "το περιτονιον," a compound of the words "περι" = around and "τεινω" = stretch; it was utilized for the first time by Hippocrates (459 or 460/375 or 351 B.C.), and afterwards, by Aristotle (384/322 B.C.), Rufus from Ephesus (first century a.d.) Aulus Cornelius Celsus (first century A.D.), Claudius Galenus (129–201), Oribasius (325–403). The word was translated into Latin as "*peritoneum*" by Celius Aurelianus (fifth century) and was used by Andrea Vesalius (1510–1564), Spigelius, Julius Pollux and Rasarius. In the Middle Ages, besides the Latin terminology, the Arabian words "*Chamel,*" "*Ziphac,*" and "*Sifac*" (Mondino de' Luzzi 1270–1326) were used. The Latin term was translated into Italian as "Peritoneo" by Della Chiesa in 1574. In the English language, the medieval Latin word "*peritoneum*" was retained

the second and third duodenal portion and the pancreas or to constitute the inflexions of the mesenteries and ligaments, limiting the *subperitoneal spaces*, where the vasculonervous structures extend.

The *visceral peritoneum* originates from the parietal peritoneal inflexions toward the abdominal cavity, surrounding the parenchymatous organs (constituting the integrative part of the fibrous capsulae) and the hollow viscera (constituting the parietal serous leaf), connecting organs and fixing them to the abdominal wall through mesenteries and ligaments.

1.1.2 Ligaments and Mesenteries

The folds extending from the abdominal wall to the various segments of the digestive canal (small intestine, colon and sigmoid) are called *mesenteries*, while those extending from the wall to the parenchymatous organs or connecting different viscera are called *ligaments* (Table 1.1).

Table 1.1. Ligaments and mesenteries

Falciform ligament and round ligament
Coronary ligament and triangular ligaments
Phrenoesophageal and phrenogastric ligaments
Lesser omentum (gastrohepatic and hepatoduodenal ligaments)
Gastrosplenic ligament
Splenorenal or splenopancreatic ligament
Gastrocolic ligament
Transverse mesocolon
Phrenocolic ligament
Greater omentum
Mesentery
Ascending and descending mesocolon
Sigmoid mesocolon

The two serous leaves extending along ligaments and mesenteries are separated by the *subperitoneal spaces*, which contain adipose tissue, blood and lymphatic vessels and nerves for the intraperitoneal viscera. These subperitoneal spaces are closely connected and constitute a network of interconnections among the intraperitoneal viscera, and between viscera and retroperitoneum.

The *arterial and venous vascularization* of the peritoneum (with the exception of the omentum, which is nourished by numerous wide vascular branches) is relatively poor and is supported by underlying visceral and parietal vessels. There are two capillary networks: one is made up of a narrow reticulum within the serosal stroma, while the other is located into the subserosal connective layer; the networks communicate through very thin branches. In contrast, there is a rich lymphatic network in the visceral and parietal subserosa, draining the lymph into the regional lymph nodes, especially at the omental and subdiaphragmatic level. The rapid reabsorption of the peritoneal liquid is attributed to this rich lymphatic structure. Furthermore, through the diaphragm the parietal lymphatic network is connected to the pleural lymphatic system, whose collectors may drain the lymph into the anterior mediastinal (internal mammary) and the hilar pulmonary lymph nodes.

Topographically, three peritoneal regions are distinguishable: the supramesocolic, the mesocolic and the submesocolic.

Supramesocolic Region (Figs. 1.1, 1.2, 1.4). At the supramesocolic level and next to the median line, the parietal peritoneum lining the abdominal part of the right diaphragmatic cupula shows a long sagittal inflexion extending to the convex face of the liver. The two peritoneal leaves adhere, to make a thick septum: *the falciform ligament* or suspensory ligament of the liver (Figs. 1.1A, B, 1.2A–D, 1.4B), which extends from the longitudinal fissure backwards to the coronary ligament. After reaching the hepatic cupula, the two leaves bend at the sides (the external on the right and the medial on the left), to cover the superior face of the liver. Anteriorly, at the level of the longitudinal fissure between the IVth and IInd segments, the two leaves separate, opening up a space that varies in width in different subjects. It communicates directly with the preperitoneal space and with the umbilical canal, between the umbilicus and the transversalis fascia. The umbilical vein (in the fetus) and the *round ligament or ligamentum teres* (in the adult) (Fig. 1.4B, C) pass through this space along their extension from the left branch of the portal vein to the umbilicus. Next to these structures, there are some accessory portal branches and hepatic lymphatic collectors, extending (with the interposition of some lymphatic stations) to the periumbilical and internal mammary lymphatic centers.

At the level of the border anterior hepatis, the parietal peritoneum extends forward along the anterior abdominal wall and adheres tightly to the transversalis fascia on the right side; from this fascia, it is separated only by the interstice of the preperitoneal adipose areolar tissue. In contrast, the visceral peritoneum bends to the back to cover (from the front backwards) the inferior face of the bowel; at the level of the hilum, it folds downward, forming the *hepatoduodenal ligament* that extends on both sides of the hilar structures.

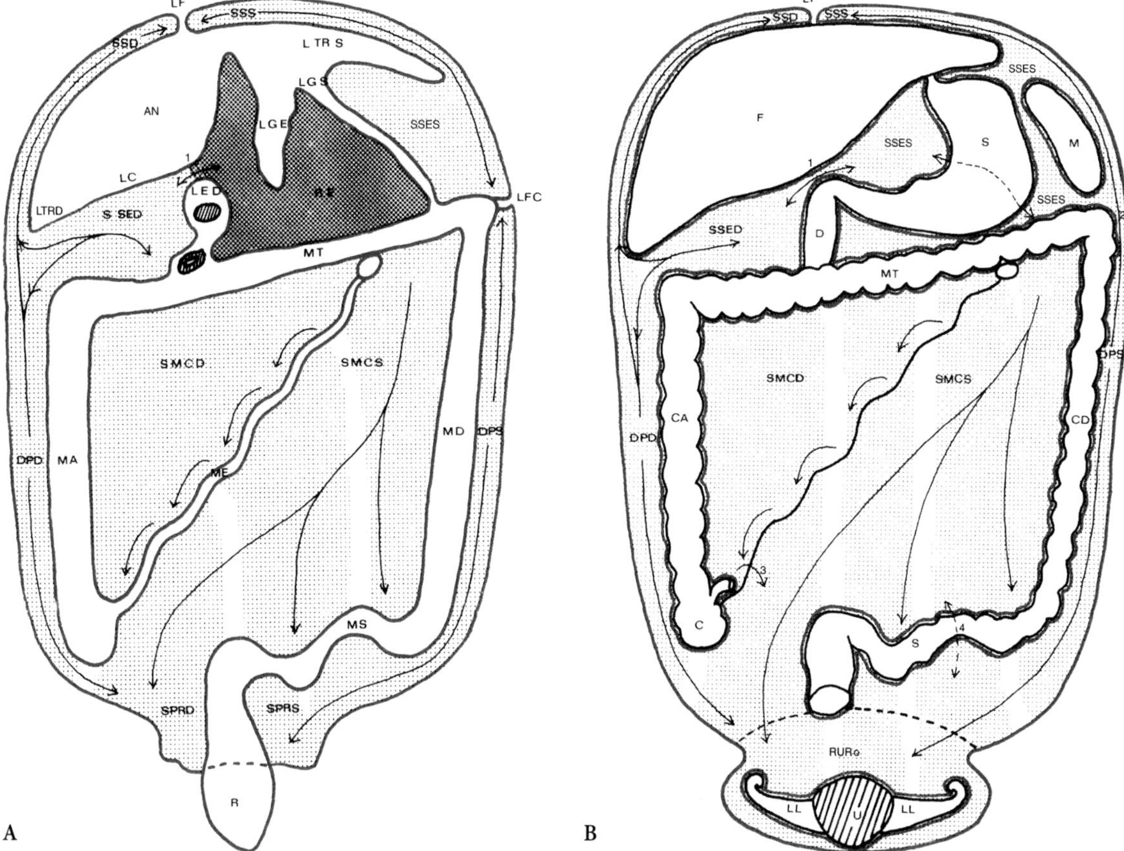

Fig. 1.1A,B. Schematic showing relative positions, in frontal section, of the posterior insertions of the ligaments and mesenteries and of the relationships and communications among spaces and recesses of the peritoneal cavity. **A** Posterior plane (ligamental insertion). At a high level, the sagittal disposition of the falciform ligament (*LF*) divides the right (*SSD*) from the left (*SSS*) subphrenic spaces. Under these spaces, the wide transverse retrohepatic bare area (*AN*), limited by the coronary (*LC*) and the triangular (*LTR*) ligaments and separating the suprahepatic from the subhepatic cavities, which communicate only on the sides. Under the bare area, the right subhepatic space (*SSED*),and the lesser sac (*RE*) which communicate through Winslow's foramen. The transverse line of the insertion of the transverse mesocolon (*MT*) divides the supramesocolic from the submesocolic cavities. On the left side, the phrenocolic ligament (*LFC*) separates the subhepatic space (*SSE*) from the paracolic gutter (*DPS*); on the right side, the supra- and submesocolic cavities communicate directly. The insertions of the ascending (*MA*) and descending (*MD*) mesocolon and the mesenteric root (ME) subdivide the submesocolic cavity in the right (*DPD*) and left (*DPS*) paracolic gutter and in the right (*SMCD*) and left (*SMCS*) inframesocolic spaces. In the pelvis, the approximately S-shaped oblique transverse insertion of the sigmoid mesocolon (*MS*) subdivides the submesocolic from the pelvic cavity; this latter cavity is represented by the right (*SPRD*) and left (*SPRS*) pararectal spaces. On either side of the sigmoid, these spaces communicate with overhanging spaces: the right paracolic gutter and the left inframesocolic spaces on the right side of the sigmoid mesocolon, the left paracolic gutter on the left side of the sigmoid mesocolon. **B** Anterior (perivisceral) plane. Direct communication between right (*SSED*) and left (*SSES*) subhepatic spaces (*1*), between the left subhepatic spaces (*SSES*) and left paracolic gutter (*DPS*) (*2*), between right (SMCD) and left (*SMCS*) inframesocolic spaces (*3*) and between the left inframesocolic space (*SMCS*) and pouch of Douglas (*4*). The peritoneum is colored red. The great cavity is *lightly dotted.* The lesser sac is *densely dotted.* The *arrows* indicate the flux of the peritoneal liquid and the communications among cavities conditioning the diffusion of collections or other pathologies through intraperitoneal pathways

At the level of the border posterior hepatis, the two leaves of the falciform ligament diverge in a rough T shape, continuing on both sides in the superior leaf of the coronary ligament.

Behind the liver, the diaphragmatic parietal peritoneum shows a double transverse inflexion; the superior inflexion joins the peritoneum that has covered the upper face of the bowel, whereas the inferior inflexion joins the peritoneum that has covered the lower face, forming the *coronary ligament* (Figs. 1.1A, 1.2A–D, 1.4A–C); this ligament fixes the posterior wall of the liver to the diaphragm.

A transverse lozenge-shaped tract of the posterior face of the liver, called the "*bare space*" or

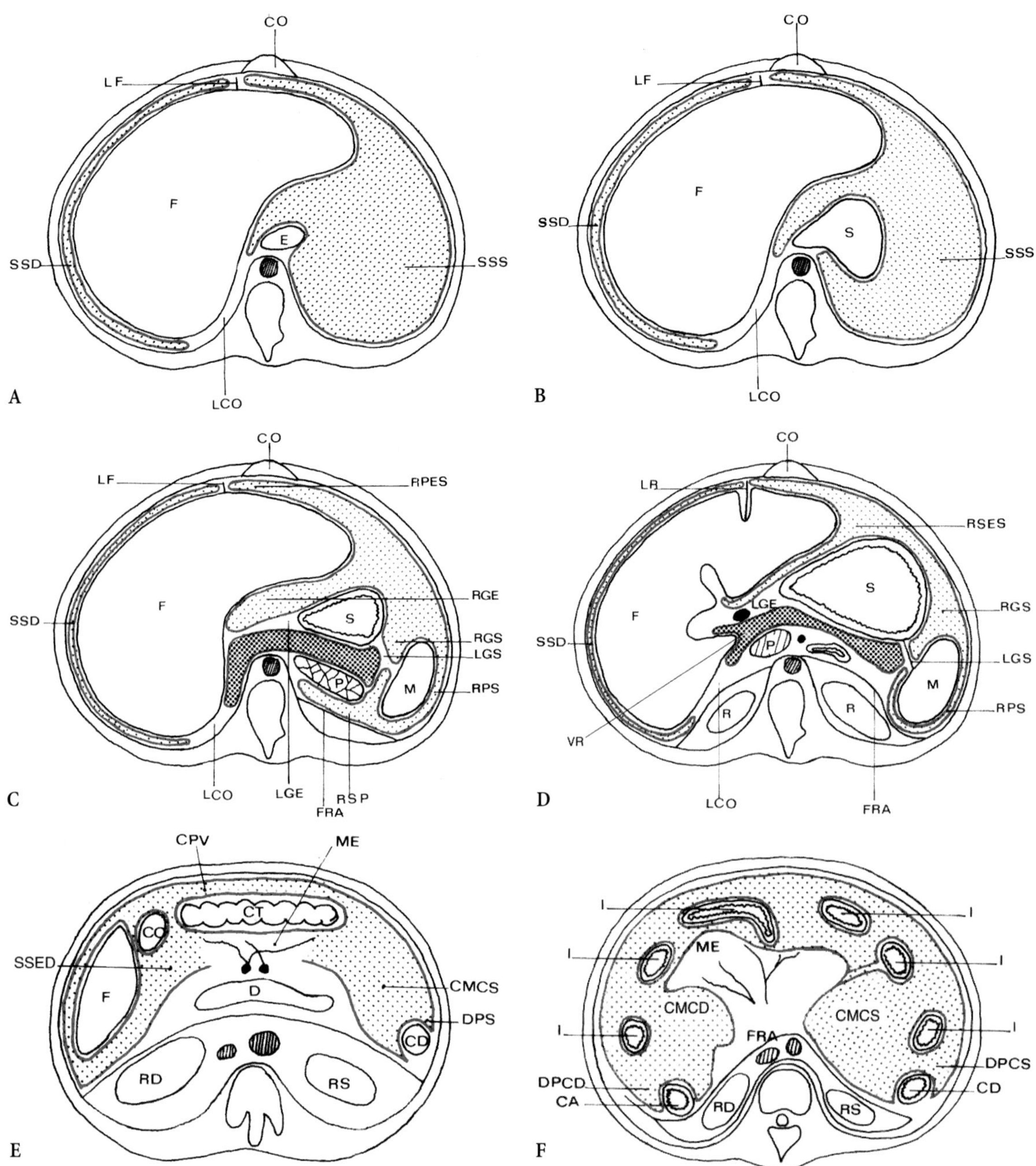

Fig. 1.2A–I. Schematic representations in transverse section of the relative positions of peritoneum, ligaments, peritoneal cavity and anterior renal fascia. **A** Superior plane: right (*SSD*) and left (*SSS*) subphrenic cavities divided by the falciform ligament (*LF*), retrohepatic bare space (coronary ligament) (*LCO*), and umbilical canal (*CO*). **B** Plane crossing the fundus ventriculi. **C** Plane crossing the cauda pancreatis and the splenic hilum: on the left side and on the median line, the prehepatic (*RPES*), gastrohepatic (*RGE*), gastrosplenic (*RGS*), splenopancreatic (*RSP*) and perisplenic (*RPS*) recesses. The lesser sac shows a transverse extension behind the stomach and the gastrohepatic ligament and in front of the pancreas and the retroperitoneum. **D** Plane crossing the hepatic hilum. The vestibular recess (*VR*) of the lesser sac shows a roughly V-shaped extension around the caudate lobe of the liver. Insertion of the gastrohepatic ligament (*LGE*) on the anterior border of the transverse fissure of the liver. **E** Plane crossing the inferior pole of the liver and the transverse mesocolon. On the *right*, the subhepatic space (*SSED*) completely surrounds the liver, without the interruptions of the coronary and falciform ligaments. **F** Umbilical plane: on the median line, the mesentery (*me*) separates the right (*CMCD*) and left (*CMCS*) inframesocolic cavities. On the sides, the prominence of the ascending (*CA*) and descending (*CD*) colon and of their mesenteries limits the right (*DPCD*) and left (*DPCS*) paracolic gutters. **G** Superior pelvic plane crossing the anterior iliac spines: disposition of the sigmoid (*S*) and of the right (*SPSD*)and left (SPSS) parasigmoidal spaces. Extraperitoneal spaces. **H** Middle pelvic plane (female) crossing the ovaries (*O*) and the fundus uteri (*U*); supravesical space (*SSV*) anteriorly and ureterorectal (*RUR*) with ovarian fossae (*FO*), retrouterine pouch or pouch of Douglas (*RUR*) and . . . → →

"bare area" (Fig. 1.1A) remains exposed between the two leaves of the ligament. This space is wider at the level of the inferior vena cava, whereas it becomes smaller on the sides where the leaves converge to blend in the *triangular ligaments* (Fig. 1.1A).

The disposition of the falciform and coronary ligaments subdivides the supramesocolic cavity into the right and left subphrenic spaces and separates both spaces from those located under the liver (Fig. 1.1A).

On the left, the parietal peritoneum covering the posterior face of the diaphragm under the coronary ligament shows an anterior inflection near the esophageal hiatus; then, it forms the two leaves covering the anterior and posterior surface of the abdominal esophagus (*phrenoesophageal ligament*) and of the stomach (*phrenogastric ligament*), respectively. These leaves continue on the two sides, under and behind the stomach, in the lesser omentum on the right (constituted by the gastrohepatic (Figs. 1.1A, 1.2C, D, 1.4C) and hepatoduodenal (Fig. 1.1A) ligaments), in the gastrocolic ligaments (Figs.1.3E, 1.4D) below and in the gastrosplenic ligament (Figs. 1.1A, 1.2C, D, 1.4D) posteriorly. These structures join the stomach to the other organs of the upper abdomen.

In particular, the continuation on the right of the two leaves covering the anterior and posterior walls of the stomach constitutes the *gastrohepatic ligament*, which joins the lesser curvature of the stomach and the subdiaphragmatic esophagus to the liver, and the *hepatoduodenal ligament*, which joins the liver to the second duodenal portion.

The superior portion of the lesser omentum is deeply inserted on the two rims of the transverse fissure of the liver (Fig. 1.2D), and below, on the second duodenal portion. Then, outside this structure, the two leaves adhere and blend. The lesser omentum divides the wide peritoneal cavity from the omental bursa; its anterior leaf constitutes the posterior wall of the great supramesocolic cavity, whereas the pos-

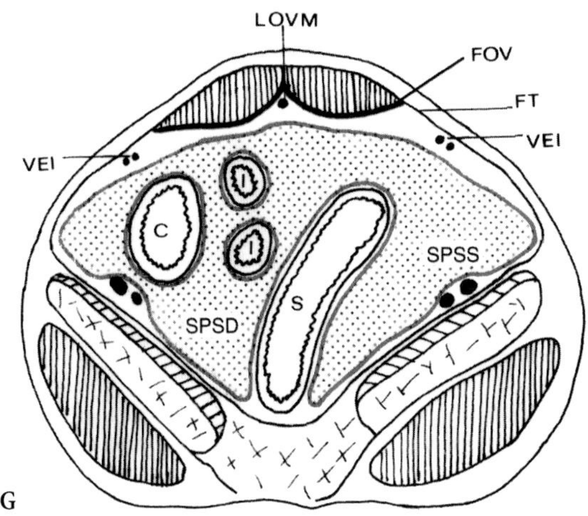

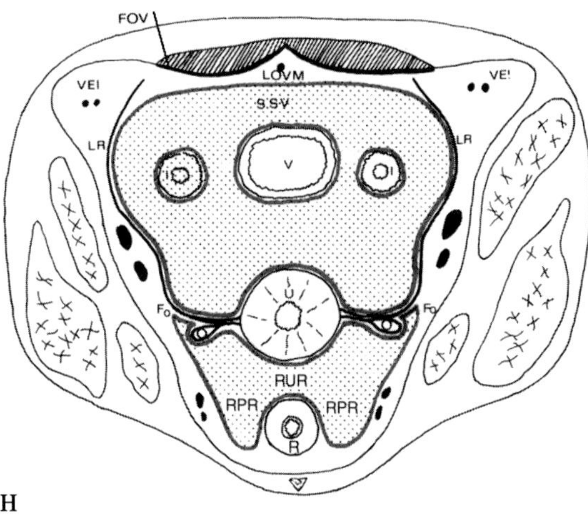

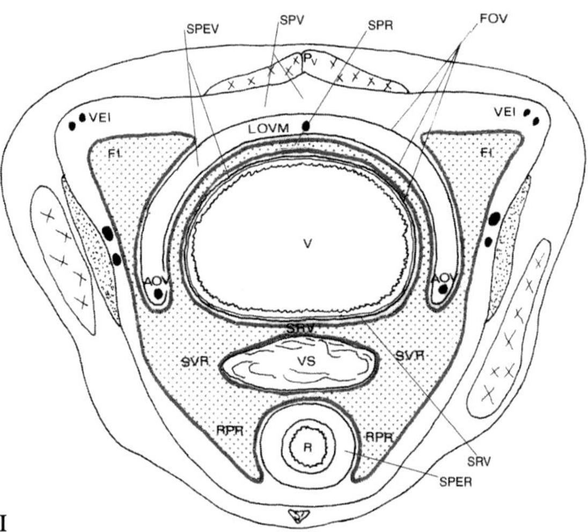

→ → . . . pararectal (*RPR*) recesses posteriorly; preperitoneal spaces with median umbilicovesical ligament (urachus) (*LOVM*) and the inferior epigastric vessels (*VEI*); lateral extraperitoneal spaces with round igaments (*VR*),external and internal iliac arteries and veins. I Middle-ow pelvic plane (male) crossing the seminal vesicles (*VS*). The pelvic cavity is subdivided by the umbilicovesical ligament and by the viscera urinary bladder (*V*), VS and rectum (*R*) into the inguinal fossae (*FI*), the perivesical (*SPV*) and vesicorectal (*SVR*) spaces, and pararectal recesses (RPR). The extraperitoneal structures also show: the umbilicovesical fascia (*FOV*), the median umbilicovesical ligament (urachus) (*LOVM*), the umbilicovesical arteries (*AOV*) (which continue the homonymous ligaments), the inferior epigastric vessels (*VEI*) and the prevesical (*SPV*), perivesical (*SPEV*), retrovesical (*SRV*), and perirectal (*SPER*) spaces. The peritoneum is colored red. The great peritoneal cavity is *lightly dotted*. The lesser sac is *densely dotted*

terior leaf constitutes the anterior wall of the omental bursa (Fig. 1.2C, D, 1.4C).

The subperitoneal spaces of the lesser omentum are closed below and on the right side by the overlapping of the two leaves, which makes up the lesser omentum, whereas they continue in the areolar tissue of the porta hepatis and, at a high level, in the areolar tissue of the longitudinal fissure.

In the subperitoneal spaces of the gastrohepatic ligament, we find: the right and left gastric arteries, extending and joining along the lesser curvature of the stomach, the veins, the lymphatic vessels, the homonymous lymph nodes and nerves, and the adipose tissue; in the subperitoneal spaces of the hepatoduodenal ligament, we find anteriorly: the extrahepatic biliary tract outside, the hepatic artery and the homonymous lymphatic vessels and lymph nodes inside, and posteriorly: the portal vein.

The *gastrocolic ligament* (Figs. 1.3E, 1.4D) connects the greater curvature of the stomach to the transverse colon; it is made up of two leaves, which, after covering the anterior and posterior walls of the stomach, extend together downwards as far as the front of the transverse colon. From this point onward, the leaflets are divided: the anterior leaflet continues downwards and becomes the anterior leaf of the greater omentum, whereas the posterior one bends backwards and continues in the superior leaf of the transverse mesocolon. The right and left gastroepiploic arteries and veins and the homonymous

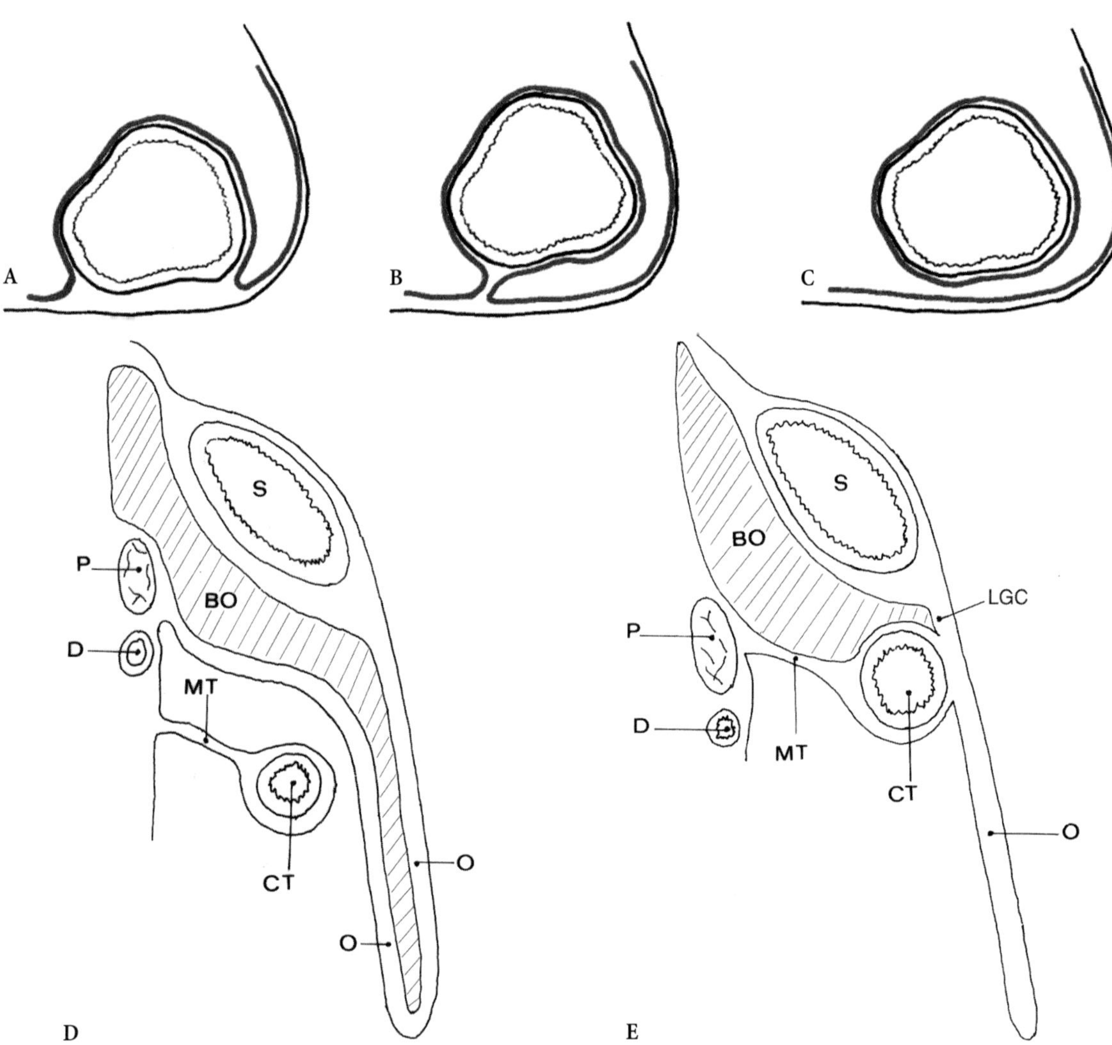

Fig. 1.3. A–C Variant arrangements of the peritoneum around the descending colon. **A** The peritoneum covers only the anterior face of the bowel. **B** The peritoneum constitutes a complete mesocolon. **C** The peritoneum completely surrounds the colon. **D** Representation (in left paramedian sagittal section) of the gastrocolic and gastrosplenic ligaments and the transverse mesocolon in the fetus. Lesser sac continues downward between the gastrocolic and gastrosplenic ligaments. **E** Representation (in left paramedian sagittal section) of the gastrocolic ligament, transverse mesocolon, and greater omentum

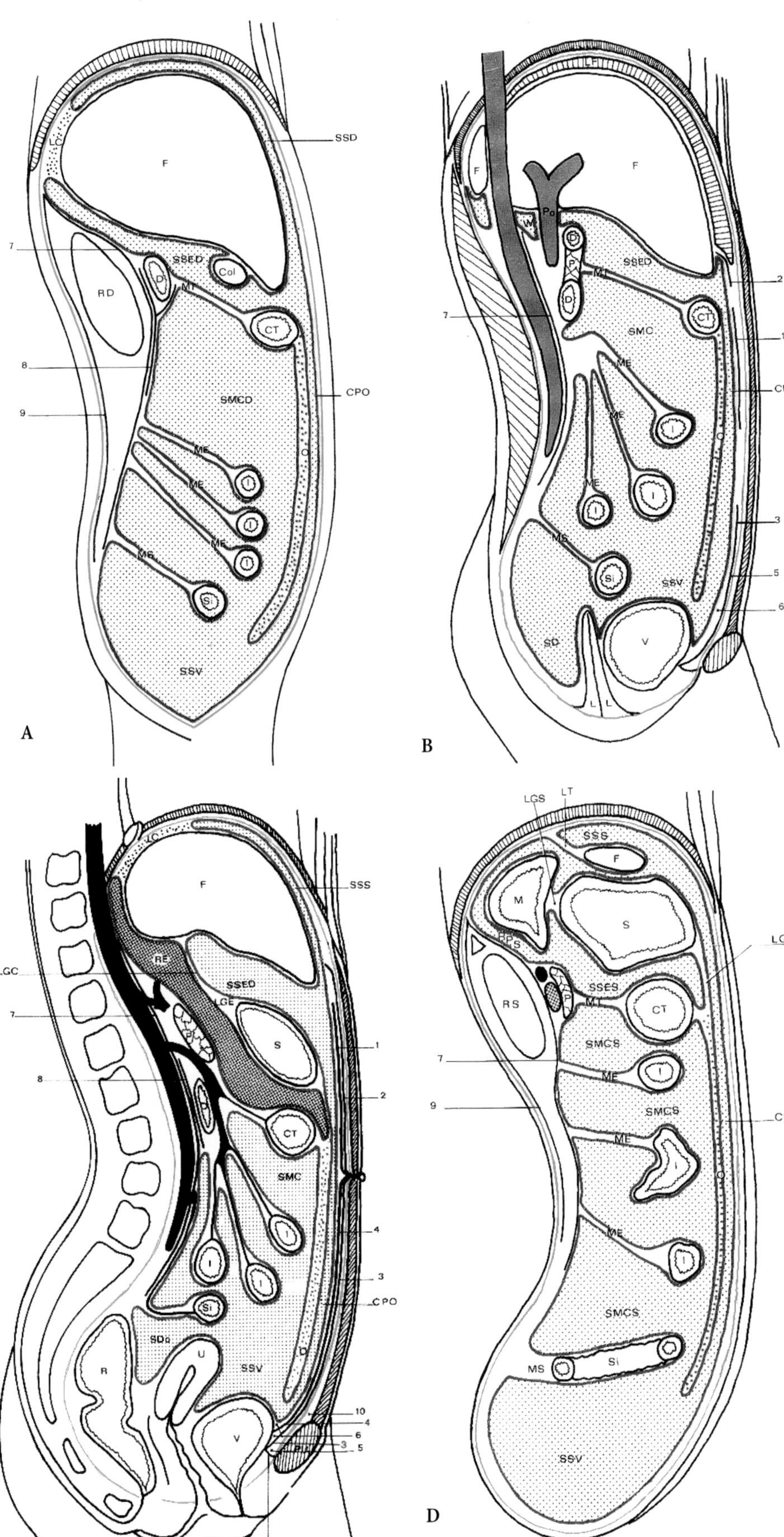

Fig. 1.4A–D. Representation in sagittal section of the arrangement of peritoneum, ligaments, peritoneal cavity and fasciae. **A** Right mediorenal plane. **B** Right paramedian plane crossing the portal trunk and the inferior vena cava. **C** Median plane crossing the abdominal aorta. **D** Left mediorenal plane. The peritoneum is colored red, and the transversalis fascia, blue. The great peritoneal cavity is indicated by a *lightly dotted* reticulum. The lesser sac is *more heavily* and *densely dotted* (*1* supraumbilical fascia, *2* round ligament (ligamentum teres), *3* umbilicovesical fascia, *4* median umbilicovesical ligament (urachus), *5* prevesical space, *6* perivesical space, *7* anterior renal fascia, *8* Toldt's fascia, *9* posterior renal fascia, *10* retromuscular space, *11* pubovesical ligament)

lymphatic vessels and nerves extend within the subperitoneal thickness of the gastrocolic ligament.

The *gastrosplenic ligament* (Figs. 1.1A, 1.2C, D, 1.4D) is made up of two parallel peritoneal leaves, with a sagittal orientation, extending backwards, in a slightly oblique direction and outside the greater curvature of the stomach, to the splenic hilum. It represents the continuation of the phrenogastrocolic ligament to the left side. The left gastroepiploic and the short gastric blood and lymphatic vessels and nerves extend in the subperitoneal space between the two leaves. The internal leaf of the ligament continues anteriorly in the peritoneum covering the posterior wall of the stomach and posteriorly in the anterior leaf of the splenopancreatic ligament, which limits the omental bursa. The external leaf continues anteriorly in the peritoneum covering the greater curvature of the stomach and posteriorly in the peritoneum covering the anterior surface of the spleen, which limits the gastrosplenic recess medially.

The *splenopancreatic* or *splenorenal ligament* connects the cauda pancreatis to the hilum of the spleen; it shows a frontal disposition and is made up of two leaves, anterior and posterior, surrounding the splenic vessels and the cauda and part of the corpus pancreatis. The anterior leaf continues medially in the posterior lamina of the lesser omentum, with which it combines to form the posterior wall of the omental bursa, and anteriorly in the internal leaf of the gastrosplenic ligament. Also, the posterior leaf extends medially behind the splenic vessels and the cauda and part of the corpus pancreatis, which it follows up to the proximities of the median line. From here, it bends backwards and then toward the left side, continuing in the parietal peritoneum that extends along the anterior renal fascia, from which it is separated by a thin layer of adipose tissue.

These inflexions of the posterior leaf of the ligament confine the splenopancreatic (or splenorenal) recess located behind the splenic vessels and the cauda and part of the corpus pancreatis (Fig. 1.2C).

The left lateral extension of the splenopancreatic ligament and of the transverse mesocolon becomes the phrenocolic ligament (or sustentaculum lienis) (Fig. 1.1A), which is inserted on the diaphragm at the level of the ninth rib and lies under the inferior pole of the spleen as a supporting "shelf" separating the spleen from the splenic flexure of the colon.

Mesocolic Region and Greater Omentum. In front of the second duodenal portion and the pancreas, the posterior peritoneum bends forwards, dividing into two parallel and coupled leaves (superior and inferior). Both leaves have a transverse disposition; next to the anterior abdominal wall, they cover the superoanterior and posteroinferior walls of the transverse colon, respectively, constituting the *transverse mesocolon* (Figs. 1.1A, 1.2E, 1.3Et, 1.4A–D).

The root of the transverse mesocolon crosses the second duodenal portion transversely and the pancreatic head medially, whereas it takes a close contact with the anterior renal fascia on the sides. This transverse disposition of the mesocolon, from the posterior to the anterior wall and from one side to the other side of the abdomen, represents a kind of large septum or diaphragm subdividing the abdominal cavity into supra- and submesocolic portions.

The middle colic branches of the superior mesenteric vessels, the nerves, and the homonymous lymphatic vessels and lymph nodes extend in the subperitoneal space of the transverse mesocolon.

Outside and under the transverse colon, the superior leaf of the transverse mesocolon blends with the posterior leaf of the gastrocolic ligament, limiting the omental bursa below. Conversely, the inferior leaf bends downwards to constitute the posterior lamina of the omentum (Figs. 1.3E, 1.4A–D).

This topographic arrangement of the gastrocolic ligament, the transverse mesocolon and the omental laminae constitutes a single wide subperitoneal compartment, which represents a route of diffusion of any inflammatory or tumoral processes originating from the hollow organs (stomach and transverse colon) that it contains.

The *greater omentum* (Fig. 1.4A–D) is a thick peritoneal "apron" extending between the transverse colon and the pubis, in front of the submesocolic intestinal hank and behind the anterior transverse abdominal fascia, from which it is separated by the virtual preperitoneal space and by the parietal peritoneum. It is made up of two pairs of peritoneal leaves combined in a single lamina ; the anterior leaves represent the continuation downwards of the gastrocolic ligament, whereas the posterior leaves are the continuation of the transverse mesocolon (Figs. 1.3E, 1.4A–D).

In the fetus, the anterior leaves are separated and extend downwards up to the proximities of the pubis, where they bend backward and upward to continue in the gastrosplenic ligament, which, after crossing the transverse colon, turns back as far as the posterior peritoneum just above the origin of transverse mesocolon. Between the two anterior and posterior leaves there is a recess representing the inferior expansion of the lesser sac (Fig. 1.3D).

At the end of fetal life the two omental leaves merge, creating the definitive greater omentum and closing the inferior expansion of the lesser sac, while the gastrosplenic ligament merges into the transverse mesocolon (Fig. 1.3E) Occasionally the recess may persist owing to failure of the two laminae to merge.

In young people, the omentum is thin and transparent. In the adult, it remains thin if the subject is lean, whereas in fat persons it may become thick as a result of adipose infiltration. It may also show variations in length and width. In extreme cases, it may appear as a thin and short band under the transverse colon; at other extreme, it may extend behind the pubis in the pelvic cavity up to the bottom of the peritoneal pouch of Douglas. Sometimes, instead of extending regularly in front of the intestinal hank, it is located on a single side, or folds and partly penetrates between the intestinal loops. In contrast to the rest of the peritoneum, it has a rich vascularization, with vertical parallel vessels coming from the gastroepiploic arcade under the greater curvature of the stomach (Figs. 1.6–1.9).

Submesocolic Region. At levels lying below the transverse mesocolon, the posterior peritoneum constitutes a series of deep anterior inflections surrounding the jejunum and the ileum: the *mesentery* (Figs. 1.1A, B, 1.2F, 1.4A–D). The insertion line of these folds or root of the mesentery has an oblique disposition from the Treitz's duodenojejunal corner, above and on the left side, to the ileocecal region, below and on the right side (Fig. 1.1A, B).

The superior mesenteric artery and vein, and the homonymous lymphatic vessels (flowing into the intestinal duct and the cisterna chyli) and nerves extend together from above downward along the median line, within the subperitoneal adipose tissue of the mesentery at the border with the retroperitoneum. The jejunoileal and ileocolic vessels, lymph nodes and nerves extend between the mesenteric folds, with a prevalent horizontal path. In the ileocecal fossa, the peritoneum bends toward the front and surrounds the cecum completely, forming a small mesentery that joins the cecum to the posterior wall: the *mesocecum* (Fig. 1.1A). At the basal level, it continues medially in the mesenteric root, whose two leaves extend upward and on the left side toward the superior mesenteric vascular axis.

The continuity of the two ileocolic peritoneal leaves into those of the mesocecum forms the inferior border of the right inframesocolic cavity, which separates it from the homonymous contralateral cavity, the right paracolic gutter, and the pelvic cavities.

The ileocolic vessels, lymph nodes, and nerves of superior mesenteric origin extend in the adipose areolar tissue of the mesocecum.

On both sides of the body, the submesocolic posterior peritoneum bends forward in a sagittal direction to become the ascending and the descending mesocolon.

The *ascending mesocolon* (Figs. 1.1A, 1.2F) is made up of posterior peritoneal folds that extend in front of the ascending colon, covering only the anterior wall, or penetrating more or less backward at the sides of the ascending colon, until they are surrounding the bowel almost completely; the vertical orientation of this mesentery separates the right paracolic gutter from the right inframesocolic space.

The right colic vessels (branches of the superior mesenteric vessels) extend within the adipose areolar tissue of the retroperitoneum, whereas their paracolic ramifications extend on the posteromedial side of the ascending colon. They are completely or partially surrounded by the mesocolon, depending on its length.

Like the ascending mesocolon, the *descending mesocolon* (Fig. 1.1A, 1.2E, F, 1.3A–C) partly or completely covers the descending colon, which may adopt an intra- or retroperitoneal position.

The left paracolic vessels and nerves of inferior mesenteric origin extend in the mesocolic adipose areolar.

Pelvic Region. At the level of the pelvis, the posterior peritoneum shows a long and deep inflection, curving like a letter S toward the abdominal cavity and surrounding the sigmoid, to form a long mesentery, the sigmoid mesocolon (Fig. 1.1A, 1.2G, 1.4A–D), which allows the bowel to move widely. It then continues downward in the serosa that covers the anterolateral wall of the rectum. Posteriorly, the sigmoid mesocolonal root follows a sinuous line from the left iliac fossa to the median line, in front of the promontory. The depth and length of the sigmoid mesocolon are very variable in different subjects, according to the sigmoidal orientation and length. When it is short, it descends directly as far as the rectum, following the left posterolateral wall of the pelvis and delineating a short arch that is open at the back; in this case, the sigmoid mobility is reduced. When it is long, it constitutes a wide loop reminiscent of a letter S and extends forward as far as where it makes contact with the anterior abdominal wall. In the right iliac fossa it is located marginally along the wall of the cecum-ascending colon; it then extends along the median line in front of the promontory.

Sometimes, it may extend not only transversely, but also in a vertical direction; in extreme situations, it becomes parallel to the descending colon, up to below the splenic flexure of the colon. A longer sigmoid mesocolon corresponds to a greater depth, and thus, to greater mobility.

The sigmoidal arteries, veins, and lymphatic vessels that are connected with the corresponding inferior mesenteric vessels are located in the subperitoneal space of the sigmoid mesocolon.

Under the sigmoid mesocolon, the *parietal peritoneum* leaving the anterior and lateral abdominal and pelvic walls bends inward and extends transversely to cover the upper part of the pelvic organs, the spaces and the connective ligaments, which separate the peritoneum from the pelvic floor. From the front backwards, it covers the urinary bladder, the uterus and the broad and round ligaments (in women) or the seminal vesicles (in men), and the anterior and lateral walls of the rectum, constituting inflections and recesses according to the underlying structures. The anterior parietal peritoneum descends as far as behind the pubis, where it bends towards the back, covering the superior face and the highest parts of the lateral faces of the urinary bladder. If the bladder is empty the peritoneum does not form pouches or recesses, whereas in the presence of a full bladder the peritoneum is raised and assumes a dome-like aspect, causing the *pubovesical, retrovesical* and *lateral recesses* (Fig. 1.2I) on the sides.

When the urinary bladder is empty in men, the parietal peritoneum has an almost complete flat extension from the retropubic region up to the sides of the rectum; in the median part of the pelvis it is interrupted by a transverse semicircular fold, with a posterior concavity, which continues on the two sides of the sacrum: the *genitosacral fold*, produced by the seminal vesicles and by the vesicosacral ligaments. This flat disposition of the peritoneum produces a single *vesicorectal cavity* (Fig. 1.2I). Posteriorly, the peritoneum bends upwards, covering the anterior face, and to varying depths the lateral faces, of the first portion of the rectum and forming the *laterorectal recesses* (Fig. 1.2I); these recesses disappear when the rectal ampulla is empty.

Behind the urinary bladder in women, the peritoneum bends inwards, transversely and upwards, constituting a deep fold (which covers the uterus on the median line) and the *broad ligaments* (Fig. 1.2H) (which contain the round ligaments, the tubes and the utero-ovarian ligaments) at the sides. This peritoneal inflection subdivides the female pelvic cavity into the *pre-* and *retrouterine compartments*, which are clearly separated.

1.1.3 Peritoneal Cavity

The peritoneal cavity is the widest extravasal space in the body, with a total surface of 1.5–2 m^2. It contains about 100 ml of citrine liquid, where some cells, mostly macrophages and lymphocytes, and rare eosinophils are present. It is closed in men, whereas in women it is open at the level of the abdominal orifice of the uterine tubes. It is subdivided by ligaments and mesenteries in secondary cavities, spaces, compartments, recesses and fossae. Topographically, it is constituted by three regions: the supramesocolic, the submesocolic (Table 1.2), which is separated by the transverse mesocolon but communicates on the sides along the paracolic gutter, and the pelvic region that communicates directly with the submesocolic region (Fig. 1.1A, B, 1.4A–D).

Table 1.2. Abdominal peritoneal cavity

Supramesocolic peritoneal cavity
Right subphrenic space
Right subhepatic space
Anterior recess
Posterior or Morrison's recess
Left subphrenic space
Suprahepatic recess
Subhepatic recess
Gastrolienal recess
Perisplenic recess
Splenopancreatic recess
Lesser sac
Submesocolic peritoneal cavity
Paracolic gutter
Inframesocolic cavities
Parasigmoidal spaces
Preomental or previsceral cavity

Supramesocolic Cavity. The supramesocolic cavity is located between the diaphragm above and the colon and transverse mesocolon below. It is divided into various spaces:

a) Right subphrenic (or interhepatodiaphragmatic) space (Figs. 1.1A, B, 1.2A–D, 1.4A). This space is located between the diaphragm and the hepatic cupula, having an anterolateral communication with the underlying subhepatic space, from which it is separated only at the back by the coronary ligament. Anteromedially, the falciform ligament divides the right from the left subphrenic space
b) Right subhepatic space (Figs. 1.1A, B, 1.4A–C). This is located between the visceral peritoneum (which covers the lower half of the right lobe of the liver and the gallbladder) and the parietal

peritoneum (which lines the anterior abdominal wall anteriorly and the renal fascia posteriorly). Below, it is closed by the transverse mesocolon, while above it communicates with the homolateral subphrenic space, except at the back, because of the interposition of the coronary ligament. Medially, it continues in the left subhepatic space, under the falciform ligament and, below and laterally, with the right paracolic gutter, outside the transverse mesocolon.

There are *two recesses*: one, the *anterior*, continues on at a high level from the homolateral subphrenic space; the *posterior* (or *Morrison's*) *recess* penetrates between the posterior wall of the liver and the superior pole of the right kidney up to the coronary ligament at a high level.

c) *Left subphrenic space* (Figs. 1.1A, B, 1.2A, B, 1.4D): it is wide and polymorphous, partly subphrenic and partly subhepatic, and is made up of five communicating recesses that are closed below by the transverse mesocolon and by the phrenocolic ligament; they are: the supra- and subhepatic, the gastrolienal, the perisplenic and the splenorenal recesses.

1) The *left suprahepatic recess* (Figs. 1.1A, B, 1.2A, B, 1.4D) is located between the diaphragm and the left hepatic lobe and is limited posteriorly by the coronary ligament and on the right side by the falciform ligament. It varies in width, according to the dimensions of the left hepatic lobe. Anteriorly, it communicates with the homolateral subhepatic recess.

2) The *left subhepatic (or gastrohepatic) recess* (Figs. 1.1A, B, 1.2C, D, 1.4D) is located between the inferior face of the left hepatic lobe and the triangular ligament above and the transverse mesocolon below, and between the anterior abdominal wall, the gastrohepatic ligament and the anterior wall of the corpus and fundus ventriculi. Anteriorly, it communicates with the homolateral subphrenic space above and the previsceral cavity below. Medially, it penetrates between the stomach and the right lobe of the liver; under the liver, it continues into the contralateral subhepatic space. Laterally, it communicates widely with the gastrolienal recess.

3) The *gastrolienal recess* (Fig. 1.2C, D) is located between the stomach and the spleen; it is limited medially by the gastrolienal ligament and anterolaterally by the parietal peritoneum, and continues backwards into the perisplenic recess.

4) The *perisplenic recess* p (Figs. 1.2C, D, 1.4C) is located between the diaphragm and the transverse mesocolon, and surrounds the spleen completely, with the exception of the hilum.

5) The *splenopancreatic* (or *splenorenal*) *recess* (Fig. 1.2C) is located behind the splenic vessels under the cauda pancreatis and in front of the anterior renal fascia, as a median posterior evagination of the perisplenic recess.

d) The *lesser sac* (or *omental bursa*) (Figs.1.1A, 1.2C, D, 1.4C) is a large flat complex space with a frontal vertical position in the median of the superior abdomen, which extends transversely from the caudate lobe of the liver to the hilum of the spleen. It is limited anteriorly by the posterior leaf of the lesser omentum, and behind by the parietal peritoneum covering the anterior renal fascia and the pancreas. It is limited on the left by the gastrophrenic, gastrosplenic and splenopancreatic ligaments, and on the right by the junction between the posterior leaf of the lesser omentum and the posterior peritoneum. Below, it is closed by the fusion of the gastrocolic ligament with the transverse mesocolon. Sometimes, in the absence of this fusion, the lesser sac may expand up to the pelvis between the leaves of the greater omentum.

It communicates with the right subhepatic recess through Winslow's foramen (Fig. 1.1A), which is located under the caudate lobe of the liver between the portal vein and the inferior vena cava over the insertion of the hepatoduodenal ligament on the bulb and the superior genu of the duodenum. The omental bursa subdivides on the median line in the right and left compartments with a deep posterior sagittal inflexion of the parietal peritoneum produced by the ascending path of the left gastric artery, which extends from the celiac trunk to the higher part of the lesser curvature of the stomach. The two compartments communicate through the foramen bursae omentalis.

The *right compartment* is made up of a vestibular and a superior recess.

The *vestibular recess* is located between the left gastric artery and the caudate lobe, which is surrounded on three sides, with a "pincer"-like aspect.

The *superior recess* penetrates upwards, between the posteromedial face of the liver and the diaphragm.

The *left compartment* is wider and more expansile than the right one, and extends from the diaphragmatic apex to the cavity formed by the junction of the posterior leaf of the gastrocolic ligament with the superior leaf of the transverse mesocolon. The left lateral extremity of this compartment penetrates the angle constituted by the gastrohepatic ligament in the front, the gastrosplenic ligament outside and the splenopancreatic ligament behind, to form the *splenic recess*.

Submesocolic Cavity. The submesocolic cavity (Fig. 1.1A, B, 1.2E–G, 1.4A–D) is located between the transverse mesocolon above, the sigmoid mesocolon below, and the parietal peritoneum.

It is subdivided by the prominence of the mesentery along the median line in the *right* and *left inframesocolic compartments*, which in turn, are separated at the sides by the introflexions of the ascending and descending colon, into the *right* and *left paracolic gutter*, respectively.

The oblique orientation of the mesenteric root (Fig. 1.1A, B) makes the right inframesocolic cavity wider at higher levels and narrow lower down; in contrast, the left cavity is narrower near the transverse mesocolon and wider below, where it expands in the right parasigmoidal space.

High up, the right paracolic gutter communicates with the homolateral subhepatic recess, whereas the left paracolic gutter is closed by the phrenocolic ligament.

The right paracolic gutter and the left inframesocolic cavity extend downward into the *right parasigmoidal space*, and through this space into the supravesical cavity.

The right inframesocolic cavity is closed below by the junction of the mesentery of the last ileal loop with the mesocecum, and communicates only in the front of this structure with the other cavities.

The left paracolic gutter continues downwards in the homolateral *parasigmoidal* and *pararectal space*, as far as the pouch of Douglas.

The *previsceral* or *preomental cavity* (Figs. 1.2E, 1.4A–D) is located between the anterior parietal peritoneum and the greater omentum; it is a thin, virtual and poorly expansile space, with direct communications with the anterior subhepatic spaces above, with the submesocolic cavity to the sides and with the pelvic spaces located under the caudal apex of the omentum.

Pelvic Cavity. The pelvic cavity (Figs. 1.1 A, B, 1.2H, I, 1.4A–D) represents the extension in the pelvis of the submesocolic cavity, with which it widely communicates. It is limited all around by the parietal peritoneum lining the abdominopelvic wall and covering the urinary bladder, the genital organs and the rectum, below. It is subdivided into compartments, spaces and recesses by vasculoligamental structures or by organs (urinary bladder, uterus, broad and round ligaments, seminal vesicles) that protrude in the direction of the peritoneal cavity.

Two compartments are can be distinguished: anterior and posterior. They are separated by the uterus and by the broad ligaments in women and by the fascia of Denonvillier in men (Table 1.3).

Table 1.3. Pelvic peritoneal compartments

Anterior
Supravesical space
Prevesical recess
Medial inguinal recesses (or fossae)
Lateral inguinal recesses (or fossae)
Retrovesical (vesicoseminal in men, vesicouterine in women) recesses
Posterior
In men: seminorectal and pararectal recesses
In women: uterorectal recess (or pouch of Douglas) and ovarian fossae and pararectal recesses

The anterior compartment (Fig. 1.2H, I) is limited by the peritoneum, which anteriorly lines the anterior abdominal wall, and posteriorly covers the uterus and the broad ligaments in women (and Denonvilliers' fascia in men). It is constituted by the supravesical space and by various recesses.

The *supravesical space* is wide; it is limited by the anterior and lateral parietal peritoneum and communicates directly with the left inframesocolic cavity and the right paracolic and parasigmoidal gutter above, and with the paravesical recesses below.

The *prevesical recess* has an arcuate extension along the median line, in front of the urinary bladder. It is more expanded on the sides and is limited by the umbilical vesical ligaments.

The *medial inguinal recesses* are located between the prominence of the umbilical vesical ligament and the incisures of the inferior epigastric vessels.

The *lateral inguinal recesses* are located outside the inferior epigastric vessels; they are mostly small and have a dome-like appearance with lateral convexity.

The *retrovesical recess* extends transversely between the posterior vesical wall and the seminal vesicles in men (*vesicoseminal recess*) and the uterus in women (*vesicouterine recess*); it communicates anteriorly with the anterior recesses and above with the supravesical space. The depth of the retrovesical recess is inversely related to the level of the vesical filling.

The posterior compartment (Fig. 1.2H, I) represents the lowest part of the peritoneal cavity; it is differently oriented in men and women.

- In *men* (Fig. 1.2I) it is made up of the large and wide *seminorectal recess*, which is produced by the inferior inflexion of the peritoneum. After covering the seminal vesicles, the peritoneum extends downward and backward, and then bends upwards in front of and at the sides of the rectum, where it forms the *pararectal recesses*. At the sides and above, it is limited by two semilunar folds (Douglas' or posterior vesical ligaments), extending from the urinary bladder to the rectum.

The seminorectal recess often continues without interruptions into the anterior recesses, constituting a single cavity: the *vesicorectal cavity*.

- In *women* (Fig. 1.2H), the *uterorectal recess* (or *pouch of Douglas*) is produced by the peritoneum, which after covering the fundus and the corpus uteri and the posterior vaginal wall, and forming the broad ligaments at the sides, bends at the base of these structures to pass upward and backward and cover the anterior and lateral walls of the first portion of the rectum. This recess is further subdivided into the *ovarian fossae* (anterolaterally) and the pararectal recesses (posteromedially) by two semilunar (right and left) peritoneal inflexions, the uterosacral ligaments, which from the uterine isthmus extend backward to the first, second, and third sacral vertebrae.

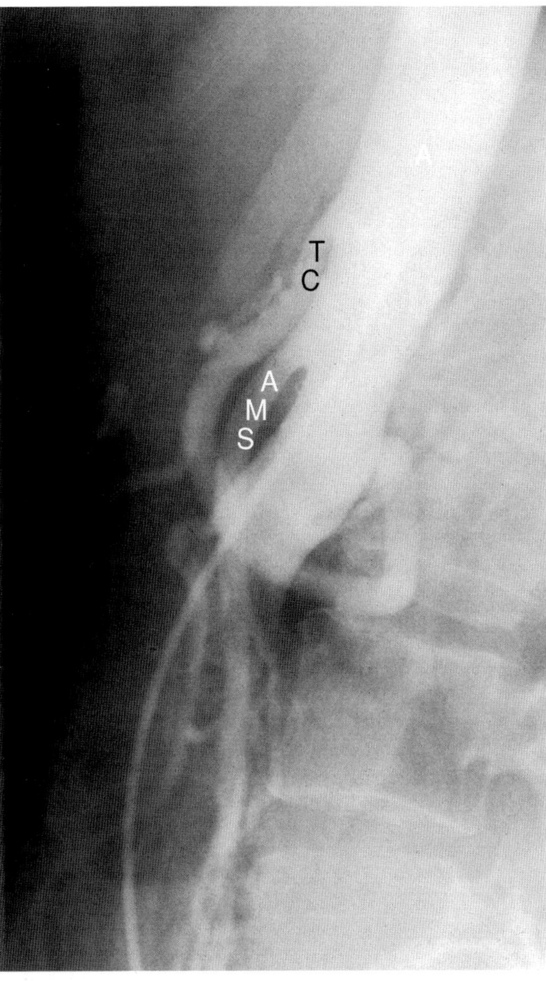

Fig. 1.5. Aortography in lateral projection. Aortic origin of the celiac trunk (*CT*) and of the superior mesenteric artery (*AMS*)

1.2 Arteries and Veins

1.2.1 Arteries

The *abdominal arterial branches* for the intraperitoneal organs extend between the two peritoneal leaves in the subperitoneal spaces, whereas the *pelvic branches* (except for the utero-ovarian arteries, which penetrate the thickness of the broad ligaments) extend in the extraperitoneal spaces.

1.2.1.1 Abdominal Visceral Arteries

1.2.1.1.1 The Celiac Trunk

The *celiac trunk* (Figs.1.5–1.9) originates from the anterior wall of the abdominal aorta, in the tract where the diaphragmatic crura constituting the crural arcade divide and extend to the sides of the aorta. The celiac trunk has a mean length of 1–1.5 cm; it extends forward and slightly toward the right side, before subdividing into three branches:

a) The hepatic artery
b) The coronarostomachic or left gastric artery
c) The splenic artery

a) The *hepatic artery* (Figs. 1.6–1.10) initially extends obliquely toward the right side, forward and downward, with a slightly sinuous path, until it is close to the pylorus; from here it bends upward and backward, extending toward the hepatic hilum, which it penetrates.

In its initial tract, the artery is located in the retroperitoneum, whereas in the ascending tract it penetrates between the leaves of the lesser omentum (hepatoduodenal ligament). In this tract, it is located in front of the portal vein and slightly inside the choledochus.

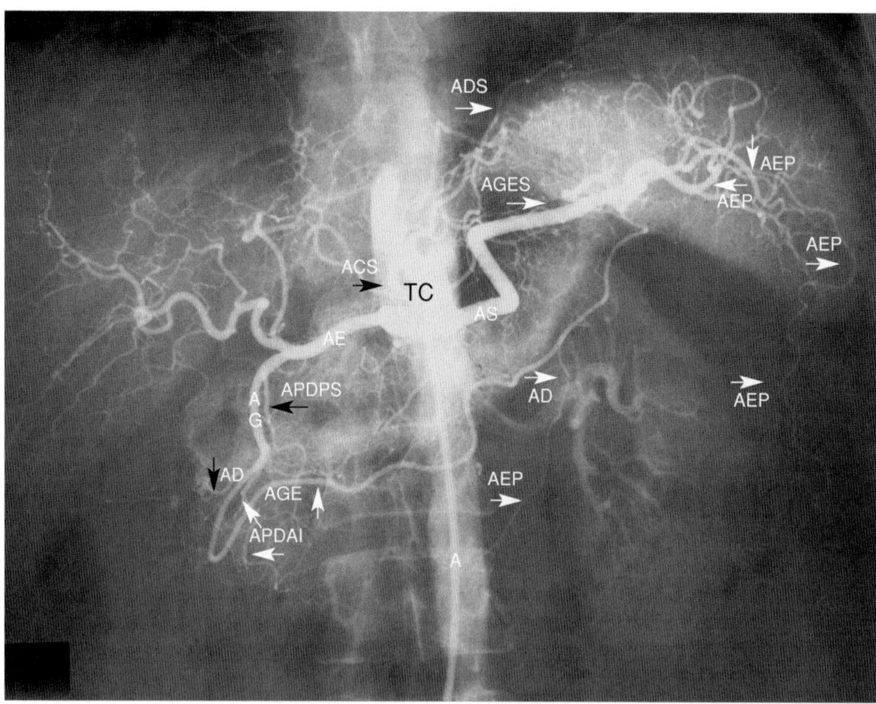

Fig. 1.6. Selective arteriography of the celiac trunk. Celiac trunk and hepatic, splenic, left gastric, gastroduodenal, gastroepiploic, superior and inferior pancreatoduodenal and duodenal arteries. Epiploic arteries from the gastroepiploic arterial arcade and from the splenic artery

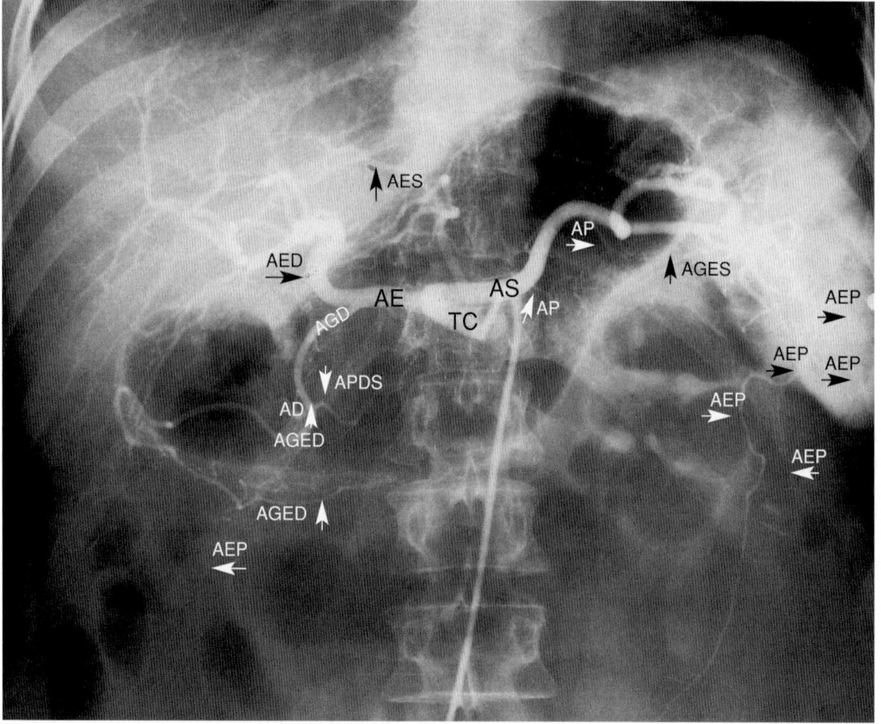

Fig. 1.7. Selective arteriography of the celiac trunk. Celiac trunk and right and left hepatic, splenic, gastroduodenal, right and left gastroepiploic, superior pancreatoduodenal and duodenal arteries. Epiploic arteries from the gastroepiploic arterial arcade and from the splenic artery. The stomach is dilated with air and is pushing the right gastroepiploic artery downwards

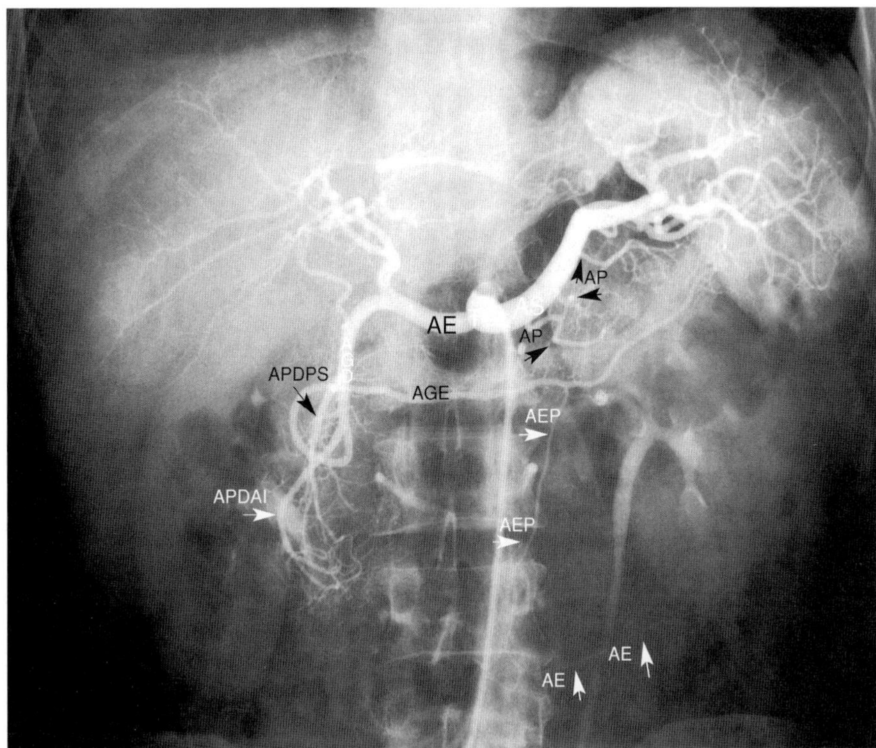

Fig. 1.8. Selective arteriography of the celiac trunk. Celiac trunk and hepatic, splenic, gastroduodenal, gastroepiploic, superior and inferior pancreatoduodenal arteries. Epiploic artery from the gastroepiploic arterial arcade and from the splenic artery. Well-developed superior pancreatoduodenal arteries

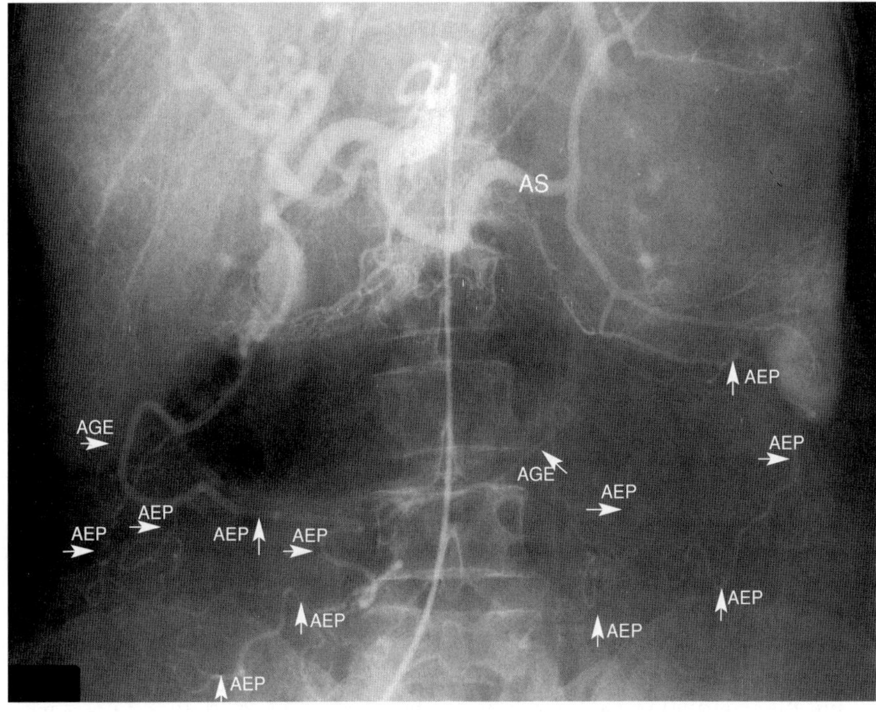

Fig. 1.9. Selective arteriography of the celiac trunk. Epiploic arteries are well developed owing to omental metastases from ovarian carcinoma. The arteries originate from the gastroepiploic and from the splenic arteries

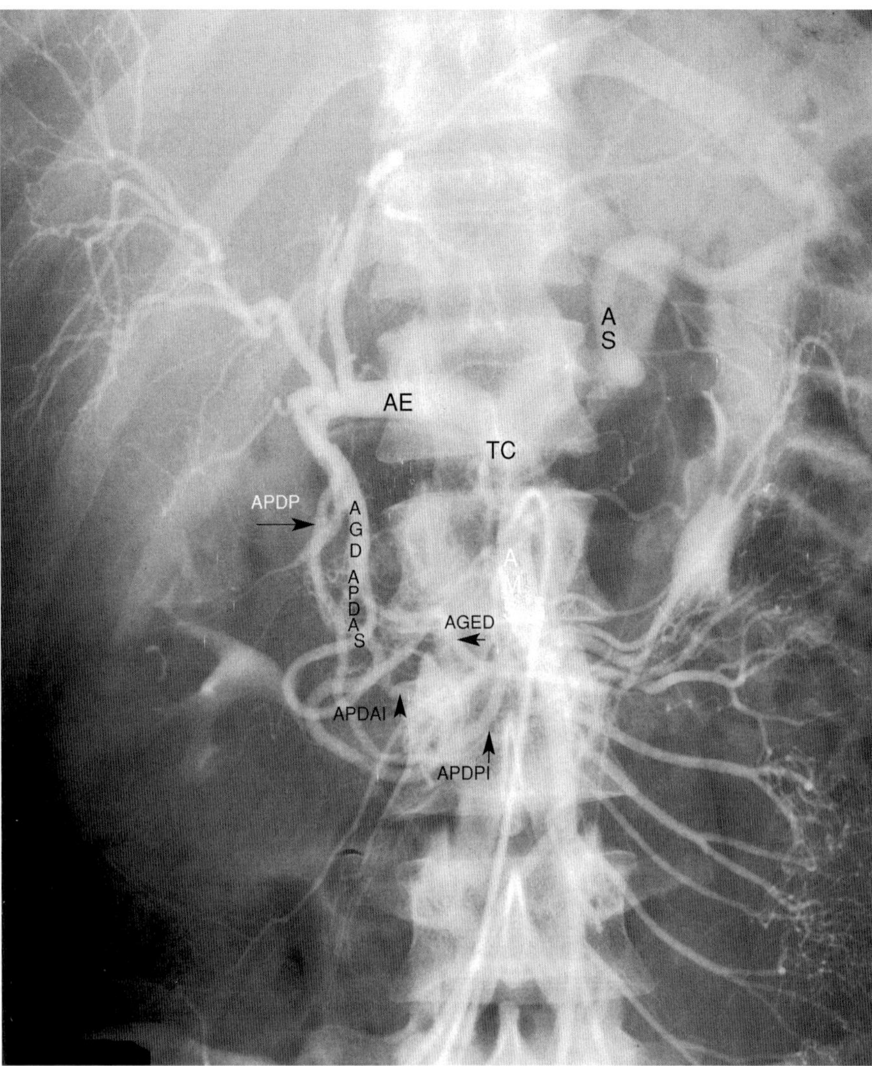

Fig. 1.10. Selective arteriography of the superior mesenteric artery. Anterior and posterior pancreatoduodenal arcades constituting a collateral circulation between the superior mesenteric artery and the branches of the celiac trunk, attributable to obstruction of the celiac trunk

The right gastric artery, the gastroduodenal artery and the cystic artery originate along the path of the hepatic artery.

The *right gastric* or *pyloric artery* is very slight; it extends downward and toward the left side, penetrating between the leaves of the lesser omentum. After reaching the superior border of the pylorus, it bends toward the left side and upward along the lesser curvature of the stomach up to the junction with the homonymous left artery.

The *gastroduodenal artery* (Figs. 1.6–1.10) extends downward and forward between the posterior wall of the first duodenal portion and the pancreatic head. Here, it subdivides into the superior pancreatoduodenal and right gastroepiploic arteries.

At 1–2 cm after its origin from the gastroduodenal artery, the *superior pancreatoduodenal artery* (Figs. 1.6–1.10) subdivides into the anterior and posterior branches, descending over the respective faces of the pancreatic head as far as the junction with the homonymous inferior branches, which extend upwards from the superior mesenteric artery; together, these branches constitute the *anterior* and *posterior pancreatoduodenal arcades* (Fig. 1.10).

The *right gastroepiploic artery* (Figs. 1.6–1.9) follows the greater curvature of the stomach from right to left between the leaves of the gastrocolic ligament, and terminates with a full canal anastomosis with the left gastroepiploic artery; together, these vessels constitute the *gastroepiploic arcade.*

The *cystic artery* originates from the hepatic artery or from its right branch at the level of the transverse sulcus; then it extends toward the infundibulum of the gallbladder, where it subdivides into two branches: superior and inferior, flowing into the cholecystic wall.

b) The *left gastric or coronarostomachic artery* (Figs. 1.6, 1.7) initially extends upward and slightly toward the left, making an impression in the peritoneum and forming a peritoneal fold that divides the vestibulum from the left recesses of the omental bursa. At the level of the right side of the cardia, it bends sharply forward and penetrates the gastrohepatic ligament; once inside the ligament it descends along the lesser curvature of the stomach up to the proximity of the pylorus, where it anastomoses with the pyloric artery.

c) The *splenic artery* (Figs. 1.6, 1.7) initially follows a sinuous path toward the left; the first tract is located in the retroperitoneum between the anterior renal fascia and the posterosuperior border of the corpus pancreatis above the homonymous vein; thereafter, it overtakes the cauda pancreatis and, together with this organ, penetrates the full thickness of the splenopancreatic ligament up to the splenic hilum. Before penetrating the spleen it subdivides into two branches: superior and inferior. As a whole, it delineates a curve with an anterior concavity identical to the curve of the body and tail of the pancreas, which it then follows along the total extension. Along its pathway, it gives origin to various arteries: particularly, the short gastric arteries and the left gastroepiploic artery from the terminal tract.

The *short gastric artery* originates from the superior branch of the splenic artery and extends within the gastrosplenic ligament up to the fundus ventriculi.

The *left gastroepiploic artery* (Figs. 1.6, 1.7) extends forward, after its origin, within the gastrosplenic ligament up to the greater curvature of the stomach, under the fundus ventriculi. From here it bends downward, extending along the greater curvature, and then terminates, with a full canal anastomosis with the contralateral gastroepiploic artery, in the thickness of the gastrocolic ligament; together, these arteries form the *gastroepiploic anastomotic arcade.*

Numerous vessels originate from the lower part of the gastroepiploic anastomotic arcade (Figs. 1.6–1.9), descending parallel and flowing into the greater omentum (Fig. 1.9): one example is the *great right epiploic branch*, extending laterally over the anterior face of the epiploic plane and then distally within the posterior lamina. It terminates with an anastomosis with the *left great epiploic branch.* This latter ramification originates from the proximal tract of the left gastroepiploic artery or from the splenic artery; it penetrates the posterior omental lamina and extends obliquely downward and toward the right side. Finally, it joins the homonymous right artery and constitutes the *Haller-Baskov subcolic anastomotic arcade* (Fig. 1.9).

1.2.1.1.2
The Superior Mesenteric Artery

The *superior mesenteric artery* (Fig. 1.5, 1.10–1.14) originates from the anterior aortic wall, at about 2 cm below the celiac trunk. Just after its origin, this artery bends downwards, extending between the aorta and the isthmus of the pancreas. After 2–3 cm, it makes an oblique forward turn, overtaking the third duodenal portion; it then penetrates the adipose areolar tissue of the mesenteric root, which it crosses from above downward up to the right iliac fossa. As a whole, it delineates a wide arch, with the concavity turned toward the right side, which terminates at the level of the junction of the last ileal loop with the cecum.

The *inferior pancreatoduodenal arteries* and some small ramifications for the duodenum and the pancreas originate from the proximal, retroperitoneal tract. Then, the anterior and posterior branches of the inferior pancreatoduodenal arteries anastomose with the homonymous superior vessels. In the case of obstruction of the celiac trunk, of a branch or of the superior mesenteric artery, this communication is an important anastomotic arcade (Fig. 1.11).

After penetrating the mesenterium, the superior mesenteric artery gives origin to the *jejunoileal arteries* (Figs. 1.11–1.14) from the convexity of its arch; about 10–20 of these vessels have a radial extension forward, downward and toward the left side, and reach the loops of the small intestine. These arteries join together (with a full canal anastomosis) and give origin to a series of parallel arcades (4 or 5, with the convexity toward the intestinal loops), which become progressively smaller and more numerous. The terminal vessels (*vasa recta*) originate from the most peripheral arcades and penetrate the intestinal walls.

At various levels, three collateral vessels originate from the concavity of the superior mesenteric artery: the middle colic, the right colic and the ileocolic arteries. These vessels show numerous variations in

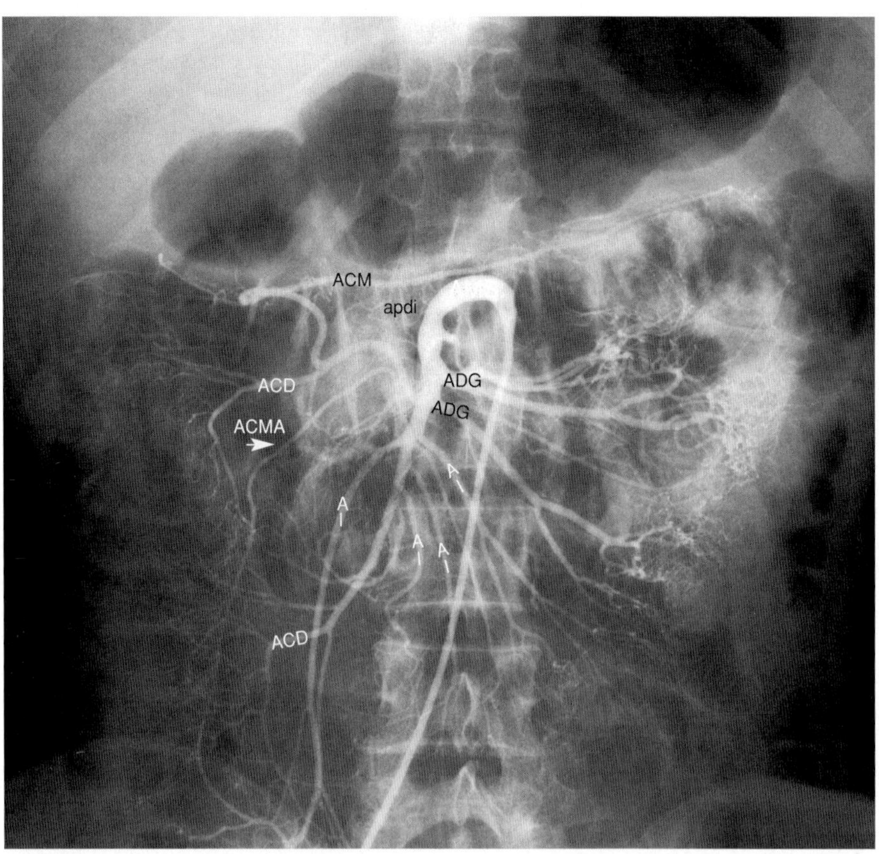

Fig. 1.11. Selective arteriography of the superior mesenteric artery. Superior mesenteric, inferior pancreatoduodenal, middle colic, jejunal, ileal, ileocolic, colic and right marginal colic arteries. Communicating arcades and vasa recta radiate in the direction of the intestinal wall

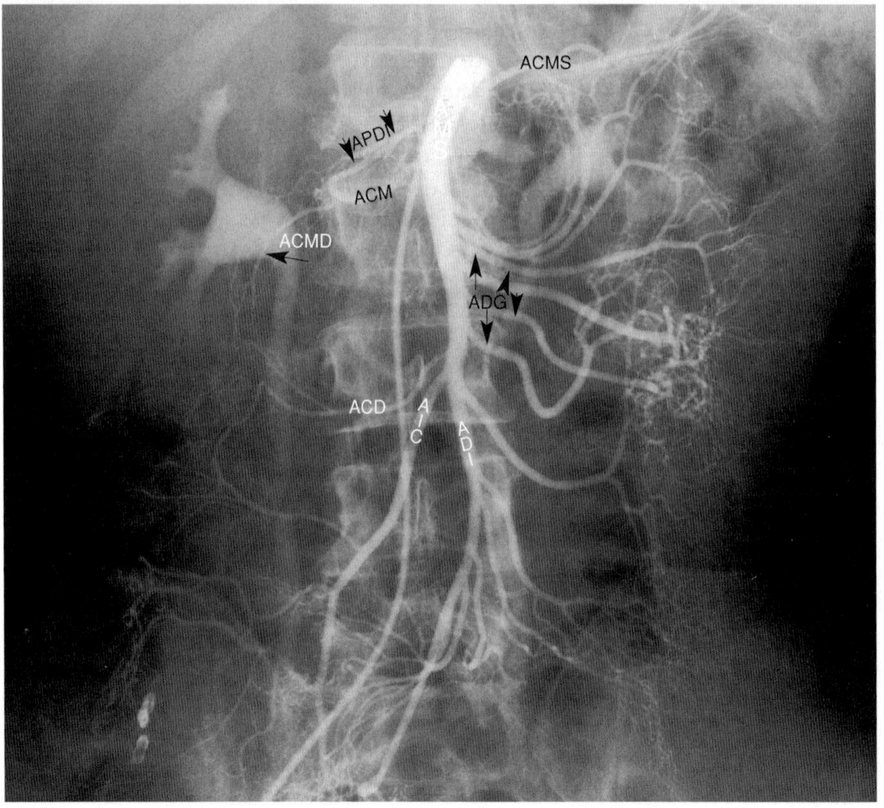

Fig. 1.12. Selective arteriography of the superior mesenteric artery. Variations in origin, size, subdivision, distribution and communications of secondary branches of the superior mesenteric artery

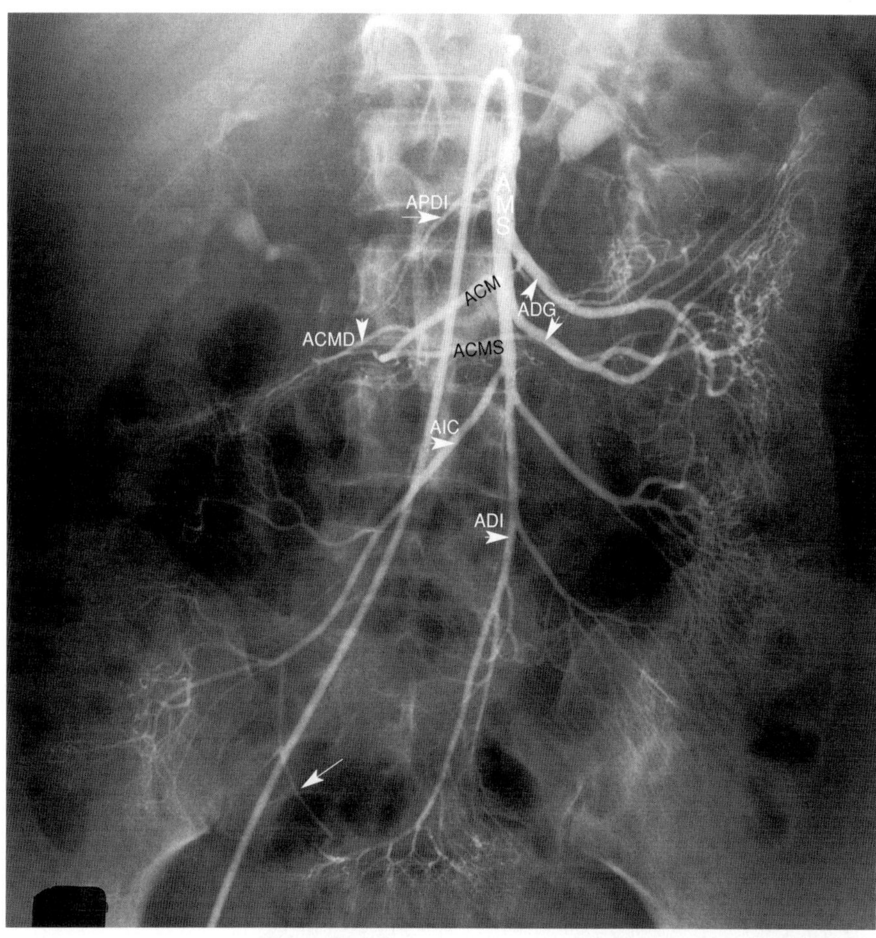

Fig. 1.13. Selective arteriography of the superior mesenteric artery. Variations in origin, size, subdivision, distribution and communications of secondary branches of the superior mesenteric artery

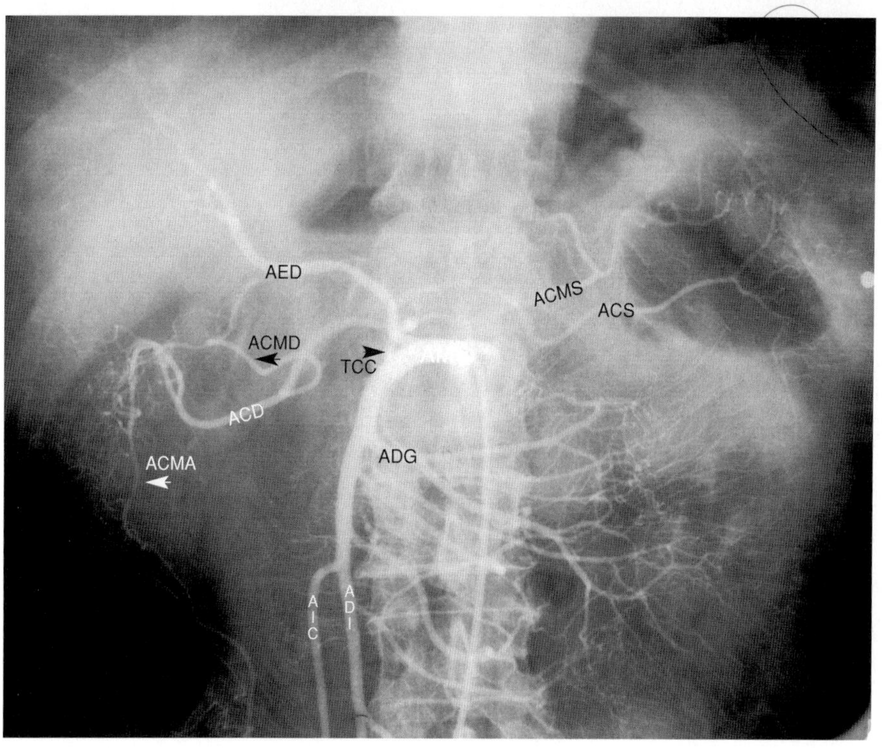

Fig. 1.14. Selective arteriography of the superior mesenteric artery. Variations in origin, size, subdivision, distribution and communications of secondary branches of the superior mesenteric artery. Right and left middle colic arteries; right colic artery with the marginal colic artery; left colic artery that continues downwards in the left marginal colic artery. The right branch of the hepatic artery originates from the superior mesenteric artery

the origin, caliber, subdivision and distribution of the single branches.

The *middle (or superior) colic artery* (Figs. 1.10–1.14) originates from the proximal tract of the superior mesenteric artery, just under the pancreas, and extends in front of the uncinate process. Then it penetrates between the leaves of the transverse mesocolon, extending forward. At a short distance from the transverse colon it subdivides into two ramifications: the left branch terminates with a full canal anastomosis with the left colic artery (inferior mesenteric artery ramification), forming *Riolan's arcade* (Fig. 1.15), the right branch extends along the transverse colon and then anastomoses with an ascending ramification of the right colic artery.)

The *right colic artery* (Fig. 1.14) originates from the superior mesenteric artery under the middle colic artery and extends toward the right side behind the posterior peritoneum up to its penetration into the ascending mesocolon. Here, it subdivides into two branches: ascending and descending. The former extends along the internal border of the ascending colon and anastomose with the right branch of the middle colic artery. The latter extends downwards and toward the ileocecal region, where it joins the ascending branch of the ileocolic artery.

The *ileocolic artery* (Fig. 1.10–1.13) constitutes the terminal tract of the superior mesenteric artery; it extends downward and outward, with an oblique path, up to the ileocecal region, where it divides into

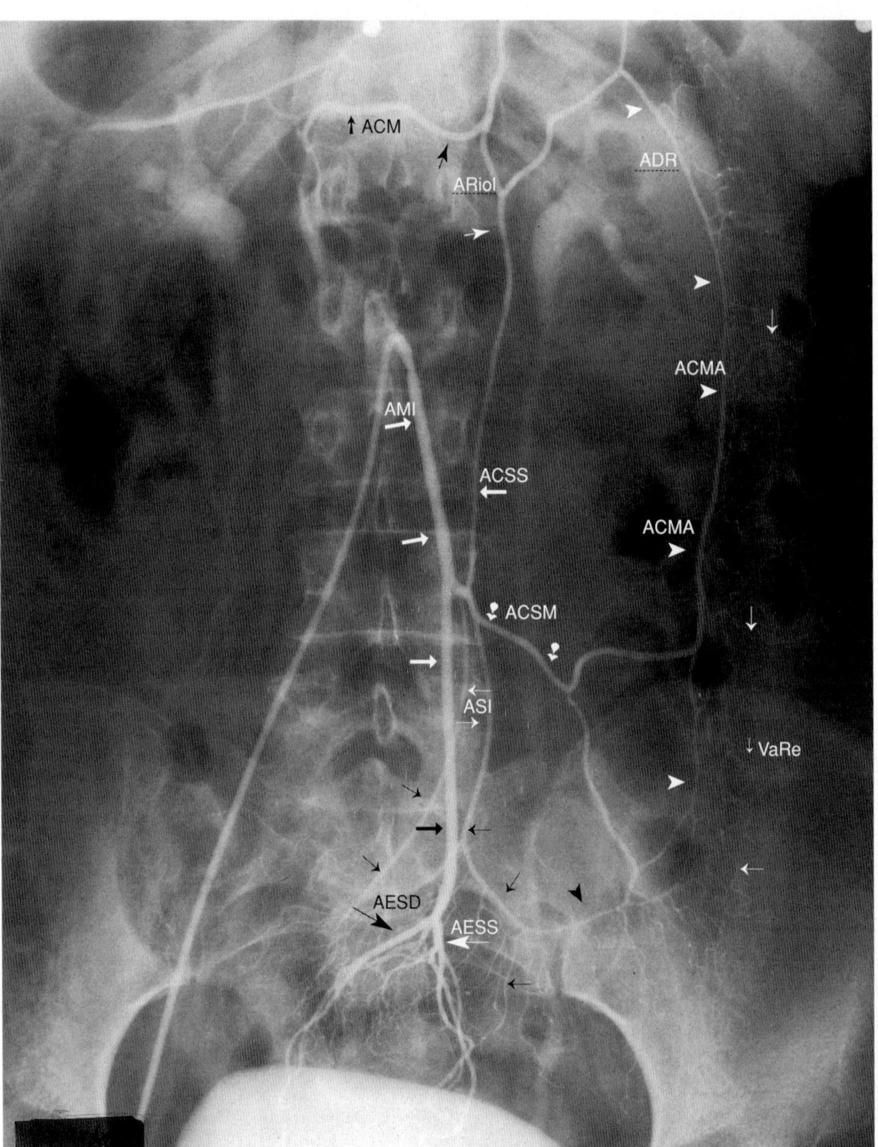

Fig. 1.15. Selective arteriography of the inferior mesenteric artery. Inferior mesenteric artery subdivides into the left colic (with the superior and median branches), sigmoidal and superior hemorrhoidal arteries. Left marginal colic artery along the mesocolic border of the descending colon, which generates the vasa recta. Riolan's arcade, links the inferior mesenteric artery to the middle colic artery. Drummond's arcade links the left marginal colic artery to the left middle colic artery

the ascending branch (which anastomoses with the descending ramification of the right colic artery) and the descending branch (which terminates with a full canal anastomosis with the last ileal arcades).

1.2.1.1.3 The Inferior Mesenteric Artery

The *inferior mesenteric artery* (Fig. 1.15) originates from the anterior face of the aorta at the level of the third lumbar vertebral body or the L3-4 space, generally at 3–4 cm under the superior mesenteric artery and 5–6 cm above the aortic bifurcation, and flows into the left and inferior part of the large intestine.

Initially, it extends downward and slightly toward the left side, between the parietal peritoneum and the anterior renal fascia, which separates this vessel from the aorta. After crossing the left common iliac vessels, it returns on the median line and continues downwards in the superior hemorrhoidal artery. Along its path, the inferior mesenteric artery generates the left colic and the sigmoidal arteries.

- The *left colic artery* (Fig. 1.15) generates an ascending branch, which extends toward the splenic flexure of the colon, where it anastomoses with the left middle colic artery, forming Riolan's arcade, and a descending branch, which extends to the median and lower tract of the descending colon.
- The *sigmoidal artery* (Fig. 1.15) penetrates the sigmoid mesocolon to reach the sigmoidal wall from above and from behind. There are numerous variations in the origin and subdivision of these two arteries: the most frequent is represented by the presence of an *intermediate colic artery* between the left colic and the sigmoidal artery.
- The *superior hemorrhoidal artery* (Fig. 1.15) represents the terminal ramification of the inferior mesenteric artery. It extends from behind and above to the rectum, which is nourished by its right and left branches.

On the side of the descending mesocolon and of the sigmoid mesocolon, the terminal ramifications of the left colic and sigmoidal arteries are connected by the *marginal colic artery* (Fig. 1.15); this latter vessel generates the *vasa recta* (Fig. 1.15) for the intestinal wall. This artery constitutes an anastomotic arcade, *Drummond's arcade*, between the branches of the inferior mesenteric artery and the left middle colic artery (Fig. 1.15).

Drummond's and *Riolan's arcades* are important anastomoses in the case of occlusion of a mesenteric artery or of a main branch.

1.2.1.2 Pelvic and Genital Arteries

The pelvic arteries can be distinguished in *parietal branches* that extend to the pelvic wall and to the structures connected to the wall, and in *visceral branches* that extend to the pelvic organs (urinary bladder, uterus and adnexae uteri, seminal vesicles and prostate, rectum).

a Parietal Branches. The *median sacral artery* (Fig. 1.16) originates from the posterior wall of the abdominal aorta, next to the bifurcation, or from the proximal tract of one of the common iliac arteries; it extends vertically downward along the median line, next to the sacrum, the coccyx and the pelvic fascia (which covers these structures) and terminates in the coccygeal glomus. On both sides of the rectum, it anastomoses with the lateral sacral arteries.

The *common iliac arteries* (Fig. 1.16) originate from the subdivision of the abdominal aorta at the level of the fourth lumbar vertebra, and extend downwards and outwards in the higher part of the extraperitoneal pelvic space. These vessels are covered over from above downward and from outside inward by the ureters, which descend vertically toward the pelvic cavity.

At the level of the sacroiliac synchondrosis, each of the common iliac arteries generates the two main branches (Fig. 1.16) that then extend downward: the anterior (*external iliac artery*) and the posterior (*hypogastric artery*). Both arteries extend within the adipose areolar tissue of the posterolateral extraperitoneal space.

In any consideration of the *branches of the external iliac arteries* (Fig. 1.16), the *inferior epigastric arteries* (Fig. 1.16) must be mentioned. These vessels originate from the inferior tract of the external iliac artery, next to the internal inguinal foramen, and initially extend medially under this structure, then upward up to the umbilical level, where they cross the transversalis fascia and penetrate the rectus abdominis muscle. Here, they anastomose with the terminal ramifications of the homolateral superior epigastric arteries. They extend into the preperitoneal space, raising the peritoneum and forming the epigastric folds that separate the lateral from the medial inguinal fossae. In the initial tract, they generate a branch extending medially toward the inguinal ring; within the inguinal canal, this branch is located near the spermatic cord in men (*spermatic or funicular artery*) and the round ligament in women (*artery of the round ligament*).

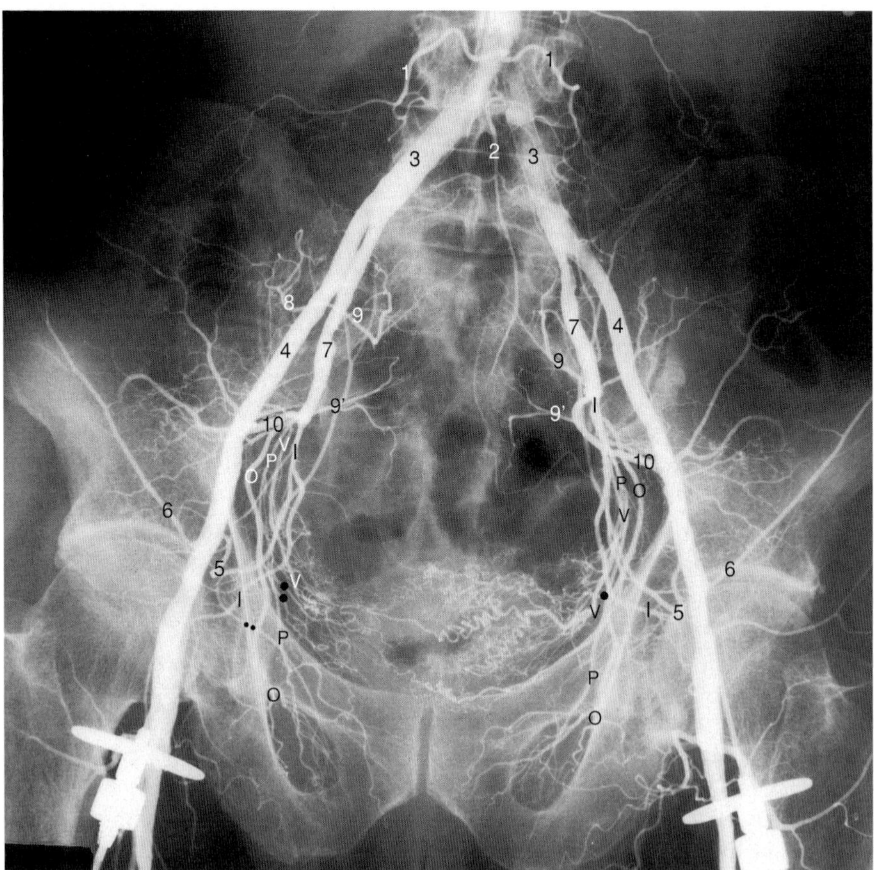

Fig. 1.16. Bilateral retrograde transfemoral pelvic arteriography. Pelvic arteries: *1* lumbar, *2* median sacral, *3* common iliac, *4* external iliac, *5* inferior epigastric, *6* iliac circumflex, *7* internal iliac, *8* ileolumbar, *9* and *9'* lateral sacral, *10* gluteal, *O* obturator, *P* internal pudendal, *V* superior vesical, *I* sciatic, • inferior vesical, •• inguinal (from the EI)

The *hypogastric or internal iliac arteries* (Fig. 1.16) extend obliquely downward and backward along the posterolateral wall of the pelvic cavity, between the peritoneum and the transverse pelvic fascia. At the level of the superior part of the greater sciatic notch, the hypogastric artery divides into several secondary branches (nine in men and eleven in women), which spread to the pelvic wall (*ileolumbar, lateral sacral, obturator, superior* and *inferior gluteal, internal pudendal arteries*) and to the intrapelvic viscera (*superior vesical* or *umbilical vesical, inferior vesical, median hemorrhoidal arteries; uterine* and *vaginal arteries*, in women).

There are numerous variations in the origin of the visceral arteries from the hypogastric artery: they may originate as single vessels or be generated from a common trunk.

The *ileolumbar arteries* (Fig. 1.16) are even and symmetrical; they extend backwards and laterally between the sacrum and the psoas muscle, subdividing after a short extension into the *lumbar branches*, which extend upward to the quadratus lumborum muscle and to the sacrospinal muscles, and into the *iliac branches* extending forward along the iliac crest in the lateral extraperitoneal space up to the homolateral iliac muscles.

The *lateral sacral arteries* (Fig. 1.16) are even and symmetrical; they extend downward in front of the alae of the sacrum, with a slightly oblique path from outside inwards to reach the piriform muscles and the levatores ani behind the rectum, where they anastomose with the median sacral artery on the median line.

The *obturator arteries* (Fig. 1.16) extend from behind forward along the lateral pelvic wall, above the homonymous veins and parallel to the innominate line. They are initially located right against the internal obturator muscle, and then extend under the parietal peritoneum, ensheathed by the sacro-recto-genito-pubic fasciae. Thereafter, they penetrate the obturator foramen, subdividing into the anteromedial (or pubic) and posterolateral branches, which extend to the muscles of the root of the thigh and to the acetabulum. They anastomose with the inferior epigastric, the femoral internal circumflex, and the sciatic arteries.

The *genital arteries* (*internal spermatic* and *ovarian arteries*) extend in the same manner in both men and women in the retroperitoneum, though within the pelvis they have a different path in each sex. They originate from the renal arteries or from the aorta just under the renal arteries and descend into the pelvis between the peritoneum and the psoas, crossing the ureters; at a low level, they overtake the external iliac vessels from outside inwards, and then veer sharply forward and slightly downwards, extending in the extra- and subperitoneal spaces.

In women, the *ovarian arteries* extend in the pelvic tract along the external side of the broad ligament, penetrating the suspensory ligaments of the ovaries and the mesovarium to reach the ovaries and terminate with a full canal anastomosis with the omolateral uterine arteries at the level of the superior uterine angle.

In men, the *spermatic arteries* continue in the subperitoneal spaces of the pelvis, extending along the pelvic wall and the psoas; initially, they extend forward, and then laterally toward the anterior abdominal wall, where they penetrate the inguinal canal, which they cross to reach the testicle.

Visceral Branches. The *superior vesical* (or *umbilical vesical*) *arteries* (Fig. 1.16) originate from the anterior face of the hypogastric arteries and extend forward along the laterosuperior vesical wall. In front of this wall they get closer; at the level of the prevesical space they bend upward and converge with an ascending path toward the umbilicus. After birth, the ascending prevesical tract becomes atrophic, transforming the arteries into the lateral umbilical vesical ligaments.

In front of the urinary bladder, they generate ramifications extending medially up to the anastomosis with their homologous contralateral branches. As a whole, the superior vesical arteries nourish the superior, lateral and anterior vesical walls.

The *inferior vesical arteries* (Fig. 1.16) extend forward to the vesical floor. In men, they generate the prostatic, urethral and deferential branches and are surrounded by the rectovesicular and rectoprostatic ligaments. In women, they generate the vaginal branches.

The *internal pudendal arteries* (Fig. 1.16) have a long, complex and tortuous pathway. They descend along the posterior pelvic wall in front of the sacral plexus, and then exit from the pelvic cavity through the inferior part of the greater sciatic foramen, under the piriform muscle. Thereafter, they delineate a wide curve, with an anterior concavity on the medial ischiatic face, extending downwards up to the greater tuberosity, and then upwards, forward and medially, along the ischiopubic blade. They terminate under the pubic symphysis in the corpora cavernosa penis (or clitoridis in women).

The *middle hemorrhoidal arteries* (Fig. 1.16) extend downward and medially toward the two sides of the rectum, where they anastomose with the superior and inferior hemorrhoidal arteries. They generate the branches for the seminal vesicles, the prostate and the posterior vesical wall in men, and the vagina in women.

It is not rare for the inferior vesical and the median hemorrhoidal arteries originate from other branches of the hypogastric artery (internal pudendal, ischiatic, superior vesical arteries).

The *uterine arteries* extend obliquely downward and forward along the lateral pelvic wall, between the parietal peritoneum and the pelvic fascia. At the level of the broad ligaments, they bend medially and extend (with a transverse path at the ligamental base) onto the sides of the portio supravaginalis cervicis. Here, they bend upward again and extend upward along a sinuous path along the sides of the uterus, between the broad ligament leaves, up to the isthmus, where they curve outward again and terminate with a full canal anastomosis with the homolateral ovarian arteries.

The *vaginal arteries* extend obliquely downwards and forward on the sides of the pelvis; then, they bend medially to reach the vagina and the vulva.

1.2.2 Veins

The following veins have an importance that is relevant in the study of the subperitoneal spaces, the mesenteries and the ligaments:

1) The portal system (portal trunk, splenic vein, superior and inferior mesenteric veins, with their main tributary veins)
2) The pelvic veins

1.2.2.1 The Portal System

The portal system is made up of the portal trunk, the splenic vein, the superior and inferior mesenteric veins and their tributary veins.

a) *The portal trunk* (Fig. 1.17) originates from the confluence of the splenic vein and the superior mesenteric vein above and outside the pancreatic head; it extends obliquely at a high level and on the right side, behind the superior genu of the duodenum, and then penetrates the hepatoduodenal ligament behind the hepatic artery and the

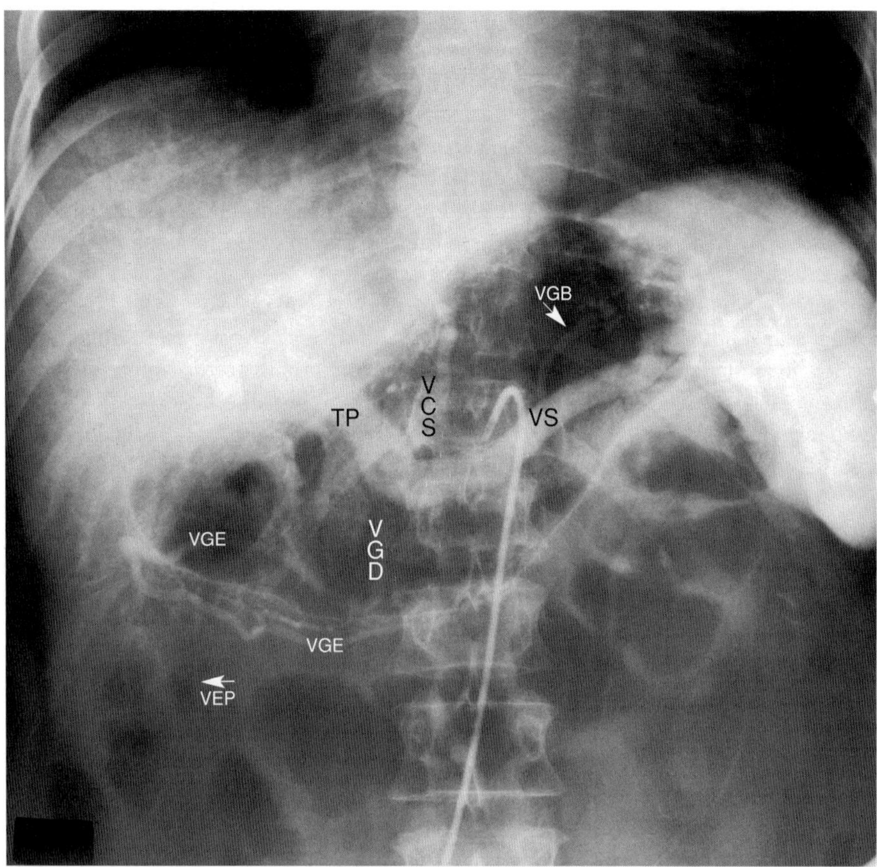

Fig. 1.17. Selective arteriography of the celiac trunk. Phase of venous drainage. Portal trunk and splenic, left gastric, short gastric, gastroduodenal, right gastroepiploic and epiploic veins

choledochus and in front of Winslow's foramen. At the level of the porta hepatis, it bends toward the right side, deeply penetrates the transverse fissure and terminates, dividing into right and left branches.

The most important tributary veins are:

- The *left gastric vein*, which is located together with the homonymous artery within the gastrohepatic ligament, which extends along the lesser curvature of the stomach.
- The *cystic vein*, which comes from the gallbladder.
- The *anterior and posterior superior pancreatoduodenal veins*, which collect blood from the upper part of the pancreatic head and the corpus pancreatis.
- The *umbilical vein* (Fig. 1.22), which extends from the left branch of the portal vein to the umbilicus, crossing the longitudinal fissure of the liver, the prehepatic preperitoneal space and the umbilical canal. In the fetus it is patent, whereas after birth it becomes the round ligament or ligamentum teres. During portal hypertension, it may open again to create hepatofugal collateral circulations.

b) The *splenic vein* (Fig. 1.17) extends downwards and inwards, with a slightly oblique path, along the superior pancreatic border, from the splenic hilum up to the confluence with the superior mesenteric vein in the portal trunk. In the initial tract, it is located in the subperitoneal space of the splenopancreatic ligament, next to the homonymous artery; in the remaining tract, it is sited in the anterior retroperitoneum.

The most important tributary veins are:

- The *left gastroepiploic vein* (Fig. 1.17); it extends parallel to the corresponding artery along the lesser curvature of the stomach, within the gastrocolic ligament, and terminates with a full canal anastomosis with the homonymous contralateral vein. Therefore, the two gastroepiploic veins constitute a wide *anteroinferior anastomotic arcade* along the greater curvature of the stomach, collecting the wide and numerous epiploic *veins of the anterior omental lamina* (Fig. 1.17), which extend parallel and upwards.

The *posterior subepiploic anastomotic arcade* is located in the posterior lamina of the greater epiploon (the thin veins of this lamina flow into this arcade) and terminates in the proximal part of the left gastroepiploic vein.

– The *short gastric veins*; these are coupled with the homonymous arteries and extend within the splenogastric ligament.

c) The *superior mesenteric vein* (Figs. 1.18, 1.19) extends vertically from below upwards along the median line, on the right of the homonymous artery, within the mesentery and next to the retroperitoneum. In the upper part, the vein progressively extends backwards up to the retroperitoneum, where it is located behind the pancreas. The most important tributary veins are:

– The *jejunoileal veins* (Figs. 1.18, 1.19), located within the mesentery and collecting the blood flowing from the small intestine.

– The *ileocolic veins* (Figs. 1.18, 1.19), located within the mesentery surrounding the cecum and the mesenteric areolar; they collect the blood flowing from the ileum and the cecum.

– The *right colic vein* (Fig. 1.19) extends from below upwards on the mesocolic side of the ascending colon and reaches the superior mesenteric vein from behind and on the right side. It terminates with a full canal anastomosis with the ileocolic veins.

– The *right and left middle colic veins* (Fig. 1.19) extend from the transverse colon between the leaves of the transverse mesocolon to the superior mesenteric vein on the median line.

– The *anterior* and *posterior inferior pancreatoduodenal veins* originate at the level of the uncinate process of the pancreas on the sides of the third duodenal portion, and extend horizontally up to the superior mesenteric vein.

– The *right gastroepiploic vein* (Fig. 1.17) extends from left to right along the greater curvature of the stomach up to the pylorus, where it bends backwards and downwards to reach the superior mesenteric vein behind the uncinate process of the pancreas.

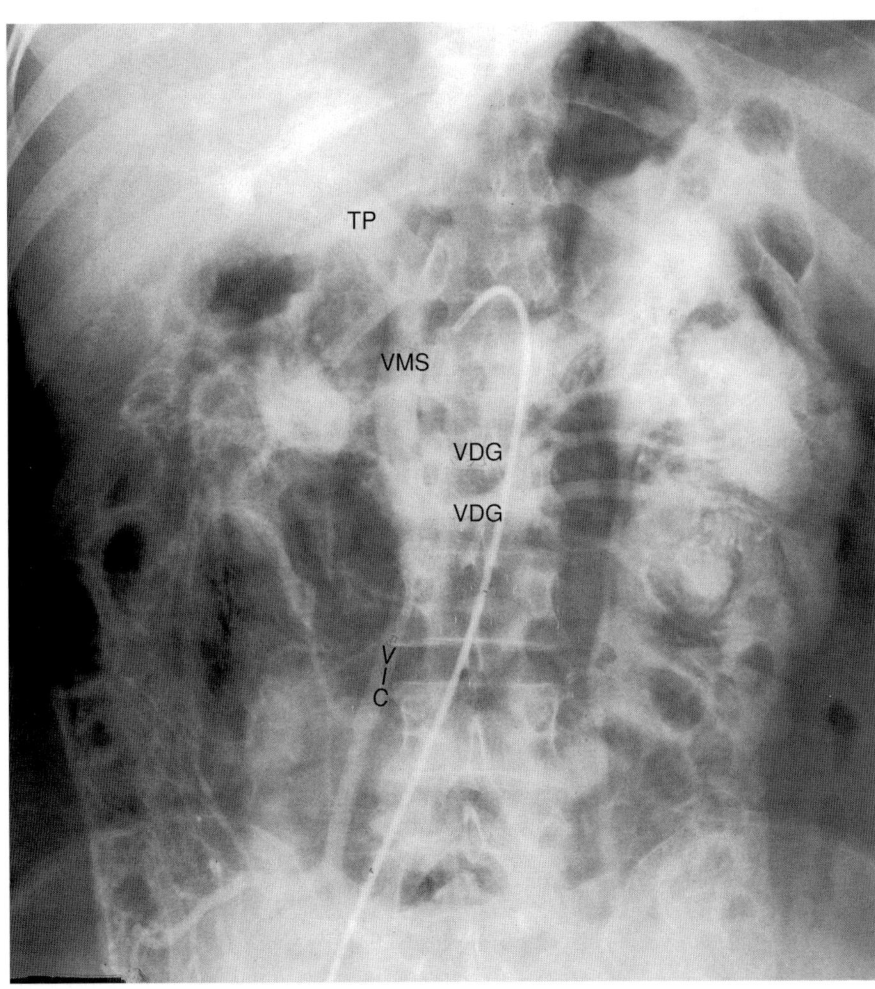

Fig. 1.18. Superior mesenteric arteriography during venous drainage phase. Superior mesenteric vein and its tributaries: jejunal and ileocolic veins

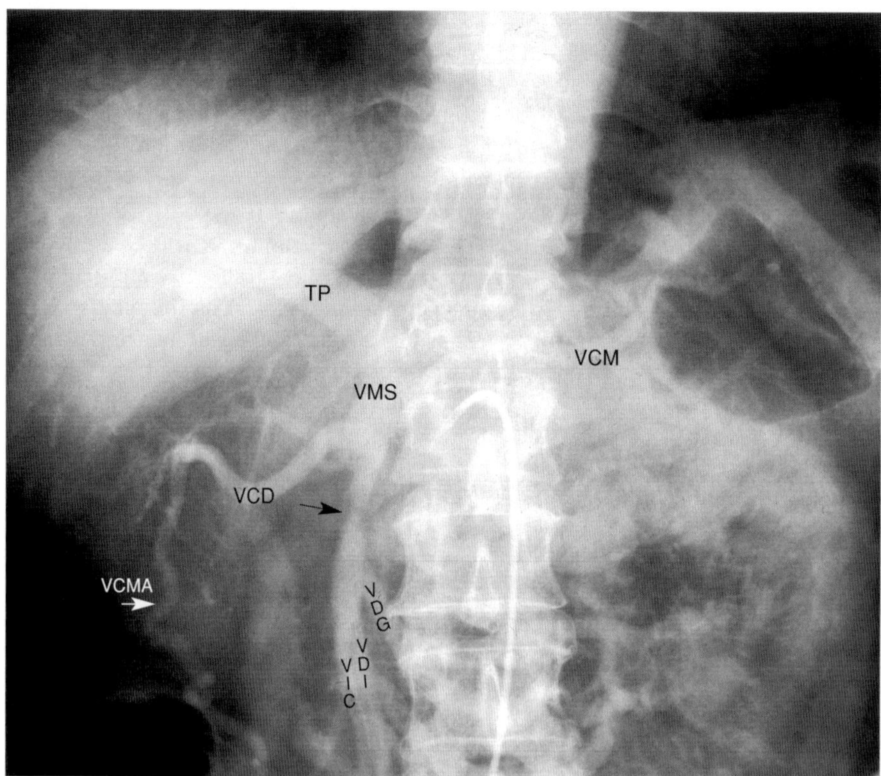

Fig. 1.19. Selective arteriography of the superior mesenteric artery during venous drainage phase. Superior mesenteric vein and its affluent veins: middle colic, jejunal, jejunoileal, ileocolic, marginal colic and right colic veins: these last veins are dilated because they constitute a collateral circulation to compensate the stenosis of the superior mesenteric vein trunk (*arrow*)

- The *subpyloric* (or *right gastric*) *vein* is short and thin; it collects the blood flowing from the gastric antrum, the pylorus and the first duodenal tract.

It is not uncommon to find the right gastroepiploic, subpyloric, right superior colic, and anterosuperior pancreatoduodenal veins joined together at the level of the right angle of the root of the transverse mesocolon in a single vessel, the *gastrocolic trunk*, which flows into the superior mesenteric vein under the splenomesenteric confluent.

The superior and inferior pancreatoduodenal veins constitute two venous arcades, one in the front and the other behind the pancreatic head, connecting (directly or through an interposed gastrocolic trunk) the portal trunk with the superior mesenteric vein.

d) The *inferior mesenteric vein* (Figs. 1.20, 1.21) extends from below upwards along the left paramedian line, from the pelvis to the left hypochondrium. It originates at a low level from the confluence of the *superior hemorrhoidal veins* with the *sigmoidal veins* and extends in anterior retroperitoneal planes in front of the iliac vessels and subsequently in front of the gonadal vessels, the left ureter and the aorta. It extends parallel to the homonymous artery, being always slightly on the left side of the aorta. In the tract above the origin of the homonymous artery from the aorta, the inferior mesenteric vein extends in planes located more anteriorly, even though it remains in the retroperitoneum; then, it crosses the left paraduodenal space outside Treitz's duodenojejunal angle and extends oblique and medially, terminating in the splenic vein next to the confluence of this vein with the superior mesenteric vein or directly into the superior mesenteric vein. Along its extension, it joins the *left colic vein* (Figs. 1.20, 1.21), which comes from the left side.

1.2.2.2 The Pelvic Veins

The parietal and visceral pelvic veins follow the disposition and path of the homonymous arteries, with the exception of the *visceral branches of the hypogastric veins*. There are twice as many of these branches as there are of the arteries, and they originate from a dense mass of interlaced and intercommunicating

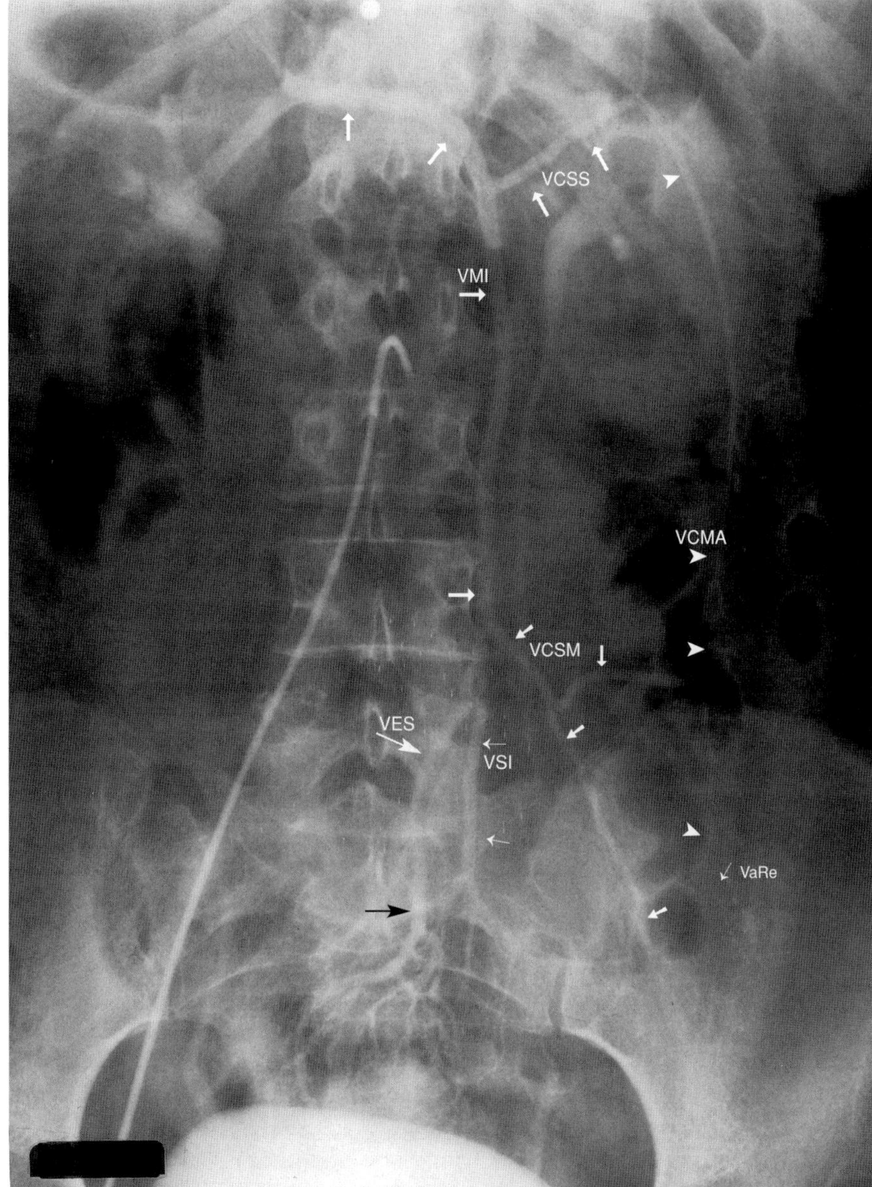

Fig. 1.20. Selective arteriography of the inferior mesenteric artery during venous drainage phase. Inferior mesenteric, sigmoidal, superior hemorrhoidal and left superior, median and marginal colic veins

veins without valves surrounding and closely adherent to the pelvic viscera: the *venous plexus*. The venous plexus are subdivided into:

- The *pelvivesical plexus*; it is located on the sides and under the urinary bladder and the seminal vesicles, and is a tributary of the vesical veins.
- The *uterovaginal plexus*; this is located on the sides of the uterus and vagina within the broad ligaments and is a tributary of the uterine and ovarian veins.
- The *hemorrhoidal plexus*; it surrounds the rectum and flows into the inferior mesenteric vein through the superior hemorrhoidal veins, into the hypogastric vein through the median hemorrhoidal veins and into the internal pudendal veins through the inferior hemorrhoidal veins.
- The *anterior sacral plexus*; it is retrorectal and retrofascial and flows into the median sacral vein.

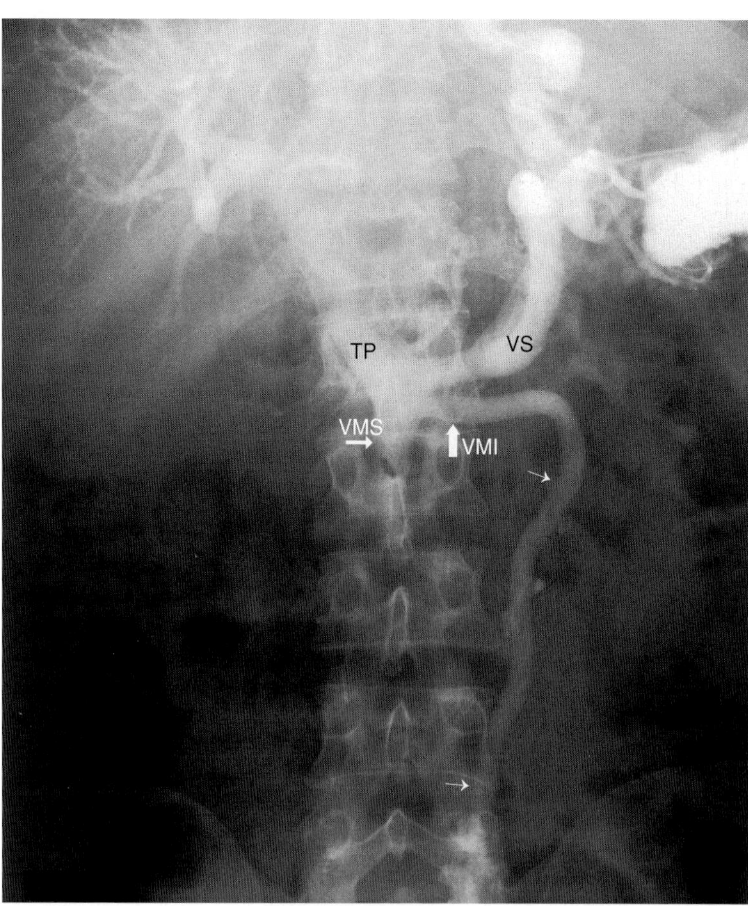

Fig. 1.21. Splenoportography in a cirrhotic patient. Confluence of the inferior and superior mesenteric veins. Inverse flux in the inferior mesenteric vein draining the blood as it cannot pass the hepatic sinusoidal obstruction

1.3 Lymphatic System

The relevant structures in the abdominal lymphatic system are represented by the subperitoneal lymphatic vessels and lymph nodes, by the lymphatic vessels of the parietal peritoneum and by their connections.

The lymph flowing from the intraperitoneal viscera is filtered by the *coeliomesenteric lymph* nodes before reaching the intestinal trunk. The number of these lymph nodes varies in a range of 15–20; they can be divided into two groups: superior (around the celiac trunk) and inferior (around the superior mesenteric artery).

The former group collects the lymph flowing from the supramesocolic organs (abdominal esophagus, stomach, duodenum, liver and spleen); the latter collects the lymph coming from the small intestine, the cecum-ascending colon and the transverse colon. The pancreatic lymphatic vessels extend to both groups.

The coeliomesenteric lymph nodes are located in the retroperitoneum in front of the anterior renal fascia, the aorta, the inferior vena cava and the left renal vein, and behind the pancreas, the duodenum and the mesenteric root. They are interconnected and are joined to the lumboaortic chains through numerous anastomotic collectors.

The lymph flowing from the intraperitoneal viscera is filtered by numerous lymph node stations before reaching the coeliomesenteric lymph nodes; the primary stations are located near the organs by which the lymph is produced, whereas the intermediate, secondary stations collect the lymph flowing from various organs. Therefore, it is very important to know the exact localization and the relationships between these lymphatic stations, and the path followed by the lymph to reach and interconnect these structures.

The *primary stations* are located along the walls of the hollow viscera, adjacent to the peripheral arterial branches or inside the hepatic and the splenic hila. The collectors follow a parallel, but inverse, path compared with that of the visceral arteries, whose extension is followed by isolated or grouped lymph nodes.

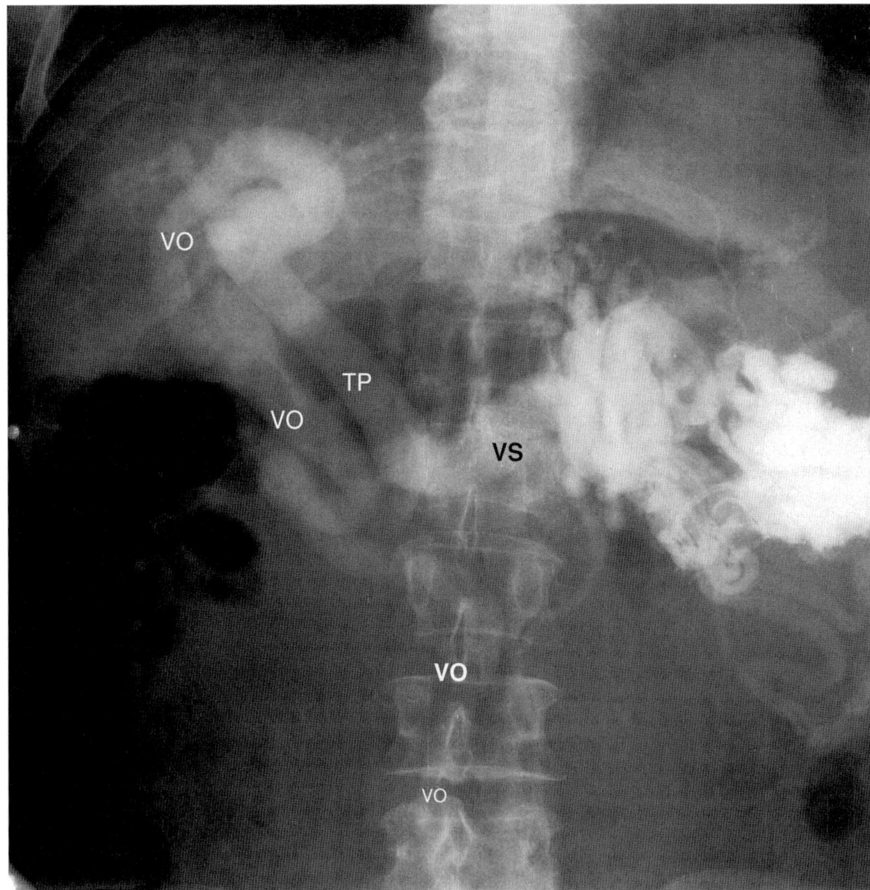

Fig. 1.22. Splenoportography in a cirrhotic patient. The umbilical vein is passable again and dilated, constituting a portocaval collateral circulation

The *main regional lymph nodes* and their relative connections can be schematically classified as follows:

- *Hepatic lymph nodes*; they are located along the extension of the homonymous artery, with the *deep* (or *primary*) *lymph nodes* (Fig. 1.23B, C) at the subdivision points of the vessels and ducts in the depth of the transverse fissure, and the *superficial* (*cystic* and *choledochal*) *lymph nodes* (Fig. 1.23C, D), located at the margin of the distal biliary tract within the hepatoduodenal ligament. The efferent collectors from the superficial hepatic lymph nodes extend to the lymph nodes of the celiac trunk (Fig. 1.23C) in a direct manner or with the interposition of the *pancreatoduodenal lymph nodes*. Collectors coming from the pylorus, the duodenum and the pancreatic head also flow into these latter lymph nodes.
- *Gastric lymph nodes*; these are located along the greater and the lesser curvature of the stomach. The former are placed between the leaves of the gastrohepatic ligament and constitute the *left gastric chain* (Fig. 1.23B–D). The latter are located within the gastrocolic ligament and constitute the *gastroepiploic chain* (Fig. 1.23A–D). The efferent collectors from the two groups extend to the *retropyloric lymph nodes* (Fig. 1.23D) next to the head of the pancreas. Collectors coming from the duodenum and the pancreatic head also flow into these latter lymph nodes.
The lymph coming from the fundus ventriculi flows into the *lymph nodes of the gastrosplenic ligament* (Fig. 1.23A) following the short gastric vessel paths; afterwards, it flows into the splenic or pancreatic lymph nodes. Furthermore, some lymph node stations (*supracardial lymph nodes*; Fig. 1.23A) are located above the cardia ventriculi; from these stations, the lymph flows into the *paraesophageal lymphatic collectors*, which extend above the diaphragm.
- *Splenic* (Fig. 1.23 B, C), *superior and inferior pancreatic* (Fig. 1.23B–E) *lymph nodes*; they are located at the splenic hilum and along the superior and inferior margins of the pancreas and collect the

lymph flowing from the spleen and from the corpus and cauda pancreatis.

- *Pancreatoduodenal lymph nodes* (Fig. 1.23E, F); they are located at the level of the pancreatic head and receive the lymph flowing from the head of the pancreas, stomach, duodenum, liver and collectors coming from splenic and superior and inferior pancreatic lymph nodes. The efferent lymphatics reach the celiac lymph nodes.
- The *superior mesenteric lymph nodes* are located between the leaves of the mesentery in three levels: the first is placed along the vascular arcades extending parallel to the intestinal wall on the mesenteric side, the second is located next to the jejunoileal and ileocolic arteries, the third surrounds the trunks of the superior mesenteric artery and vein. In turn, these latter are placed in two planes: one in the front and the other behind the vessels. The mesenteric lymphatics flow into the lymph nodes located in front and on the sides of the origin of the superior mesenteric artery from the aorta. Numerous anastomoses connect them to the celiac and lumboaortic lymph nodes.
- The *mesocolic lymph nodes*; analogously to the mesenteric lymph nodes, they are located in three levels:

  a) *Paracolic* or *marginal lymph nodes* (Fig. 1.23A–G); they are located in the mesocolon, relatively to each tract (ascending, transverse) along the extension of the marginal colic arteries.

  b) *Intermediate lymph nodes*; they are located along the middle colic (Fig. 1.23F) and the right colic (Fig. 1.23G) branches of the superior mesenteric artery.

  c) *Superior mesenteric lymph nodes* (Fig. 1.23D–G); they are located on the sides of the homonymous vessels. Also the jejunoileal and ileocolic collectors (Fig. 1.23F, G) flow into these lymph nodes.
- *Inferior mesenteric lymph nodes.*

The *primary* or *marginal lymph nodes* (Fig. 1.23C–G) collect the lymph flowing from the descending colon, sigmoid and superior tract of the rectum. They are located within the mesenteries, inside, behind or on the sides of these viscera, respectively. Their collectors flow into *intermediate lymphatic stations* located along the extension of the left colic (Fig. 1.23E), sigmoidal (Fig. 1.23H) and superior hemorrhoidal (Fig. 1.23I) arteries. From these stations, the lymph flows into the *distal lymph nodes* (Fig. 1.23E, G), located along the extension of the inferior mesenteric artery, and then, into the lumboaortic lymph nodes placed in front and on the left side of the subrenal aorta.

Some *lymphatic collectors* do not extend along the artery, but rather *along the inferior mesenteric vein*, up to the lymph nodes located into the left paraduodenal space. Thereafter, they reach the inferior pancreatic lymph nodes, and then, the celiac lymph nodes.

There is a rich lymphatic network within the *greater omentum*, prevalently located in the anterior lamina. These lymphatics are very dense and numerous and extend upwards along the arterial branches; most of them reach the lymph nodes of the subpyloric group, whereas a lower number of lymphatics flow into the lymph nodes of the gastroduodenal arcade. Thereafter, both groups reach the celiac lymph nodes. Some small lymph nodes are located along the extension of the omental collectors.

The lymphatics placed into the posterior lamina are sparse and thin; they flow into the lymph nodes of the pancreatosplenic chain and then into the celiac lymph nodes.

The *lymphatics of the parietal peritoneum* extend upwards along various pathways: one group follows the retrosternal pathway to reach the superior mediastinal lymph nodes, whereas another group crosses the diaphragm next to the inferior vena cava and the phrenic nerves, and flows into the pulmonary hilar lymph nodes.

Fig. 1.23A–I. Scheme showing positions of the abdominal lymph nodes relative to each other and to the vascular organs and structures in axial section. **A** Subdiaphragmatic level. Supracardial (*SC*), left gastroepiploic (*GES*) and marginal colic (*CMA*) lymph nodes. **B** Level of the hepatic hilum. Deep hepatic (*EP*), left gastric (*CS*), splenic (*S*), gastroepiploic (*GES*) and left marginal colic (*CM*) lymph nodes. **C** Celiac level. Deep (*EP*) and superficial (*ES*) hepatic lymph nodes; node of Winslow's hiatus (*W*); splenic (*S*), coronarostomachic (*CS*), gastroepiploic (*GES*), left marginal colic (*CM*), celiac (*C*) and lumboaortic (*LA*) lymph nodes. **D** Level of the body and tail of the pancreas. Cystic and choledochal (*CI*), right gastroepiploic (*GED*), right left gastric (*CS*), superior mesenteric (*MS*), parapancreatic (body and tail) (*PA*), posterior pancreatoduodenal (*PDP*), and marginal colic (*CM*) lymph nodes. **E** Level of the pancreatic head. Pancreatoduodenal (*PD*), pancreatic (*PA*), marginal colic (*CM*), inferior mesenteric (*MI*), left colic (*CSI*) and omental (*O*) **F** Level of the transverse mesocolon. Middle colic (*CME*), superior mesenteric (*MS*), jejunal (*DI*), anterior (*PDA*) and posterior (*PDP*) pancreatoduodenal (*PDA* and *PDP*), left marginal colic (*CM*) and omental (*O*) lymph nodes **G** Mesenteric level. Superior mesenteric (*MS*), ileal (*I*), right colic (*CD*), marginal colic (*CM*), omental (*O*), left colic (*CSI*), inferior mesenteric (*MI*) lymph nodes. **H** Sigmoidal (high pelvic) level. Paracecal (*CE*), sigmoidal (*S*) and external iliac (*IE*) lymph nodes. **I** Level of the fundus uteri. Vesical (*V*), utero-ovarian (*UO*), superior hemorrhoidal (*EMS*) and external (*IE*) and internal (*II*) iliac

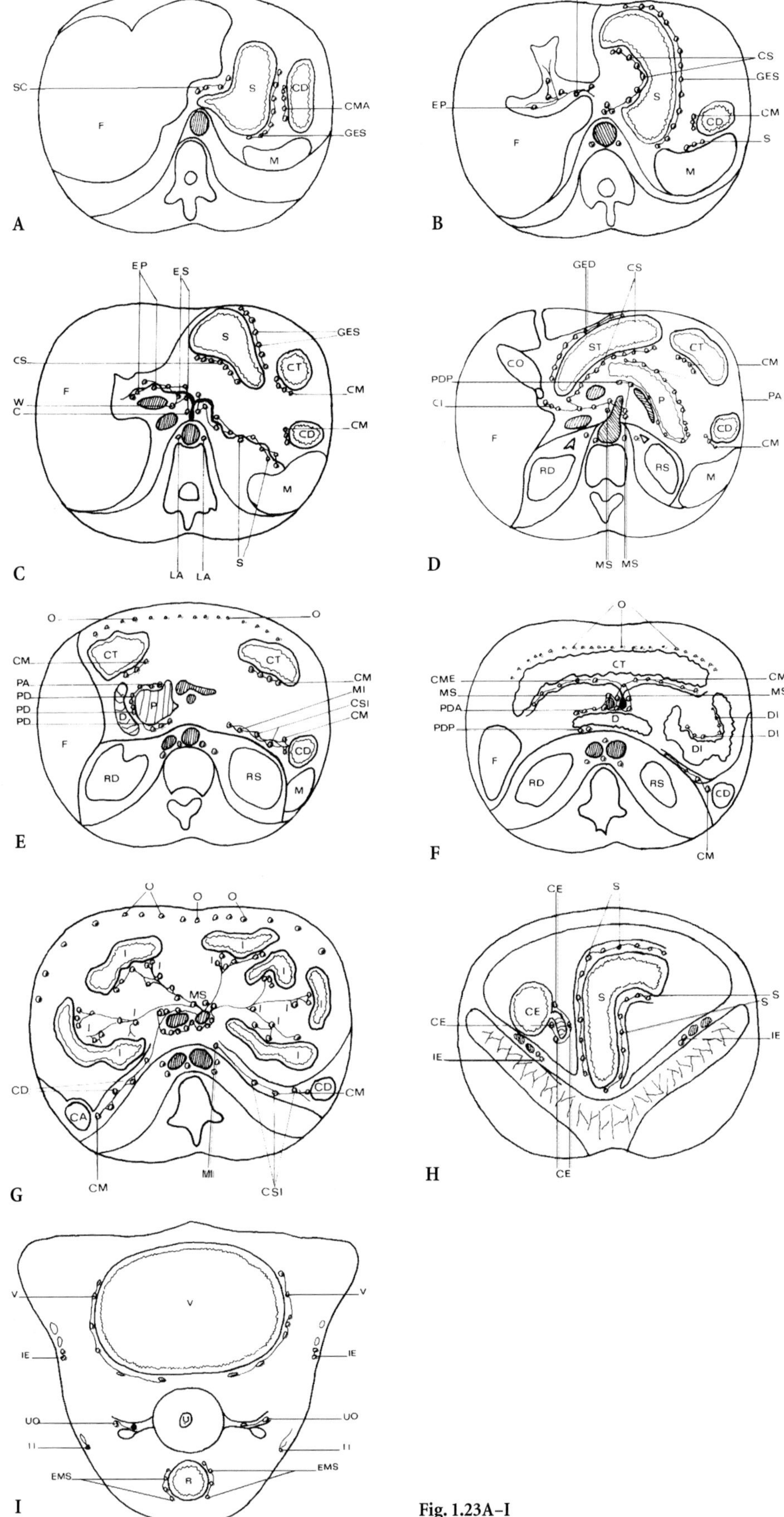

A
SC
F
S
CD
CMA
GES
M
B
EP
CS
GES
CM
CD
S
M
C
EP
ES
GES
CS
CT
CM
W
C
CM
CD
M
S
LA
LA
D
GED
CS
ST
CT
CM
PDP
CO
PA
CI
P
CD
CM
RD
RS
M
MS
MS
E
O
O
CM
CT
CT
CM
PA
PD
MI
PD
CSI
PD
CM
CD
RD
RS
M
F
O
CT
CME
CME
MS
MS
PDA
DI
PDP
DI
DI
RD
RS
CD
CM
G
O
O
O
MS
CD
CD
CM
CA
CM
MI
CSI
H
CE
S
CE
S
S
CE
IE
IE
CE
I
V
V
IE
IE
UO
UO
EMS
EMS
R

Fig. 1.23A–I

Other lymphatics directly reach the thoracic duct and the cisterna chyli, at various levels; finally, some posterior lymphatics flow into the gastric, pancreatic and renal lymph nodes.

1.4 Nervous System

The abdominal nervous system comprises the sympathetic system and the spinal nervous plexus.

1.4.1 Abdominal Sympathetic System

In the abdomen, the sympathetic system extends in two levels:

1. At a posterior level, nervous cords continue without interruption from the first cervical to the last coccygeal vertebra, anterolaterally to the vertebral bodies and medially to the iliopsoas insertions, behind the inferior vena cava on the right side and the abdominal aorta on the left side. Along their extension, the cords show fusiform ganglial enlargements: four lumbar, four sacral and one or two coccygeal.
2. At an anterior prevertebral level, a plexiform structure is formed by knotting of nervous fibers coming from the thoracic ganglia through the greater and the lesser splanchnic nerves and from the abdominal ganglia. It is located behind and on the sides of the abdominal aorta along its total extension. Numerous nervous branches originate from this plexus; they extend in front of the aorta and surround the origin of the main arterial trunks with masses of nervous and ganglial fibers, constituting the celiac (or solar), lumboaortic and hypogastric prevascular plexuses.

1.4.1.1 Celiac or Solar Plexus

The celiac plexus is located in front of the proximal tract of the abdominal aorta around the celiac trunk and the superior mesenteric artery. It is connected with the secondary plexus, which extends along the ramifications of these vessels up to their terminations, having the same names, disposition and distribution. Along their extensions, they generate small ganglia.

Following the origin and the extension of the abdominal vessels from above downwards, we find the following peripheral plexuses:

a) *Phrenic* or *inferior diaphragmatic plexuses*; they are even and symmetrical, and are located just under the diaphragm. These plexuses generate branches for the adrenal glands.
b) *Coronostomachic or superior gastric plexuses.*
c) *Hepatic plexuses*, with the pyloric, gastric, gastroduodenal and right gastroepiploic secondary plexuses;
d) *Splenic plexuses*, with the pancreatic, left gastroepiploic and short gastric secondary plexus.
e) *Superior mesenteric plexus*, with the mesenteric plexus of the right and transverse mesocolon.
f-h) *Adrenal, renal, spermatic and utero-ovarian plexuses*, which are even and symmetrical.

1.4.1.2 Lumboaortic Plexus

The lumboaortic plexus is located under the solar plexus, in front and on the sides of the subrenal aorta. It generates:

a) The *inferior mesenteric plexus*, which in turn generates the left colic, the sigmoidal and the superior hemorrhoidal plexuses
b) The *common and external iliac plexuses*, which are bilateral and symmetrical
c) The *hypogastric plexus*, which is located medially and represents the continuation of the lumboaortic plexus. It bifurcates to follow the two (right and left) hypogastric arteries, which in turn generate the secondary plexus

1.4.1.3 Pelvic or Sacral Plexus

At the pelvic level, the sympathetic cords extend in front of the sacrum, medially to the anterior sacral foramina and on the sides of the rectum. Four sacral ganglia and one or two coccygeal ganglia are located along these cords. A series of ramifications originate from these ganglia. After joining some nervous fibers coming from the sacral nerves, these branches form the *hypogastric plexus* (on the sides of the pelvic viscera within the subperitoneal pelvic space), which are made up of dense and complex knots of nervous fibers with numerous ganglia.

The hypogastric plexuses terminate in four secondary plexuses, which are even and symmetrical and follow the extension of the branches of the hypogastric artery and distribute to the pelvic viscera, constituting:

a) The *median hemorrhoidal plexus* on the sides of the rectum

b) The *inferior vesical plexus* for the fundus vesicae, the urethra and the terminal part of the ureter
c) The *prostatic plexus* on the sides of the prostate, which extends forward, continuing in the cavernous plexus of the penis
d) The *vesiculodeferential plexus* around the seminal vesicles and the deferent duct
In women, instead of the prostatic and vesiculodeferential plexus, we observe:
e) The *uterine plexus*, which is located within the broad ligaments on the sides of the uterus
f) The *vaginal plexus*, which is located on the sides of the vagina and continues forward into the cavernous plexus of the clitoris

1.4.2 Lumbosacral Plexus of the Spinal Nerves

The lumbosacral plexus consists of the complex of the radicular plexus formed by the anterior branches of the lumbar and sacrococcygeal nerves.

It generates the nerves for the inferior part of the trunk, the pelvic viscera and the lower limbs. Topographically, it is subdivided into the lumbar and the sacrococcygeal plexus.

1.4.2.1 Lumbar Plexus

The primary and bilateral lumbar plexus is made up of the anterior blades of the first, second, third and fourth lumbar nerves interconnected by anastomotic arcades; it extends vertically into the paravertebral gutter of both sides within the thickness of the psoas, between its insertions on the transverse process and on the vertebral body. It has a triangular shape, with a posterior base at the level of the conjugation foramina and the apex constituted by the femoral nerve extending downwards and laterally. It is covered by the parietal pelvic fascia, by which it is separated from the renal fascia and from the peritoneum.

Communicating branches join the lumbar to the sympathetic plexus, which is located inside and extends in front of the anterolateral part of the vertebral body.

At various levels, the lumbar plexus generates a series of branches. In particular, we distinguish four collateral branches, placed as follows (from above downwards):
1) Greater abdominogenital (or ileohypogastric) nerve
2) Lesser abdominogenital (or ileoinguinal) nerve
3) Femorocutaneous nerve (or lateral cutaneous nerve of the thigh)
4) Genitocrural (or genitofemoral or external spermatic) nerve

and two terminals:
a) The obturator nerve
b) The femoral or crural or lumboinguinal nerve

Besides these long branches, short ramifications for the intertransversarii laterales, the psoas and the quadrati lumborum muscles originate from the lumbar plexus.
1) The *greater abdominogenital* (or *ileohypogastric*) nerve originates from the anterior branch of the first lumbar nerve and extends behind the muscular bundles of the psoas up to the level of the transverse apophysis of L-2; thereafter, it extends laterally, downward and forward between the transversalis fascia and the aponeurosis of the transverse muscle, and then between this latter muscle and the internal oblique muscle. At the level of the anterosuperior iliac spine, it divides into the abdominal and genital branches. The former extends medially between the internal and external oblique muscles and terminates anteriorly in the rectus abdominis muscle. The genital branch extends downward and backward between the oblique muscles up to the inguinal canal, which it penetrates.
2) The *lesser abdominogenital* (or *ileoinguinal*) *nerve* has the same origin, path and distribution as the greater abdominogenital nerve.
3) The *femorocutaneous nerve* (or *lateral cutaneous nerve of the thigh*) originates from the anterior branch of the second and partly of the third lumbar nerve. Initially, it extends oblique behind the psoas, and subsequently downwards, outwards and forward, up to the front of the quadratus lumborum muscle and then of the iliac muscle; after this, it penetrates between this latter muscle and the pelvic transversalis fascia. Coming out from the pelvis between the two anterior iliac spines, it subdivides into the gluteal and femoral branches, which spread to the skin of the anterolateral face of the thigh and the lateral part of the buttock.
4) The *genitocrural* (or *genitofemoral or external spermatic*) *nerve* originates from the second lumbar nerve, alone or together with the lumboinguinal nerve. Together with this latter nerve, it extends forward in the thickness of the psoas up to the promontory. After crossing the muscular aponeurosis, it descends oblique and forward, overtakes

the common iliac vessels, and extends in front of the external iliac vessels and the internal spermatic vessels, medial to the ureter, within the adipose areolar tissue that is located among the transversalis fascia, the peritoneum and the pelvic organs.

Anteriorly, it subdivides into: a genital branch, that extends along the spermatic vessels in the inguinal canal and distributes to the scrotal skin and a crural branch, that follows the external iliac artery in the crural canal. In the Scarpa's triangle, it is located in front of the femoral artery. It innervates the skin of the anterior part of the thigh.

a) The *obturator nerve* originates from the fusion of the anterior roots of the second, third and fourth lumbar nerves. Initially, it extends within the thickness of the psoas, medially to the crural nerve; thereafter, it extends on the internal side of the muscle, behind the common iliac vessels. It remains in a extrafascial site and descends forward, following the obturator vessels along the lateral wall of the pelvis. It then penetrates the obturator canal under the pubis. It is separated from the hypogastric vessels and from the ureter by the pelvic fascia. It terminates with the innervation of the adductor muscles of the thigh.
b) The *femoral* (or *crural* or *lumboinguinal*) nerve originates from the anterior root of the second, third and fourth lumbar nerves. Initially, it is located deep in the thickness of the greater psoas, and then extends outward and downward along the gutter constituted by this muscle and by the iliac muscle. It descends beyond the femoral ring up to the insertion of the psoas on the lesser trochanter.

In the abdominopelvic tract, the nerve is constantly located outside the transversalis fascia, by which it is separated from the ureter and from the common and external iliac vessels. Furthermore, the psoas extends between these vessels and the nerve for its total length.

At the inguinal level, it is located laterally to the femoral vessels. It terminates with the generation of motor branches for the anteromedial muscles of the thigh and for the skin of the anterior face of the thigh, the knee and the medial region of the leg and of the foot.

1.4.2.2 Sacrococcygeal Plexus

The sacrococcygeal plexus is formed by the complex of the anastomoses interconnecting the fifth lumbar nerve and the sacral and coccygeal nerves before their peripheral distribution. It is triangular, with the base located at a high level (at the level of the conjugation foramina) and an inferolateral apex at the converging point of the five branches (at the level of the greater sciatic incisure). It is located deeply in the posterointernal part of the pelvis, within the space between the anterior face of the pyramidal muscle and the parietal pelvic fascia, the hypogastric vessels, the laterorectal extraperitoneal areolar tissue, the perirectal fascia, the rectum and the peritoneum being located in front of the parietal pelvic fascia.

The sacrococcygeal plexus generates collateral branches, being divided into an anterior and a posterior branch (which extend downward and outward toward the greater sciatic incisure and distribute to the muscles of the pelvic girdle, to the genital organs and to the perineal skin and muscles), and a terminal branch, the *greater sciatic nerve*, innervating the posterior part of the lower limb.

Furthermore, the visceral branches originate from the anterior face of the sacrococcygeal plexus; they extend forward, on the sides of the pelvic cavity, up to the junction with the sympathetic branches. Together, these ramifications constitute the *hypogastric plexus* posteriorly, and the *pelvic plexus* anteriorly, along the homonymous branches of the hypogastric artery, on the sides of the viscera (see sympathetic system).

1.5 Extraperitoneal Structures Connected with the Peritoneum

In order to provide a more complete description, we are now adding a section about the juxtaperitoneal structures that are closely connected with the peritoneum and the subperitoneal spaces. These structures deserve particular attention during diffusion of the inflammatory and tumoral processes involving the peritoneum.

a) The preperitoneal space of the superior abdomen, the supraumbilical fascia and the umbilical canal
b) The preperitoneal subumbilical space
c) The subperitoneal pelvic space
d) The anterior and lateroconal renal fasciae and the anterior pararenal space
e) The transversalis fascia

There is no general agreement among anatomists on the existence of the supra- and subumbilical fasciae; furthermore, there is no agreement on their position (anterior or posterior) relative to vessels and cords crossing the preperitoneal space and converging toward the umbilicus, or even on their names.

This disagreement probably depends on the great variability in the existence, extension and connection of these fasciae and in the subdivision of the preperitoneal spaces that are crossed by these fasciae.

In the anatomical description of these fasciae and of the limited spaces, we have taken into account a fundamental element: their correspondence with the CT representations. This correspondence agrees with the description made by the old, but still valid text by Testut (1905).

1.5.1 Preperitoneal Space of the Superior Abdomen. (Supraumbilical Fascia and Umbilical Canal)

The areolar connective tissue located between the transversalis fascia and the peritoneum is thin on the sides and wider on the median line between the ensiform apophysis and the umbilicus; it constitutes a space with a biconvex lenticular shape: *Richet's space* or *umbilical canal* (Figs. 1.2A–D, 1.4B, C). The thickness (1–3.4 cm) and width (2–12 cm) of this space vary in different subjects; it is occupied by adipose tissue, by the ensiform vessels (terminal branches of the internal mammary vessels and/or of the superior epigastric vessels) and by the vestiges of the funiculus umbilicalis (ligamentum teres or round ligament) or by the umbilical vein.

This space is limited posteriorly by a thin lamella of transverse fibers, the *supraumbilical fascia*, which is frequently, but not constantly located anteriorly and in close contact with the parietal peritoneum. The thickness and width of this lamella is very variable in different subjects; on the left side and below (at the umbilical level), it joins the transversalis fascia, whereas on the right side and above it blends with the peritoneum.

The *ligamentum teres* or *round ligament* (vestige of the funiculus umbilicalis) extends from the umbilicus to the intersegmental fissure of the left hepatic lobe. Just after its umbilical origin, it is initially located along the median line within the umbilical canal, where it takes contact with the transversalis fascia; thereafter, it extends upward and progressively backward. At the level of the free margin of the falciform ligament it bends toward the right side at an angle of 30°–40°. After a short extension between the transversalis fascia and the parietal peritoneum, it penetrates between the laminae of the falciform ligament into the intersegmental fissure of the left hepatic lobe, up to the junction with the left branch of the portal vein.

1.5.2 Subumbilical Preperitoneal Space

The subumbilical preperitoneal space is located between the posterior wall of the linea alba and of the rectus and obliquus abdominis muscles and the peritoneum. From the front backward (Figs. 1.2G–I, 1.4B, C) it comprises:
1) The transversalis fascia
2) The umbilicoprevesical space
3) The umbilicovesical fascia
4) The umbilicoperivesical space

At a high level under the umbilicus, the *transversalis fascia* (Fig. 1.4) is thick and closely adherent to the rectus and obliquus abdominis muscles; it is formed by the superimposition and fusion of the posterior aponeuroses of these muscles. Below, from the semicircular Douglas' arcade, it becomes very thin, being composed just of the posterior sheath of the rectus muscle. In this tract, it moves away from this muscle and extends progressively downward to insert at the superointernal border and the posterior side of the pubis and to merge with the pubovesical ligament on the median line, then continuing downward in the pelvic fascia. A triangular space, with a superior apex occupied by adipose tissue, the *suprapubic* or *retromuscular space* (Fig. 1.4B, C) is located between the rectus abdominis muscle, which inserts at the anterosuperior border of the pubis and the transverse fascia.

At the level of Douglas' semicircular line, the transversalis fascia is symmetrically crossed from behind forward on both sides by the inferior epigastric vessels and nerves for the rectus muscle.

The *umbilicoprevesical space* is a wide abdominopelvic space. In the abdominal tract, it takes the form of a thin layer of adipose tissue, contained between the transversalis and the umbilicovesical fasciae and between the umbilicus and the pelvic fascia; at the sides it communicates with the lateral extraperitoneal spaces and through these spaces with the retroperitoneum. In the pelvic tract, it expands, constituting anteriorly (in the presuprapubic region) a space occupied by adipose tissue (Retzius' prevesical or Scarpa's preperitoneal space), which continues with a cuneiform shape on the sides of the urinary bladder, between the umbilicovesical fascia inside and the sacro-recto-genito-pubic fascia outside (see subperitoneal pelvic spaces).

The *umbilicovesical fascia* (Fig. 1.4B, C) is a thin abdominopelvic fascia; in the abdominal tract it has a triangular shape with a superior apex (which inserts in the inferior part of the umbilical cicatrix) and expands, as it extends progressively downward. It is limited at the sides by the diverging umbilicovesical ligaments. At the pelvic level, it extends backward, delineating a semicircle with posterior concavity in front and to the sides of the urinary bladder, to which it becomes closely adherent. Below, it inserts and blends with the internal margin of the pubovesical ligament on the median line and with the superior fascia of the pelvic diaphragm on the sides of the uterine cervix (or of the prostatoperitoneal fascia) and of the rectum (see subperitoneal pelvic spaces). It subdivides the subumbilical preperitoneal adipose tissue into the pre- and perivesical spaces.

The *umbilicoperivesical space* (Figs. 1.2G–I, 1.4B, C) is a very thin interstice located between the umbilicovesical fascia and the anterior and pelvic parietal peritoneum. The median umbilicovesical ligament and the medial or lateral umbilicovesical ligaments extend within this space.

The *median umbilicovesical ligament* (Figs. 1.2G–I, 1.4B, C) is a residual cord of the atretic urachus; it extends from the umbilicus to the vesical dome.

The *medial* or *lateral umbilicovesical ligaments* (Figs. 1.2G–I, 1.4B, C) (fibrous residual cords of the atretic homonymous arteries) descend on both sides of the median ligament, from the umbilical to the retropubic region, moving away from the median ligament, as they extend progressively downward. Next to the pubis, they bend back, extending along the two sides of the urinary bladder, and continue in the superior vesical arteries up to the origin of these from the hypogastric arteries.

In the pelvic tract, these ligaments make impressions in the peritoneal folds, limiting the *median inguinal fossae* (between the median umbilicovesical ligament and the lateral umbilicovesical ligaments) and the *lateral inguinal fossae* [between these latter ligaments and the inferior epigastric vessels (Fig. 1.21)].

1.5.3 Subperitoneal Pelvic Space

The subperitoneal pelvic space (Figs. 1.24, 1.25) is located between the inferior parietal peritoneum, the

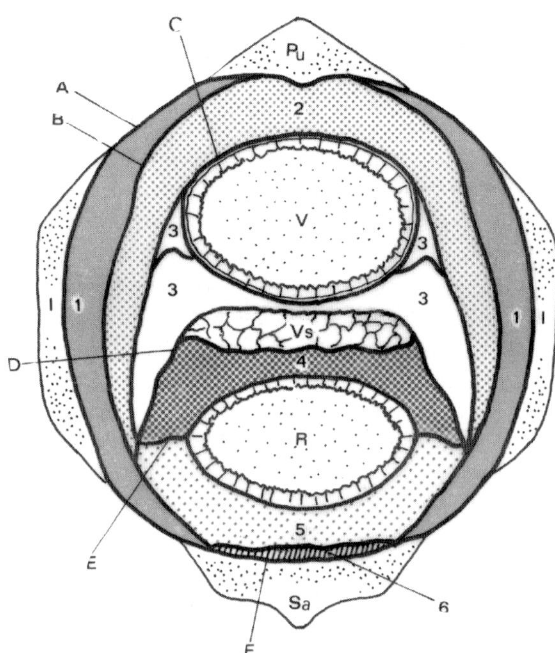

Fig. 1.24. Subperitoneal pelvic space (in men). Axial section (*A* pelvic fascia, *B* sacro-recto-genito-pubic ligament (visceral pelvic fascia), *C* umbilicovesical ligament, *D* vesicosacral ligament, *E* lateral ligament or ala recti, *F* presacral fascia, *1* laterorectal space, *2* prevesical space, *3* peri- and retrovesical space, *4* prerectal space, *5* retrorectal space, *6* presacral space)

pelvic fascia covering the perineal (internal obturator, piriform, elevator ani and ischiococcygeal) muscles and the parietal skeletal structures. Within this space, the pelvic organs (urinary bladder, uterus or seminal vesicles and prostate, rectum) are located along the median line, whereas the vasculonervous structures extend on the sides, surrounded by adipose tissue.

This space is subdivided into compartments or secondary spaces, which are clearly limited by thick and resistant fibrovascular laminae produced by the increased density and thickness of the subperitoneal areolar tissue surrounding the vessels, which they follow along the total extension. Together with these vessels, the laminae extend around the viscera, constituting fibrous sheaths supporting the viscera and maintaining their position (Testut 1905).

The laminae are distinguished as follows (Figs. 1.24, 1.25):

1) The sacro-recto-genito-pubic ligaments
2) The umbilicovesical fascia
3) The lateral umbilicovesical ligaments
4) The genital ligaments in women:
   a) The broad and round ligaments
   b) The vesicogenital ligaments

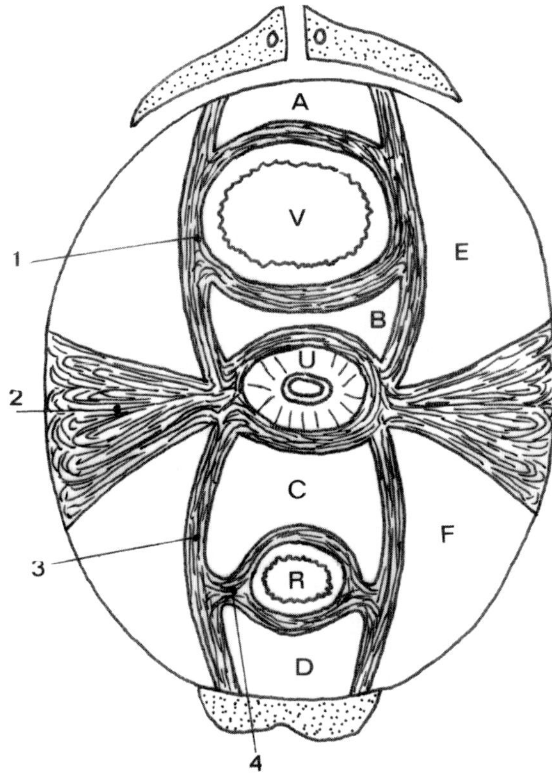

Fig. 1.25. Female pelvis at the level of the uterine cervix; subperitoneal ligaments and spaces. Axial section (*1* vesicouterine ligament, *2* cardinal ligament, *3* uterosacral ligament, *4* lateral ligament or ala recti, *A* prevesical space, *B* vesicouterine space, *C* uterorectal space, *D* retrorectal space, *E* paravesical space, *F* pararectal space)

c) The cardinal or transverse cervical ligaments
d) The uterosacral and uterolumbar ligaments

5) The genital ligaments in men:
   a) The vesicosacral ligaments
   b) Denonvilliers' prostatoperitoneal fascia
6) The lateral ligaments of the rectum

The *sacro-recto-genito-pubic ligaments* (or visceral pelvic fascia; or Delbet's fascia) (Fig. 1.24) are symmetrical and have a sagittal disposition; they extend from the pubis to the sacral foramina on the sides of the pelvic organs, along the lateral sacral artery (posteriorly) and the internal obturator artery (anteriorly). They separate the external (or laterorectal) from the median pelvic spaces. Posteriorly, they raise the peritoneum, constituting two folds (Douglas' folds) limiting the homonymous peritoneal fossa. These folds are more easily distinguished in women and are therefore also called uterosacral ligaments.

The *umbilicovesical fascia* (see also subumbilical preperitoneal space and fasciae) (Fig. 1.24) extends from the umbilicus to the pelvis up to behind the pubis, where it bends back to delineate a semicircle in front and on the sides of the urinary bladder, to which it becomes closely adherent; it then continues backward at the sides of the uterus (or of the seminal vesicles) and of the rectum, following the superior vesical (or umbilicovesical) artery up to the hypogastric artery. Below, it joins the pelvic fascia.

The *lateral umbilicovesical ligaments* (Figs. 1.2I, 1.24) extend across the pelvis from behind forward, on the sides of the median organs; they then converge in front of the urinary bladder, where they bend upward and continue in the abdominal preperitoneal space, terminating on both sides of the umbilicus. They are constituted by the superior vesical vessels and by their prevesical prolongation, surrounded by a prevalently fibrous connective tissue. They make symmetrical impressions in the anterior pelvic peritoneum, separating the median from the lateral inguinal fossae.

The *broad ligaments* (Fig. 1.2H) are made up of two wide transverse peritoneal laminae, anterior and posterior, which adhere to one another and are strengthened inside by smooth muscular fibers. They cover the two uterine faces and extend laterally up to the pelvic wall. At the sides of the uterus, the two laminae adhere together, with the sole interposition of a thin layer of adipose tissue; at the sides they diverge, with one of them bending forward and the other backwards. These laminae limit a triangular space with a lateral base, where venous plexuses, arteries, lymphatics and nerves are surrounded by adipose areolar tissue.

Also at a low level, the two peritoneal leaves diverge, with one of them bending forward to cover the posterosuperior face of the urinary bladder, and the other backward to surround the anterolateral wall of the rectum.

In the upper part, the broad ligament thickness contains the round ligaments, the tubes and the ovaries anteriorly, medially and posteriorly, respectively.

The *round ligaments* (Fig. 1.2H) extend from the anterolateral margin of the uterus to the lateral wall of the pelvis; from here they bend forward, toward the internal orifice of the inguinal canal, which they penetrate up to the base of the labia majora pudendi. Under this ligament, the ovarian vessels extend transversely within the thickness of the broad ligaments.

At the base of the broad ligaments, the adipose areolar tissue becomes thicker, denser and more compact, adopting the character of fibrous tissue and knotting with the muscular tracts that extend everywhere, and continues in the subperitoneal areolar tissue.

Under the isthmus, the uterine cervix is firmly connected to the pelvic wall and to the adjacent organs by six ligaments placed symmetrically: two anteriorly, the vesicogenital ligaments, two laterally, the cardinal ligaments, and two posteriorly, the uterosacral ligaments.

The *vesicogenital ligaments* (Fig. 1.25) (formed of the vesicouterine ligaments above and by the vesicovaginal ligaments below) connect the posterolateral vesical wall to the anterolateral border of the uterine isthmus and to the fundus vaginae.

The *cardinal ligaments* (Fig. 1.25) are made up of two transverse laminae joining the lateral borders of the uterine cervix to the lateral pelvic wall.

The *uterosacral ligaments* (*Douglas' folds*) (Fig. 1.25) are made up of two adherent laminae with a semicircular disposition on the two sides of the rectum, joining the posterior wall of the uterine cervix to the anterior face of the first, second and third sacral vertebrae, just inside the sacroiliac synchondrosis. They raise the peritoneum, constituting the lateral walls of the pouch of Douglas (uterosacral folds).

Vallin-Hugnier's uterolumbar ligaments (inconstant) are located just above the uterosacral ligaments; they join the posterior face of the uterine cervix to the fifth lumbar vertebra.

In men, the *vesicosacral ligaments* (Fig. 1.24) (bilateral and symmetrical) extend with an arcuate shape from the lateral vesical borders, to which they are closely adherent, to the rectum, to which they are joined through its lateral ligaments. They fix these organs to the wall of the pelvis: anteriorly on the posterior face of the pubis and posteriorly on the sacrum. Fibrous extensions join these ligaments to the lateral borders of the seminal vesicles and of Denonvilliers' fascia. At a lower level, they continue in the sacro-recto-genito-pubic (or Delbet's) fascia.

Denonvilliers' prostatoperitoneal fascia (Fig. 1.24) unsheathes the seminal vesicles, the ejaculatory ducts and the vesiculodeferential vessels and nerves, constituting a transverse septum firmly fixed on the prostatic base, which divides the retrovesical from the prerectal subperitoneal spaces. At the sides, the fascia inserts on the vesicorectal fasciae, extending slightly backwards along the path of the vesiculodeferential vessels, which extend from the hypogastric vessels to the seminal vesicles and to the prostate.

The anterior subperitoneal space is crossed by the pelvic portion of the *deferent ducts*, extending from the internal inguinal orifice up to behind the urinary bladder, along and inside the inferior epigastric and external iliac vessels and laterally to the obturator vessels. They pass under the superior vesical arteries and extend along the inferoexternal border of the urinary bladder up to the rectovesical septa. After penetrating these septa, they bend in almost a U-shape, to reach the seminal vesicles at the bottom of the urinary bladder from behind forward and crossing behind the ureter.

The deferent ducts are reached by the deferential vessels, which are branches of the superior vesical arteries and which follow them from the seminal vesicles through the inguinal canal up to the scrotum.

The umbilicovesical ligaments, the deferent ducts and the broad and the round ligaments are constantly covered by the pelvic parietal peritoneum, which these structures raise and make impressions in, constituting the borders of the pelvic recesses.

The *lateral ligaments* or *alae recti* (Figs. 1.24, 1.25) are thin transverse laminae joining the lateral wall of the rectum to the sacro-recto-genito-pubic ligaments, surrounding the median hemorrhoidal vessels and subdividing the perirectal space into anterior and posterior parts.

The various ligaments subdivide the pelvis into well-separated compartments occupied by septate adipose tissue that resembles the fat surrounding the kidneys.

These compartments or secondary spaces comprise (Figs. 1.24, 1.25):

- The laterorectal spaces
- The prevesical space
- The perivesical space
- The perirectal space

The *laterorectal spaces* (Figs. 1.24, 1.25) expand symmetrically and sagittally on the two sides of the pelvic cavity, between the sacro-recto-genito-pubic ligament and the pelvic fascia; they represent the inferior continuation of the lateral extraperitoneal spaces and contain the external iliac vessels, nerves, lymphatics and lymph nodes anteriorly, the ureters in an intermediate position and the hypogastric (with the relative obturator, pudendal, etc. branches) vessels, nerves, lymphatics, and lymph nodes posteriorly.

The other pelvic subperitoneal spaces are located inside the laterorectal spaces with a transverse or prevalently transverse disposition. From the front backward, we find:

a) The *prevesical space* (Figs. 1.24, 1.25); it extends like a bridge in front and on the sides of the urinary bladder, the internal genital organs and the rectum; it is located between the transversalis fascia anteriorly, the umbilicovesical fascia and ligaments medially and the sacro-recto-genito-pubic fascia laterally. Below, it is closed by the pubovesical and puboprostatic ligaments in men and by the pubovaginal ligaments in women. It continues above in the homonymous abdominal space (see subumbilical preperitoneal spaces). It is wider anteriorly, at the sides of the urinary bladder, and becomes smaller (taking a cuneiform aspect) posteriorly, where it is closed by the confluence of the lateral and medial ligaments at the level of the rectum.

b) The *perivesical space* (Fig. 1.2H, I) represents the adipose space located in front and on the sides of the urinary bladder, which continues backward on the sides of the uterine cervix and of the vagina in women and of the seminal vesicles in men, up to the proximity of the rectum. Anteriorly and at the sides, it is limited by the umbilicovesical fascia (that is laterally strengthened by the lateral umbilicovesical ligaments), and medially by the urinary bladder (anteriorly) and by the vesicosacral ligaments in men and by the uterosacral and vaginosacral ligaments in women. Posteriorly, it is closed by the confluence of these ligaments with the vesicoumbilical ligaments. It continues upwards and anteriorly in the homonymous spaces between the umbilicovesical fascia and the peritoneum. The umbilicovesical ligament (urachus) extends anteriorly along the median line within the perivesical adipose tissue.

c) The *perirectal space* is located among the posterior wall of the uterine cervix and the vagina in women (Fig. 1.25) (or of the seminal vesicles and Denonvilliers' fascia in men) anteriorly, the sacro-recto-genito-pubic fascia (strengthened by its fusion with the vesicosacral and uterosacral ligaments) at the sides, and the sacrum posteriorly. It is occupied by adipose tissue, which surrounds the total circumference of the rectum and contains the perirectal vessels, nerves and lymph nodes; it is subdivided transversely on the sides of the rectum by the lamina of the alae recti in the pre- and retrorectal spaces.

A thin small transverse band, located posteriorly between the sacral insertion of the sacro-recto-genito-pubic ligament, further subdivides the retrorectal space from the presacral space (Fig. 1.24.1.25) (where the median sacral vessels and nerves extend).

The prevesical, laterorectal and perirectal pelvic spaces communicate directly with the overhanging extra- or retroperitoneal spaces. In the past, this communication has been utilized for diagnostic purposes; in fact, a gas introduced as a lucent contrast into pelvic spaces expands in the retroperitoneum and in the mediastinum, giving a clear radiographic representation of the organs contained in these spaces. Analogously, suprapubic, perirectal or laterorectal collections diffuse into the overhanging extraperitoneal spaces, and particularly into the retroperitoneal spaces, where expansion is easier because these spaces are wide and the sides easily cease to adhere to each other; on the other hand, preperitoneal or retroperitoneal collections may diffuse downwards into the prevesical spaces.

1.5.4 Anterior Renal and Lateroconal Fasciae and Anterior Pararenal Space

The *anterior renal fascia* (Figs. 1.2C–F, and 1.4A–D) is a thin, but well-formed fibrous lamina, which is difficult to penetrate. It extends transversely from the diaphragm to the pelvis in front of the kidney and the adrenal glands on the sides, and to the aorta, the lumbar veins, the lumbar lymphatic duct and the inferior vena cava on the median line. It always maintains a position posterior to the thoracic duct and the cisterna chyli. At a high level, it blends on the right side with the inferior leaf of the coronary ligament, which is strengthened. Above the ligament, it takes a direct contact with the posterior wall of the liver at the level of the bare area, between the reflections of the coronary and triangular ligaments. After its fusion with the lateroconal fasciae (Fig. 1.2E, F), the anterior renal fascia continues at the sides in the right and left posterior renal fasciae. The lateroconal fasciae are two thin laminae of connective tissue joining the renal fascia to the posterolateral parietal peritoneum and blending with both structures. Together with the posterior peritoneum and the anterior renal fascia, they contribute to limit the lateroconal compartments (Fig. 1.2E, F).

At a low level, the anterior renal fascia becomes progressively thinner upward, to disappear in the pelvic areolar connective tissue.

Anteriorly, it is strengthened by Treitz's retroduodenopancreatic fascia on the right side and by Toldt's retropancreatic fascia on the left and on the median line (Fig. 1.4A, C).

The retroduodenopancreatic fascia continues forward in a leaf surrounding the duodenum and the pancreatic head, and then penetrates medially between these organs and the posterior peritoneum.

The *anterior pararenal space* (Figs. 1.2C–F, 1.4A–D) is located between the posterior parietal peritoneum and the anterior lamina of the renal fascia. At the sides, it is closed by the lateroconal fasciae, which connect these two structures. Depending on the presence or absence of organs inside, it varies in thickness: in the superior planes it is very thin, virtual to allow for close contact of the peritoneum (which posteriorly covers the liver, the spleen, the esophagus and the stomach) with the anterior renal fascia, with or without the interposition of adipose tissue. At a lower level, the space becomes wider, constituting the pancreatic compartment on the median line and the lateroconal compartments on the sides, whereas a virtual space remains in the two intermediate tracts.

The pancreatic compartment is complex; it contains:

1) The celiac trunk.
2) The portal venous axis, with the splenic vein (which extends transversely from the left to the right along the superoposterior border of the pancreas) and the superior mesenteric vein.
3) The pancreas, with an arcuate transverse disposition in front and on the left side of the greater abdominal vessels.
4) The superior mesenteric artery along the median line; it extends initially between the pancreas and the anterior renal fascia, then in front of the third duodenal portion, and finally at the border between the mesentery and the anterior pararenal space.
5) The second duodenal portion on the right side of the pancreatic head.
6) The third duodenal portion, with a transverse extension just under the pancreas, from which it is separated by the superior mesenteric artery.
7) The thoracic duct and the cisterna chyli.
8) The inferior mesenteric artery on the median and left paramedian line.
9) The celiac-mesenteric lymph nodes.

The *lateroconal compartments* are located at the sides and are triangular. Their wall is constituted by the posterior peritoneum, the lateroconal fascia and the anterior renal fascia. The lateroconal compartments contain the ascending and the descending colon on the right and left side, respectively.

In the submesocolic inferior planes, the anterior pararenal space is thin; it is occupied by adipose tissue and by the inferior mesenteric vessels, nerves and lymphatics. At the level of the mesenteric roots, the anterior pararenal space continues forward in the subperitoneal spaces.

1.5.5 Abdominal Transversalis Fascia

The abdominal transversalis fascia (Fig. 1.4A–D) is a thick lamina of connective elastic collagen lining the internal abdominal wall and covering the aponeuroses of the rectus, obliquus, transversus, quadratus lumborum muscles and iliopsoas and the spinal column. At various levels, it blends with other structures: the diaphragmatic crura, the aponeuroses of the psoas, the posterior renal fasciae.

After covering the pubis anteriorly and the sacrum posteriorly, and after blending with the aponeurotic fasciae of the internal obturator muscles on the sides, the transversalis fascia terminates caudad in the pelvic aponeurotic fascia which lines the perineum inside. The subperitoneal pelvic space is located between this fascia and the peritoneal serosa.

Bibliography

Bruni AC (1948) Compendio di anatomia descrittiva umana. Vallardi, Milan
Castiglioni A (1948) Storia della medicina. Mondatori, Milan
Galeno C (1991)Ανατομικαι εγχειρησεισ. Procedimenti anatomici. Bur Rizzoli, Milan
Williams PL, Warwick R, Dyson M, Bannister LH (eds) (1980) Gray's anatomy, 36th edn. (Revised by the editors) Longman Group / Zanichelli, Bologna
Gullino D (1988) Chirurgia del peritoneo e del sottoperitoneo. In: Paletto G (ed) Tecnica Chirurgica. UTET, Turin
Hyrtl J (1970) Onotomatologia anatomica. Georg Olms, Hildesheim New York
Mascagni P (1787) Vasorum linfaticorum corporis humani historia et iconografia. Senis ex Tipografia Pazzini Carli
Netter FH (1989) Atlas of human anatomy. Novartis for Ciba Medical Education Division, Milan
Ottaviani G (1969) Manuale di Anatomia Topografica. L'Ateneo Parmense, Parma
Pensa A, Favaro G (1935) Trattato di anatomia sistematica. UTET, Turin
Rabaiotti A, Rossi L, Prevedi G (1956) Arteriografia addominale e delle estremità. Minerva Medica, Turin
Reuter SR, Redman HC (1977) Gastrointestinal angiography. Saunders, Philadelphia
Ritcher E, Feyerabend T (1991) Normal lymph nodes topography CT atlas. Springer, Berlin Heidelberg New York
Rossi L (1963) Metodica, valore, limiti e indicazioni nello studio radiologico dell'apparato linfatico mediante linfografia. IDOS, Milan
Rouvière H (1979) Anatomie humaine descriptive et topographique. Masson, Paris
Testut L (1902) Trattato di anatomia umana. UTET, Turin
Testut L (1905) Anatomia topografica. UTET, Turin
Testut L, Latarjet A (1971) Trattato di anatomia umana. UTET, Turin

2 Physiology and Physiopathology of the Peritoneum

CONTENTS

The particular structure of the peritoneum provides its membranes with the peculiar possibility to secrete, absorb and filtrate, and gives them antibacterial, plastic and supporting properties. Therefore, we believe that it can be useful to recollect some physiological or physiopathological elements for a better evaluation of the mechanisms underlying generation, blockade and diffusion of the pathological processes affecting the peritoneal leaflets, the subperitoneal spaces, and the intraperitoneal organs.

2.1 Physiology

The peritoneum secretes a citrine serous liquid (specific weight: 1,015), where proteins (3 µg/100 ml; mainly albumin) and some cells (lymphocytes and macrophages, and rare eosinophils and mast cells) are present. The liquid *secretion* into the peritoneal cavity keeps the peritoneal laminae soft and elastic and gives to the peritoneal organs the capability of sliding to accommodate to different individual body positions and during the various phases of digestion and respiration.

The peritoneal liquid (about 100 cc) diffuses everywhere within the cavity and is continuously renewed; in fact, a turnover of 5 ml per 24 h has been calculated. It flows upward into the subphrenic recesses, where the intraperitoneal hydrostatic pressure is lower (–30 mmH_2O in comparison with 0 mmH_2O in the pelvic spaces) and the reabsorption is more active (Salkin 1934).

The liquid reabsorption is promoted by the peritoneal property to function as a dialyzing membrane, particularly at the diaphragmatic and omental level; here, in contrast with other areas of the peritoneum, there is a rich hematic and lymphatic vascularization and a fenestrated mesothelial structure, which allows direct communication between the vasculostromal skeleton and the peritoneal cavity.

Furthermore, the peritoneal *reabsorption* is favored by the respiratory activity, because of the pumping effect of the diaphragmatic movements; therefore, every condition that increases respiratory rhythm, and thus intraperitoneal and thoracic pressure, stimulates this reabsorption, and vice versa.

Experimental studies have demonstrated that the reabsorption is *selective*, *hematic* or *lymphatic*, according to the characteristics of the absorbable substances: aqueous solutions (e.g., methylene blue) follow the hematic pathway, whereas colloid or insoluble substances are absorbed through the lymphatic pathway (Courtile and Steinbeck 1951).

The peritoneal reabsorption through the lymphatic pathway has been demonstrated by radiological means with the use of stabilized colloidal thorium (Thorotrast, Toriofanina) (Cavallaro 1932; Menville and Anée 1932; Held 1932; Capua 1934). In fact, intraperitoneally administered contrast medium accumulates in the subphrenic recesses; afterwards, the lymphatic system of the inferior diaphragmatic face and the internal mammary lymphatic vessels and lymph nodes become opaque. Occasionally, this reabsorption occurs through posterior mediastinal paratracheal collectors converging into the bronchomediastinal trunk, and then flowing into the thoracic duct.

However, the reabsorption is not limited to liquids and solutes, but includes toxic substances and bacteria, which are also selectively absorbed by the stomal fissures. Therefore, these structures also exert an *antibacterial, defensive activity*. This function is enhanced by the presence of macrophages (histiocytes), which may accumulate together with lymphocytes, plasma cells and mast cells in the milk spots (lymphoreticular structures with a vascular glomus-like architecture), where they exert an intense activity of phagocytosis.

Gases are also rapidly absorbed by the peritoneum; in this case too, reabsorption times depend on composition. The reabsorption time is quicker for oxygen (1–2 days) than for carbon dioxide. The complete reabsorption time of air remaining within the peritoneum after surgery is variable: CT evaluations showed that air was still present in the peritoneal cavity in 87% of cases after 3 days, and in 50% of cases after 6 days.

The peritoneum has a notably *plastic* quality, which provides the possibility of quick regeneration and adhesion to any injured surface, with the formation of adhesions plugging the perforations, blocking and isolating the inflammatory processes, the foreign bodies, the hematic collections and the invasive processes.

The interconnections among intraperitoneal viscera and between viscera and retroperitoneum (which is made up of the peritoneum itself, the subperitoneal spaces and the relative vessels) allows three functions: *support–fixation*, *sliding–mobilization* and *nourishment* of the organs located inside.

2.2 Physiopathology

There are different methods of diffusion of the abdominal pathological processes, because both peritoneum and subperitoneal structures may represent diffusion pathways or obstacles to expansion (Meyers 1970, 1973, 1992; Meyers et al. 1978; Oliphant and Berne 1982; Oliphant et al. 1986).

In the peritoneal cavity, the collections may be limited by an active peritoneal reaction and remain within the recess where they have been generated or may expand into the total peritoneal cavity. The subperitoneal collections extend into the cellular tissue adjacent to the organ in which they have been generated; hence, they diffuse, ungluing the perivascular fat of the ligaments, whose extension they may follow right up to the retroperitoneum.

The position, nature, composition and density of the collections are determinant factors in their diffusion. Therefore, intraperitoneal exudate and transudate effusions that have higher fluidity and lower capacity to stimulate the peritoneal reactivity move more quickly toward the lowest recesses and spaces than do purulent, hematic, biliary and urinary collections, which the peritoneum tries to surround with a protective barrier. In the subperitoneal spaces, these latter fluids are initially limited by the shoots and networks of the adipose cellular tissue; then, they pass over these structures and expand along connections among the subperitoneal spaces and between these spaces and the retroperitoneum. Therefore, subperitoneal collections (such as those caused by appendicitis and diverticulitis) diffuse into the retroperitoneum and vice versa (for example, necrotic-hemorrhagic collections formed during pancreatitis penetrate the transverse mesocolon, the mesentery and the gastrosplenic and splenopancreatic ligaments). The peritoneum exerts stronger resistance to the expansion of the collections and to their penetration into the cavity. In the case of fluid diffusion, the serosa develops an intense reactive hyperemia and produces an exudate that is rich in leukocytes, antibodies, and fibrin. In a few hours, the exudate induces the constitution of adhesions between the peritoneal leaflets, which merge, limiting collections and simultaneously favoring selective reabsorptions.

When the lesion passes this barrier, because of the elastic characteristics of the serosa, the collection first expands into the lowest spaces (Morrison's space, pouch of Douglas, paracolic gutter); thereafter, it eventually spreads into the other compartments.

When pathologic conditions induce a greater accumulation of fluid (i.e., ascites) because of an altered metabolism, the possible causes are:

1. Increased secretion as a result of irritation and stimulation of the mesothelial membrane induced by inflammatory or tumoral processes
2. Stasis induced by venous or lymphatic load (as in portal hypertension)
3. Fall in the osmotic-colloidal pressure as a result of low albumin concentrations and consequent imbalance of the Starling's factors (as in cirrhosis)
4. Sodium retention by the kidney and relative expansion of the plasmatic volume (as in nephrosis)

The routes of distribution and diffusion of the excessive amount of intraperitoneal liquid are conditioned by anatomical (disposition of ligaments and mesenteries, communications among peritoneal spaces at various levels), functional (intraperitoneal pressure, tendentiously upward-directed flux, gravity) and physiopathological (site of penetration, density, speed of accumulation, amount of fluid) factors.

The *main* and *preferential flux* and *diffusion pathways* (Fig. 2.1A, B) can be summarized as follows:

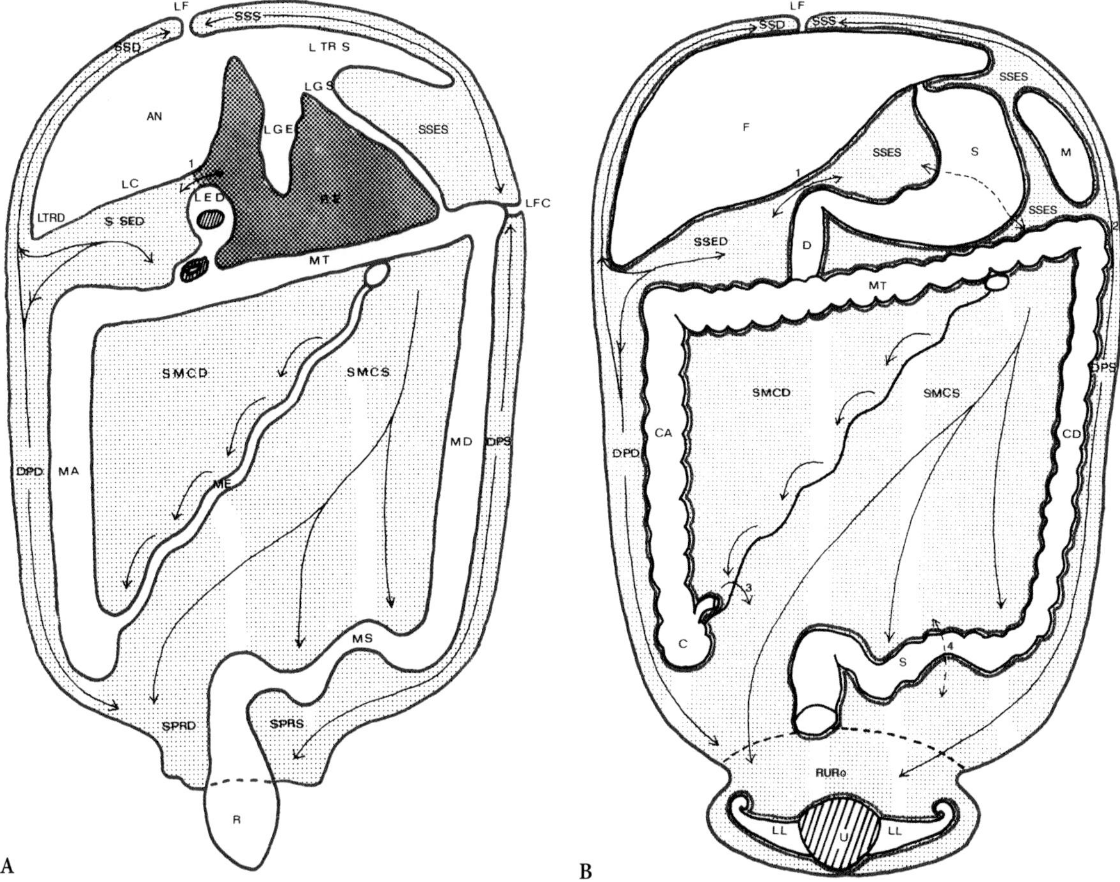

Fig. 2.1 A, B. Communication pathways between spaces and recesses in the peritoneal cavity. **A** Posterior plane (ligamental insertion). **B** Anterior (perivisceral) plane. *Right:* main communication between the subphrenic, subhepatic, paracolic gutter, parasigmoidal and pelvic spaces. *Left:* communication between subphrenic and subhepatic spaces and between parasigmoidal and pelvic spaces. On this side the phrenocolic ligament is obstructing communication between the supra- and submesocolic spaces, so that communication is possible only anterior to this ligament (**B***2*). The communication between the right and left subphrenic spaces is closed by the falciform ligament. There is a direct communication of the left space with the right one (**B***1*), and through this with the right highway. Communication between lesser sac and the right subhepatic space (**A***1*). The left inframesocolic space communicates with the pelvic cavity directly through the right parasigmoidal spaces or via the sigmoid (**B***4*). The right inframesocolic space is closed by the folds of the mesentery and the colon. Passing over the last ileal loop it may communicate with the right paracolic gutter, parasigmoidal space and pelvic cavity (**B***3*). The peritoneum is colored red. The large cavity is *thinly dotted*. The lesser sac is *darkly dotted*. The *arrows* indicate the flux of the peritoneal liquid and the communications among cavities conditioning the diffusion of collections or other pathologies through intraperitoneal pathways

a) There is a free liquid exchange between the supra- and submesocolic compartments through communications between the right paracolic gutter, Morrison's recess and the right subphrenic recess. Therefore, a wide and easy communication on the right side allows the movement of collections from the right subphrenic space to the pelvis and vice versa (Figs. 4.18, 4.19, 4.21).
b) The collections in the right and left supramesocolic compartments and those in the right paracolic submesocolic compartments tend to flow into the Morrison's subhepatic recess.
c) The direct exchange of liquids between the right and left subphrenic cavities is blocked by the falciform and the coronary ligaments (Figs. 4.18–4.21).
d) The subhepatic cavities freely communicate (with a preferential flux that is generally directed from the left to the right side) through a direct communication under the falciform ligament (Figs. 4.16, 4.17, 4.22).
e) The lesser sac communicates with the Morrison's recess through the Winslow's foramen (Fig. 4.16).

f) The left subphrenic and submesocolic cavities are separated by the transverse mesocolon and the phrenocolic ligament constituting a barrier, which it is difficult for the small and medium-sized collections to pass (Figs.4.16, 4.18, 4.21).
g) The left paracolic gutter and the pelvic cavities communicate widely on the left side of the sigmoid mesocolon (Fig. 4.18, 4.19).
h) From the left inframesocolic space the collections spread into the pelvis, through the right parasigmoidal space, or in an anterior direction (Fig. 4.18–4.21).
i) The collections of the right inframesocolic space are initially located within the folds of the mesentery, and then spread downward in a cascade up to the recess constituted by the insertion of the last ileal loop on the cecum (Fig. 4.18). After passing over this structure, the fluids slide on the right side of the sigmoid mesocolon and reach the pelvis, where they occupy the pouch of Douglas and then the paravesical and laterorectal recesses.

The peritoneum, the peritoneal cavity, the interstices and the blood and lymphatic vessels of the subperitoneal spaces may represent a pathway of growth and diffusion of *tumors of visceral* origin (see detailed descriptions in the specific section). The major obstacle is set by the lymph nodes, which function as interposed filters between the tumors and the general circulation.

Bibliography

Capua A (1934) Iniezioni di thorotrast colloidale nella cavità peritoneale per lo studio della diffusione del mezzo di contrasto per le vie linfatiche. Radiol Med 21:289

Cavallaro M (1932) Il biossido di Torio per via endoperitoneale. Riforma Med 48:1507

Courtice FC, Steinbeck AW (1951) Absorption of protein from peritoneal cavity. J Physiol 114:336–355

Courtice FC, Steinbeck AW (1951) The effects of lymphatic obstruction and posture on the absorption of protein from the peritoneal cavity. J Exp Biol Med Sci 29:451

Dunnick NR, Jones RB, Doppman JL, Speyer J, Myers CE (1979) Intraperitoneal contrast infusion for assessment of intraperitoneal fluid dynamics. AJR Am J Roentgenol 133:221

Duranteau M, Oury F, Proux C, Leger R (1955) Essais de limphographie abdomino-thoracic par injection intraperitoneal des substances iodées. Presse Med 63:1986

Efskind L, Ortliche X (1940) Veränderungen bei intraperitonealer Injektion von Thoriumdioxid (thorotrast). Acta Chir Scand 84:79

Feldman GB, Knapp RC (1974) Lymphatic drainage of the peritoneal cavity and its significance in ovarian cancer. Am J Obstet Gynecol 119:991–994

Held J (1932) Die Resorption von kolloidalen Thorium (Thorotrast) aus der Bauchhoehle. Z Exp Med 80:819

Holm-Nielsen P (1953) Pathogenesis of ascites in peritoneal carcinomatosis. Acta Pathol Microbiol Scand 33:10–21

Leak LV, Rahil K (1978) Permeability of the diaphragmatic mesothelium: the ultrastructural basis for stomata. Am J Anat 151:557–594

Mavroudis C, Malangoni MA, Katzmark SL, et al (1988) Comparative clearance rates of the pleural and peritoneal cavities (abstract). Radiology 168:292

Menville LJ, Anée JN (1932) Roentgen-ray study in absorption of Thorium dioxide from the peritoneal cavity of the albino rat. Proc Soc Exp Biol Med 30:28

Meyers MA (1970) The spread and localization of acute intraperitoneal effusions. Radiology 95:545–547

Meyers MA (1973) Distribution of intraabdominal malignant seeding: dependency on dynamics of flow and ascites fluid. AJR Am J Roentgenol 119:198–206

Meyers MA (1992) Radiologia dinamica dell'addome. Verduci, Rome

Meyers MA, Oliphant M, Berne AS, Feldberg MAM (1978) The peritoneal ligaments and mesenteries: pathways of intraabdominal spread of disease. Radiology 163:593–504

Micera O (1993) La fisiologia del peritoneo. Paper presented at the 10th National Congress of SIRM, Gastroenterological Radiology Section, Naples

Oliphant M, Berne AS (1982) CT of subperitoneal spaces: demonstration of direct spread of intraabdominal diseases. J Comput Assist Tomogr 6:1127–1131

Oliphant M, Berne AS, Meyers MA (1986) Subperitoneal spread of intra-abdominal disease. In: Meyers MA (ed) Computed tomography of the gastrointestinal tract. Springer, New York Heidelberg Berlin

Procaccini D, Querques M, Tappi A (1988) Peritoneal clearances. Long-term study. ASAIO Trans 34:437–440

Proto AV, Lane EJ, Marangola JP (1976) A new concept of ascitic fluid distribution. AJR Am J Roentgenol 126:974–980

Raval B, Lakmi N (1987) CT demonstration of preferential routes of the spread of pelvic disease. Crit Rev Diagn Imaging 26:17–48

Recklinghausen FT (1869) Van zur Filtresorption. Virchows Arch 26:172–208

Rotondo A, Grassi R, Contino A, Smaltino F (1991) Spazi peritoneali. In: Dal Pozzo G (ed) Compendio di tomografia computerizzata. UTET-USES, Verona

Salkin D (1934) Intra-abdominal pressure and its regulation. Am Rev Tubercul 30:436–457

Vecchioli A, Bonomo L, Renda F (1984) Fisiopatologia del peritoneo. Report to the XXXIst National Congress of the National Society for Medical Radiology (SIRM). Monduzzi, Bologna

3 CT Technique

An efficient technique is indispensable if clinically relevant information is to be obtained.

The necessity of utilizing helical scanners or, at least, short scan times, providing high-level spatial and densitometric resolution and a wider gray-scale range allowing images that are both soft and detailed is well known and does not need to be stressed; furthermore, the prints of the images should not present any substantial loss compared with the monitor pictures.

The parameters must be selected according to the diagnostic purpose; in the absence of specific questions a standard abdominal program should first be performed (for example a consecutive series with 7.5- to 10-mm collimation and 7.5- to 10-mm image spacing) for preliminary information, followed by a series with thinner collimation and image spacing (3.5 mm) to obtain better anatomical and pathologic definition.

A *nonionic iodate i.v.*-administered *contrast agent* should be systematically used, because the contrast enhancement of the vessels, parenchymatous organs, intestinal walls and (slightly) peritoneum increases the difference in density between these and the lucency of sub- or retroperitoneal fat, fluids and nonvascularized or poorly vascularized structures, favoring their identification and permitting characterization of the pathologic processes (e.g., the peripheral enhancement of abscesses within solid structures, or conversely, the lack of attenuation changes in cystic structures or necrotic areas).

We suggest using the *dynamic helical* technique with *automatic injector* for accurate analysis of the structures (particularly of the vascular ones) and of the visceral profiles, and for an optimal multiplanar reconstruction. The following may represent an examination scheme of this technique:

1) *Digital abdominal radiography* followed by *precontrast helical scans* performed with 7.5- to 10-mm collimation and image spacing.
2) Further *biphasic helical scanning after rapid i.v. injection of contrast medium*: the first phase 30–40 s after the beginning of the injection (arterial phase); the second 60–120 s after, in the venous or equilibrium phase. Contrast agent, 100–150 ml, preferably nonionic, is administered i.v. with an automatic injector and 16–18G needle at a rate of 2–3 ml/s. Helical parameters included 3.5-mm collimation, 3.5-mm image spacing and 3.5-mm/s table speed. This technique improves the resolution, eliminates false recording and even permits high-quality multiplanar reconstruction.

A series of deep inspirations before the scans are started (to obtain pulmonary hyperventilation) helps patients to hold their breath throughout the total time needed for scanning.

To achieve optimal depiction of the intestinal wall (thickness, profile) and to identify and evaluate the extent of the intestinal abnormalities, it is very useful for the stomach or the colon to be filled with water (Baert et al.1980, 1989; Angelelli et al. 1987; Angelelli and Macarini 1988) or with low-density contrast agents (meglumine diatrizoate saline solution – Gastrografin or Iopamidolo-Gastromiro) (Megibow 1986), orally or by administration as an enema. Water is safe, economical, and physiological and does not entail discomfort or risk to the patient. Having a slight hypotonic effect, lukewarm water also reduces spasms and peristaltic activity. To distend the stomach, the duodenum and the jejunum, not less than 500 ml of fluid, perhaps given in two administrations close together, is needed. For an enema 1,000–1,500 ml of contrast material is the optimal amount for distension of the colon, except in the case of strictures or intestinal occlusions, when the smallest amount that can effect distension should be given.

The administration of contrast agents by mouth should also be avoided in the presence of congestive heart disease or chronic renal failure, since the ingestion of large amounts of fluid can cause problems with renal output.

We believe that the administration of *low-concentration (2%–3%) iodate contrast agents* orally or by nasogastric tube should be limited to the investigation of intestinal perforations and dehiscence of digestive anastomoses, or to the evaluation of the path and extent of intestinal fistulae. Occasionally, it can be used to distinguish lymph nodes or subperitoneal collections from intestinal loops distended by liquids or stool.

Enema contrast agents should not be used in patients with suspected intestinal infarct, ulcerative rectocolitis or toxic megacolon. We do not like the use of diluted barium as a contrast medium (Hatfield et al. 1980) in the study of small bowel or colonic pathology, because the increased differences in density between lumen, intestinal wall and perivisceral fat do not provide optimal images of these structures. In addition, in the case of an intestinal perforation, whether occult or produced by the contrast enema itself, relevant complications may even occur. Finally, the contrast medium may stagnate owing to parietal hypokinesis or the presence of obstacles caused by absorption of the liquid component and inspissation of the barium, and a secondary obstruction may then occur.

To obtain visualization and correct evaluation of the diffusion and activity in Crohn's disease, Rollandi et al. (1991) suggest injecting 2–3 l of 2% *carboxymethylcellulose* into the jejunum through a nasojejunal tube as a low-density contrast medium for the small intestine, in association with injection of a nonionic iodate contrast agent, 80 ml i.v., which can make the intestinal wall opaque. The intravenous contrast medium should be given at 37% concentration and a speed of 3 ml/s. Spiral CT should be used; scans should be taken 30 s after injection of the contrast medium.

When urinary collections are suspected, we suggest first performing an unenhanced scan and then continuing up to complete filling of the urinary bladder and finishing with postmicturition digital radiograph.

CT peritoneography may be useful in the search for small metastases (Rotondo et al. 1991) that are not detectable with standard CT techniques, especially in the absence of peritoneal collections, and in patients being treated with peritoneal dialysis (Brown et al. 1987; Maxwell et al. 1990; Scanziani et al. 1992) to evaluate the spread of liquid into the peritoneal spaces and any complications. This technique consists in the intraperitoneal infusion through a catheter of 100–200 ml of a 30% nonionic contrast agent diluted in 500–2000 ml normal saline solution; the patient must subsequently adopt different positions to make it easier for the contrast medium to spread into the whole of the peritoneal cavity.

Caseiro-Alves et al. (1995) proposed the use of *pneumoperitoneum* to improve the sensitivity of CT in the detection of peritoneal carcinosis. This technique made it possible for them to visualize the subphrenic spaces and the paracolic gutter with particular accuracy, while the pelvic cavity could never be clearly visualized. This meant that peritoneal nodes (even smaller than 2 cm) and synechial bridles could be correctly individualized. However, we believe that images obtained with this technique are worse in quality than those observed after intraperitoneal administration of a water-soluble contrast medium. On the other hand, we believe that the administration of a normal *saline solution* into the peritoneal cavity, as in the dialysis technique used by nephrologists, is a useful alternative.

The extrahepatic biliary tract can be investigated with the aid of *intravenous* (Furukawa et al. 1997; Gillams et al. 1994; Stockberger et al. 1994; van Beers et al. 1994) or *oral hyopanoic acid contrast agent* (Caoili et al. 2000; Chopra et al. 2000; Soto et al. 1999; Stabile Ianora et al. 2000) *cholangiography* associated with spiral CT, with or without three-dimensional volume reconstruction.

Oral cholangiography is used in patients who are candidates for laparoscopic cholecystectomy and for diagnosis of choledochal cystic dilatation and assessment of where surgical clips are positioned (Stabile Ianora et al. 2000), whereas for detection of posttraumatic or postsurgical biliary duct ruptures and bile leakage i.v. cholangiography is preferable.

The *high-resolution technique* is sometimes useful as a complementary method for the study of the abdominal pathology; in fact, it may show details that are not visible with the standard technique.

This technique is also useful to:

1) Recognize the smallest structures by enhancement of particular elements
2) Evaluate tumoral spread outside the organ from which the tumor has originated when the profile of the organ affected in not clearly defined.
3) Visualize individual extraorganic pathologies in the absence of cleavage planes in extremely lean subjects or in patients with very little intra-abdominal adipose tissue (Fig. 3.1).

An important role is exerted by *coronal* (Figs. 4.15, 4.20, 4.23, 4.36, 4.69, 4.70, 4.90) and *sagittal* (Figs. 4.21, 4.24, 4.37, 4.68, 4.91) and *volumetric* (Fig. 4.73) *reconstructions* when a topographical demonstration of liquid-containing peritoneal cavities and a better representation of prevalently vertically extended structures

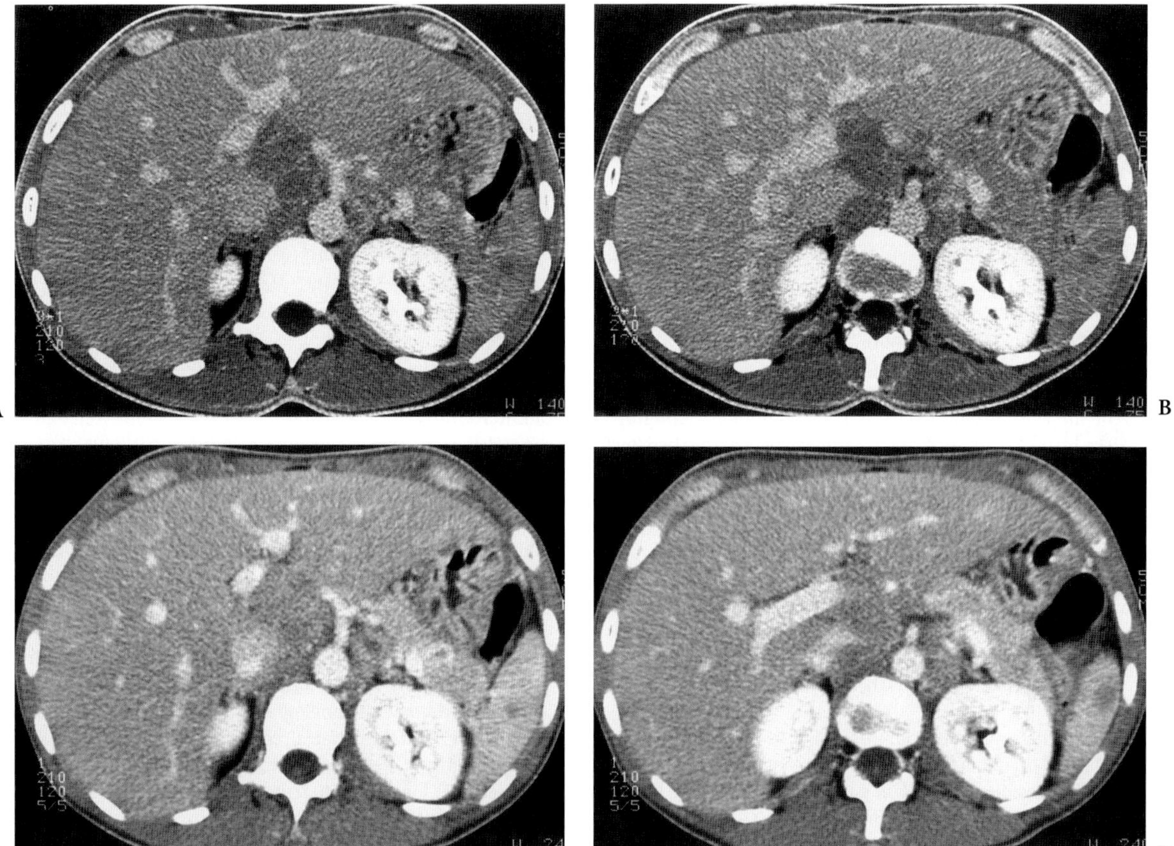

Fig. 3.1. A, B High resolution shows up the visceral profile and the differences in density of the structures, making the hepatic, celiac and retroperitoneal lymph nodes clearly visible [they are only hypothesized after standard CT, or even a thin (5-mm) section technique (**C, D**)] in a patient in whom the absence of adipose cleavage planes does not facilitate distinction among the various abdominal structures

(vessels, extrahepatic biliary tract, ureters, ligaments) and of relationships between organs, ligaments and cavities are needed. Thin (5 mm or less) contiguous scans are needed to obtain optimal reconstructions.

A good choice of *window* by which the images are printed is also important; it must be chosen according to the information needed.

Optimal reproduction and storage of the images require the use of *laser printers* and *optical disks*. At present, *dry printers* worsen both definition and contrast of the images.

Bibliography

Angelelli G, Macarini L (1988) CT of the bowel: use of the water to enhance depiction. Radiology 169:848–849

Angelelli G, Macarini L (1992) TC del tratto gastroenterico. Minerva Medic, Turin

Angelelli G, Macarini L, Frazzle A (1987) Use of the water as an oral contrast agent for CT study of the stomach (letter). AJR Am J Roentgenol 149:1084

Aronberg DJ (1983) Techniques. In: Lee JKT, Sagely SS, Stanley RJ (eds) Computed body tomography. Raven Press, New York

Baert AL, Rex G, Wills G, Marshal G, Deschepper C (1980) Computed tomography of the rectum with water as contrast. Gastrointest Radiol 14:345–348

Baert AL, Roex L, Marchal G, Hermans P, Dewilde G, Wilms G (1989) Computed tomography of the stomach with water as an oral contrast agent: technique and preliminary results. J Comput Assist Tomogr 13:633–636

Brown DL, Johnson JB, Kraus AP, Duke RA, Barrett MR (1987) Computed tomography with intraperitoneal contrast medium for localization of peritoneal dialysis leaks. J Comput Assist Tomogr 11:276–278

Caoili EM, Paulson EK, Heyneman LE, et al (2000) Helical CT cholangiography with three-dimensional volume rendering using an oral biliary contrast agent: feasibility of a novel technique. AJR Am J Roentgenol 174:487–492

Caseiro-Alves F, Goncalo M, Abraul E, et al (1995) Induced pneumoperitoneum in CT evaluation of peritoneal carcinomatosis. Abdom Imaging 20:52–57

Cronin EB, Belville JS, Tumeh SS (1988) New low-density contrast agent for evaluation of the rectosigmoid with CT. Radiology 169:405

Dunick NR, Jones RB, Doppman JL, Speyer J, Myers CE (1979) Intraperitoneal contrast infusion for assessment of intraperitoneal fluid dynamics. AJR Am J Roentgenol 133:221–223

Furukawa H, Sano K, Kosuge T, et al (1997) Analysis of biliary drainage in the caudate lobe of the liver: comparison of three-dimensional CT cholangiography and rotating cine cholangiography. Radiology 204:113–117

Gillams A, Gardener J, Richards R, et al (1994) Three-dimensional CT cholangiography: a new technique for biliary tract imaging. Br J Radiol 67:445–448

Gossios KJ, Tsianos EV, Demou LL, et al (1991) Use of water or air as oral contrast media for computed tomography study of the gastric wall: comparison of the two techniques. Gastrointest Radiol 16:293–297

Hatfield KD, Segal SD, Tait K (1980) Barium sulfate for abdominal computed assisted tomography. J Comput Assist Tomogr 4:570–572

Johansen GJ (1978) Assessment of a nonionic contrast medium (Amipaque) in the gastrointestinal tract. Invest Radiol 523:13–15

Kivisaari L, Kormano M (1982) Comparison of diatrizoate and barium sulfate bowel markers in clinical CT. Eur J Radiol 2:33–35

Maxwell AJ, Boggis CRM, Sambrook P (1990) Computed tomographic peritoneography in the investigation of abdominal wall and genital swelling in patients on continuous ambulatory peritoneal dialysis. Clin Radiol 41:100–104

Megibow AJ (1986) Techniques of gastrointestinal computed tomography. In: Megibow AJ, Balthazar EJ (eds) Computed tomography of the gastrointestinal tract. Mosby, St Louis

Megibow AJ, Zerhouni EA, Hulnick DH, Bezanbaum R, Balthazar EJ (1984) Technical note. Air insufflation of the colon as an adjunct to computed tomography of the pelvis. J Comput Assist Tomogr 8:797–800

Mitchell DG, Bjorgvinsson E, Termeulen D, et al (1985) Gastrografin versus dilute barium coloni CT examination: a blind, randomized study. J Comput Assist Tomogr 9:451–453

Raptopoulos V, David MA, Davidoff A, et al (1987) Fat-density oral contrast agent for abdominal CT. Radiology 164:653–656

Raptopoulos V (1989) Technical principles in the CT evaluation of the gut. Radiat Clin North Am 27:631–651

Rollandi GA, Curone PF, Pastorino C, et al (1991) Gastromiro vs Gastrografin vs Prontobario TAC per tomografia computerizzata. Radiat Med 82:295–302

Rotondo A, Grassi R, Contino A, Smaltino F (1991) Spazi peritoneali. In: Dal Pozzo M (ed) Compendio di tomografia computerizzata. UTET-USES, Verona

Scanziani R, Dozio B, Caimi F, De Rossi N, Magri F, Surian M (1992) Peritoneography and peritoneal computed tomography (CT) in the diagnosis of subcutaneous leaks sites during continuous ambulatory peritoneal dialysis (CAPD). Perit Dial Bull 4:163–166

Solomon A, Michowitz M, Papo J, et al (1986) Computed tomographic air enema. Gastrointest Radiol 11:194–196

Soto JA, Velez SM, Guzman J (1999) Choledocholithiasis: diagnosis with oral-contrast-enhanced CT cholangiography. AJR Am J Roentgenol 172:943–948

Stabile Ianora AA, Scardapane A, Midiri M, Rotondo R, Angelelli G (2000) Studio pre- e postoperatorio delle vie biliari con tomografia computerizzata spirale. Radiol Med 100:152–159

Stockberger SM, Wass JL, Sherman S, et al (1994) Intravenous cholangiography with helical CT: comparison with endoscopic retrograde cholangiography. Radiology 192:675–680

Stork J (1985) Intraperitoneal contrast agents for computed tomography. AJR Am J Roentgenol 145:300

Van Beers BE, Lacrosse M, Trigaux JP, et al (1994) Noninvasive imaging of the biliary tree before or after laparoscopic cholecystectomy: use of three-dimensional spiral CT cholangiography. AJR Am J Roentgenol 1962: 1331–1335

Winter TC, Ager GD, Nghiem HV, Hill RS, Harrison SD, Freeny PC (1996) Upper gastrointestinal tract and abdomen: water as an orally administered contrast agent for helical CT. Radiology 201:365–370

Zerhouni EA, Fishmann EK, Jones B (1988) Principles and techniques. In: Fishman EK, Jones B (eds) Computed tomography of the gastrointestinal tract. Churchill Livingstone, New York

4 CT Anatomy

CONTENTS

4.1 Peritoneum, Ligaments, Mesenteries and Peritoneal Cavity

4.1.1 Peritoneum

Usually, in normal subjects the peritoneum is not detectable on CT, because it is extremely thin. Only occasionally, and in particular regions, do both parietal and visceral peritonea appear as a dense thin linear image with uniform thickness, when it is limited on both sides by adipose tissue and is vertically oriented. This condition occurs in the case of the parietal peritoneum at the abdominal level, when it is compressed between preperitoneal space fat and omental fat (Fig. 4.1), and at the pelvic level, where it is limited on both sides by intra- and extraperitoneal adipose tissue (Figs. 4.5, 4.6, 4.8–4.11). Furthermore, it can be detected as a linear image produced by the reciprocity between peritoneum and fasciae, as in the case of the anterior renal fascia or for the umbilical fasciae, which are closely adherent to the peritoneum (Fig. 4.11).

On the other side, the visceral peritoneum is sometimes visible where it constitutes the mesenteries on the sides of the submesocolic adipose areolar tissue (Fig. 4.7).

In paraphysiological conditions in elderly subjects the mesenteric peritoneum is sometimes seen as serpiginous lines crossing the mesentery at the sides of vessels.

In pathologic conditions, when the peritoneum is thickening (Fig. 4.2–4.4) or in the case of effusions in the peritoneal cavity (Fig. 4.3), it is possible to visualize it and sometimes to distinguish between parietal and visceral components (Fig. 4.4).

The entire *pelvic peritoneum* can be visualized only in the presence of fluid in its cavity (Fig. 4.20, 4.32–4.34). In the absence of liquid, the peritoneal profile is not constant: it is visible only in subjects with abundant adipose areolar tissue, in whom it can be seen as a thin line extending behind the anterior abdominal wall and the transversalis fascia. These structures are parallel to the peritoneum, but are separated from it by an interposed space occupied by adipose tissue; in this space the punctiform images of the umbilicovesical ligament can be seen along the median line and the images of the lower epigastric vessels, at the sides (Fig. 4.6–4.11). This line continues upward with the hypogastric parietal peritoneal line and at the sides, behind and inside, it follows the pelvic wall, being separated from it by the low-density adipose tissue of the extraperitoneal spaces, where the images of the external and internal iliac vessels stand out (Fig. 4.16, 4.20).

Behind the arcuate transversal line of the anterior parietal peritoneum, the transparency of the omental adipose tissue shows up the small dots of the omental vessels (Fig. 4.17).

Going downward, the peritoneal profile is still visible at the sides, whereas in the middle it merges with that of the anterior vesical wall. At this level, the pelvic fasciae and ligaments (umbilicovesical, large and round) and the organs (urinary bladder, uterus, seminal vesicle and rectum) start to be obvious; the peritoneum folds over these structures and adheres to them, becoming unrecognizable on CT images.

4.1.2 Ligaments and Mesenteries

Ligaments and mesenteries can be recognized by the transparency of the adipose areolar tissue contained by them; the vessels crossing them and their positions relative to abdominal organs are useful for their correct localization.

Ligaments supporting parenchymatous organs have a constant position, whereas those connecting hollow viscera to each other or the abdominal wall to viscera vary in position, length and width according to constitutional type, longilineal types being longer and lower while the brevilineal types are shorter and higher. Furthermore, both replenishment of viscera and a lying position of the patient

A

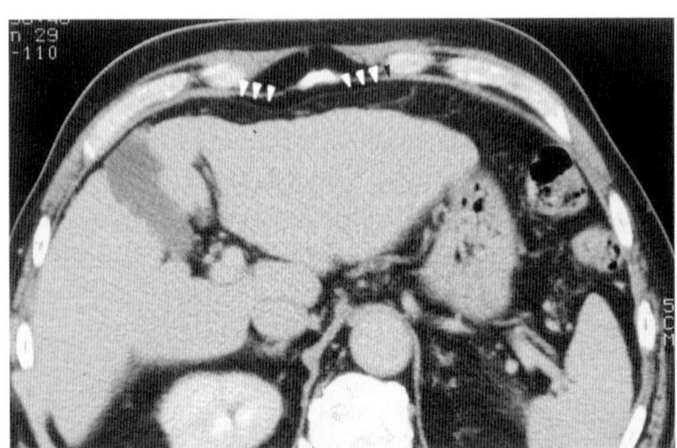

B

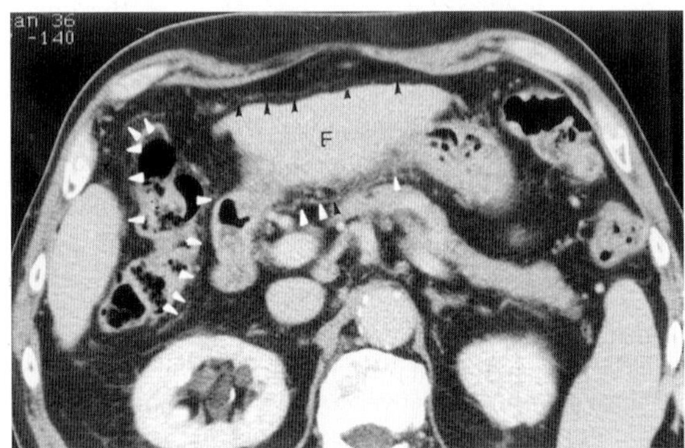

Fig. 4.1. Supramesocolic peritoneum. Anterior parietal peritoneum (*arrowheads*) limited by the preperitoneal and omental fat

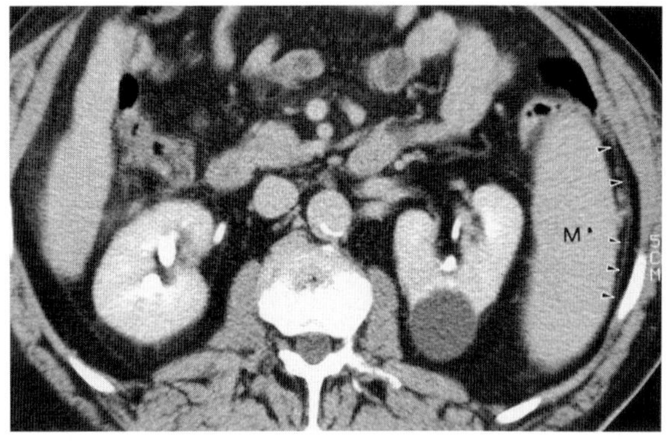

Fig. 4.2. Supramesocolic peritoneum. Thickening perisplenic peritoneum (*arrowhead*) in a patient affected by cirrhosis with splenomegaly Dilatation of the perisplenic veins between peritoneum and spleen

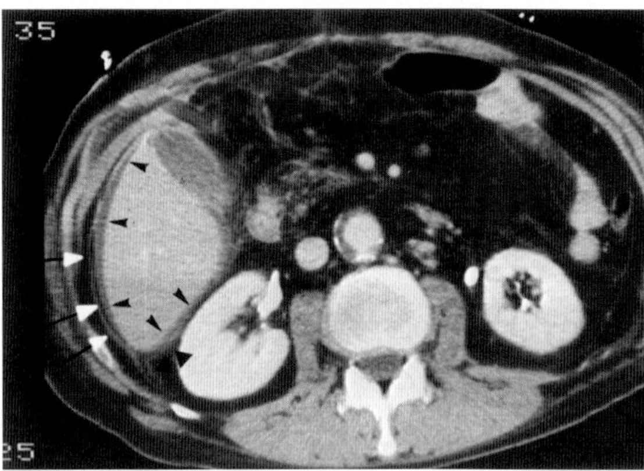

Fig. 4.3. Perihepatic supramesocolic peritoneum. *Outside* to *inside*: the extrafascial adipose areolar tissue, the lateroconal fascia (*white arrows*), the interstice occupied by extraperitoneal adipose areolar tissue, the parietal peritoneum, a thin intraperitoneal effusion (*arrowheads*), the visceral peritoneum adherent to the liver

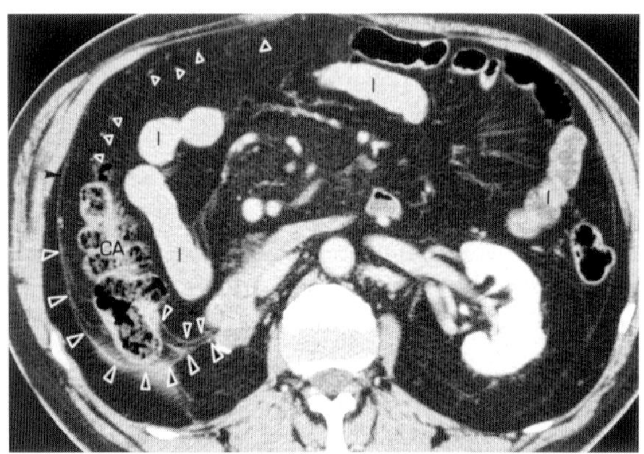

Fig. 4.4. Submesocolic peritoneum. Right posterolateral parietal peritoneum, thickened for an inflammatory process and adherent to the lateroconal fascia at the side and to the anterior renal fascia posteriorly (*arrowheads*). Visceral peritoneum (*small arrowheads*), thickening at the pericecal level

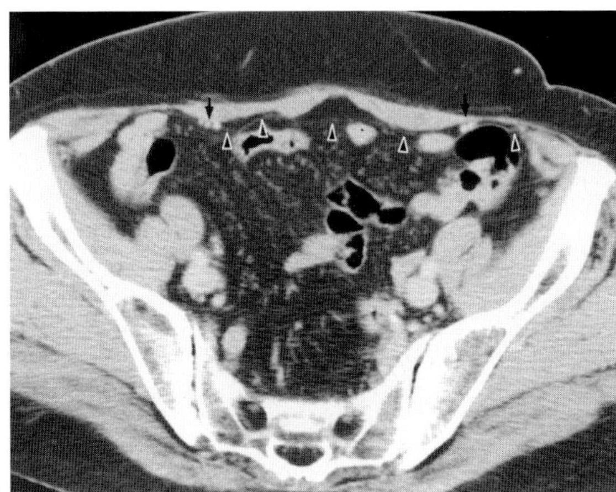

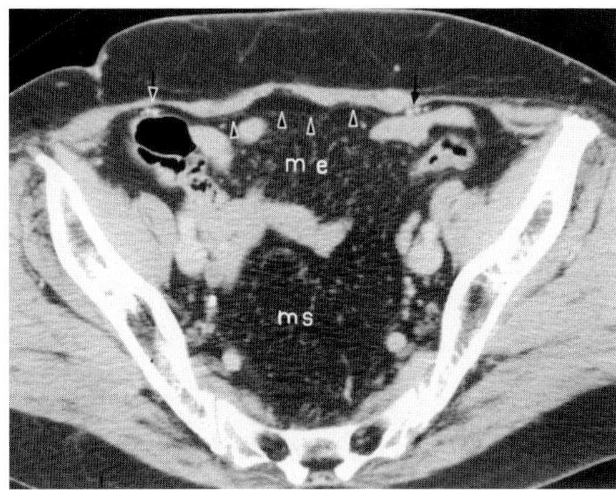

Fig. 4.5A, B. Submesocolic parietal peritoneum. Thin dense anterior transverse line of the peritoneum (*arrowheads*) parallel to the abdominal wall, from which it is separated by the interstice occupied by the adipose areolar tissue of the umbilicovesical preperitoneal space This space is more expanded in the recesses of the abdominal wall on the sides of the musculi recti and behind the linea alba. Symmetrical hyperdense punctiform images of the right and left inferior epigastric vessels (*arrows*). In planes posterior to the peritoneum, the mesentery (*me*) is seen, studded by the punctiform images of transverse sections of the distal ileal branches, and at the back, the sigmoid mesocolon (*ms*), where the vessels follow the sigmoidal sinuosity

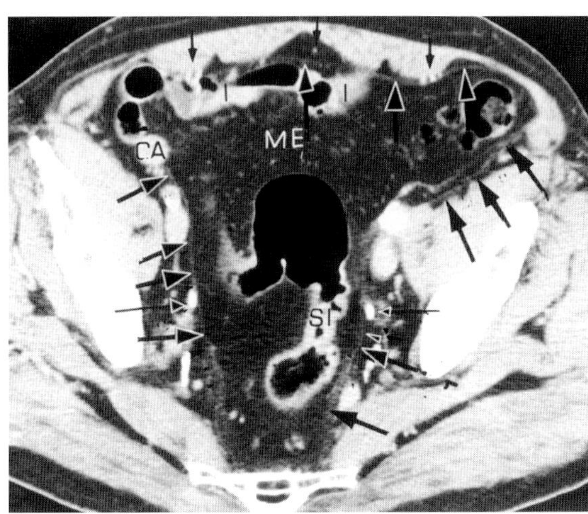

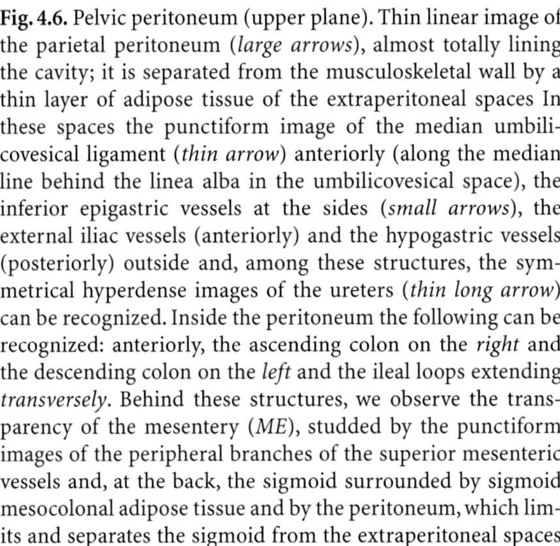

Fig. 4.6. Pelvic peritoneum (upper plane). Thin linear image of the parietal peritoneum (*large arrows*), almost totally lining the cavity; it is separated from the musculoskeletal wall by a thin layer of adipose tissue of the extraperitoneal spaces In these spaces the punctiform image of the median umbilicovesical ligament (*thin arrow*) anteriorly (along the median line behind the linea alba in the umbilicovesical space), the inferior epigastric vessels at the sides (*small arrows*), the external iliac vessels (anteriorly) and the hypogastric vessels (posteriorly) outside and, among these structures, the symmetrical hyperdense images of the ureters (*thin long arrow*) can be recognized. Inside the peritoneum the following can be recognized: anteriorly, the ascending colon on the *right* and the descending colon on the *left* and the ileal loops extending *transversely*. Behind these structures, we observe the transparency of the mesentery (*ME*), studded by the punctiform images of the peripheral branches of the superior mesenteric vessels and, at the back, the sigmoid surrounded by sigmoid mesocolonal adipose tissue and by the peritoneum, which limits and separates the sigmoid from the extraperitoneal spaces

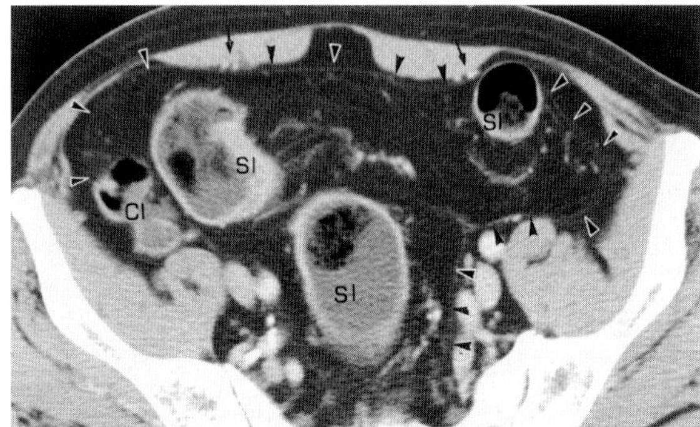

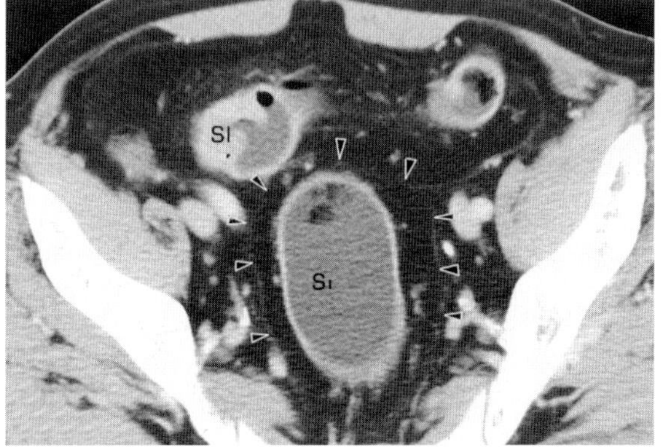

Fig. 4.7A, B. Pelvic peritoneum (middle plane). **A** Thin dense line of the anterior parietal peritoneum, extending along the abdominal wall, from which it is separated by adipose tissue of the preperitoneal space (*arrowheads*). **B** Thin dense line of the peritoneum constituting the sigmoid mesocolonal wall (*arrowheads*), located in front and on the sides of the sigmoid. The punctiform or sinuous hyperdense images of the sigmoidal vessels stand out between the peritoneum and the bowel in the transparency of the sigmoid mesocolonal adipose areolar tissue

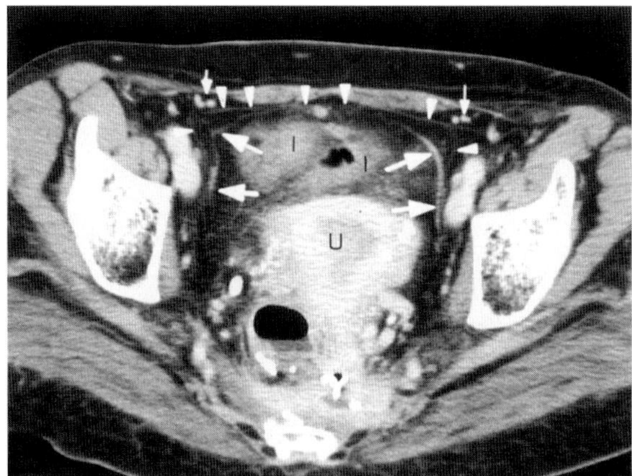

Fig. 4.8. Pelvic peritoneum (supravesical plane). Thin transverse line of the anterior parietal peritoneum (*arrowheads*), which limits the preperitoneal space posteriorly. This is wider along the median line and at the sides, at the level of the inferior epigastric vessels (*small arrows*), and thin behind the expansion of the musculi recti. Behind the peritoneum, the supravesical and medial inguinal spaces appear to be separated by the lateral umbilicovesical ligaments (*thick arrows*). The ileal loops sink in the supravesical space (*I*)

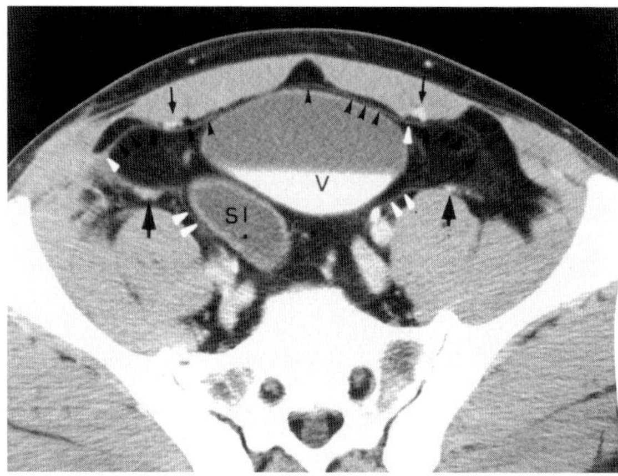

Fig. 4.9. Pelvic peritoneum (vesical plane). Thin dense line of the parietal peritoneum (*arrowhead*) extending along the anterior abdominal wall, from which it is separated by adipose tissue of the preperitoneal space The punctiform hyperdense images of the inferior epigastric vessels (*arrows*) are located on the sides of this space Then, the peritoneum passes downward, following the lateral wall of the pelvis The spermatic vessels (*large arrows*) are recognizable on the sides in front of the psoas and between the psoas and the peritoneum

A

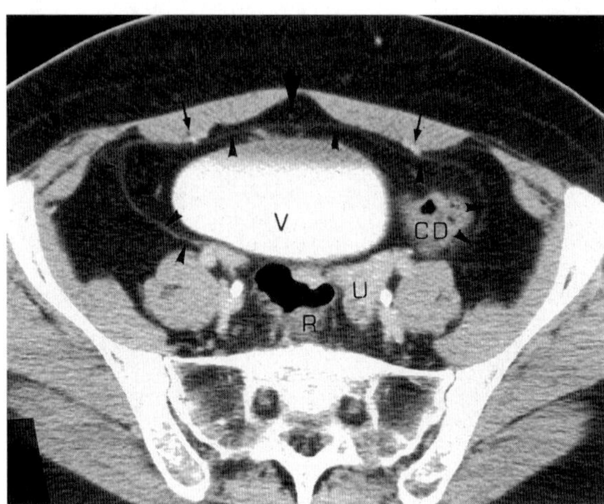

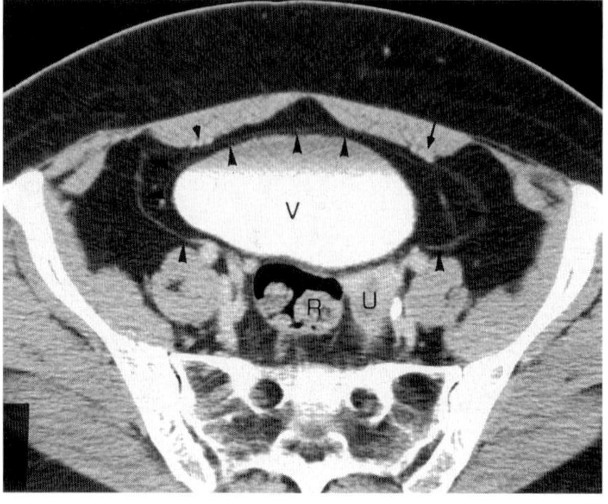

B

Fig. 4.10. Pelvic peritoneum (vesical plane). Thin circular line (*arrowhead*) of the parietal peritoneum, well visible for the thick layer of the pre- and intraperitoneal adipose tissue surrounding the urinary bladder and the colonsigmoidal junction (*CD*). The peritoneum limits the preperitoneal space, where the punctiform images of the inferior epigastric vessels (*small arrows*), on the sides, and the median umbilicovesical ligament (urachus) (*large arrowheads*), along the medial line, are recognizable

can cause the position of ligaments and mesenteries to change.

Using the same sequence as is used to delineate normal anatomy, we now describe the CT aspects of single ligaments and mesenteries.

The *falciform ligament* (Figs. 4.16–4.18, 4.20, 4.21) is visible only in the case of effusions in the right and left subphrenic spaces, when it is seen as a thin lamina that is slightly arcuate and is oblique from left to right and from front to back; it joins the anterior abdominal wall to the left lobe of the liver, between the II and IV segments.

In normal conditions, the *coronary ligament* (Figs. 4.16, 4.17, 4.19, 4.20, 4.22) is not visible on CT, whereas in the presence of fluid in the perihepatic spaces it corresponds to the posteromedian border, where no collection is present. The lack of fluid penetration above the posteromedian border of the liv-

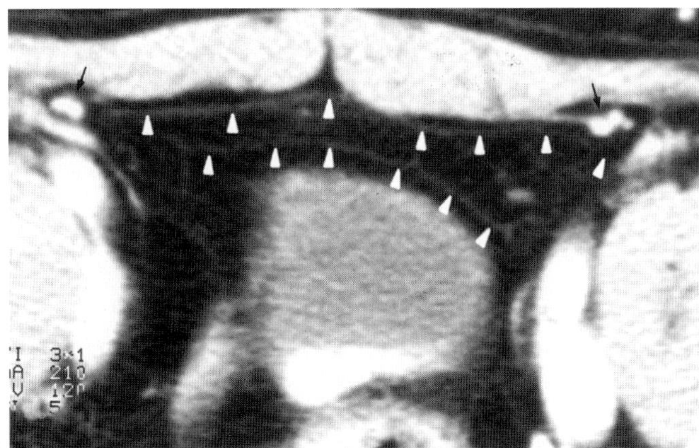
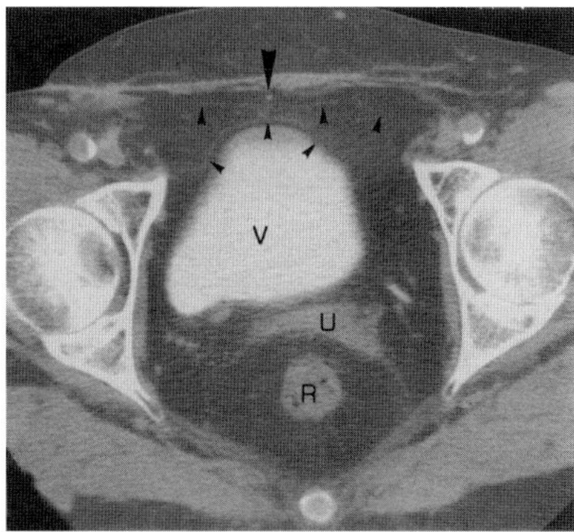

A B

Fig. 4.11A, B. Pelvic peritoneum (low vesical plane). The anterior pelvic parietal peritoneum (*arrowheads*) sinks into the suprapubic space behind the anterior abdominal wall. It then follows an upward path, extending in front of and above the urinary bladder. Therefore, it appears as a double linear image, made up of an anterior transverse and a prevesical posterior semicircular component The intraperitoneal adipose tissue is located between these two parts. Between the transverse peritoneal line and the anterior abdominal wall, we observe the umbilicovesical or prevesical space, where the punctiform image of the median umbilicovesical ligament (*large arrowhead*) stands out. The interstice containing adipose tissue and located between the curved line and the vesical wall corresponds to the perivesical space

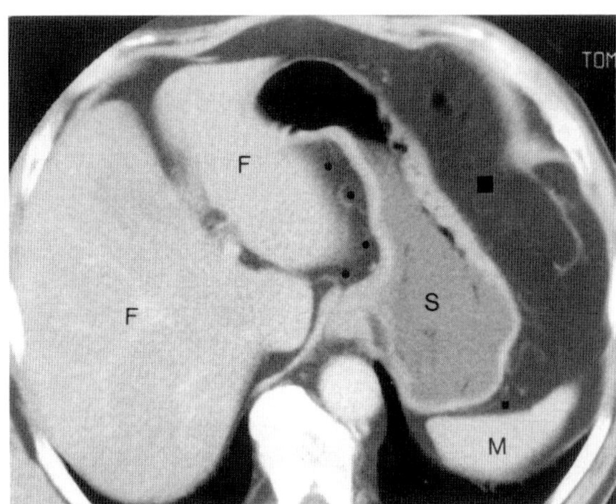

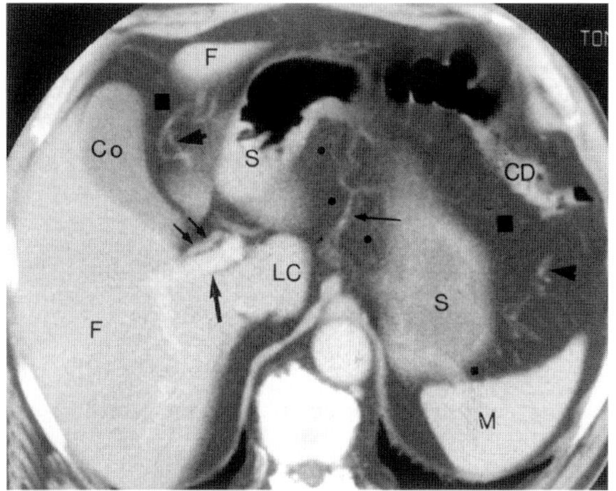

A B

Fig. 4.12A, B. Supramesocolic ligaments. **A** Gastrohepatic ligament (*round dots*) between stomach and left hepatic lobe, crossed by the coronarostomachic vessels and extending into the transverse fissure of the liver. Gastrocolic ligament (*squares*) outside the greater curvature of the stomach. Gastrosplenic ligament (*small square*) between stomach and spleen, crossed by the short gastric vessels. **B** Gastrohepatic ligament (round dots) and coronarostomachic artery (*long thin arrow*). Gastrocolic ligament (*square*) on the right side outside the greater curvature of the stomach (with the right gastroepiploic vessels (*arrowhead*), and on the left side between the greater curvature of the stomach and the descending colon (with the left gastroepiploic vessels (*arrowhead*). Hepatoduodenal ligament in front of the caudate lobe of the liver, with the hepatic artery (*thin arrows*) and the portal trunk (*large arrow*) inside

er makes it possible to distinguish peritoneal collections (Figs. 5.1–5.3) from pleural effusions, which spread medially up to the front of the diaphragmatic crura (Fig. 5.4–5.6), and from subcapsular hepatic collections, which diffuse before the coronary ligament. Furthermore, the ligament divides the right subphrenic from the subhepatic cavity.

Occasionally, the presence of liquid may allow visualization of both the *left triangular ligament* (Figs. 4.19, 4.20), which then appears as a thin transversal band crossing the subphrenic space from the apex of the left hepatic lobe, and the *phrenogastric ligament* (Figs. 4.16–4.19), seen as a transparent sagittal band between the left hemidiaphragm and the fornix of the stomach, which is limited at the sides by the liquid in the left subphrenic cavity.

The *gastrohepatic ligament* (Figs. 4.12, 4.13, 4.15, 4.16, 4.20, 4.22, 4.26) appears as a transparent space

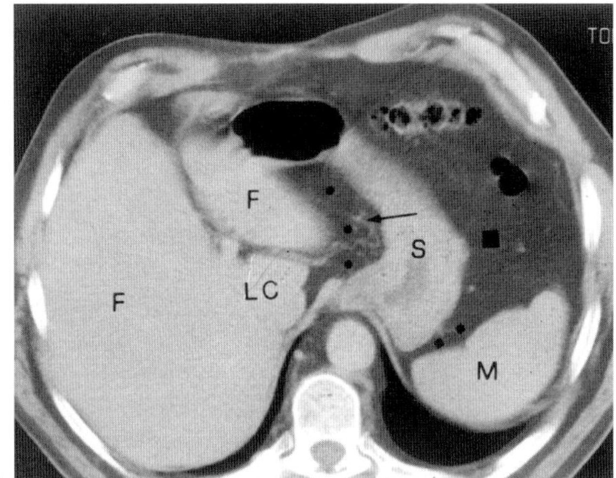

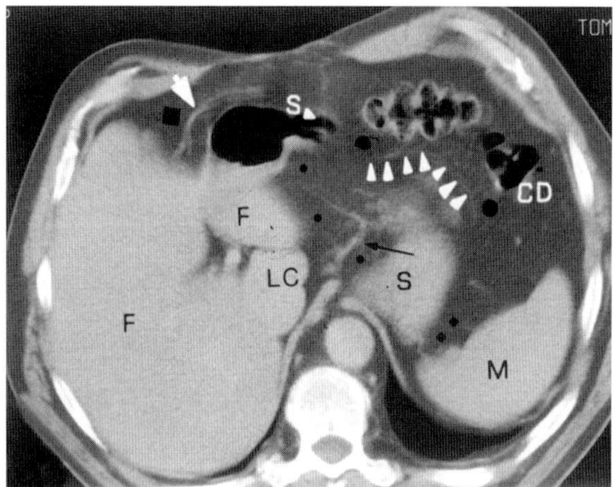

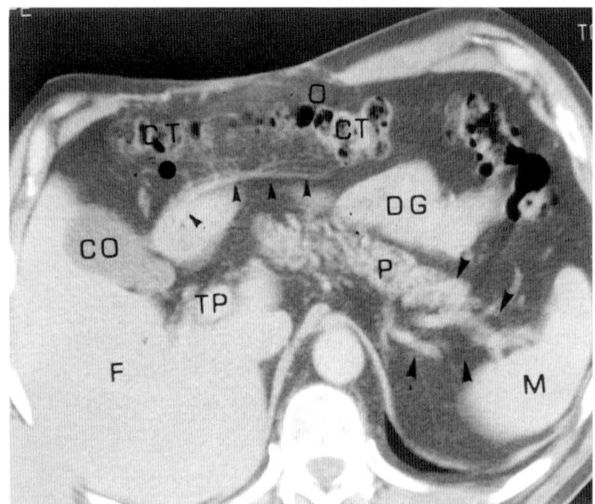

Fig. 4.13A–C. Supramesocolic ligaments. **A** Gastrohepatic ligament (*round dots*), between stomach and liver, crossed by the coronarostomachic vessels (*long thin arrow*); the ligament penetrates the transverse fissure of the liver. Gastrocolic ligament (*square*) between stomach and splenic flexure of the colon. Gastrosplenic ligament (*small squares*) between fundus ventricoli and spleen, with the short gastric vessels. **B** Gastrohepatic ligament (*round dots*), with the coronarostomachic artery (*long arrow*), which extends behind the lesser curvature of the stomach. Gastrocolic ligament (*square*) on the right, with the gastroepiploic vessels (*large arrowhead*), extending anteriorly along the gastric antrum. Left transverse mesocolon (*large round dots*), with the median colic vessels (*small arrowhead*). **C** Right transverse mesocolon (*large round dots*), with the middle colic vessels (*arrowhead*). Splenopancreatic ligament around the cauda pancreatis and the splenic hilum (*large arrowhead*). Omentum (*O*) studded with the punctiform images of its vessels in front of the transverse colon

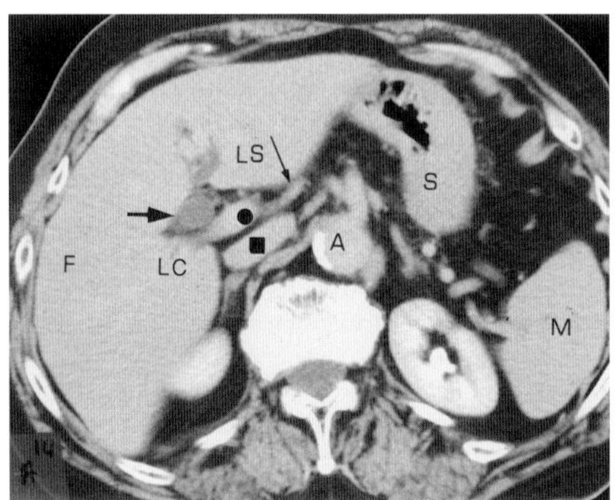

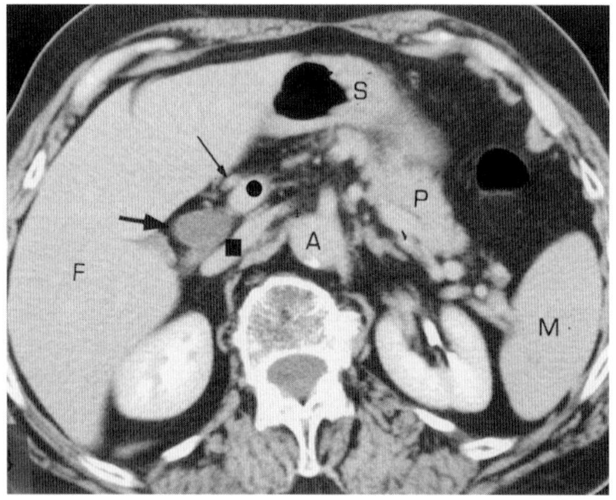

Fig. 4.14A, B. Supramesocolic ligaments. **A** Hepatoduodenal ligament (mediohepatic plane) between the left lobe in the front, and the caudate lobe and the inferior vena cava (*square*) behind, in the transverse fissure of the liver, where the hepatic artery (*thin arrow*), the portal trunk (*large round dots*) and the dilated hepatocholedochus (*arrow*) are recognizable. **B** The hepatoduodenal ligament (subhepatic plane) between liver and inferior vena cava

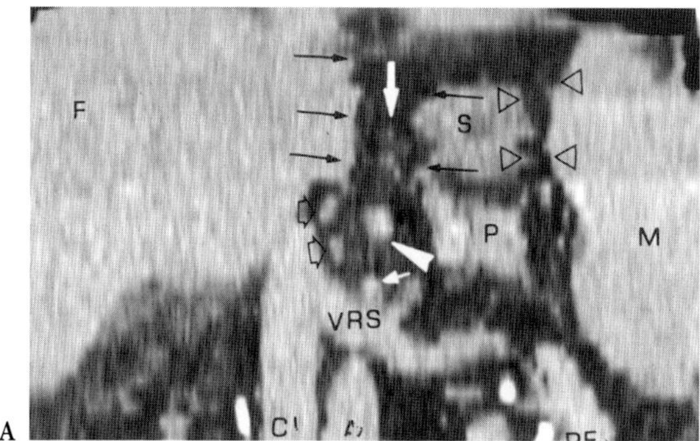

A

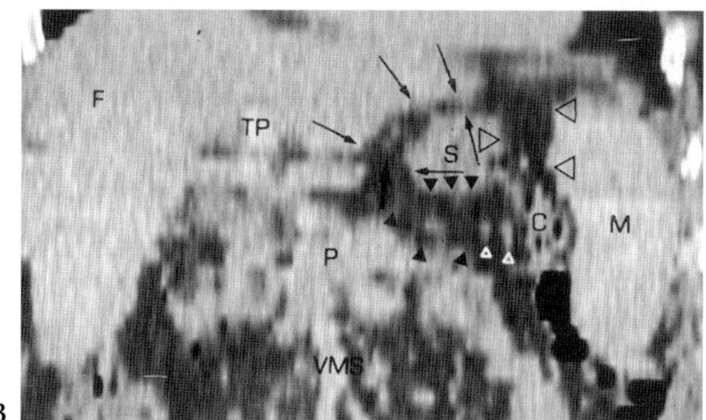

B

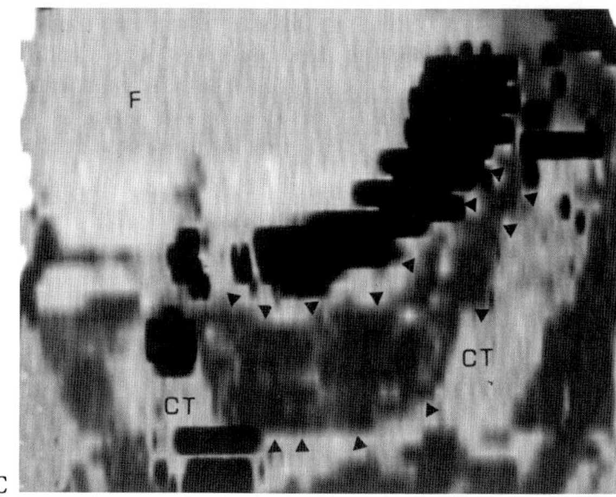

C

Fig. 4.15A–C. Supramesocolic planes. Coronal reconstructions from back to front. **A** Plane crossing the large vessels. Gastrohepatic ligament (*long arrows*) between stomach and liver, with the coronarostomachic vessels (*thick arrow*) and, at a lower level, the superior mesenteric vein (*arrowhead*) and the artery (*short arrow*) On the *right*, the retropancreatic vessels (*open arrows*); gastrosplenic ligament (*open triangles*) between stomach and spleen. **B** Plane 3 cm in front of that of the previous picture. Besides the above-mentioned structures, we observe the gastrocolic ligament (*triangles*), with the gastroepiploic vessels transversely sectioned (*open small triangles*), the portal trunk (*TP*) and the superior mesenteric vein (*VMS*). **C** Anterior plane. The total extension of the gastrocolic ligament (*triangles*) between stomach (expanded by gas) and transverse colon is visible

in the upper abdominal planes on the median line in front of the diaphragmatic crura, between the lesser curvature of the stomach and the liver; it is crossed from behind forward by the sinuous left gastric artery, which can frequently be detected from its origin up to the proximal parts of the pylorus. The ligament continues on the right outward in the intersegmental fissure of the liver, between the left and the caudate lobes (Fig. 4.26), at a high level in the longitudinal fissure and at a low level under the hepatic hilum, within the *hepatoduodenal ligament* (Figs. 4.12, 4.14, 4.20). In the transparency of the adipose tissue of the latter ligament, anteriorly the hepatic artery on the left and the main biliary tract on the right, medially the portal trunk, and posteriorly, behind the retroperitoneum, the inferior vena cava can be distinguished. Between the portal trunk and the inferior vena cava it is sometimes possible to detect a small transverse band made up of the peritoneal folds that limit Winslow's foramen; alternatively, this space may be penetrated by the papilliferous process of the caudate lobe.

The *gastrosplenic ligament* (Figs. 4.12, 4.13, 4.15, 4.16, 4.18–4.20, 4.29, 4.31) is located as a transparent space extending from the front backward and from right to left between the greater curvature of the stomach and the upper half of the spleen. Within this ligament, we distinguish the short gastric and the left gastroepiploic vessels, which have a sinuous and multipunctiform aspect. The gastrosplenic ligament constitutes the left wall of the lesser sac and limits collections that may diffuse inside; it continues downward and forward with the gastrocolic ligament and, medial to the splenic hilum, with the splenopancreatic ligament.

The *splenorenal* or *splenopancreatic ligament* (Figs. 4.13, 4.16, 4.20, 4.31) is visible as a transparent space behind the pancreatic tail around the vessels of the splenic hilum. Mostly it shows a triangular shape, wider at the sides and becoming progressively thinner and less easily visible as we move more and more inward. It constitutes the posterior wall of the omental bursa. It is easier to identify the ligament when some fluid is present in this cavity or in the splenopancreatic recess.

The *gastrocolic ligament* (Figs. 4.12, 4.13, 4.15–4.17) continues the gastrosplenic and gastrohepatic ligaments downward, connecting stomach and transverse colon. It is represented by the transparent space between these two viscera, where the right and left gastroepiploic vessels extend parallel to the greater

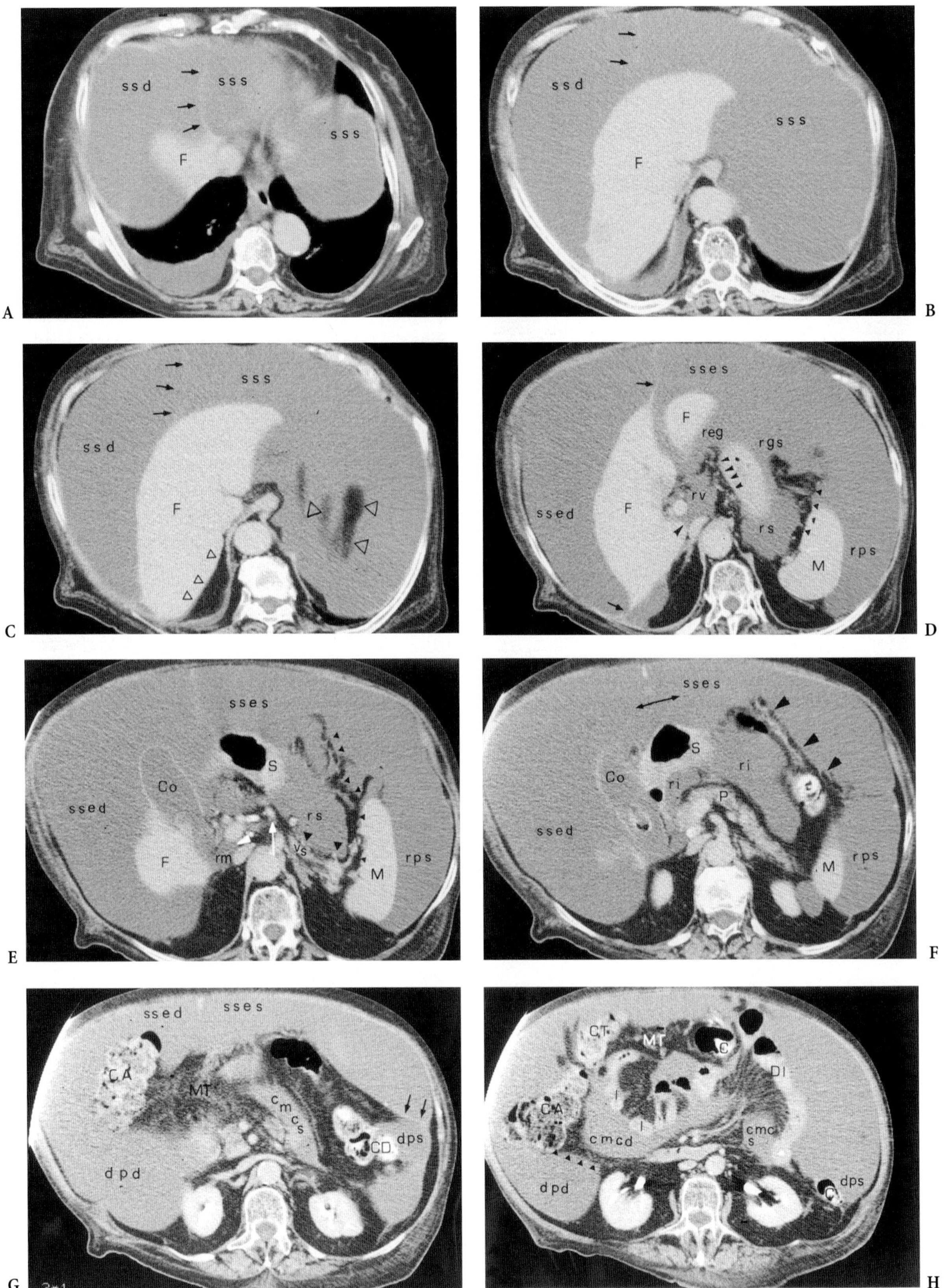

Fig. 4.16A–N. Ligaments and peritoneal cavities. Abundant ascites in peritoneal carcinosis for sigmoidal carcinoma. Axial sections from the diaphragm to the pelvis. **A, B** Subdiaphragmatic plane. The liver is displaced downward, medially and away from the diaphragm The right and left subphrenic spaces are hyperexpanded by fluid and separated by the falciform ligament (**A–D**); fortuitously, it is almost completely recognizable in this section (*thin arrows*). **C** 1 cm lower than the previous section. The transparency of the phrenogastric ligament (*open triangles*) begins to be visibile. The bare area is located on the posteromedian border of the liver, between the leaves of the coronary ligament, which prevents fluid diffusion between liver and diaphragm (*open small triangles*). **D** 4 cm under the previous section. The right and the left subhepatic spaces are separated by the falciform ligament (*small arrows*) .... →→

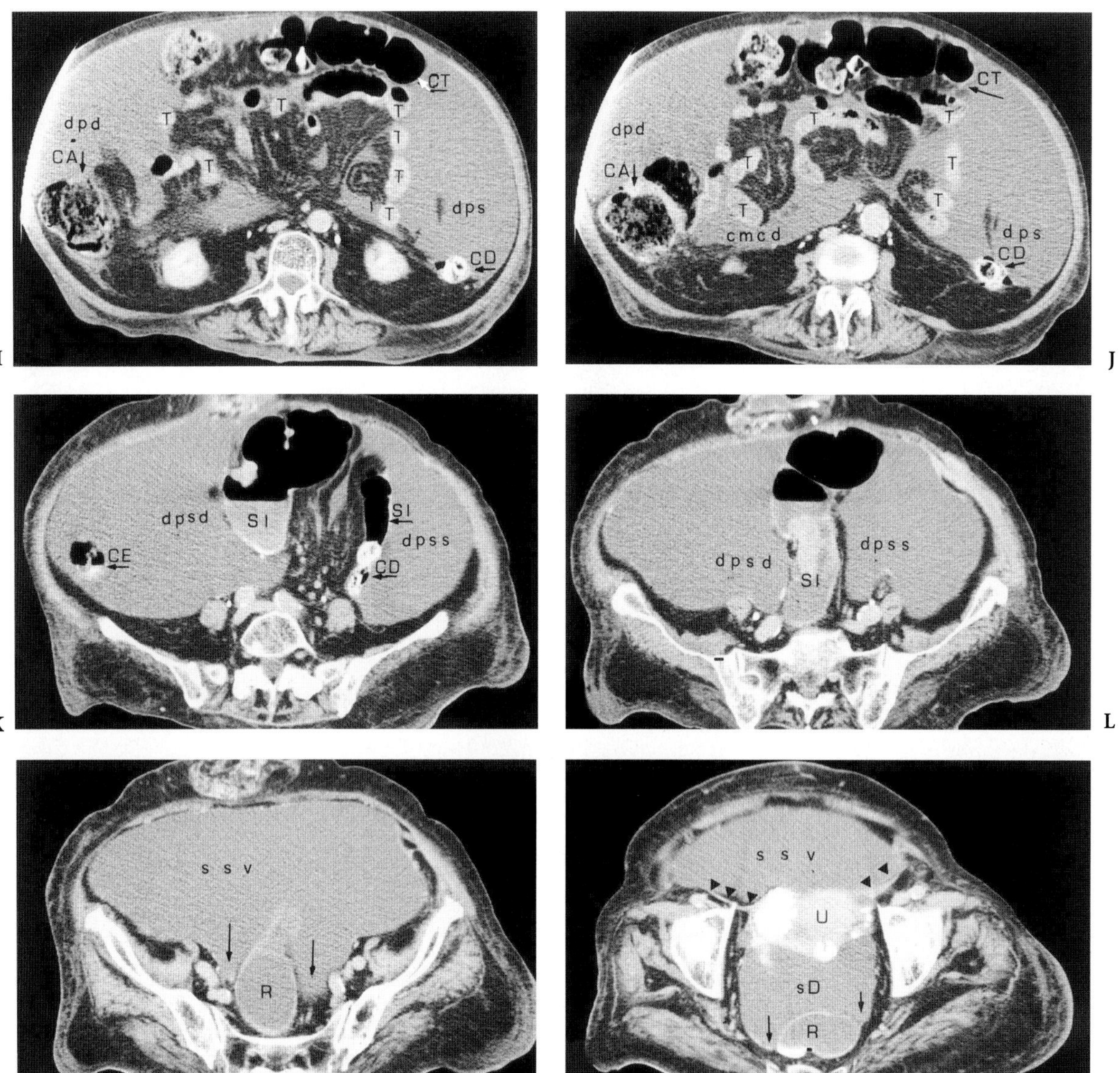

.... → → The gastrohepatic (*arrowhead*) and gastrosplenic (*small triangles*) ligaments subdivide the left cavity in hepatogastric (*reg*), gastrosplenic (*rgs*) and perisplenic (rps) recesses. Omental bursa with vestibular (*rv*) and splenic (*rs*) recesses, separated by the left gastric artery incisure Winslow's foramen (*large arrowhead*) between portal vein and vena cava, by which the vestibular recess communicates with Morrison's space. **E** 3 cm under the previous section. Right subhepatic space surrounding the cholecystic wall with adherent visceral peritoneum. Winslow's foramen (*white arrowhead*) and its communication with Morrison's posterior subhepatic recess. Phrenicocolic ligament (*small triangles*), splenopancreatic ligament with the splenic vein (*large triangles*), and gastrohepatic ligament with the left gastric artery (*thin arrow*), all of which limit the splenic recess of the omental bursa. **F** Pancreatic plane. Right and left subhepatic spaces communicating under the liver because of the absence of the falciform ligament at this level. Inferior expansion of the omental bursa recesses (*ri*) limited anteriorly by the peritoneum [surrounding the posterior wall of the stomach on the right and constituting the medial leaf of the gastrocolic ligament (*arrowhead*) on the left] and by the gastrosplenic ligament, and closed behind by the posterior parietal peritoneum. **G** Transverse mesocolic plane. Right subhepatic space, which continues downward with the right paracolic gutter (outside) and insinuates itself behind the ascending colon. The left subhepatic space is separated from the paracolic gutter by the phrenicocolic ligament (*arrows*). The left inframesocolic cavity begins to be visible along the median line. **H** High mesenteric plane. On the sides, the paracolic gutters, and centrally the inframesocolic cavities, separated by the ascending and descending colon and mesocolon. **I** Middle mesenteric plane. Fan-like disposition of the mesentery and of its vessels. **J**) Horizontal disposition of the transverse colon in the anterior planes, with the paracolic gutters on the sides Posteriorly on the median line, the inframesocolic cavities are separated by the mesentery and by the ileal loops. **(K, L)** High pelvic plane. Median and left paramedian expansion of the sigmoid and of its mesentery, with the right and left parasigmoidal gutters on the sides Cecal fundus completely surrounded by the peritoneum. **K** Middle pelvic plane. Unique wide supravesical space, where the peritoneal cavities converge Pronounced pararectal recesses (*arrows*). **L** Inferior pelvic plane. Empty urinary bladder and fibromatous uterus. Supravesical space and pouch of Douglas separated by the uterus and by the broad and round ligaments (*triangle*) The right laterorectal recess (*arrows*) is very pronounced

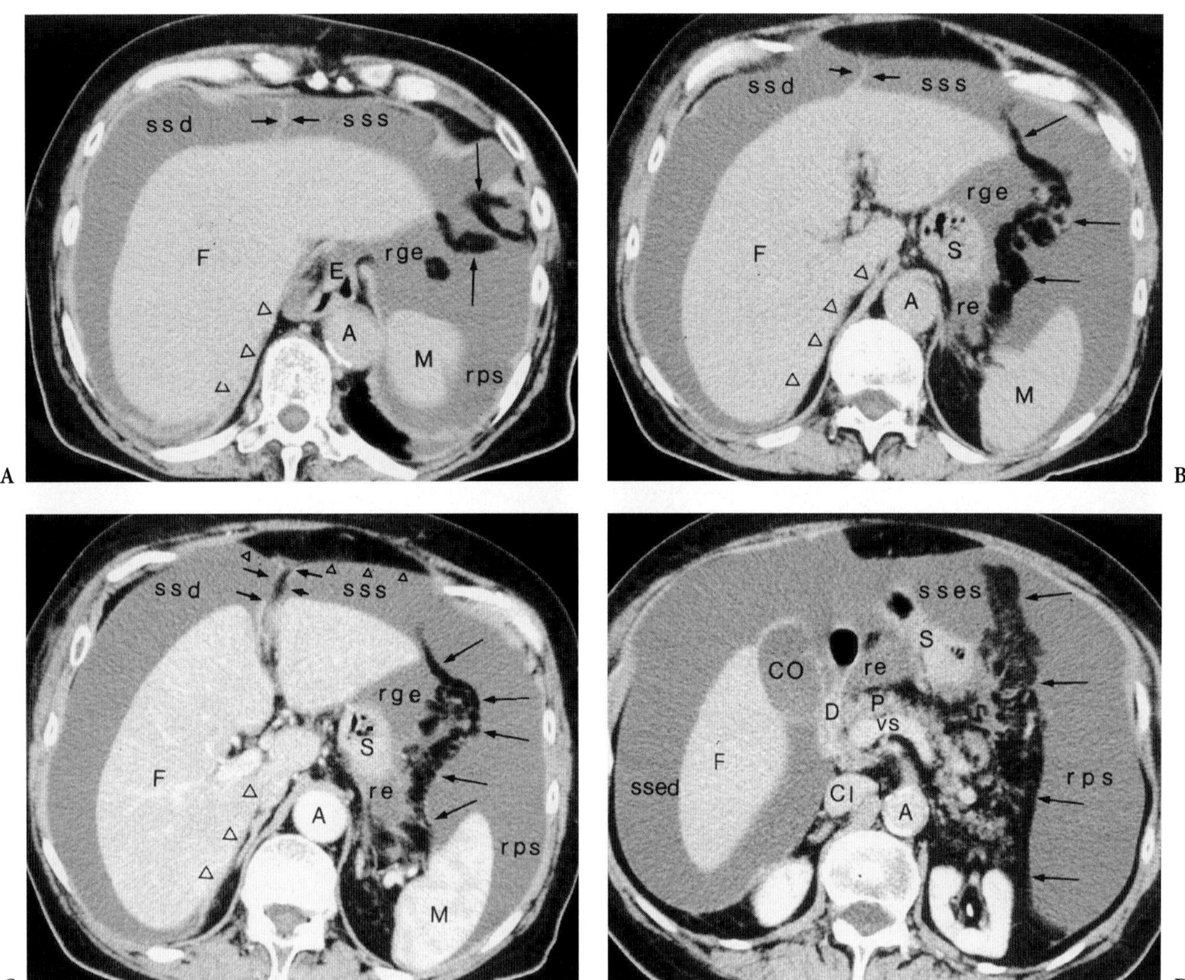

Fig. 4.17A–J. Ligaments and peritoneal cavities. Peritoneal carcinosis with omental metastases due to endometrial carcinoma. Axial scans from the diaphragm to the pelvis. **A–C** Right and left subphrenic spaces divided by the falciform ligament (*thin arrows*). The phreno-gastro-spleno-colic ligament (*long arrows*) subdivides the left subphrenic space into the suprahepatic (anteriorly), gastrohepatic and perisplenic recesses, and separates these recesses from the lesser sac (*rge*). Retrohepatic bare area (*open triangles*) corresponding to the coronary ligament; it separates the right subphrenic space from the subhepatic recess. Anteriorly and medially (**B, C**), fat density biconvex lens-like structure of the umbilical canal communicating with the longitudinal fissure of the liver in the point where the leaves of the falciform ligament diverge to insert on both sides of the fissure (**C** *small open triangles*). **D** Pancreatic plane. Right subhepatic space surrounding the inferior pole of the right hepatic lobe and the gallbladder. Anteriorly, the right and left subhepatic spaces communicate without the interposition of the falciform ligament. The wide sagittal band of the gastro-spleno-colic ligament (*long arrows*) joins the transverse mesocolon and the mesenteric root posteriorly, and penetrates between the left subhepatic and the perisplenic recess. **E** Plane of the root of the transverse mesocolon. Right paramedian transparency of the root of the transverse mesocolon (*small triangles*), where the superior mesenteric vessels and the gastrocolic venous trunk (*small square*) stand out. On the left, the gastrocolic ligament (*long arrows*) continues in the transverse mesocolon and in the omentum, which is thickening because of metastases, and posteriorly in the left phrenicocolic ligament (*arrowhead*). The supramesocolic cavities are swelled by liquid and expand downwards and on the sides. On the left, the inframesocolic cavity and the paracolic gutter, separated by the splenic flexure of the colon (*FS*) and by its mesentery, begin to be visibile. Anteriorly, the umbilical canal becomes progressively thinner along its extension toward the umbilicus. **F, G** The wide median fan-like expansion of the transparency of the mesentery separates the right from the left inframesocolic cavities, and the posterior inflexions of the ascending and descending colon, with their respective mesenteries, divide these cavities from the corresponding paracolic gutters. The omentum is thickening and denser because of metastases. The previsceral cavity is delineated in front of viscera and omentum. Thickening of the leaves of the mesenteric peritoneum extending in a sagittal direction on the sides of the ileal vessels (**G**). **H, I** Superior pelvic plane. Left median and paramedian expansion of the sigmoid mesocolon (*large arrowhead*); the sigmoid and the sigmoidal vessels are recognizable within its transparency. The expansion separates the wide right parasigmoidal recess, where the right paracolic gutter and the left inframesocolic cavity converge, from the left paracolic gutter and parasigmoidal recess. **J** Middle pelvic plane. Supravesical space and pouch of Douglas, separated transversely by the uterus and by the broad ligaments

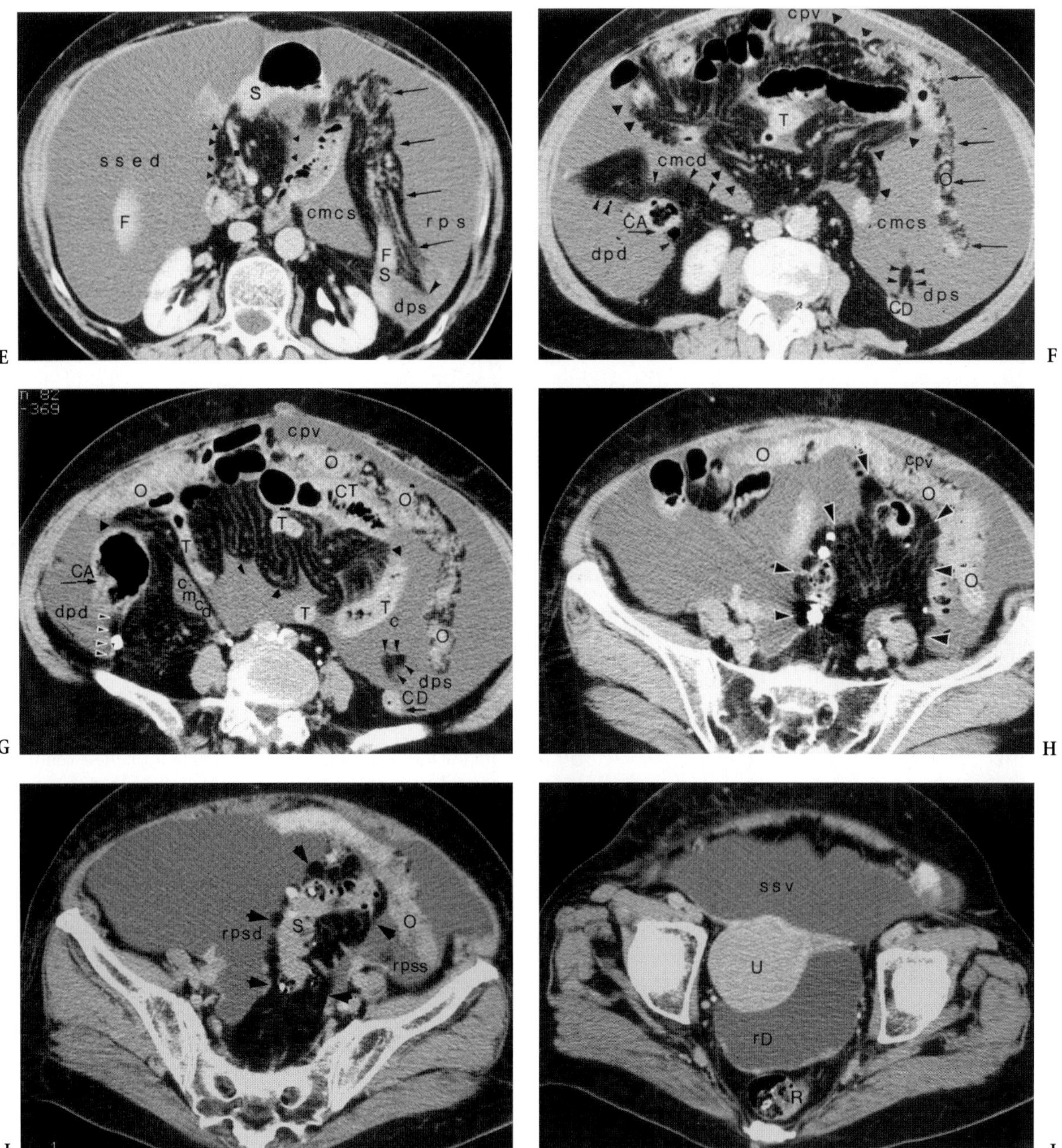
E
S
s s e d
F
cmcs
r p s
F
S
dps
F
cpv
T
cmcd
CA
dpd
cmcs
O
dps
CD
G
n 82
-369
cpv
O
CT
O
O
T
T
CA
c
mcd
dpd
T
Tc
O
dps
CD
H
O
cpv
O
O
I
S
rpsd
O
rpss
J
ssv
U
rD
R

Fig. 4.17E–J.

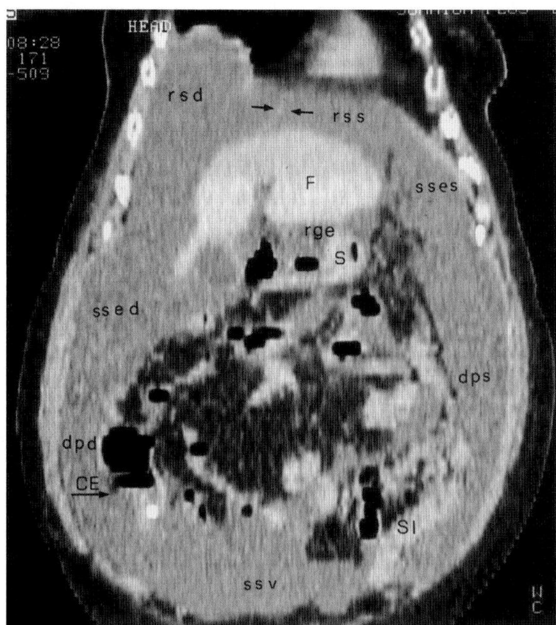

A

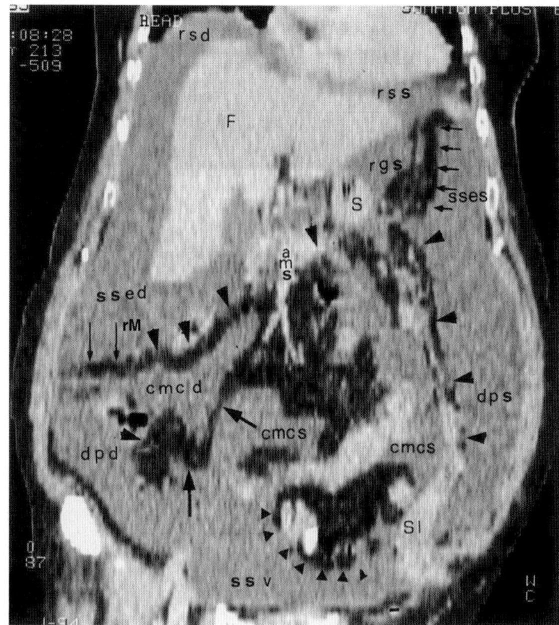

B

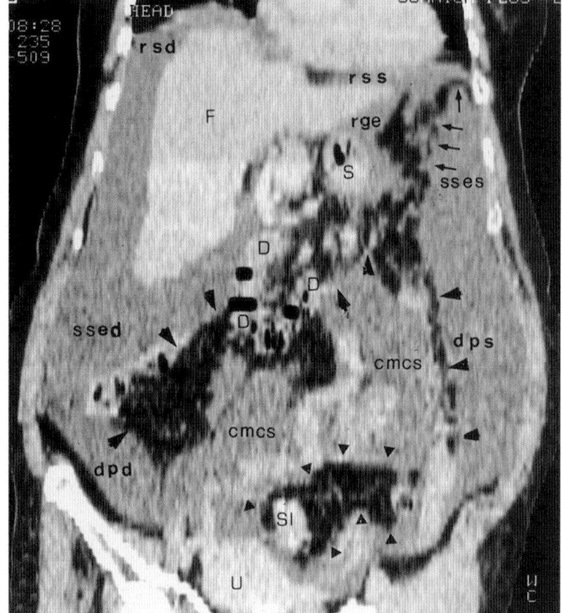

C

Fig. 4.18A–C. Ligaments and peritoneal cavities. Coronal reconstructions from the front backwards. **A** Plane at 7 cm from the anterior abdominal wall. We recognize at a high level the right and left subphrenic spaces, divided by the falciform ligament (*arrows*), which have a direct communication with the underlying subhepatic space, and through this space, with the homolateral paracolic gutters. In turn, these continue in the supravesical pelvic spaces. In a central position, the transparency of the mesentery, limited on the sides by the ascending and descending colon, stands out. **B** Plane located at 4.5 cm behind the previous plane. The total extension of the posterior insertions of the phreno-gastro-spleno-colic ligament (*arrows*), of the mesocolon (*arrowhead*) and of the sigmoid mesocolon (*triangles*) begin to be visible. At a high level, the subphrenic and subhepatic spaces surround the liver. The right phrenicocolic ligament (*long thin arrows*) separates Morrison's recess (*rM*) from the right paracolic gutter and inframesocolic cavity. In a central position, the transparency of the mesenteric root is crossed vertically by the superior mesenteric artery. At a low level on the right, the confluence of the inferior mesenteric tract with the mesocecum (*large arrows*) closes the bottom of the right inframesocolic cavity and separates it from the left cavity and from the underlying pelvic spaces. At a low level on the left, the sigmoid and its mesentery (*triangles*) separate the left inframesocolic cavity from the supravesical space. **C** Plane located at 2 cm behind the previous plane. Total extension of the posterior insertion of the phreno-gastro-spleno-colic ligament (*arrows*), of the mesocolon (*arrowhead*) and of the sigmoid mesocolon (*triangles*). The left inframesocolic cavity appears in a central position, inside the transparency of the descending mesocolon and above the sigmoid mesocolon; this cavity continues downwards on the right in the pelvic recesses and joins the right paracolic gutter. On the *left*, the paracolic gutter continues through the parasigmoidal gutter in the pelvic recesses, maintaining its separation from the inframesocolic cavity because of the presence of the descending mesocolon and the sigmoid mesocolon

curvature of the corpus ventriculi and the gastric antrum. The position of this ligament shows maximal variations according to the constitutional type, gastric filling and colic distension . Therefore, it has various possible locations: between stomach and transverse colon in a high position in the same section plane between these two viscera in brachytypical subjects, and below the stomach, between this bowel and the transverse colon in a low position in longitypical subjects. The gastrocolic ligament can be distinguished from the underlying transverse mesocolon only by the vessels crossing it: gastroepiploic vessels in the case of the gastrocolic ligament and middle colic vessels in the case of the transverse mesocolon. These vessels are recognizable by their pathways: the gastroepiploic vessels extend from above downward and on the left side of the corpus ventriculi above the transverse colon; the middle colic vessels extend from the upper mesenteric vascular bundle.

Owing to its mainly horizontal position, extending from behind forward, and its scant thickness, the *transverse mesocolon* (Figs. 4.13, 4.17–4.22) is not easy to recognize and must be identified by reference to the abdominal structures and confirmed by the finding of the middle colic vessels extending inside its thickness. Therefore, it is necessary to search along a line extending from right to left in front of the median tract of the second duodenal portion and the head of the pancreas and in front of the lower border of the corpus pancreatis and the pancreatic tail, under the spleen and between the aforementioned organs and the transverse colon. This latter bowel section may be in a high position, with the transverse mesocolon located in the same plane of the organ (Fig. 4.23), or in a low position, with the mesocolon extending obliquely downward and from behind forward. Inside the transverse mesocolon, the middle colic vessels extend horizontally in the adipose tissue located between the lower pancreatic and the upper transverse colon profiles, diverging from the upper mesenteric vessels on the median line toward the two sides. When the transverse colon is high, under the diaphragm, as frequently occurs at the level of the splenic flexure, the mesocolon and the middle colic vessels are located in lower planes than the transverse colon. Conversely, when the transverse colon is low, as it often is in the median tract, both mesocolon and middle colic vessels are located above the bowel.

The *phrenicocolic ligament* (Figs. 4.16–4.19, 4.21) is the lateral continuation of the transverse mesocolon. It can be recognized only when it is limited by a peritoneal effusion, when it appears as an arcuate line or a transparent band linking the splenic flexure of the colon with the lateral abdominal wall under the spleen and precluding communication in either direction between the spaces located above and those sited under the mesocolon.

The *greater omentum* (Figs. 4.13, 4.17, 4.19, 4.20, 4.22) appears as a transparent arcuate band behind the anterior abdominal wall in front of the transverse colon and the ileal loops. Inside, omental vessels stand out as small dots that are often coupled. Omental thickness varies both from person to person and in the same person: it is greater in individuals with abundant fat deposits, whereas it is thinner in lean subjects; often it is different on the two sides of the body. It is not rare for it not to cover the whole of the previsceral space, but it can cluster on one side or penetrate partly or completely among the ileal loops, or fold upward, adopting a position under the diaphragm in front of the liver and the stomach. Its length is also very variable: it can be short and limited to coverage of the transverse colon and the first loops of the small bowel, or wide, extending downward as far as the front of the urinary bladder. When it is pathologic, especially in case of secondary neoplastic localizations, the omentum increases in thickness and density (Figs. 4.17, 4.19).

The *mesentery* (Figs. 4.5, 4.16–4.22, 4.24) corresponds to the wide median abdominal space occupied by adipose tissue; it opens like a fan from behind forward, is limited by small intestinal loops and is crossed by vascular branches converging in the upper mesenteric vessels in a medioposterior plane and continuing backward without interruption in the adipose areolar tissue of the anterior retroperitoneum. In the case of a peritoneal effusion, the mesenteric position and borders become very sharply delineated and are limited by the peritoneal cavities expanded by the fluid. Therefore, it is possible to follow the extension of the mesentery from its root at the level of the duodenojejunal flexure, where it joins the transverse mesocolon, up to the right iliac fossa, and to observe the fan-like unfolding (Figs. 4.17, 4.18) in front of the mesenteric areolar tissue and vessels and the peripheral location of the duodenojejunal loops.

The *mesocecum* (Figs. 4.18, 4.19) corresponds to adipose tissue crossed by ileocecal vessels, which extend from the left side of the bowel medially toward the upper mesenteric vascular axis with small dots or thin sinuous lines, and by right marginal colic vessels continuing upward along the internal side of the ascending colon. The adipose tissue located around the cecum may have a higher density than the adjacent retroperitoneal fat, and the peritoneum

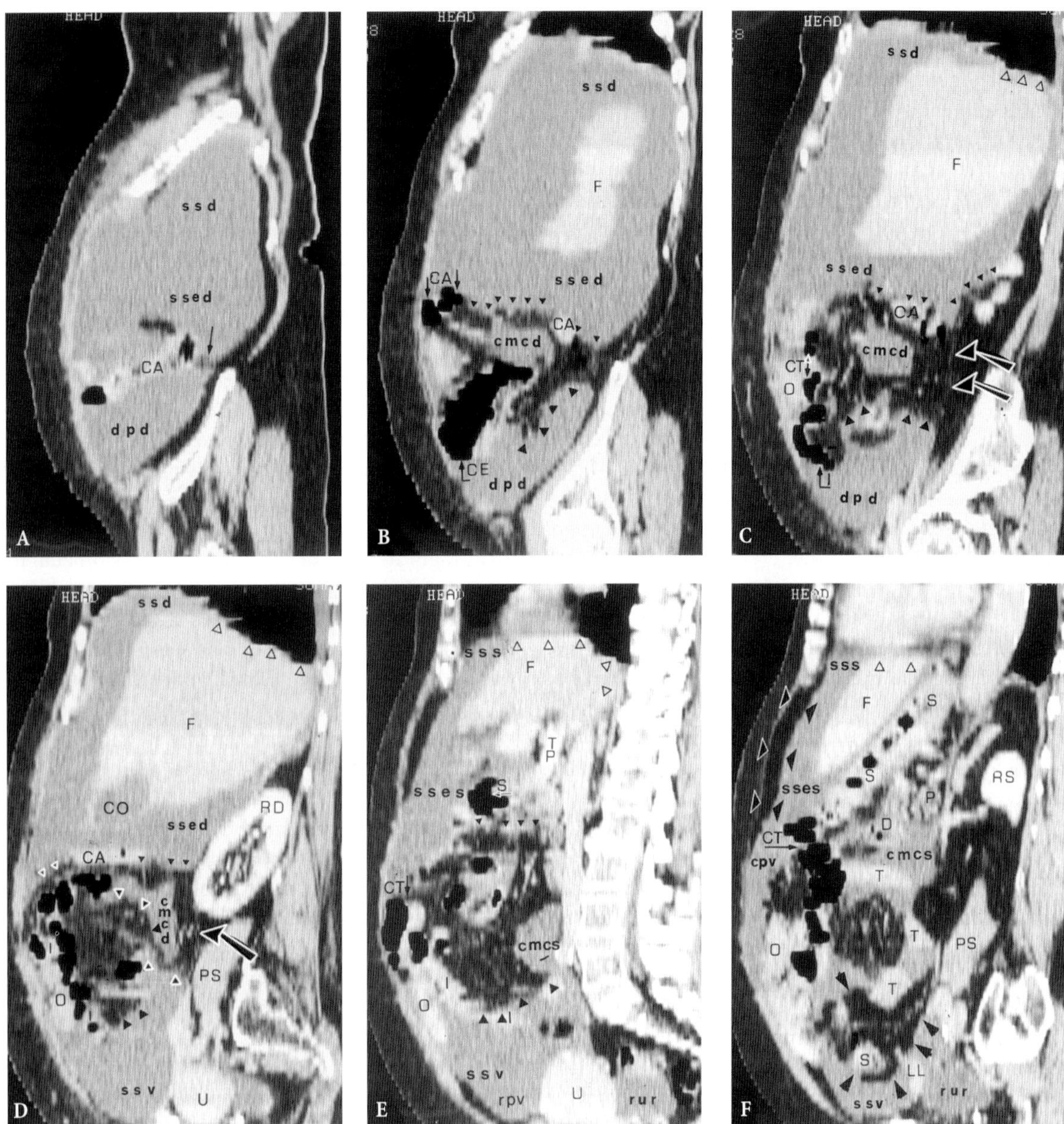

Fig. 4.19A–J. *Ligaments and peritoneal cavity.* Sagittal reconstructions from right to left. **A** Plane outside the liver. Unique right subphrenic and subhepatic space, separated anteriorly from the right paracolic gutter by the ascending colon and mesocolon, and posteriorly by the right phrenicocolic ligament (*arrow*) The transparency of the adipose tissue in the pararenal compartments is visible behind the profile of the posterior parietal peritoneum and of the adherent anterior renal fascia. **B, C** At 35 and 6 cm inside. At a high level, the right subphrenic and subhepatic spaces, located around the liver, freely communicate in the lateral plane (**B**), whereas they are separated in the medial planes (**C–F**) by the coronary ligament (*open triangles*), which allows the penetration of liquid between liver and diaphragm. These spaces are closed below by the ascending colon and its mesentery and by the transverse mesocolon (*small triangles*), which cuts the abdomen horizontally. Under these structures, the right inframesocolic cavity are recognized, which is limited in the front by the cecum-ascending colon and its mesentery, and posteriorly by the mesentery (*large triangles*) The mesenteric adipose tissue continues with the anterior pararenal fat. The anterior renal fascia (*large curved arrows*) separates them from the pararenal compartment. The right paracolic gutter is located below. **D** Right mediorenal plane. Under the mesocolon (*small triangles*), we observe from the front backwards the dense and thickening omentum, the ileal loops, the mesentery (*large triangles*), the right inframesocolic cavity, the anterior pararenal space, the renal fascia (*large curved arrow*) and the parirenal compartment. Below, the supravesical spaces appear to be greatly expanded, and are displacing the uterus backwards. **E** Caval plane passing medially to the falciform ligament. At a high level, we observe the left subphrenic and subhepatic spaces, which communicate in front of the liver and the antrum of the stomach; below, they are closed by the transverse mesocolon (*small triangles*) and by the transverse colon. Under this, the thick anterior vertical band of the omentum and the wide central ransparent expansion of the mesentery (big triangles) are limited inferiorly by the arch constituted by the ileal loops Behind the mesentery, we observe the left inframesocolic cavity. At a low level, the supravesical space, the paravesical recesses, the uterus tand the uterorectal recess are easily visible. .... →→

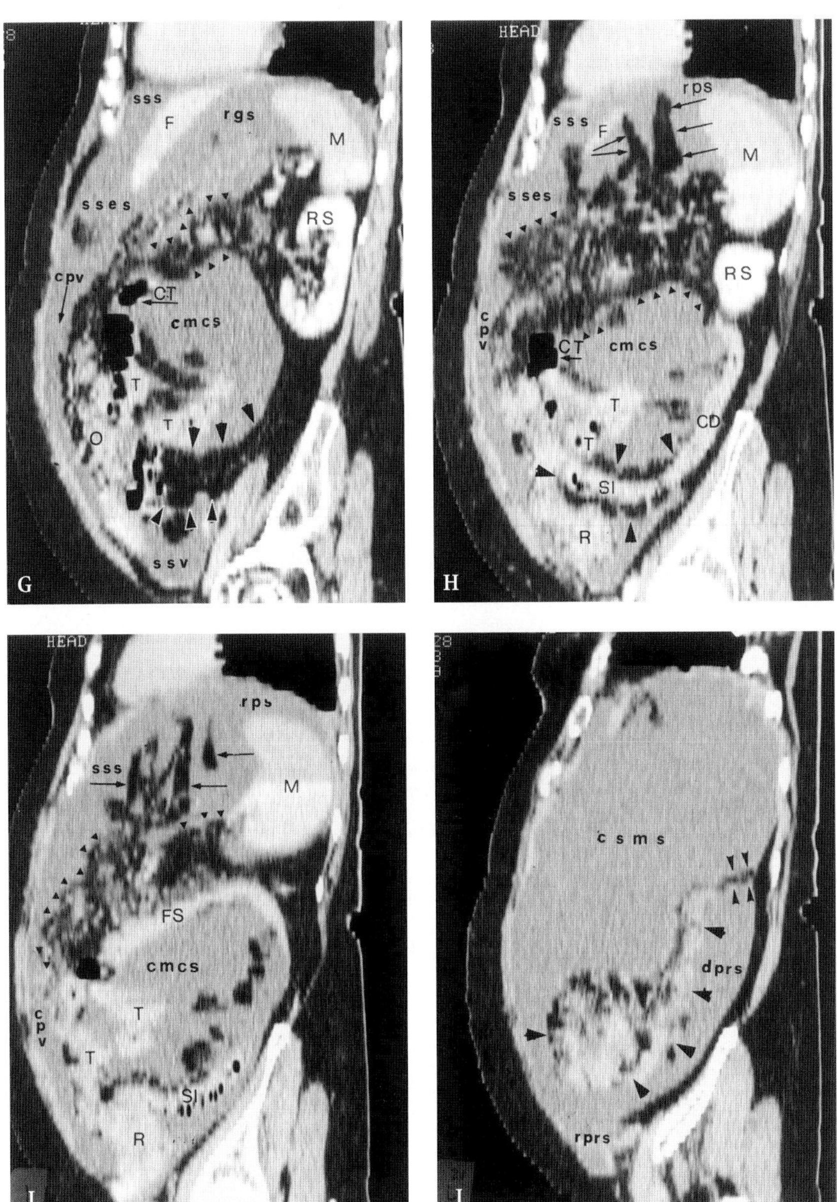

→ →... **F** Left paravertebral plane The left subphrenic and subhepatic spaces are separated by the coronary ligament at a high level, whereas they join below. The subhepatic space is limited behind by the stomach and continues downwards, in front of the transverse colon and the omentum, in the previsceral cavity. The mesentery is observed in a central position, as is the left inframesocolic cavity, which extends among the loops of the small intestine. Below, the sigmoid mesocolon (*large arrowhead*) is crossed by the sigmoidal vessels and separates the left inframesocolic cavity from the pelvic spaces. The vertical band of adipose tissue of the umbilical canal (*flat triangles*) is visible behind the anterior abdominal wall, between the ensiform apophysis and the umbilicus; it is limited posteriorly by the parietal peritoneum. The vertical hypodense band of the adipose tissue located in the umbilicovesical space is visible in the suprapubic region, between the abdominal wall and the peritoneum. **G** Left mediorenal plane The left subphrenic space is separated from the gastrosplenic recess by the liver and by the triangular ligament at a high level, and continues below in the subhepatic space and in the prevesical or preomental cavity: In a central position, the left inframesocolic cavity shows its maximal expansion; it is limited by the transverse mesocolon (*small triangles*) above, by the sigmoid mesocolon (*large arrowhead*) below, by the omentum, the transverse colon and the ileal loops at the front and by the posterior peritoneum, the renal fascia and the anterior pararenal space at the back. **H, I** At 2 and 35 cm to the left of the previous plane. Point of confluence of the phreno-gastro-spleno-colic ligament (*long arrows*), with the root of the transverse mesocolon and the superior tract of the mesentery (*small triangles*). At a high level, the phreno-gastro-splenic ligament separates the subhepatic from the perisplenic recess. The left inframesocolic cavity and the wide dense arch constituted by the splenic flexure, the descending colon and the proximal tract of the sigmoid stand out under the transparency of the mesenteries Anterior continuity of the peritoneal cavity from the diaphragm to the pelvis. **J** Left lumbar region The left phrenicocolic ligament (*small arrowhead*), the descending mesocolon and the sigmoid mesocolon (*large arrowhead*) separate the wide supramesocolic cavity from the left paracolic gutter, converging at a lower level in the left pararectal recess

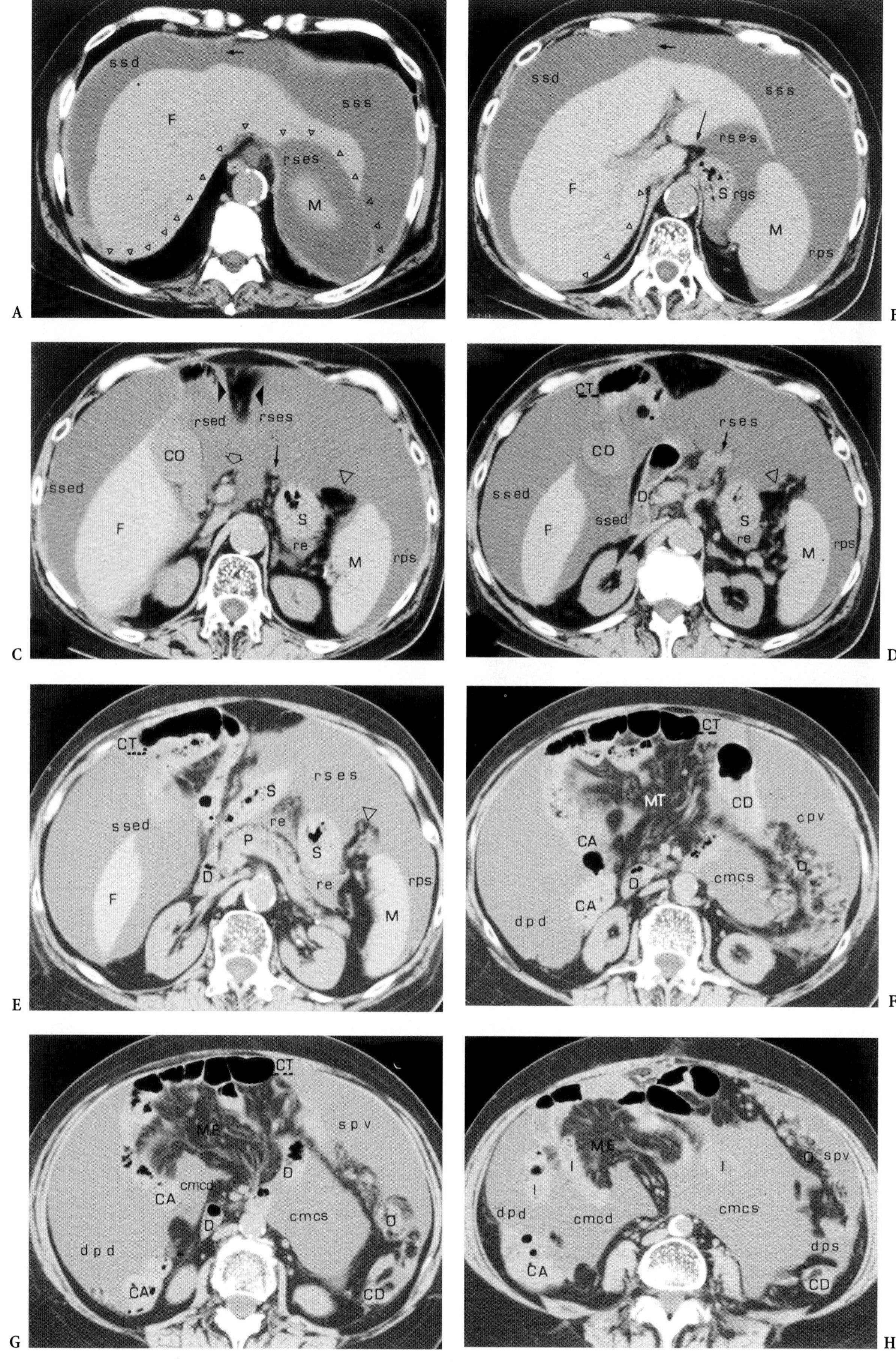

A
ssd
F
sss
rses
M
B
ssd
sss
rses
F
S rgs
M
rps
C
rsed
rses
CO
ssed
F
S
re
M
rps
D
CT
rses
CD
ssed
D
F
ssed
S
re
M
rps
E
CT
rses
S
ssed
re
P
S
D
re
F
rps
M
F
CT
MT
CD
cpv
CA
O
D
cmcs
CA
dpd
G
CT
ME
spv
D
cmcd
CA
D
cmcs
O
dpd
CA
CD
H
ME
O spv
I
I
I
dpd
cmcd
cmcs
dps
CA
CD

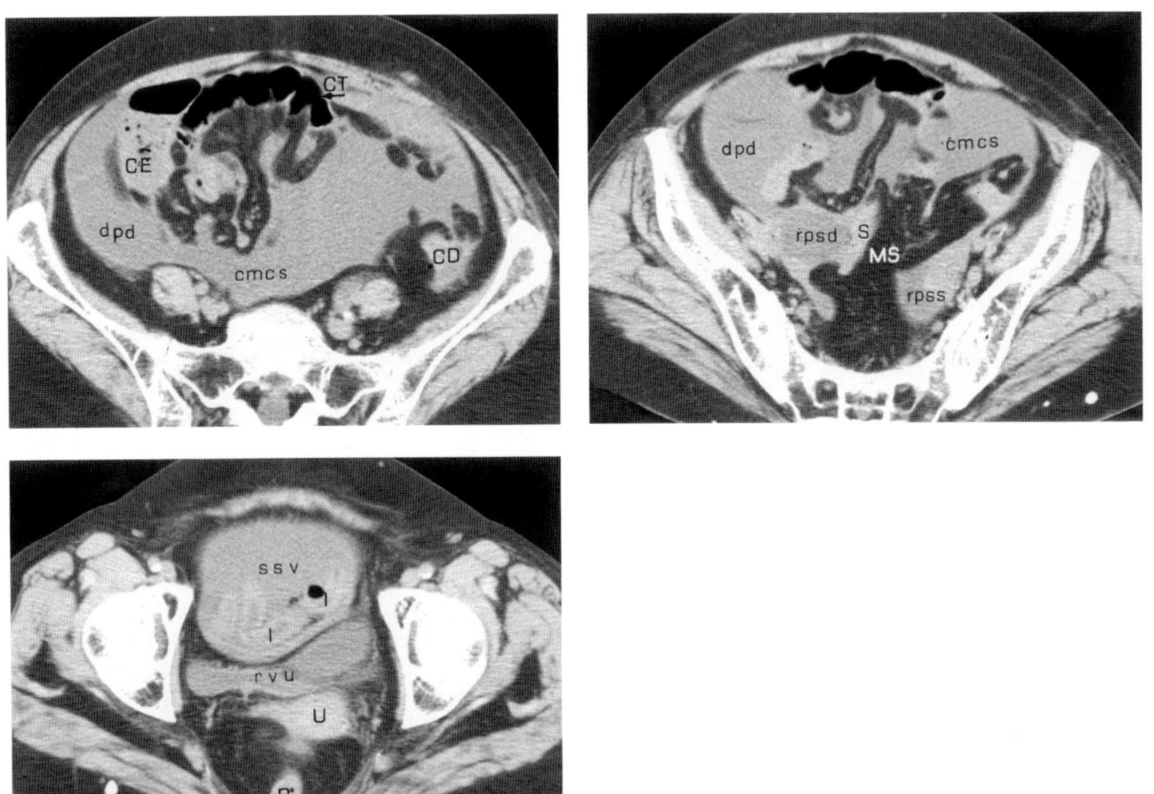

Fig. 4.20A–K. Ligaments and peritoneal cavity in the presence of a carcinomatous ascites. Axial sections from the diaphragm to the pelvis. **A** Right and left subphrenic spaces divided by the falciform ligament (*arrow*). The left subphrenic space and subhepatic recess are separated by the left lobe of the liver and by the left triangular ligament The latter can be followed from the left (where its diaphragmatic insertion is located) to the right [where it continues in the coronary ligament (*open triangles*)]. **B** Besides the abovementioned spaces and ligaments, we observe the perisplenic and gastrosplenic recesses and the insertion of the gastrohepatic ligament in the transverse fissure of the liver (*arrow*). **C–E** The right subhepatic space around the liver and the gallbladder is closed posteriorly by the parietal peritoneum, adherent to the anterior renal fascia, and medially by the lateral leaf of the hepatoduodenal ligament (*open arrowhead*) Inside this space, we recognize the portal trunk, the hepatic artery and the superior genu of the duodenum. Communication on the median line, under the falciform ligament (*triangles*), between the right and left subhepatic recesses. The gastrohepatic (*thin arrow*) and gastrosplenic (*open triangle*) ligaments and the recesses of the left subhepatic cavity are well recognizable Left recess of the lesser sac (*re*) among stomach, gastrosplenic, splenopancreatic and gastrohepatic ligaments. **F** The right subhepatic space continues without interruption in the underlying paracolic gutter, which is distented, displacing the ascending colon medially The transparency of the transverse mesocolon (limited at the front and the sides by the colic loops) shows a fan-like expansion on the median line On the left, the previsceral cavity pushes the omentum backward and medially The left inframesocolic cavity is visible behind the omentum. **G** Besides the cavities described above, the right inframesocolic cavity is beginning to be visible The mesentery separates the right and left inframesocolic cavities on the median line. **H** Maximal extension of the inframesocolic cavities. The mesentery is expanded on the right side, where the ileal vessels are easily recognizable. On the left, the omentum divides the inframesocolic from the previsceral cavity. **I** The left inframesocolic cavity and the right paracolic gutter communicate under the cecum and the last ileal loop. **J** Posteriorly and along the median line, the transparency of the sigmoid mesocolon separates the right and left parasigmoidal recesses. At the front and the sides, the inferior expansion of the right paracolic gutter and of the left inframesocolic cavity are observed. The right paracolic gutter directly communicates with the homolateral parasigmoidal recess. **K** Anteriorly, the supravesical space, where the ileal loops float; posteriorly, the vesicouterine recess

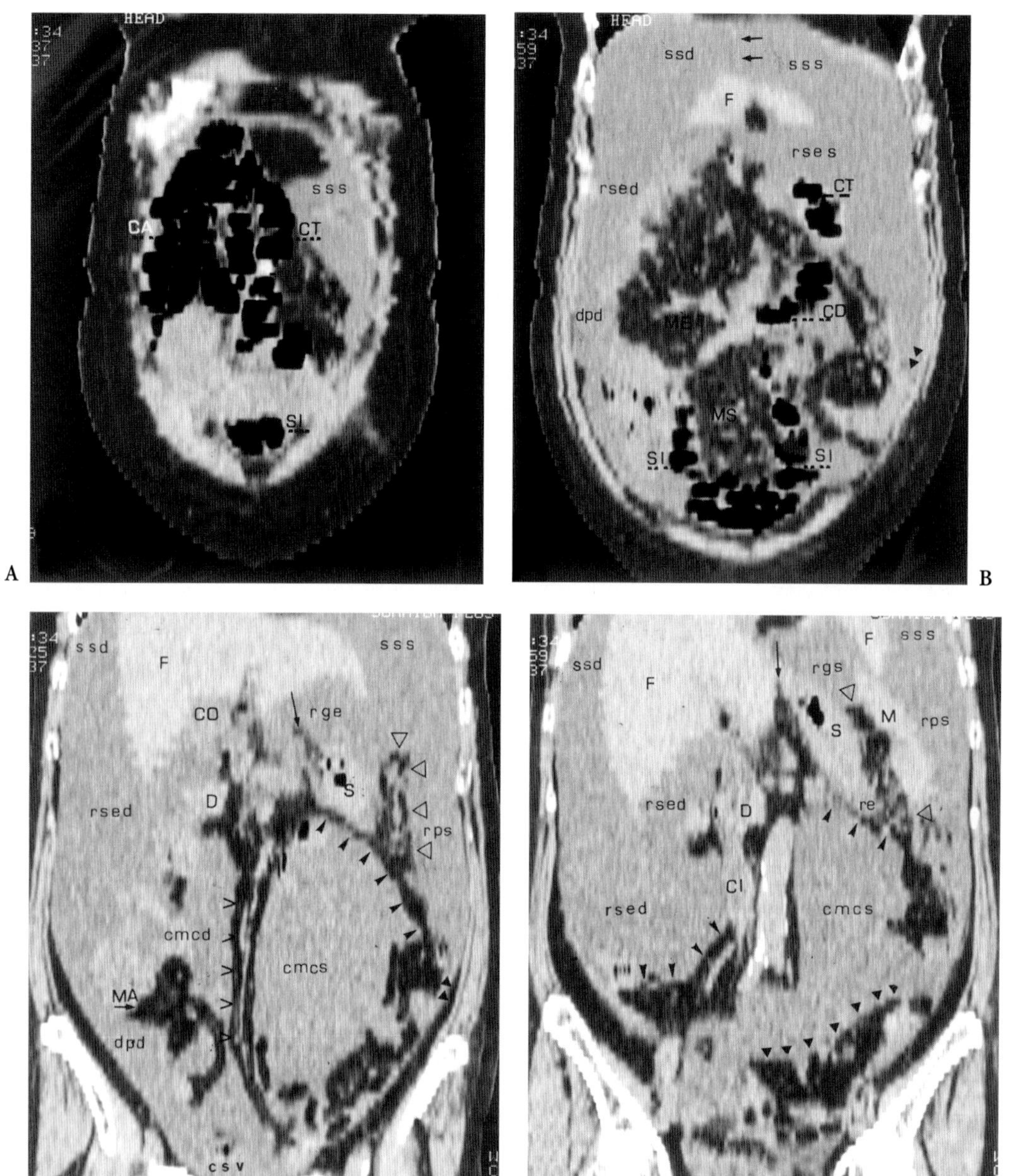

Fig. 4.21A–D. Peritoneal cavity and ligaments. Coronal reconstructions from the front backwards. **A** Colic and sigmoidal loops expanded by gas. The splenic flexure and the transverse colon are displaced forward on the right and downward by the liquid contained in the left subphrenic space. **B** Along the median line and from above downward, the falciform ligament (*thin arrows*), the left lobe of the liver, the mesentery, the sigmoid mesocolon and the sigmoid are visible. On the left paramedian line the transverse colon is recognizable; at the sides, the right and left subphrenic spaces are observed at a higher level and the right and left subhepatic spaces, at a lower level. The right subhepatic space extends downward in the homolateral paracolic gutter. On the left, the subhepatic space is closed below by the phrenicocolic ligament (*small triangles*). **C** On the right, from above downward the wide communication among the subphrenic space, the subhepatic recess, the paracolic sulcus, and the supravesical cavity are visible. On the left, the subphrenic space and the gastrohepatic and gastrosplenic recesses are recognizable; they are closed below by the transverse mesocolon (*arrowhead*) and by the phrenicocolic ligament (*triangles*) The gastrosplenic ligament (*empty triangles*) penetrates between the gastrohepatic and gastrosplenic recesses and continues downwards in the transverse mesocolon. The mesenteric root is located on the median line; within its transparency, the artery and a tract of the superior mesenteric vein separate the right from the left inframesocolic cavities. In turn, the ascending mesocolon (*arrow*) divides the right inframesocolic cavity from the homolateral paracolic gutter. **D** On the right, the subphrenic space and the subhepatic recess are visible. The latter is hyperexpanded by liquid and is pushing the transverse mesocolon (*arrowhead*) downward. On the left and at a high level, the subphrenic, gastrosplenic and perisplenic recesses are separated from the left inframesocolic cavity by the transverse mesocolon. Outside, this cavity is separated by the interposition of the descending mesocolon from the paracolic gutter, whereas at a lower level, it continues in the right parasigmoidal cavity above the sigmoid mesocolon (*triangles*), where the right paracolic gutter also converges The gastrohepatic ligament (long thin arrow) and the big abdominal vessels extend along the median line. The gastrosplenic ligament extends between stomach and spleen (*open triangles*) and joins the transverse mesocolon at a lower level

of the limiting mesentery may appear as a thin dense pericecal curved line.

The *ascending mesocolon* (Figs. 4.16–4.19, 4.21) is located on the medial posterior side of the ascending colon and of the cecum. Within the transparent shape it is seen as, it is possible to observe the right paracolic and the colic vessels, which extend in parallel and appear as small dots or sinuous lines.

The *descending mesocolon* (Figs. 4.16, 4.18, 4.19, 4.22) is located on the medial and posterior side of thedescending colon. Within its transparency, we can recognize the paracolic and left colic vessels extending in parallel, prevalently vertically and mostly with a punctiform aspect. However, it is sometimes possible to follow the left colic vessels from the paracolic branches to the lower mesenteric vessels in the same plane within the mesenteric and retroperitoneal thickness.

In the presence of effusions in the paracolic gutters and in the mesenteric colic cavities, the peritoneal position around ascending and descending colon and respective mesenteries is very obviously visible. These constitute a posterolateral inward curve that extends continuously from above downwards, discontinuing the linear posterior profile of the peritoneal cavity.

In order to distinguish the *sigmoid mesocolon* (Figs. 4.16–4.22, 4.37), two elements can be examined: sigmoid and sigmoidal vessels. The extension of this mesentery is related to the length and position of the sigmoid. If the sigmoid is short, it makes an arch that opens posteriorly between the left iliac fossa and the median line in front of the promontory. A long sigmoid occupies the width of the hypogastrium transversely and deeply, following an approximately S-shaped line, first extending forward up to where it makes contact with the anterior abdominal wall and then extending on the right side up to the iliac fossa, where it makes contact with the ascending cecum; finally, it takes a backward turn toward the median line and joins the rectum.

The sigmoid mesocolon appears as a transparent band of adipose tissue, varying in size in different subjects; on its sides, we can observe the double linear image of the peritoneum, i.e., its walls. Within the transparency of the mesentery, we observe the sigmoidal vessels extending from the lower mesenteric vessels as sinuous lines above sigmoid loops. In favorable conditions, the subdivisions of these vessels can be seen up to where they make contact with the visceral wall; they have a linear or Y-shaped aspect or look like dense punctiform 'rain,' according as whether they are arranged horizontally or craniocaudad.

4.1.3 Peritoneal Cavity

In normal conditions, the peritoneal cavity is not visible on CT, because of its virtual character; however, it becomes easily recognizable when it contains a certain amount of fluid. In this case, each single space can be clearly recognized and easily distinguished because of its site, its orientation and its position relative to organs, ligaments, mesenteries, and vascular structures.

In keeping with the subdivisions used to describe normal anatomy, we will examine the supra- and submesocolic and the pelvic regions separately, describing the CT aspects of the various spaces analytically.

Supramesocolic Cavity. The supramesocolic cavity, extending from the diaphragm and the transverse mesocolon, is divided by ligaments into the following spaces:

a) Right subphrenic space
b) Right subhepatic space
c) Left subphrenic space
d) Lesser sac

a) Right Subphrenic Space (Figs. 4.16–4.22). This space can be easily identified as an arcuate image between the liver and the diaphragm in the planes located immediately under the diaphragm; it is separated from the contralateral subphrenic space by the thin sagittal line connecting the anterior contour of the liver to the diaphragm on the right paramedian line, which corresponds to the falciform ligament. The inferoposterior limit of this space is constituted by a zone from which fluid is absent, corresponding to the upper leaf of the coronary ligament and to the retrohepatic bare area.

b) Right Subhepatic Space (Figs. 4.16–4.22). This space extends right round the lower pole of the liver and is made up of two recesses, anterior and posterior. The *anterior recess* communicates directly with the homolateral subphrenic space above and at the sides, whereas below it continues at the side with the right paracolic gutter.

The scanograms show the junction between the right subhepatic space and the paracolic gutter at the

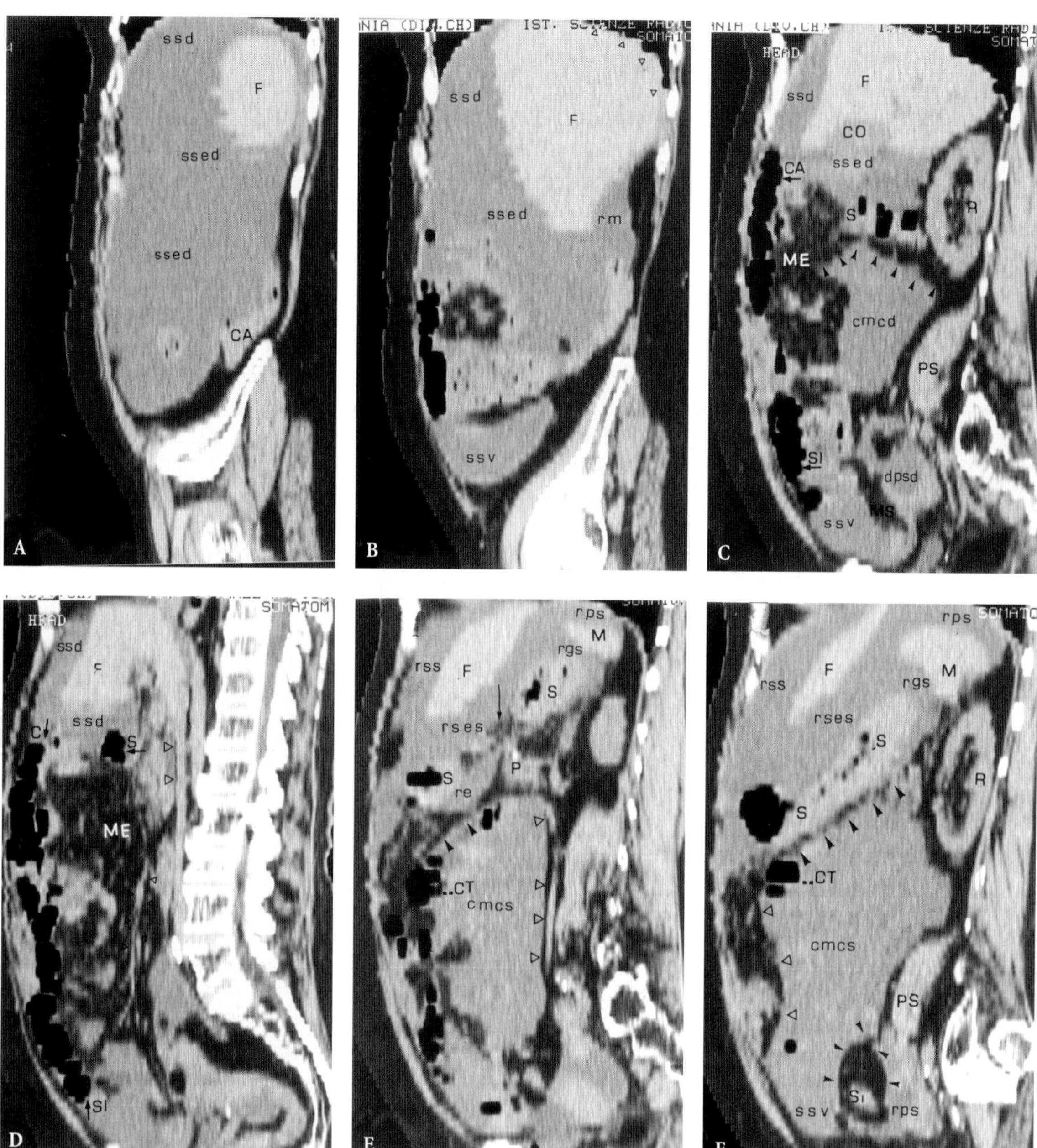

Fig. 4.22A–H. Ligaments and peritoneal cavity. Sagittal reconstructions from right to left. **A** Widely communicating right subphrenic and subhepatic spaces. **B** Right subphrenic and subhepatic spaces, with the posterior Morrison's recess; retrohepatic bare area (*open triangles*); supravesical space. **C** Right mediorenal plane At a high level, the right subphrenic and subhepatic spaces are separated from the homolateral inframesocolic cavity by the transverse mesocolon (*arrowhead*); at a low level, the supravesical space is separated from the right parasigmoidal gutter by the sigmoid mesocolon. **D** Caval plane: wide expansion of the mesentery crossed from above downwards by the superior mesenteric vessels (*open small triangles*). **E** Left paravertebral plane. At a high level, from the front backwards the subphrenic space, the left subhepatic recess, and the gastrosplenic and perisplenic recesses are observed. The lesser sac is limited above and anteriorly by the stomach and by the gastrohepatic ligament (*arrow*), posteriorly by the pancreas and below by the transverse mesocolon (*arrowhead*). The expansion of the left inframesocolic cavity is visible under the transverse mesocolon. In the adjacent retroperitoneal spaces, the inferior mesenteric vein (*open triangles*) for a long tract. **F** Left mediorenal plane Maximal expansion of the supra- and submesocolic cavities, which are separated by the transverse mesocolon (*arrowhead*) In anterior submesocolic planes, the transparency of the omentum (*open triangles*) extends vertically At a low level, the sigmoid mesocolon (*small arrowhead*) separates the supravesical space from the left parasigmoidal recess. (**G, H** see next page)

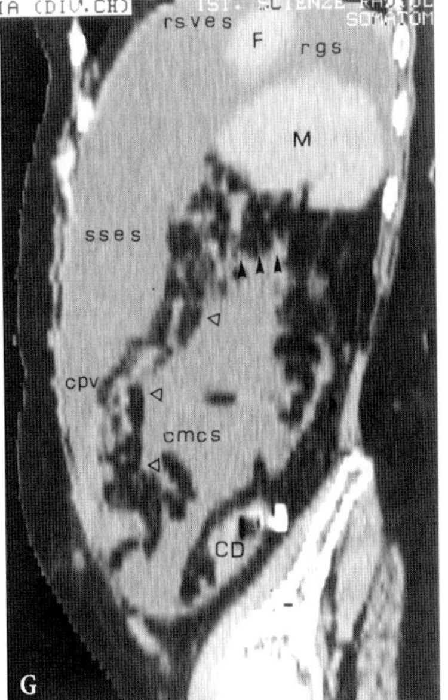

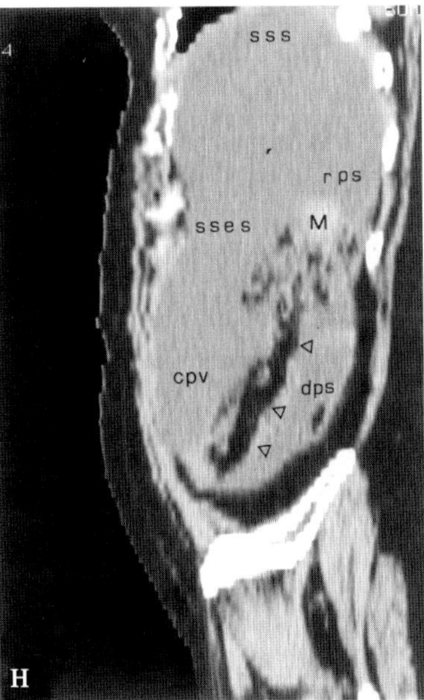

Fig. 4.22A–H. (Continued)
G Continuity of the left supramesocolic cavities with the previsceral cavity in front of the omentum (*open triangles*). **H** Left lateral plane. Continuation of the subphrenic space with the left subhepatic and perisplenic recesses and the previsceral cavity. The descending mesocolon (*open triangles*) separates the previsceral cavity from the left paracolic gutter

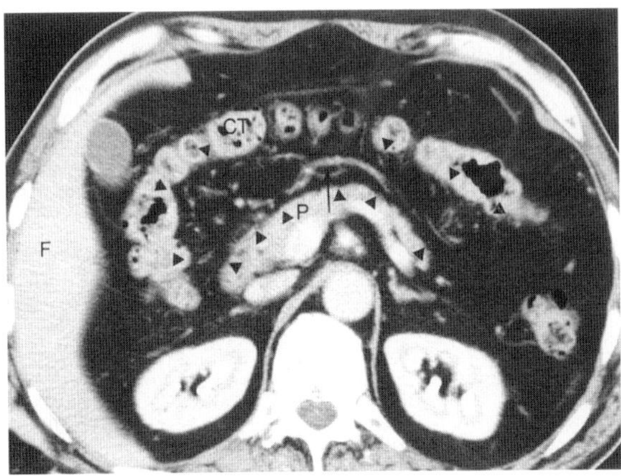

Fig. 4.23. The transverse mesocolon (*triangles*) is crossed by the middle colic vessels (*arrow*); it is located among the transverse colon extending as an arch in the anterior part of the abdomen, and the duodenum and pancreas posteriorly

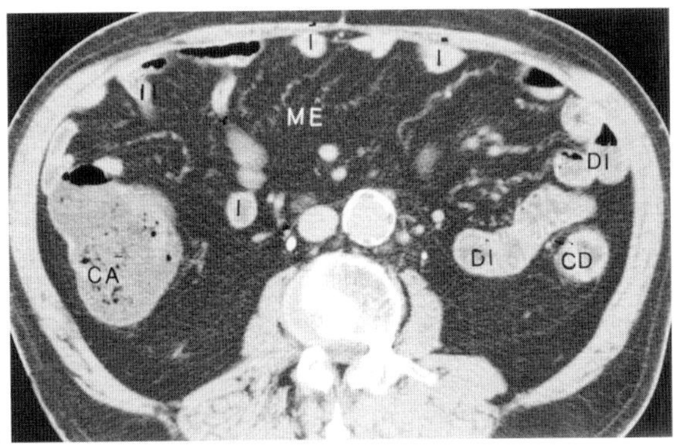

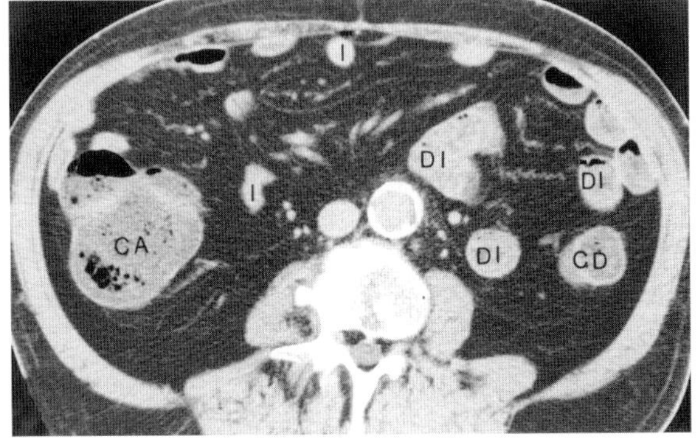

Fig. 4.24. A, B. The mesentery (*ME*) is crossed by the superior mesenteric vessels between the ascending and descending colon on the sides and is limited anteriorly by the jejunoileal loops. Posteriorly, it continues directly with the retroperitoneal adipose tissue

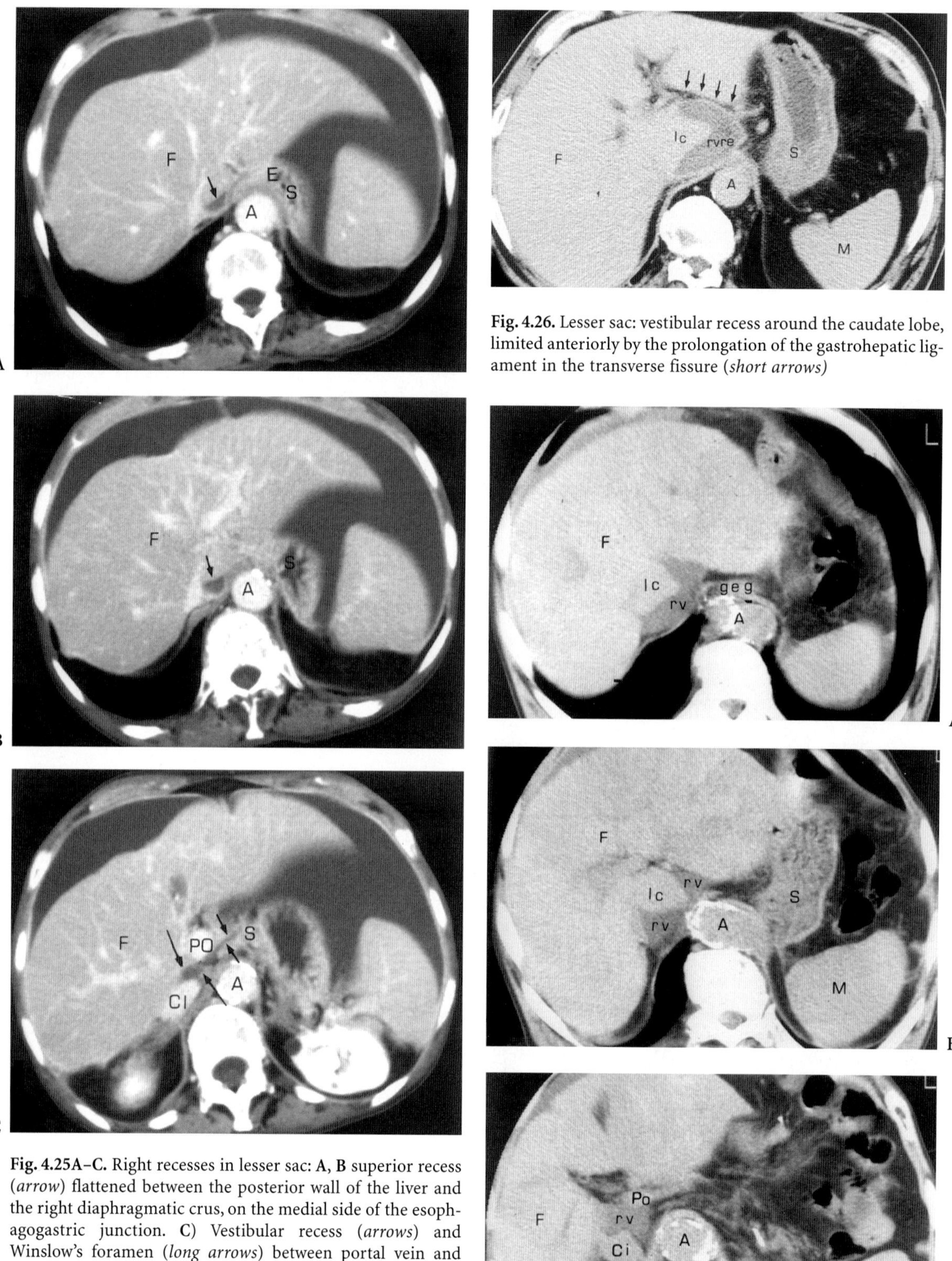

Fig. 4.25A–C. Right recesses in lesser sac: **A, B** superior recess (*arrow*) flattened between the posterior wall of the liver and the right diaphragmatic crus, on the medial side of the esophagogastric junction. **C**) Vestibular recess (*arrows*) and Winslow's foramen (*long arrows*) between portal vein and inferior vena cava

Fig. 4.26. Lesser sac: vestibular recess around the caudate lobe, limited anteriorly by the prolongation of the gastrohepatic ligament in the transverse fissure (*short arrows*)

Fig. 4.27A–C. Lesser sac: vestibular recess. **A, B** V-like arrangements around the caudate lobe. **C** Inferior and median expansion

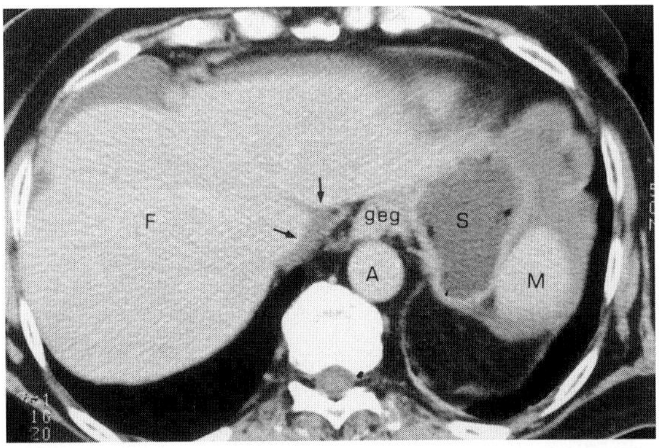

Fig. 4.28A–E. Right and left compartments of lesser sac. **A–C** Right compartment (*small arrows*): superior recess between liver and right diaphragmatic crus, **D** vestibular recess around the caudate lobe, and **E** Winslow's foramen between portal vein and vena cava. The left compartment (*long arrows*) is located behind the stomach, between the left gastric artery (*large long arrow*) medially, and the gastrosplenic ligament (*large arrows*) outside, in front of the cauda pancreatis and the splenic vessels (**D**). It extends up to the hilum of the spleen, constituting the splenic recess Below, it is closed by the inferior recess (**E**)

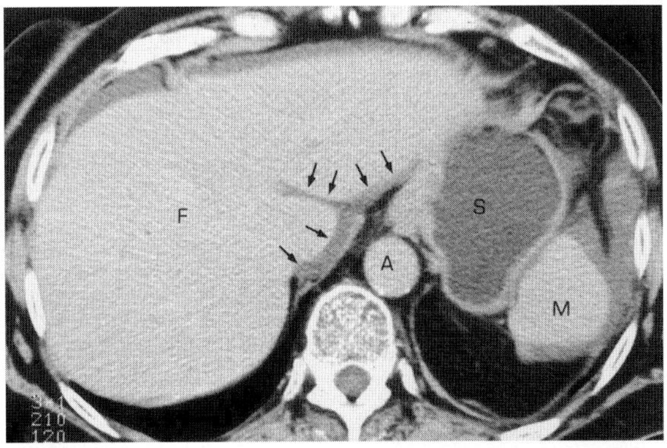

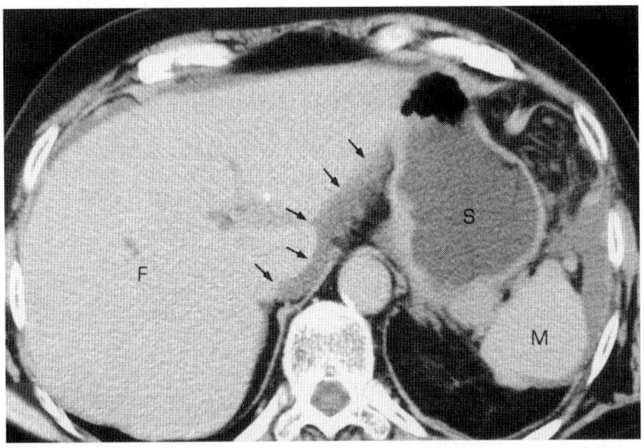

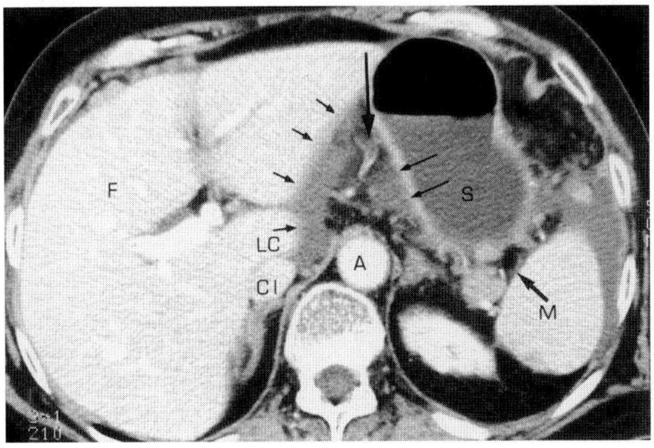

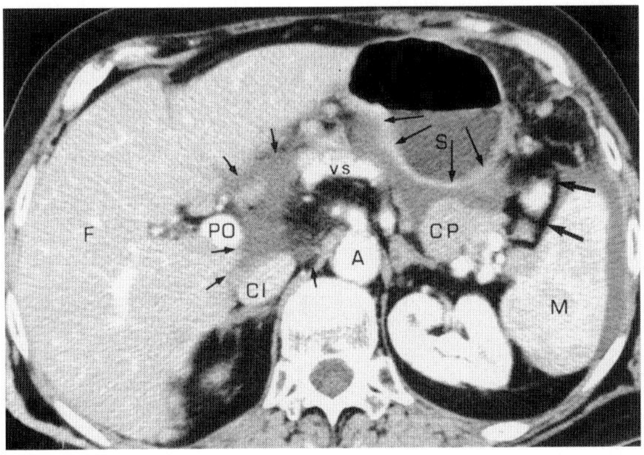

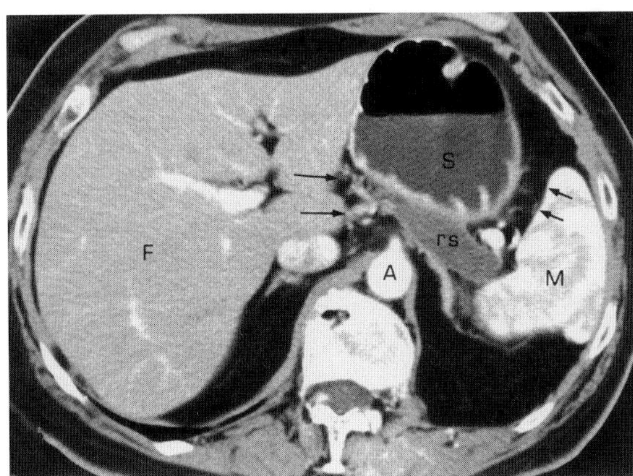

Fig. 4.29. Left compartment of lesser sac: superior and splenic expansion of the left compartment, extending transversely between the stomach and the diaphragmatic crus, limited on the right by the lesser omentum (*long arrows*), where the coronarostomachic artery is visible, and outside by the gastrosplenic ligament with the short gastric and left gastroepiploic vessels (*short arrows*)

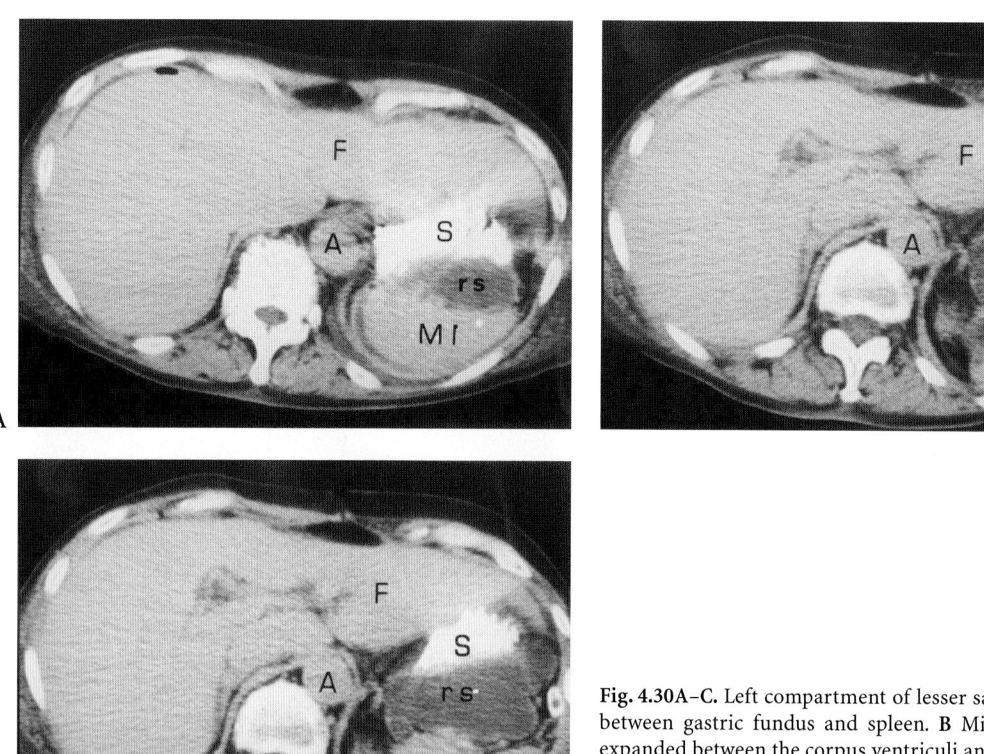

Fig. 4.30A–C. Left compartment of lesser sac. A Superior part between gastric fundus and spleen. B Middle part is more expanded between the corpus ventriculi and the spleen; it has a thin and well-designed peritoneal wall and is located between the coronarostomachic vessels medially and the gastrosplenic ligament laterally. C Inferior expansion between stomach, pancreas and inferior pole of the spleen

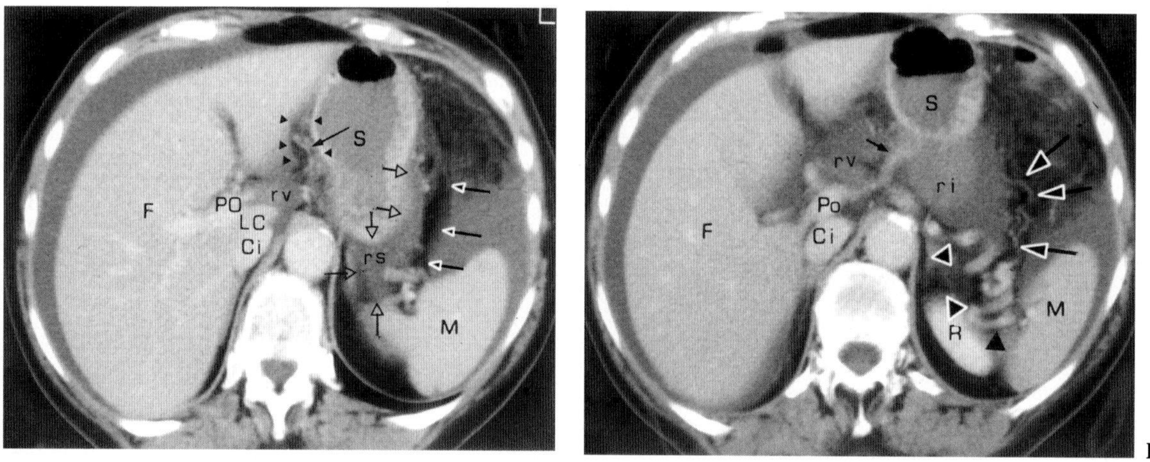

Fig. 4.31A, B. Right and left compartments of lesser sac. A Vestibular recess located around the caudate lobe. Left compartment, located behind and on the left side of the stomach between the gastrohepatic ligament (*small triangles*), coronarostomachic vessels (*long arrow*) medially and gastrosplenic ligament (*white arrows*), extending posteriorly in the splenic recess (*open arrow*) up to the proximities of the splenic hilum. B Right and left recesses separated by the trunk of the left gastric artery (*arrow*) Left inferior recess located among stomach, gastrosplenic ligament [with the left gastroepiploic vessels (*large white arrows*)] and splenopancreatic ligament [with the splenic vessels (*large white triangles*)]

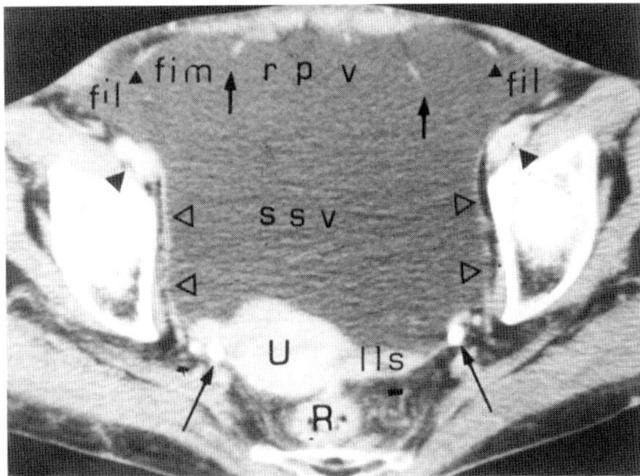

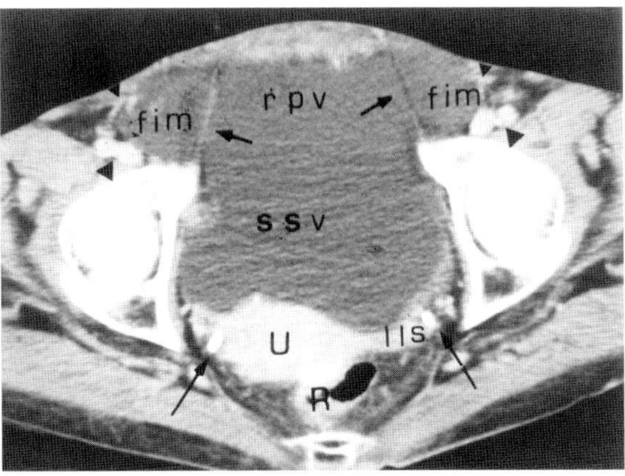

Fig. 4.32A, B. Pelvic cavities. Supravesical space (woman with an empty urinary bladder) limited and completely surrounded by the peritoneum lining the anterolateral pelvic wall, the broad and round ligaments (*empty triangles*) and the uterus. At the front and medially, there are depressions in the peritoneum at the sides made by the symmetrical incisures made by the lateral vesicoumbilical ligaments (*arrows*) and laterally by the inferior epigastric vessels (*small triangles*), which subdivide the supravesical space into the prevesical recess on the median line, medial inguinal fossae in an intermediate position, and lateral inguinal fossae on the outside. Between the peritoneum and the lateral pelvic wall, the transparency of the extraperitoneal fat [with the external iliac vessels ahead (*triangles*)] and the ureters (*long arrows*) behind the broad ligaments

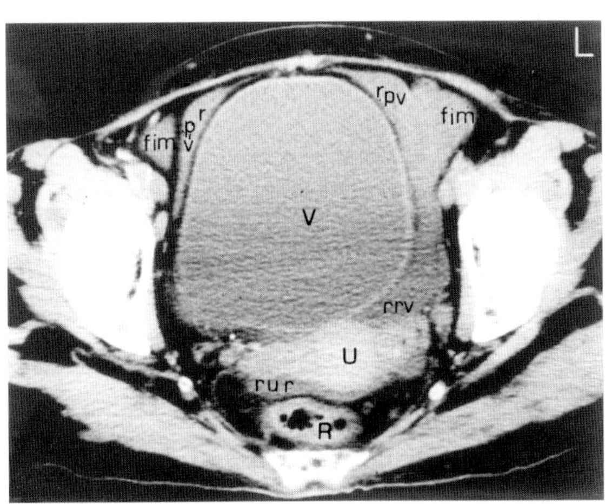

Fig. 4.33. Anterior compartment of pelvic cavities: woman with a full urinary bladder. Prevesical recess and medial inguinal fossae separated by the umbilicovesical ligaments. On the left side, the medial inguinal fossae are continued in the retrovesical recess. The uterorectal recess is visible behind the uterus. The transparencies of the umbilicovesical fascia and of the perivesical space show a semicircular form between the urinary bladder and the paravesical recesses. The punctiform image of the median umbilicovesical ligament stands out in the anterior part of this space

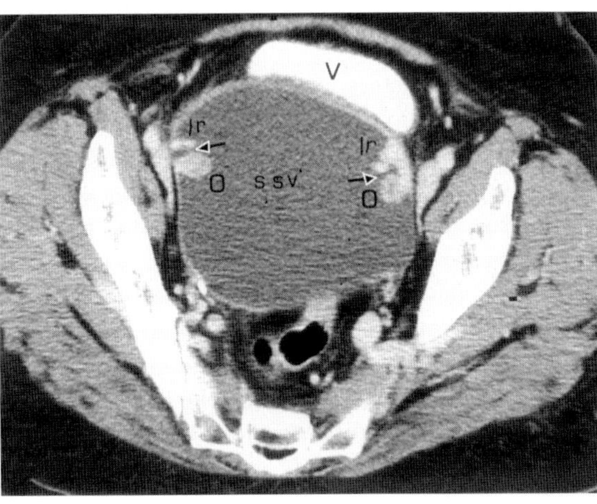

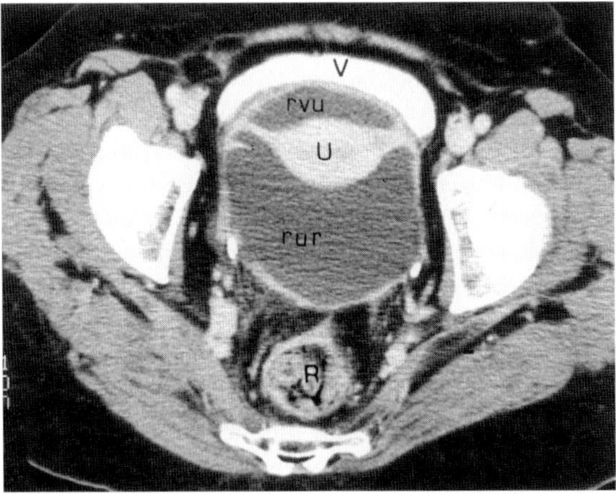

Fig. 4.34A, B. Retrovesical and uterorectal recesses (pouch of Douglas). **A** Superior pelvic planes: unique retrovesical cavity between urinary bladder and rectum; the ovaries and the round ligaments stand out on the sides of this cavity. Between these latter structures, we observe the ovarian fossae (*arrows*). **B** Middle pelvic plane The space is divided by the peritoneal fold surrounding the uterus and the broad ligaments in the vesicouterine and uterorectal recesses

side as the restricted point between the two cavities; in coronal reconstructions it can be recognized by its hourglass-like appearance (Fig. 4.18). When the fluid in the anterior recess is abundant, it also spreads around the gallbladder, with the exception of the infundibulum, the cystic duct and the small mesentery joining the gallbladder to the inferior hepatis face.

The *posterior recess (Morrison's)* extends from the coronary ligament to the transverse mesocolon behind the posterior wall of the liver and in front of the upper pole of the right kidney; it is closed below by the transverse mesocolon. It is the lowest portion of the supramesocolic cavity, where minimal ascitic effusions tend to collect.

Medially, the right subhepatic space continues with the contralateral subhepatic space and communicates with the omental bursa through the foramen of Winslow. This latter structure appears (Figs. 4.16, 4.25, 4.28) as a thin layer between the inferior vena cava and the portal vein, medial to the caudate lobe.

c) Left Subphrenic Space (Figs. 4.16–4.22). This space extends from the left hemidiaphragm to the transverse mesocolon and is divided into the *supra-* and *subhepatic, gastrolienal, perisplenic* and *splenopancreatic recesses.* Each of these recesses is recognizable from its position relative to the liver, stomach, and spleen and the falciform, phrenogastric, gastrohepatic, gastrocolic, gastrosplenic and splenopancreatic ligaments. However, when there is abundant fluid in the left subphrenic peritoneal cavity, a single wide cavity develops, in which no individual recesses can be distinguished.

The *left suprahepatic* (or *anterior*) *recess* can be distinguished in the upper planes immediately under the diaphragm, above and in front of the left hepatic lobe; it is limited on the right by the falciform ligament and continues downward and forward in the underlying gastrohepatic (medially) and gastrosplenic (laterally) recesses. This communication is more easily visible when the peritoneal effusions are particularly abundant.

The *left* (or *gastrohepatic*) *subhepatic* (or *posterior*) *recess* extends from the stomach and the posterior border of the left hepatic lobe up to the flexure of the venous ligament, in front of the gastrohepatic ligament and, at a lower level, up to the gastrocolic ligament. At the side, it continues into the gastrosplenic recess and medially and below with the contralateral homologous recess, since the limitation of the falciform ligament is missing at this level.

At a lower level, the transverse mesocolon and the left phrenicocolic ligament separate this space from the submesocolic cavities. Occasionally, it is possible to observe its continuation with the previsceral cavity anteriorly; however, this cavity always expands with difficulty.

The *gastrosplenic recess* must be distinguished specifically between the greater curvature of the stomach and the anteromedial border of the spleen; it is limited medially by the transparent homonymous ligament and laterally by the parietal peritoneum lining the left abdominal wall. When the effusion is abundant, it is possible to observe its continuation forward with the supra- and subhepatic recesses and, posteriorly, with the perisplenic space. The downward expansion of this space is stopped by the transverse mesocolon and by the left phrenicocolic ligament.

The *perisplenic recess*, because of its perisplenic position, is easy to pinpoint, even when only a small amount of fluid is present. In the reflection point of the splenopancreatic ligament on the posteromedial border of the spleen, it is sometimes possible to observe a short tract where the fluid does not penetrate: the *splenic bare area.*

The *splenopancreatic recess* extends from the splenic vessels and the posterior visceral leaf of the homonymous ligament, which functions as its anterior wall, to the parietal peritoneum, which limits the recess posteriorly. Medially, it is closed by the reflection of the posterior peritoneal leaf of the splenopancreatic ligament toward the left posterior parietal peritoneum and represents a median evagination of the perisplenic recess. The fluid collection diffuses as a thin linear transverse fluid behind the vessels of the splenic hilum and the corpus and cauda pancreatis, in front of the anterior pararenal fascia; it may sometimes simulate a retroperitoneal collection.

It is possible to recognize the fluid's position correctly by careful evaluation of the images of the over- and underlying planes: a retroperitoneal collection tends to spread outward, downward and backward in the lateroconal spaces, or medially, around the pancreas and the splenic vessels; in contrast, a collection into the splenopancreatic space rarely reaches the median line, and laterally it continues in the perisplenic cavity without expanding downward, because it is limited by the transverse mesocolon.

Very occasionally, the splenopancreatic recess extends medially behind the pancreas to enclose the organ completely, which then becomes intraperitoneal. This condition occurs when the embryonal peritoneal recess persists, whereas it is usually obliterated in adulthood, because the dorsal mesogastrium blends with the posterior parietal peritoneum (RUBENSTEIN et al. 1983).

The splenopancreatic recess can be distinguished from the lower cavity of the lesser sac by its position, which is further in the posterior direction than those of the splenic vessels and the corpus and cauda of the pancreas. In fact, collections in the omental bursa are located in front of these structures.

When the supramesocolic cavities are expanded by an abundant effusion, the fluid pushes the transverse mesocolon, the colic flexures and the phrenicocolic ligament downward and penetrates at the sides, simulating collections in the paracolic gutter. However, careful examination of the scan sequence shows the lower prolongations of the supramesocolic cavities, because they assume a funnel-like shape on both sides outside the colic loops; this aspect is more easily visible in coronal reconstructions (Figs. 4.20, 4.23).

d) Lesser sac (omental bursa) (Figs. 4.16, 4.17, 4.20, 4.22, 4.25–4.31). The lesser sac appears as a transverse band extending on the median plane from the stomach to the gastrohepatic and hepatoduodenal ligaments in the front and to the pancreas behind, and from the caudate lobe on the right to the gastrosplenic ligament on the left. In the center, the left gastric artery, which divides the bursa into right and left compartments, is always easily recognized.

In the *right compartment*, we distinguish two recesses: vestibular and superior. The *vestibular recess* (Figs. 4.25–4.28, 4.31) extends transversely from the caudate lobe on the right to the coronarostomachic artery incisure on the median line. It has a characteristic orientation around the caudate lobe, which extends in a cuneiform shape toward this recess, and occupies a site peculiar to itself, posterior to the portal trunk, the hepatic artery and the hepatocholedochus.

The *superior recess* (Figs. 4.25, 4.28) appears as a thin fluid between the posteromedian border of the liver and the crus of the right hemidiaphragm; at its highest level, it spreads up to the esophagogastric junction on the right side.

The *left compartment* (Figs. 4.28–4.31) must be searched for between the coronarostomachic artery incisure and its surrounding adipose tissue on the median line and the transparent sagittal band of the gastrosplenic ligament on the left side, where it is in close contact with the posterior wall of the stomach. It assumes different aspects according to the amount of fluid that it contains; therefore, it may appear as a thin transverse band of retrogastric fluid or as a wide cavity displacing the stomach forward and the gastrosplenic ligament laterally, extending downward in front of the pancreas up to the mesocolon and the transverse colon. It penetrates posteriorly on the left side up to the splenic hilum, constituting the *lienal recess* medial to the hilum (Figs. 4.28, 4.30, 4.31).

When the gastrocolic ligament and the transverse mesocolon fail to merge, the omental bursa may continue downward and forward between the omental leaves, extending up to the pelvis under the colon and the transverse mesocolon, but this is rare.

In contrast with those on the right, the recesses on the left are widely expansible, and they can therefore contain significant amounts of fluid.

e) Submesocolic Cavity. The submesocolic cavity develops between the transverse mesocolon and the pelvis and between the anterior abdominal wall and the anterior pararenal space. Its anterior profile is sharp and arcuate, and it extends parallel to the abdominal wall, whereas the posterior profile is sinuous and is furrowed by the incisures of the ascending and descending mesocolon at the sides and by the wide prominence of the mesentery centrally.

Both mesentery and ascending or descending mesocolon subdivide the submesocolic cavity into paracolic gutters and right and left inframesocolic cavities.

The *paracolic gutters* (Figs. 4.16–4.21) extend at the sides from the ascending or descending colon to the abdominal wall. Both gutters continue in the pelvis, on the right or on the left of the sigmoid and its mesentery, respectively. Their widths and depths depend on the arrangement of the peritoneum around the colon. They may be just slightly defined when the peritoneum limits only the anterior colic wall, or wide and deep when the peritoneum constitutes a real mesentery surrounding the colon on the sides.

The *right paracolic gutter* continues upward with the anterior recess of the subhepatic space, outside the transverse mesocolon; a slight stricture indicates the crossing point between the two cavities.

The *left paracolic gutter* is closed above by the phrenicocolic ligament, which is easily visible owing to its transversal position.

An analytical description of the various aspects of the right and left inframesocolic cavities is not possible; in fact, these cavities are extremely variable, depending on the amount of the mesenteric adipose tissue and on the positions of the ileal loops

(Figs. 4.16–4.22). Usually, they are located on both sides of the mesentery, but they may sometimes have an anterior position between the mesentery and the omentum or a posterior one with the peritoneum adhering to the anterior renal fascia; or, finally, they may penetrate medially between the small intestine loops, with wide polymorphism. At the sides, they continue with their respective right and left paracolic gutters, from which they are separated by the prominence of the ascending and descending colon and their respective mesenteries.

The mesenteric root (Figs. 4.18, 4.21), extending obliquely from left to right and from above downward, divides the right inframesocolic cavity from the left one. This makes the right inframesocolic cavity wider in its upper part than the contralateral one. The right inframesocolic cavity is closed below by the mesenteries surrounding the last ileal loop and the cecum. The lower part of the left inframesocolic cavity continues into the right paracolic gutter; it then continues together within the pelvic cavity on the right side of the sigmoid (Fig. 4.21). However, the continuation of the submesocolic into the pelvic cavity is conditioned by the length and disposition of the sigmoid. In fact, this bowel segment can be short, protruding only slightly toward the abdominal cavity and located on the median line and on the left side; in contrast, it can extend forward up to the proximities of the anterior abdominal wall and, on the right side, to the iliac fossa, forming a long sinuous loop. In the first case, the parasigmoidal recesses are wide and make it possible for the submesocolic cavities to establish a wide communication with the underlying pelvic cavities, both in front and laterally (Fig. 4.18). In contrast, a long and prominent sigmoid reduces the peritoneal cavity anteriorly to a virtual space, forming a diaphragm-like structure between the submesocolic and pelvic cavities and limiting their communications to the sides only: on the right, between the inframesocolic recesses and the right paracolic gutter with the anterior pelvic cavities; on the left, between the paracolic gutter and the pararectal recesses (Figs. 4.17, 4.20, 4.21).

The *previsceral cavity* (Figs. 4.17, 4.19, 4.20, 4.22) is visible only in the presence of an abundant peritoneal effusion, such as fluid interposed between the anterior abdominal wall and the omentum. The cavity is wider at the sides, where it continues into the inframesocolic cavities and the paracolic gutter, whereas it is very thin and often not visible on the median line. However, its aspect changes according to the extension and position of the omentum; when this is short and thin, the perivisceral and the inframesocolic cavities together make up a single compartment; in contrast, when the omentum is wide and thick, the two cavities are clearly separated. Inferiorly, the previsceral cavity extends into the anterior pelvic compartment at different levels, according to the omental length.

f) Pelvic Cavity. The CT aspect varies according to sex, vesical and rectal distension, and prominence of vasculo-ligamentary structures. The pelvic cavity is divided into two compartments: anterior and posterior, subdivided transversely by the uterus and the broad ligaments in women and by Denonvilliers' fascia in men.

The *anterior compartment* (Figs. 4.16–20, 4.22, 4.32–34, 4.36, 4.37) is subdivided into the supravesical space, pre- and retrovesical recesses, and medial and lateral fossae inguinales.

The *supravesical space* (Figs. 4.16–4.20, 4.22, 4.32, 4.37) occupies the upper part of the pelvic cavity and expands only when the remaining parts of the compartment are filled with fluid.The limiting anterior parietal peritoneum shows the symmetrical inflexions of the lateral umbilicovesical ligaments and the inferior epigastric vessels on the sides and the urachus on the median line. Inside this space, there are the ileal loops, the cecum and the sigmoid rectum, which extends outward from behind, constituting the *right* and *left parasigmoid recesses* (Figs. 4.17, 4.20–4.22).

The underlying recesses and fossae extend in front and on the sides of the urinary bladder; they are more visible when the bladder is full and are subdivided into:

a) Prevesical recess
b) Fossae inguinales mediales
c) Fossae inguinales laterales
d) Retrovesical recess (vesicouterine or vesicovesicular)

a) The *prevesical recess* (Figs. 4.19, 4.32, 4.33) has a semicircular shape and is located in front of the urinary bladder; it is limited outside by the umbilicovesical ligaments and is more easily visible when the urinary bladder is full.

b) The *fossae inguinales mediales* (Figs. 4.32, 4.33) are located symmetrically on the sides of the prevesical recess between the inflexions of the umbilicovesical ligaments inside and the inferior epigastric vessels outside.

c) The *fossae inguinales laterales* (Figs. 4.32, 4.33) have a triangular shape and are poorly expansible; they are located outside the fossae inguinales medi-

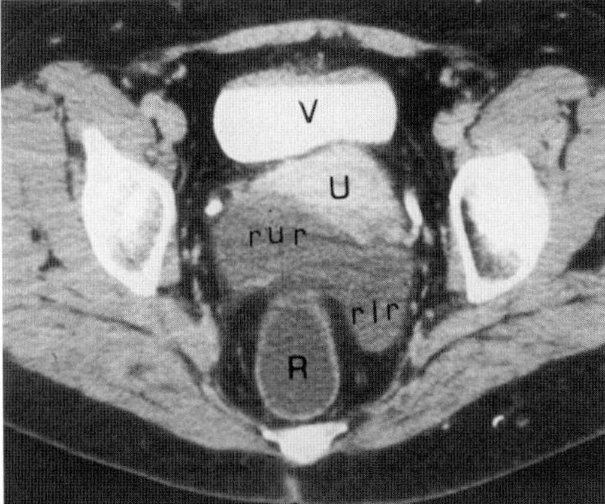

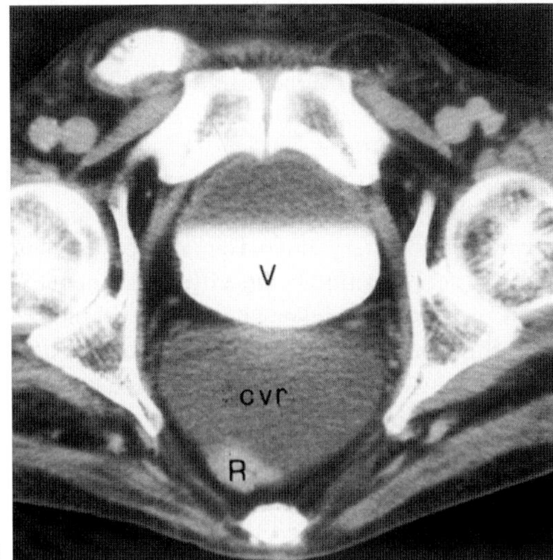

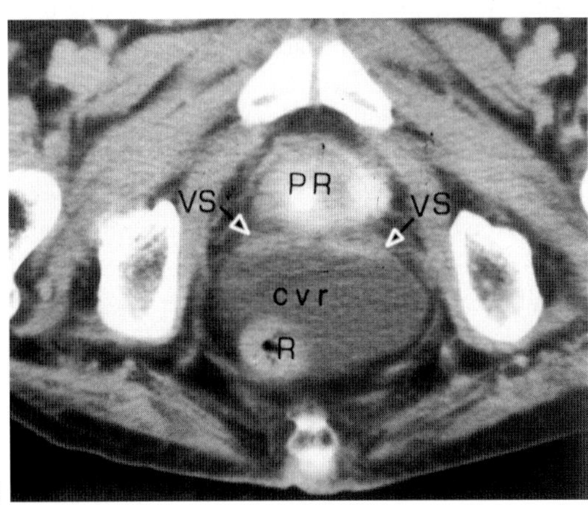

Fig. 4.35A–C. Pelvic cavity: posterior compartments. **A** In women. Uterorectal (pouch of Douglas) and left laterorectal recesses limited by the peritoneum, that surrounds the posterior wall of the uterus and the broad ligaments anteriorly and the anterolateral facies of the rectum posteriorly. **B, C** In men. **B** Middle pelvic plane. Unique cavity between urinary bladder and rectum. **C** Inferior pelvic plane. Blind pouch between fascia of Denonvillier, seminal vesicles, prostate and rectum; it extends on the sides of these structures, forming the pararectal recesses

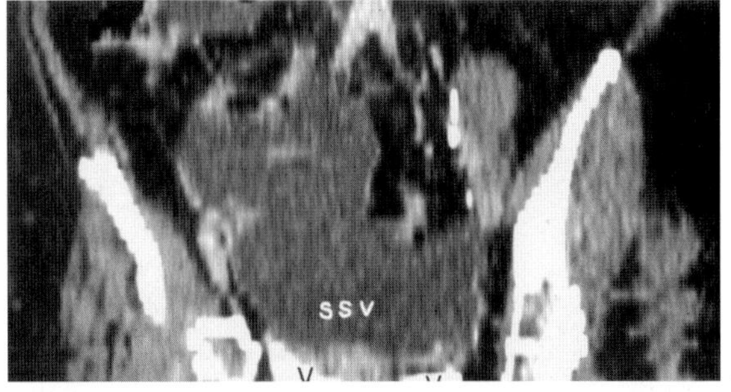

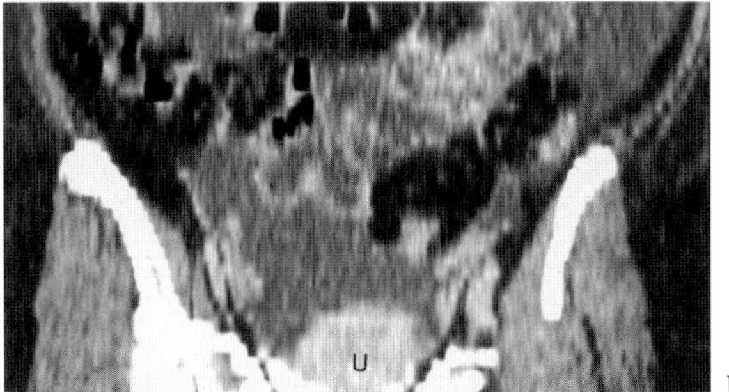

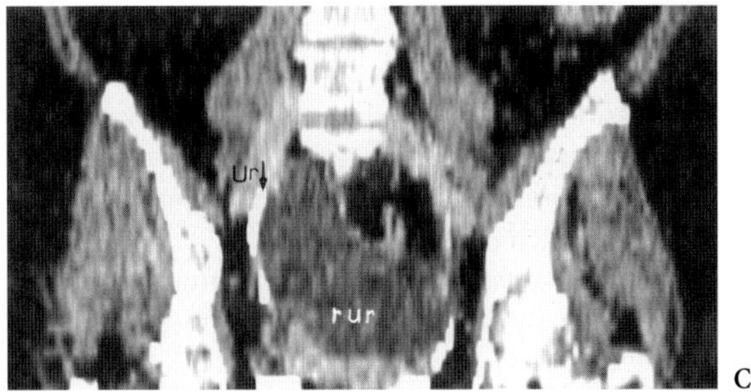

Fig. 4.36A–C. Pelvic cavity. Coronal reconstructions (woman). **A** Anterior plane: supravesical space limited by the peritoneum on the sides. **B** Middle plane (uterine): the pelvic cavity extends above and to the sides of the uterus. **C** Posterior plane: uterorectal recesses limited by the peritoneum on the sides Outside, we recognize the extraperitoneal space, where the ureters extend

ales and the inferior epigastric vessels, in front of the external iliac vessels, in the site where these vessels enter the femoral canal.

d) The *retrovesical recess* is located transversely behind the urinary bladder, between the latter and the uterus and the broad ligaments (*vesicouterine recess*) in women (Figs. 4.20, 4.34, 4.37) and Denonvillers' fascia in men.

The *posterior compartment* (Figs. 4.16, 4.17, 4.19, 4.34–4.37) is not divided further, and it is located medially among organs, genital structures and the rectum; it expands laterally up to the proximities of the pelvic wall, from which it is separated by a thin interstice of adipose tissue. In men, it may be a sin-

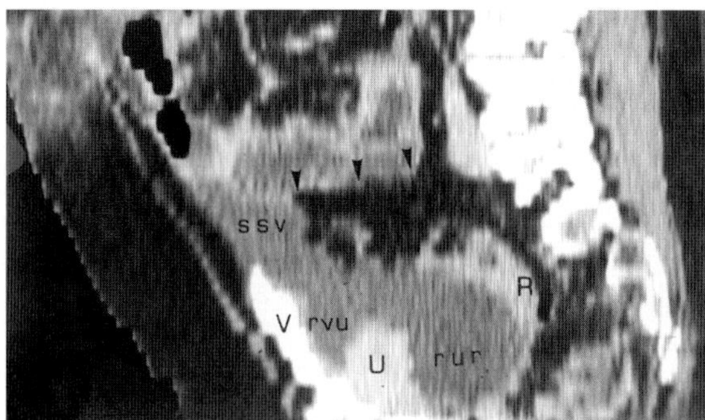

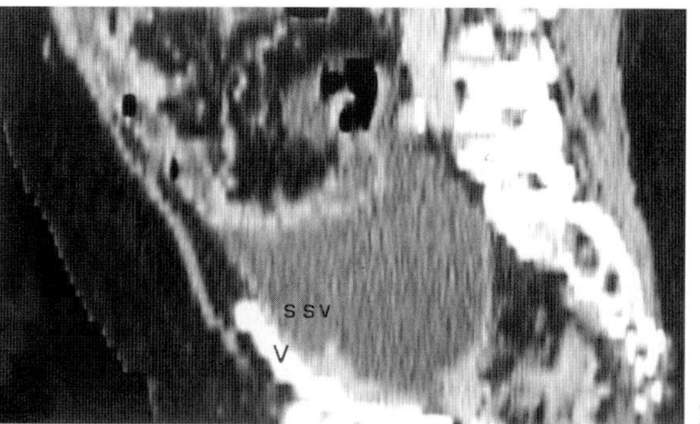

Fig. 4.37A, B. Pelvic cavity. Sagittal reconstructions (woman). **A** Middle plane: vesicouterine and uterorectal recesses divided by the dome-shaped prominence of the uterus, limited at a high level by the sigmoid mesocolonal transparency (*arrowhead*). Anteriorly and above, the two recesses continue in the supravesical space. The urinary bladder is compressed against the anterior abdominal wall by the fluid collection. Anteriorly, the transparency of the adipose tissue contained in the prevesical space (extending from the umbilical region downwards to the front of the urinary bladder) stands out between the dense line of the musculus rectus abdominis and the profile of the parietal peritoneum and of the umbilicovesical fascia. **B** Right paramedian plane: wide unique supravesical space extending from the anterior to the posterior wall of the abdomen

gle space incorporating the retrovesical and the anterior recesses. Posteriorly, it may penetrate one or both the sides of the rectum, forming the *pararectal recesses* (Figs. 4.16, 4.35), or may have only a slight impression made by the rectum itself.

Minimal amounts of fluid collect preferentially at the lowest point of this compartment (*pouch of Douglas*) (Figs. 4.16, 4.34–4.37).

When a conspicuous amount of fluid collects in this compartment, it is possible to observe further subdivisions in secondary recesses, such as the anterolateral and posteromedial recesses produced by the uterosacral (in women) and vesiculosacral (in men) ligaments.

In women, it is possible to identify two additional small recesses in the anterolateral corners: the ovarian fossae (Fig. 4.34), which are limited anteriorly by the broad and round ligaments and, posteriorly, by the ovaries and by the peritoneum surrounding these organs and the meso-ovary.

4.2 Arteries and Veins

The high-tech nature of the CT instruments is making it possible to detect the arteries and veins on images from the origin up to their thinnest branches with increasing frequency.

The CT representation of vessels depends on their pathway: if it is craniocaudal or caudocranial, the vascular image seen is round or punctiform; in contrast, when vessels extend along the transversal section plane, they show a tubular or linear appearance.

Frequently, an artery and a vein are coupled and appear as a double round or linear image, where the artery is usually the smaller and denser vessel and the vein the larger vessel with lower density.

The images of some vessels are constant in appearance and position; other vessels that empty into mobile viscera, such as the alimentary canal, show variable images according to the position and distension of the bowel. In the former condition it is not difficult to recognize the vessels, whereas in the latter situation doubts may persist. (For example, in longilineal subjects with gastroptosis and low transverse colon there might be some doubt about whether a transverse linear image under the stomach should be interpreted as a gastroepiploic vessel or a middle colic vessel.) However, following the retrograde extension toward its original trunk usually makes it possible to achieve clear identification of the vessel.

Great care is needed in the study of the arteries, because it is not rare for them to vary in origin, extension, subdivision and distribution.

4.2.1 Arteries

The arteries emptying into organs and peritoneal or subperitoneal structures originate from the *abdominal aorta*, which is located in a retroperitoneal position, in front and just to the left of the vertebral spine, and the CT shows a circular aspect.

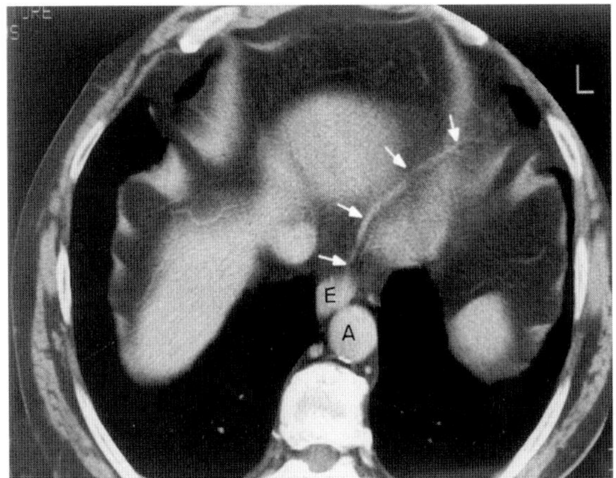

A

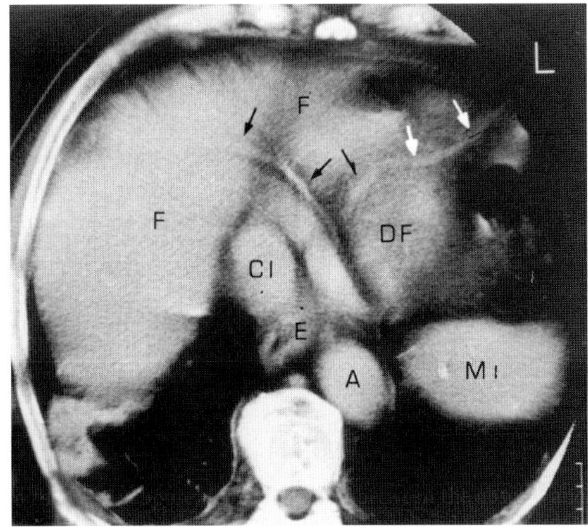

B

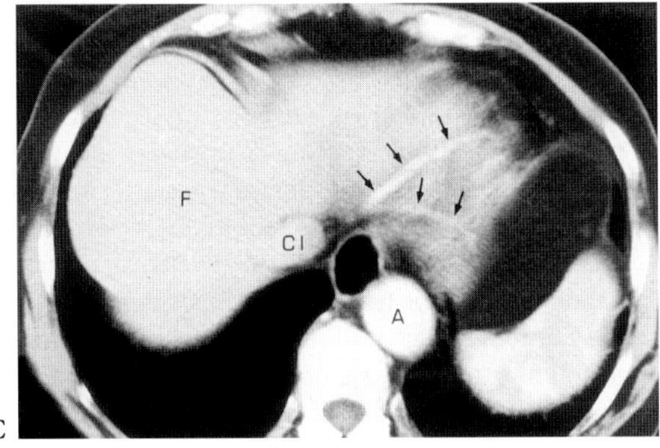

C

Fig. 4.38A–C. Diaphragmatic vessels. **A** Left inferior diaphragmatic artery (arrows) extending from the aorta forward and below the diaphragm, between the transverse fascia and the peritoneum. **B** Right and left inferior diaphragmatic veins (*arrows*) extending to the inferior vena cava. **C** Left diaphragmatic veins (*arrows*) converging in the inferior vena cava

4.2.1.1
Visceral Arteries

The *inferior diaphragmatic arteries* (Fig. 4.38) can be identied within the adipose tissue interposed between the diaphragmatic cupola and the superior parietal peritoneum. It is possible to follow their linear pathway from behind forward on the median line and to distinguish their opening as an arch on the sides under the hemicupolae.

4.2.1.1.1
Celiac Trunk

The celiac trunk (Figs. 4.39, 4.47, 4.49, 4.51, 4.68) is constantly visible in a single plane or in two contiguous planes for its horizontal extension from behind forward and above the pancreas. It leaves the anterior wall of the abdominal aorta in the point where the diaphragmatic crura subdivide and extend on its sides. It has a linear or slightly arcuate aspect, a horizontal length of 0.8–2 cm, and a caliber ranging between 6 and 8 mm. In young subjects it has a mainly rectilinear extension, whereas with aging it tends to become slightly curvy and to increase in caliber. Extending forward, it opens as a Y or a T or withan appearance reminiscent of a seagull with open wings, continuing with the hepatic artery on the right and with the splenic artery on the left. In front of the division in the celiac trunk, it is possible to observe the round image of the left gastric artery, extending upward up to the lesser curvature of the stomach at the level of the cardias, where it leans forward, following the lesser curvature.

There are many variations in the origin, disposition and subdivision of the celiac trunk. The most common are: the isolated origin of one or more branches directly from the aorta (Figs. 4.43, 4.44), or the common origin with the superior mesenteric artery (Fig. 4.42).

a) The *left gastric* or *coronarostomachic artery* (Figs. 4.12, 4.13, 4.15, 4.39, 4.40, 4.47, 4.51) must be searched for in its initial tract as a round image extending from the celiac trunk upward in front of the aorta and the diaphragmatic crura up to the level of the cardias. Here, it veers forward, downward and toward the right side, extending along the internal border of the lesser curvature of the stomach, which it follows along a sinuous track with a tubular aspect up to the proximity of the pylorus.

b) The *hepatic artery* (Figs. 4.14, 4.39–4.44, 4.47, 4.51) commonly originates from the celiac trunk; because of its tortuous and oblique path, it cannot be easily followed along its total length and must be studied by examining various contiguous layers. In the first tract, it extends obliquely toward the right side and slightly forward; in one or more planes, it shows a rectilinear aspect up to the vicinity of the liver. From that point on, it shows a punctiform aspect extending vertically upwards into the hepatoduodenal ligament up to the hepatic hilum.

In the first tract, it overtakes the splenic vein from behind toward the front next to the splenomesenteric confluent and the head of the pancreas. In its ascending tract and in the hepatic transversal fissure it is located in front of the portal trunk on the right side of the choledochus and has a linear (Figs. 4.12, 4.14) or a punctiform appearance.

It is not rare to find a variation represented by the origin of the hepatic artery from the superior mesenteric artery (Fig. 4.42). This variation is recognizable not only by its origin, but especially by the extension of the horizontal tract of the artery behind rather than in front of the portal trunk. Analogously, also the origin of the sole right branch from the superior mesenteric artery may be recognized by its retrocaval path, whereas the left branch may appear as a thin ramification extending horizontally from the left gastric artery to the right toward the hepatic hilum (Fig. 4.41).

A further possibility is the separation of the right and left branches before crossing the splenic vein; the right branch extends between the portal trunk and the inferior vena cava, whereas the left one extends along the usual path of the hepatic artery (Fig. 4.40).

Favorable conditions may also allow recognition of the secondary branches of the hepatic artery, such as the right (or pyloric) gastric artery, the gastroduodenal artery and its continuation in the superior pancreatoduodenal arteries, the right gastroepiploic artery and, occasionally, the cystic artery.

- The *right* (or *pyloric*) *gastric artery* (Figs. 4.39, 4.47) is recognizable in the first tract from its punctiform aspect and its position between the trunk of the hepatic artery and the pylorus; afterwards, it has a linear and sinuous path along the lesser curvature of the gastric antrum and continues toward the left side with the left gastric branch coming downwards from the cardias.
- The *gastroduodenal artery* (Figs. 4.42, 4.47, 4.48) appears as a small hyperdense punctiform image because of its vertical path, which extends downwards; it is located between the pancreatic head medially and the superior duodenal genu laterally; generally, this branch of the hepatic artery is the most visible and may also show some of its secondary ramifications:
- The *superior pancreatoduodenal artery* (Fig. 4.42, 4.48), which represents the downward continuation of the gastroduodenal artery, is divided into two branches, anterior and posterior. These ramifications also have a punctiform aspect and extensions: the former on the right side of the pancreatic head (between this structure and the duodenal second portion and inferior genu), the latter behind the head of the pancreas and the choledochus. Sometimes, the posterior branch appears as a thin sinuous line extending inside.
- The *right gastroepiploic artery* (Figs. 4.12, 4.40, 4.46, 4.47) is located in an anterior plane compared with the pancreatoduodenal artery and has a punctiform aspect in its initial tract; afterwards, it is linear and arcuate along the greater curvature of the gastric antrum. The artery extension may be followed on the left up to the inosculation with the homonymous contralateral artery. According to the position of the stomach, it may be located under or in front of the bowel and sometimes above.
- The *cystic artery* (Figs. 4.40, 4.45) originates from the common hepatic artery next to the longitudinal hepatic fissure and extends forward through a linear path that is parallel to the median border of the gallbladder.

c) The *splenic artery* (Figs. 4.39, 4.43, 4.44, 4.47, 4.49–4.51) is recognizable by its sinuous extension in different planes. Its initial tract is the left branch of the celiac trunk; it has a tubular aspect and extends horizontally for 3–6 cm. The aspect of the intermediate tract is characterized by multiple close dots; it is located on the sides of the homonymous vein. The terminal tract subdivides at the splenic hilum into two branches; it then gives origin to four branches that extend transversely. When the stomach is full, it tends to exend in a unique horizontal plane and presents an arcuate aspect with the anterior cavity (Fig. 4.50).

It is frequently possible to observe its main collateral branches, which originate from the proximy of the splenic hilum, the short gastric arteries and the left gastroepiploic artery.

- The *short gastric arteries* (Figs. 4.12, 4.13) extend from their origin to the upper part of the gastrosplenic ligament, between the fundus ventriculi and the spleen. Mostly they have a punctiform

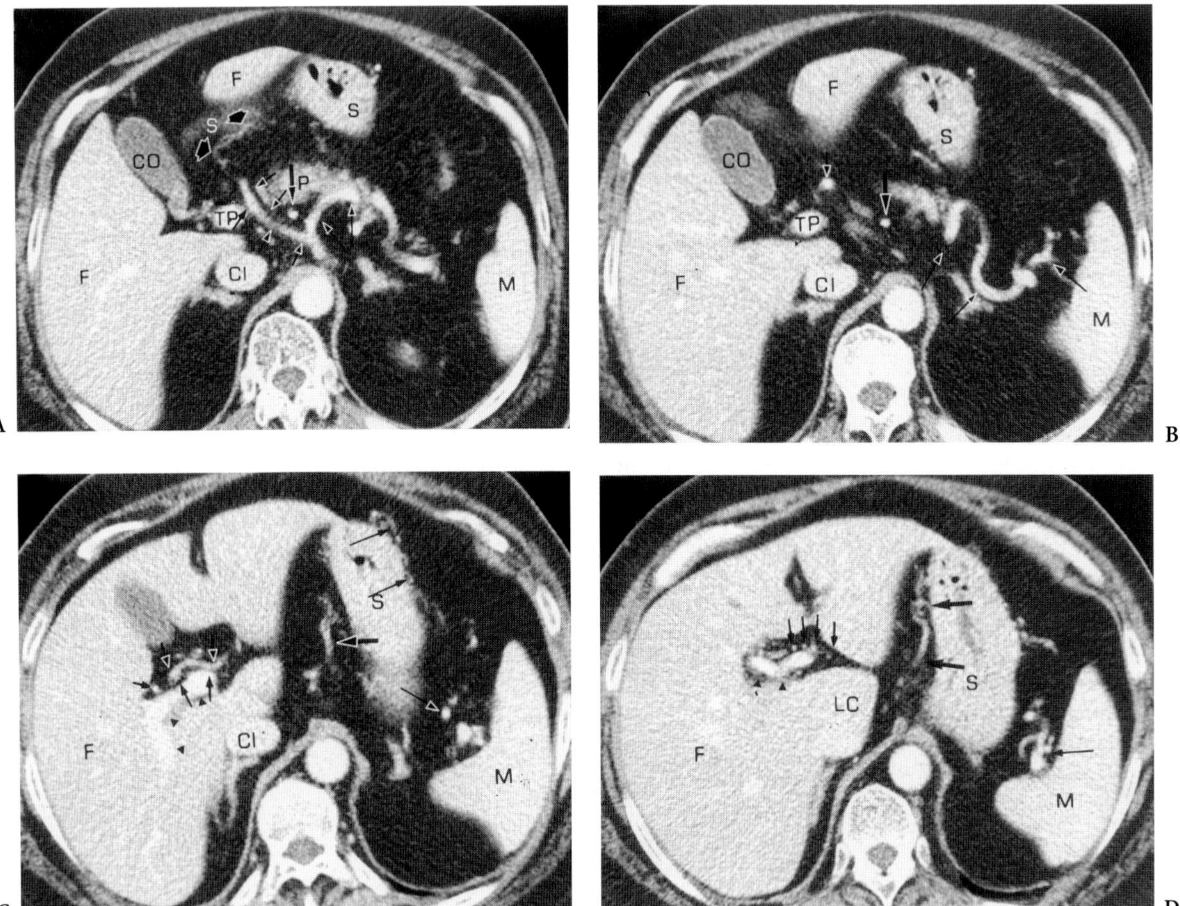

Fig. 4.39A–D. Supramesocolic arteries. Sequence of scans from below upward. **A** Celiac trunk with its three branches: common hepatic artery (*arrows*) extending to the right, splenic artery (*long arrows*) toward the left side and left gastric artery (*thick arrow*) upward. The pyloric branch (right gastric artery) (*stubby arrow*) originates from the hepatic artery. **B** Punctiform images of the common hepatic (*arrow*) and left gastric (*thick arrow*) arteries extending upwards Sinuous aspect of the splenic artery (*long arrows*). **C** On the median white line, the left gastric artery (*thick arrow*) located in the gastrohepatic ligament. The hepatic artery (*short arrows*) follows a slightly sinuous path and is located within the transverse fissure of the liver, in front of the right branch of the portal vein (*triangles*). The punctiform hyperdense images of its secondary branches for the left and the right lobes are located in the front and inside the hepatic artery The sinuosity of the left gastroepiploic artery (*long arrows*) can be followed along the greater curvature of the stomach. **D** The left gastric artery on the median line. Deep in the transversal fissure of the liver, at the sides of the left branch of the portal vein (*triangles*), hyperdense punctiform arterial branches for the left lobe anteriorly and for the caudate lobe posteriorly. At the level of the splenic hilum, the left gastroepiploic vessels (*long arrow*) within the gastrosplenic ligament

appearance, because of their predominantly ascending path.

- The *left gastroepiploic artery* (Figs. 4.12, 4.39, 4.51) extends along the greater curvature of the stomach, and its position is therefore closely related to that of the stomach and varies according to the subject's habitus and the height at which the transverse colon and its mesentery are sited. In the initial tract, after the origin of the splenic artery, the vessel's appearance is round because of the ascending extension toward the high part of the greater curvature of the corpus ventriculi in the gastrosplenic ligament. On rare occasions only, it may appear as a sinuous strand, which extends forward with a slight medial direction. After reaching the greater curvature of the stomach, between fundus and corpus ventriculi, it appears as a sinuous and slightly arcuate line extending from left to right along the greater curvature of the stomach in the gastrocolic ligament, up to the junction with the homonymous right artery.

  In brachytypical subjects, whose stomach is in a high position, the gastroepiploic artery extends in front of the stomach, between the bowel and the anterior abdominal wall, whereas in longitypical subjects, whose bowel is long and extends down-

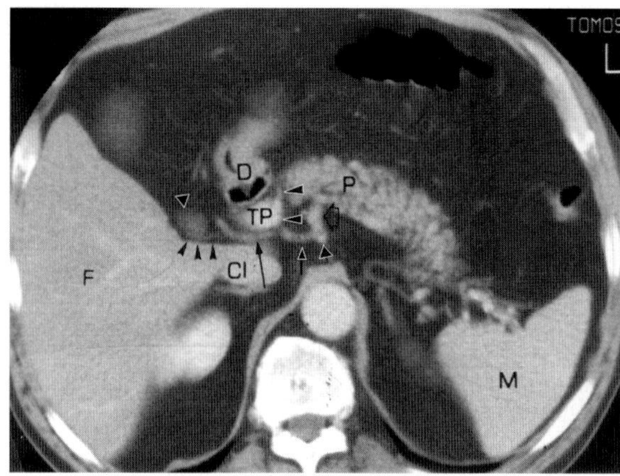

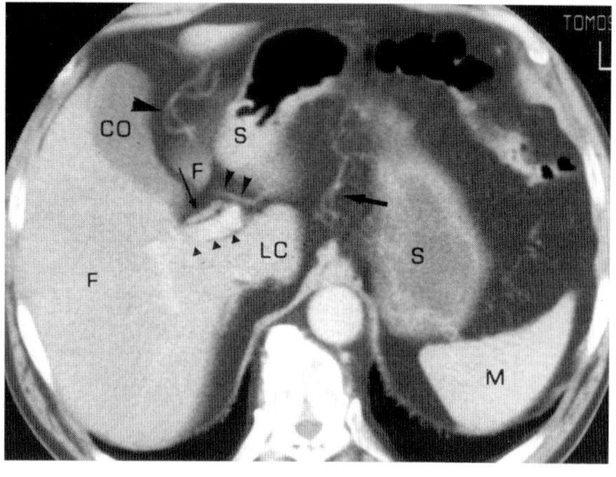

Fig. 4.40A, B. Supramesocolic arteries: anatomical variants. **A** The hepatic artery (*small arrow*) subdivides precociously. The left branch (*large arrowhead*) extends in front of the portal trunk, whereas the right branch (*long thin arrow*) passes between the portal trunk and the inferior vena cava. The cystic artery (*small arrowhead*) originates from the latter branch and extends outside toward the cholecystic infundibulum (*triangle*). The punctiform left gastric artery (*short arrow*) extends upward; the splenic artery (*open thick arrow*) extends toward the left. **B** Plane 2 cm higher than in **A**. The left gastric artery (*thick arrow*) on the median line within the gastrohepatic ligament extending along the lesser curvature of the stomach. At the level of the hepatic hilum, in the upper part of the hepatoduodenal ligament, the right (*long arrow*) and the left (*arrowhead*) hepatic arteries are sited in front of the portal vein (*small triangles*). The right gastroepiploic vessels are located within the gastrocolic ligament, near the greater curvature of the gastric antrum (*large arrowhead*)

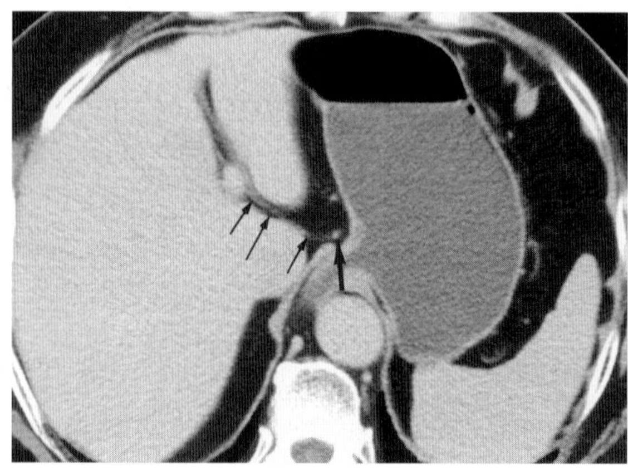

Fig. 4.41. Supramesocolic arteries: anatomical variants. Left branch of the hepatic artery (*thin arrows*) coming from the coronarostomachic artery (*thick arrow*)

ward, the vessel is located below the stomach.

The *epiploic* or *omental vessels* originate from the convexity of the arches of the right and left gastroepiploic arteries (Fig. 4.13) and their number varies in different subjects. Because of their vertical disposition, they always present a punctiform aspect in the transparency of the greater omentum, behind the anterior abdominal wall, and extend along a single line or are grouped, according to the position or extension of the omentum.

4.2.1.1.2
Superior Mesenteric Artery

The superior mesenteric artery (Figs. 4.15, 4.21, 4.22, 4.47, 4.52, 4.53, 4.68, 4.69, 4.72, 4.73) is visible, when conditions are favorable, along its total path, from the origin up to terminal ramifications. The trunk of the vessel has a diameter ranging between 0.8 and 2 cm and originates from the aortic anterior wall just under the celiac trunk, with a spur-like aspect. After its origin, it immediately veers downward, behind the pancreatic isthmus; thereafter, it crosses in front of the third duodenal portion and comes up by the side of the homonymous vein. Afterwards, it extends vertically within the adipose areolar tissue of the mesenteric root, coupled with the homonymous vein, with a round aspect. Around the perivascular adipose areolar tissue, it is possible to observe a thin circular lamella separating vessels from mesenteric adipose tissue (Fig. 4.52). Sometimes there is also a

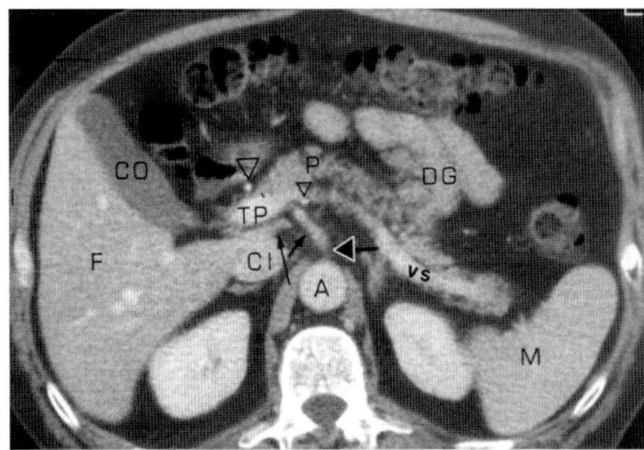

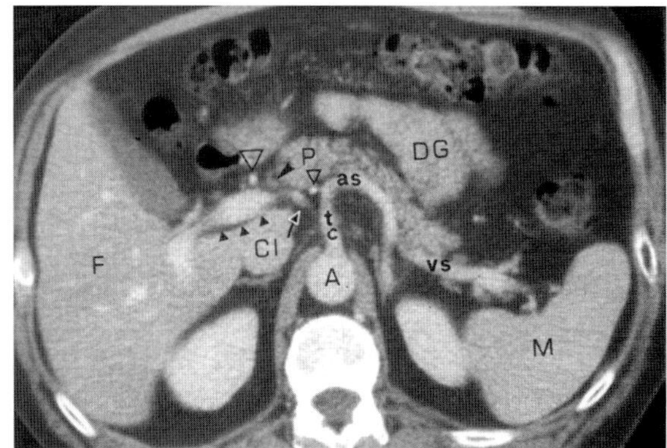

Fig. 4.42A, B. Supramesocolic arteries: anatomical variants. The hepatic artery (*short arrow*) originates from the superior mesenteric artery (*thick arrow*) and extends upwards and on the right. At the level of the portal trunk, it subdivides into a right branch (*long arrow*), passing between the portal vein and the vena cava, and a left branch extending in front of the portal vein (**B**) (*arrowhead*). In addition, the gastroduodenal (*large open triangle*) and posterior pancreatoduodenal (*small open triangle*) arteries are recognizable

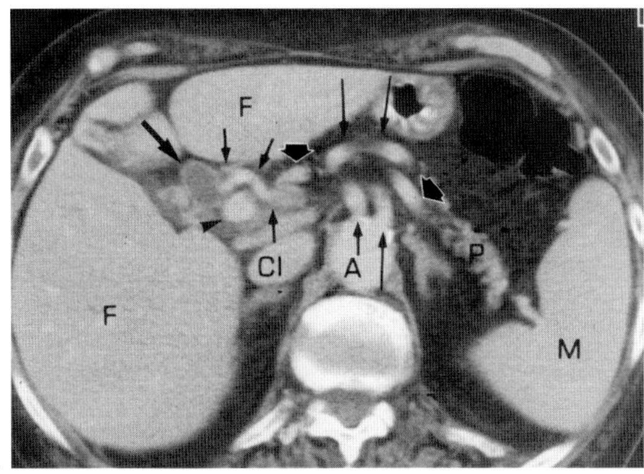

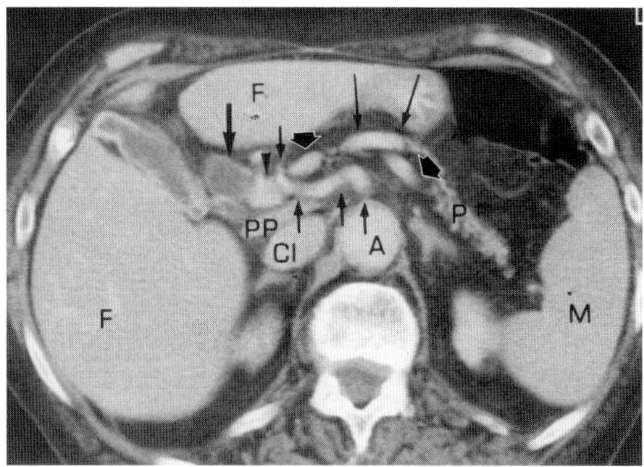

Fig. 4.43A, B. Supramesocolic arteries: anatomical variants. Separate origins of the hepatic (*arrows*) and splenic (*long arrows*) arteries from the aorta (**A**). The hepatic artery veers to the right (**B**) and extends in front of the portal trunk (*arrowhead*) and the dilated choledochus (*long thick arrow*). The papillary process of the caudate lobe penetrates transversely between the portal vein and the vena cava. Splenic vein is also shown (*stubby arrow*)

slight difference in density between the adipose tissue surrounding the mesenteric vessels and the subperitoneal fat outside the fascia (Fig. 4.52).

Besides the superior mesenteric artery trunk, its collateral branches are often visible at various levels.

The *inferior pancreatoduodenal artery* (Figs. 4.47, 4.48, 4.53, 4.56, 4.57) is the first branch originating from the superior mesenteric artery in the point where it leans forward to overtake the duodenum. Its image is punctiform according to its ascending path, and initially it is located behind the superior mesenteric artery, by which it is separated anteriorly from the inferior pancreato-duodenal vein.

In an upper plane, behind the pancreas, the two inferior pancreato-duodenal vessels come closer together. Further branches of the artery are recognizable behind the pancreatic head and the corpus pancreatis, where the artery maintains a punctiform aspect whereas the vein flattens. At this level, it is difficult to distinguish the superior from the inferior pancreatoduodenal vessels and, often, the veins from the arteries, these vessels are followed in subsequent planes from below upward and vice versa.

Just after the origin of the inferior pancreatoduodenal artery from the anterior wall of the superior mesenteric artery, the middle colic artery comes out (Figs. 4.13, 4.23, 4.53, 4.57), extending forward in the transparenct transverse mesocolon in the planes located between pancreas and transverse colon. This artery, which is mostly linear and slightly arcuate,

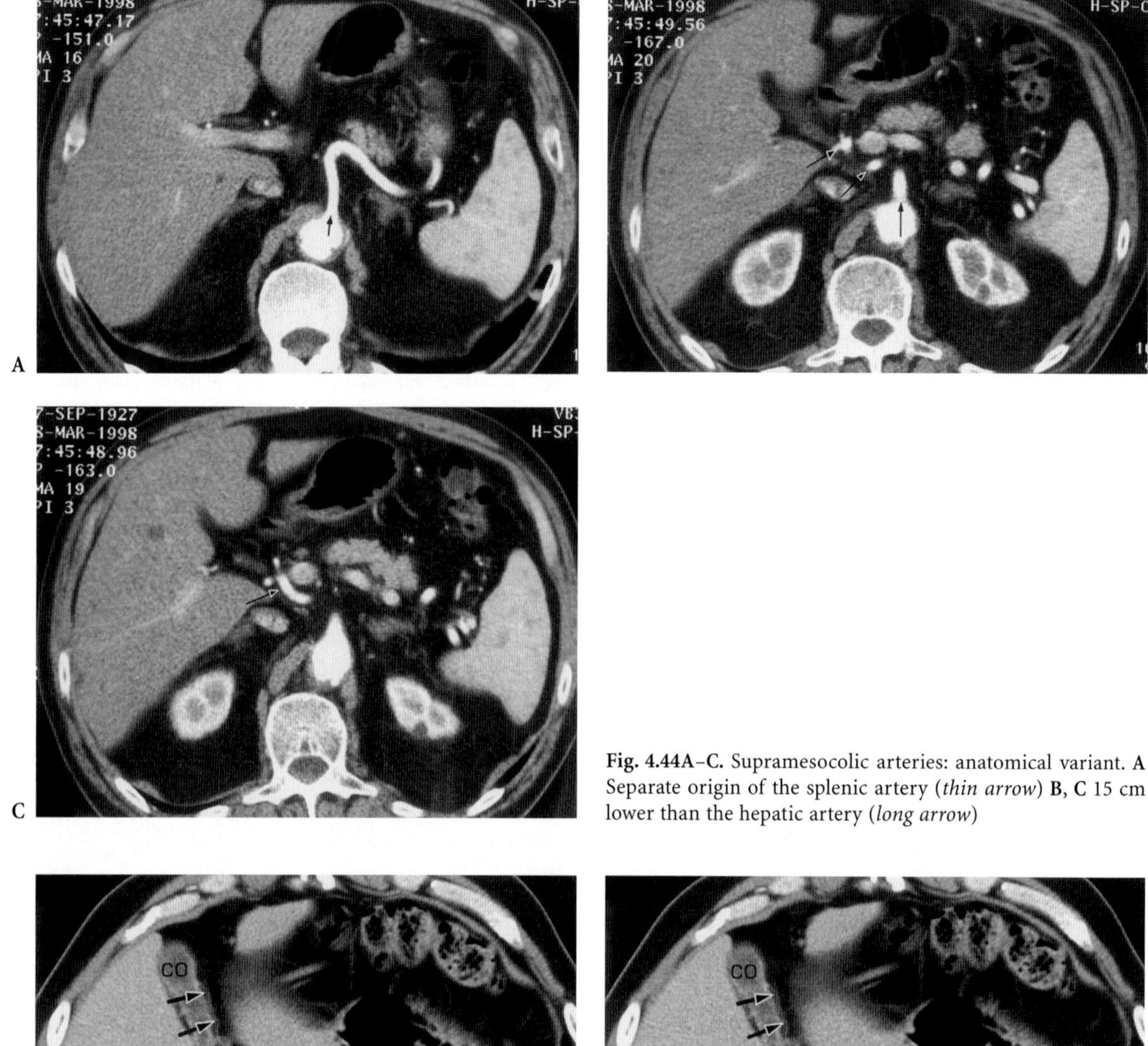

Fig. 4.44A–C. Supramesocolic arteries: anatomical variant. **A** Separate origin of the splenic artery (*thin arrow*) **B, C** 15 cm lower than the hepatic artery (*long arrow*)

Fig. 4.45A, B. Supramesocolic vessels. **A** Cystic artery (*thick arrows*) and **B** vein (*thin arrows*) extending along the medial border of the gallbladder

subdivides into right and left branches, extending along the mesocolic border of the transverse colon (Fig. 4.56).

When conditions are favorable, the trunk and the branches of the middle colic artery may become visible in a single plane, with an appearance reminiscent of a bird's wing.

Going downward, the superior mesenteric artery subdivides into the jejunoileal and ileocolic branches (Figs. 4.52, 4.53), which extend at the side of the homonymous veins, with a punctiform aspect, first parallel and close to the median line, and afterwards progressively diverging. The ramifications extending on the right (ileocolic branches) and on the left side

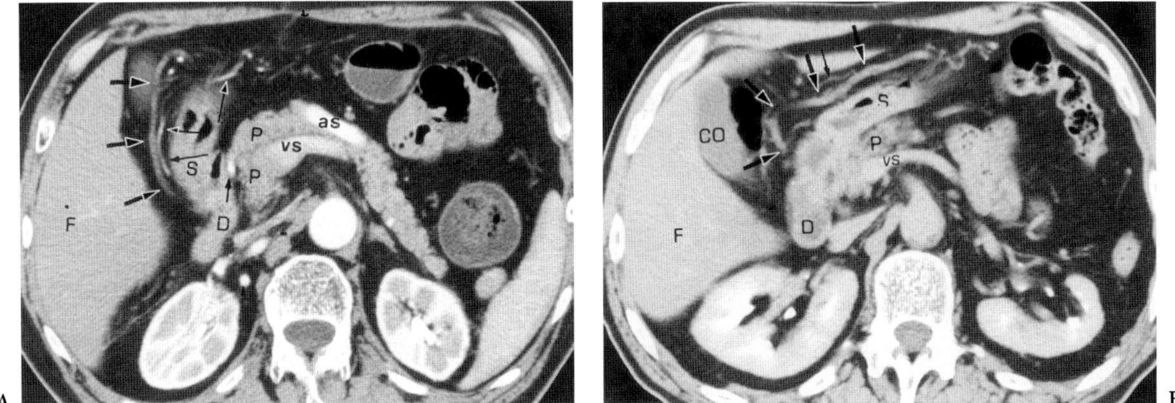

Fig. 4.46A, B. Supramesocolic vessels. The gastroepiploic vessels extend along **A** the greater curvature of the antrum and **B** of the corpus ventriculi within the gastrocolic ligament. (*Large arrows* gastroepiploic vein, *long thin arrows* gastroepiploic artery, *short thin arrow* gastroduodenal artery). Splenic vein is also observed

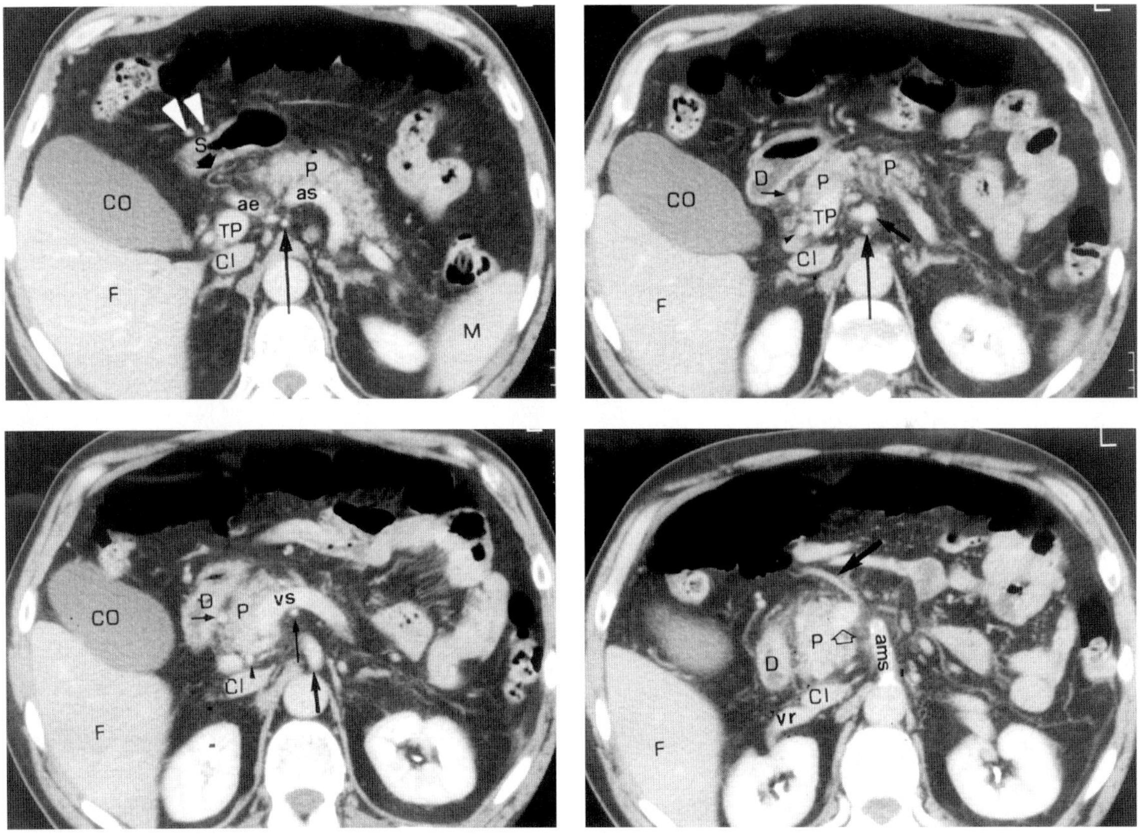

Fig. 4.47A–D. Supramesocolic vessels. Sequence from above downward: **A** Hepatic artery (*ae*), proximal tract of the splenic artery (*as*) and left gastric artery (*long arrow*) after their separation from the celiac trunk. The thin and short branch of the right gastric artery (*stubby arrow*) originates from the hepatic artery; this branch is located behind the pylorus and the gastric antrum In the front of this structure, we observe the round images of the right gastroepiploic artery and vein (*large white arrowhead*). **B** Gastroduodenal artery (*short arrow*) between the duodenum (*D*) and the pancreatic head (*P*), superior pancreatoduodenal vein (*arrowhead*) on the posteromedian side of the pancreatic head, along the margin of the portal trunk (*TP*), and celiac trunk (*large arrow*) on the median line, in front of the left gastric artery (*long arrow*). **C** The inferior pancreatoduodenal artery (*thin arrow*) extends upward from the superior mesenteric artery (*large arrow*) along the median line, behind the splenic vein (*vs*). **D** Trunk of the superior mesenteric artery; gastrocolic venous trunk (*thick arrow*) emptying into the superior mesenteric vein (*open arrow*)

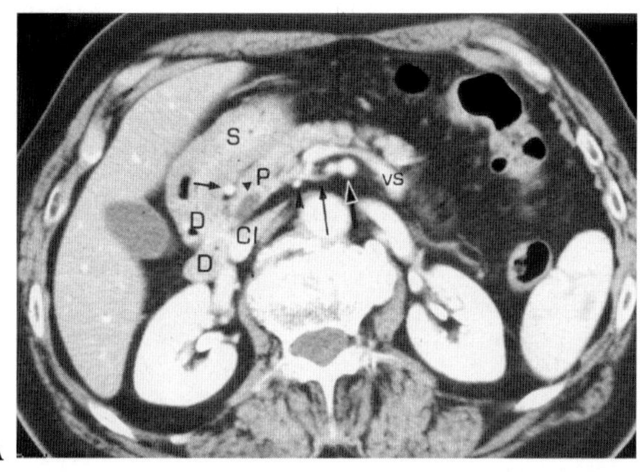

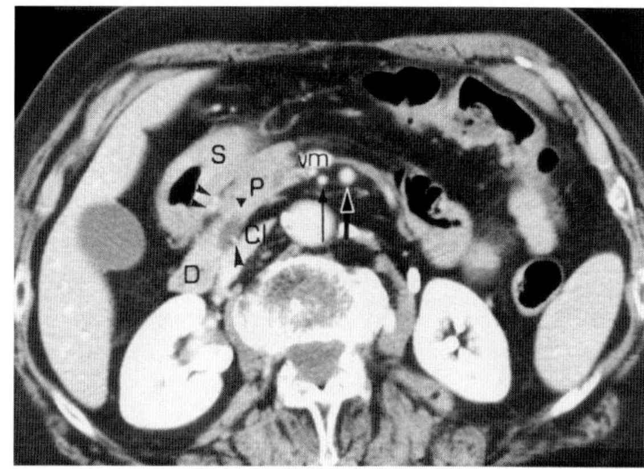

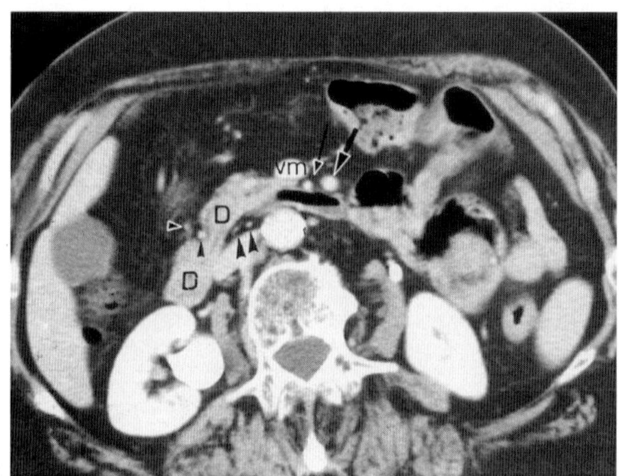

Fig. 4.48A–C. Supramesocolic vessels. **A** The gastroduodenal artery (*arrow*) extends between the anterolateral border of the pancreatic head and the superior genu of the duodenum The inferior pancreatoduodenal artery (*long arrow*) is linear: it originates from the superior mesenteric artery (*large arrow*). The inferior pancreatoduodenal vein appears punctiform behind and on the right side of the homonymous artery (*arrowhead*). Choledochus (*triangle*) is also observed. **B** The superior pancreatoduodenal artery and vein extend outside the pancreatic head (*small arrowhead*) The inferior pancreato-duodenal artery (*long arrow*) is located on the right of the superior mesenteric artery (*large arrow*); its terminal branch (*arrowhead*) is located behind the choledochus (*triangle*). **C** Anterior (*small arrow points*) and posterior (*large arrowhead*) arterial duodenal branches On the median line, we observe the superior mesenteric vein and artery (*large arrow*) and the inferior pancreatoduodenal artery (*long arrow*)

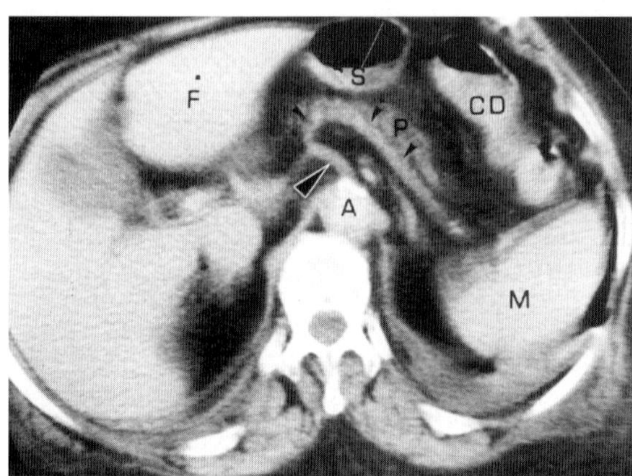

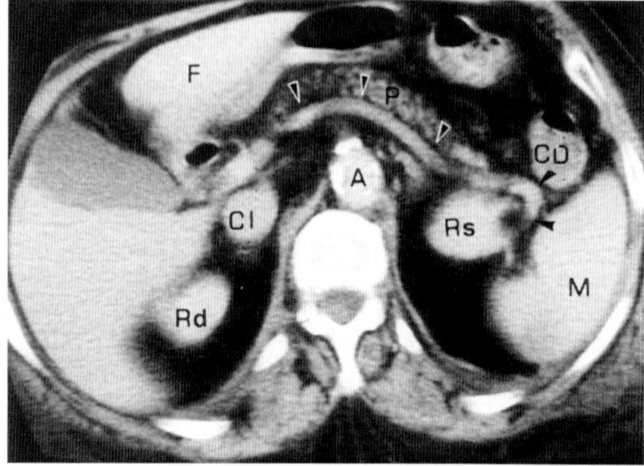

Fig. 4.49A, B. *Supramesocolic vessels.* **A** The splenic artery (small arrowhead) is located above and slightly behind the corpus and cauda pancreatis; the celiac trunk (big arrow) extends in a unique plane. **B** The splenic vein (*arrowhead*) extends from the hilum of the spleen to the splenomesenteric confluence

(jejunoileal branches) become progressively thinner and more numerous. Also, around the trunks of these vessels, adipose areolar tissue is sometimes visible; it is denser and is surrounded by an even denser thin annular lamina.

- The *jejunal* and *ileal arteries* (Figs. 4.52, 4.53, 4.59, 4.69) come out at various levels from the trunk of the superior mesenteric artery and extend to the intestinal loops: the jejunal branches at a higher level on the left side, with a main-

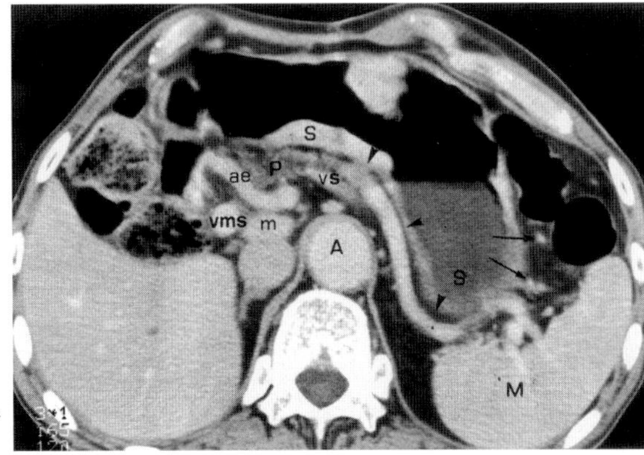

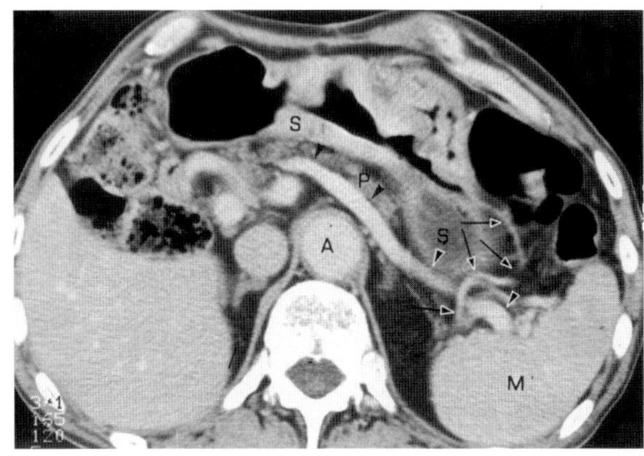

Fig. 4.50 A, B. Supramesocolic vessels.y Splenic vessels (stomach is distended by water and air) in a patient with a gastric tumor. **A** The splenic artery (*arrowhead*) is pushed backward and is only visible in one tomogram; it follows the lesser curvature of the stomach Round images of the left gastroepiploic vessels (*thin arrows*) outside the greater curvature. **B** The splenic vein (*arrowhead*) extends from the hilum of the spleen to the confluence with the superior mesenteric vein. A portion of the left gastroepiploic vein (*thin arrow*) is visible above the hilum of the spleen

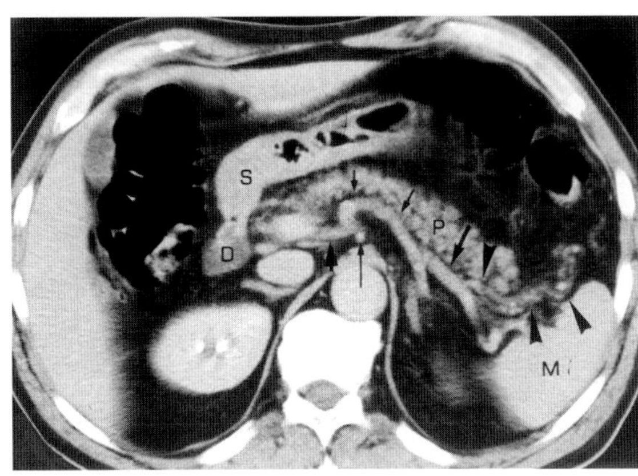

Fig. 4.51. Supramesocolic vessels. Left gastroepiploic artery and vein (*large arrowhead*). Trifurcation of the celiac trunk: hepatic artery (*arrowhead*), splenic artery (*small arrows*) and coronarostomachic artery (*long thin arrow*)

la transverse extension and a linear aspect. At a lower level, the ileal branches open forward and to the sides with a fan-like apearance toward the intestinal loops. They may appear tubular or punctiform, according to their course. Finally, the terminal vascular branches of the ileal loops (Fig. 4.58) extending forward have a serpiginous spoke-like aspect from the center to the periphery, whereas those extending downward toward the pelvis have a dense punctiform aspect that is visible in the transparent mesenteric adipose areolar tissue.

- The *right colic artery* comes out just below the origin of the median colic artery on the right side of the superior mesenteric artery (Figs. 4.52, 4.53) and divides into two branches, ascending and descending, that extend to the marginal arteries of the hepatic flexure and of the ascending tract of the colon, respectively. The right colic artery is recognizable by its origin, extension on the right side and curvilinear strip aspect with the concavity turned toward the intestinal loops.
- The *ileocolic artery* (Figs. 4.52–4.54) originates in front of the third duodenal portion and extends obliquely downward, toward the right iliac fossa. It has a round appearance and is located in the retroperitoneum along the mesenteric root, in front of the renal fascia. Along its extension, it gives origin to several branches, with a prevalently tubular and sinuous appearance. These ramifications insinuate themselves between the mesenteric layers and show a spoke-like distribution to the ileal loops. Occasionally, it is possible to observe the *vasa recta ilii*, which come out from the marginal branches and penetrate the intestinal wall with a Y or V configuration.

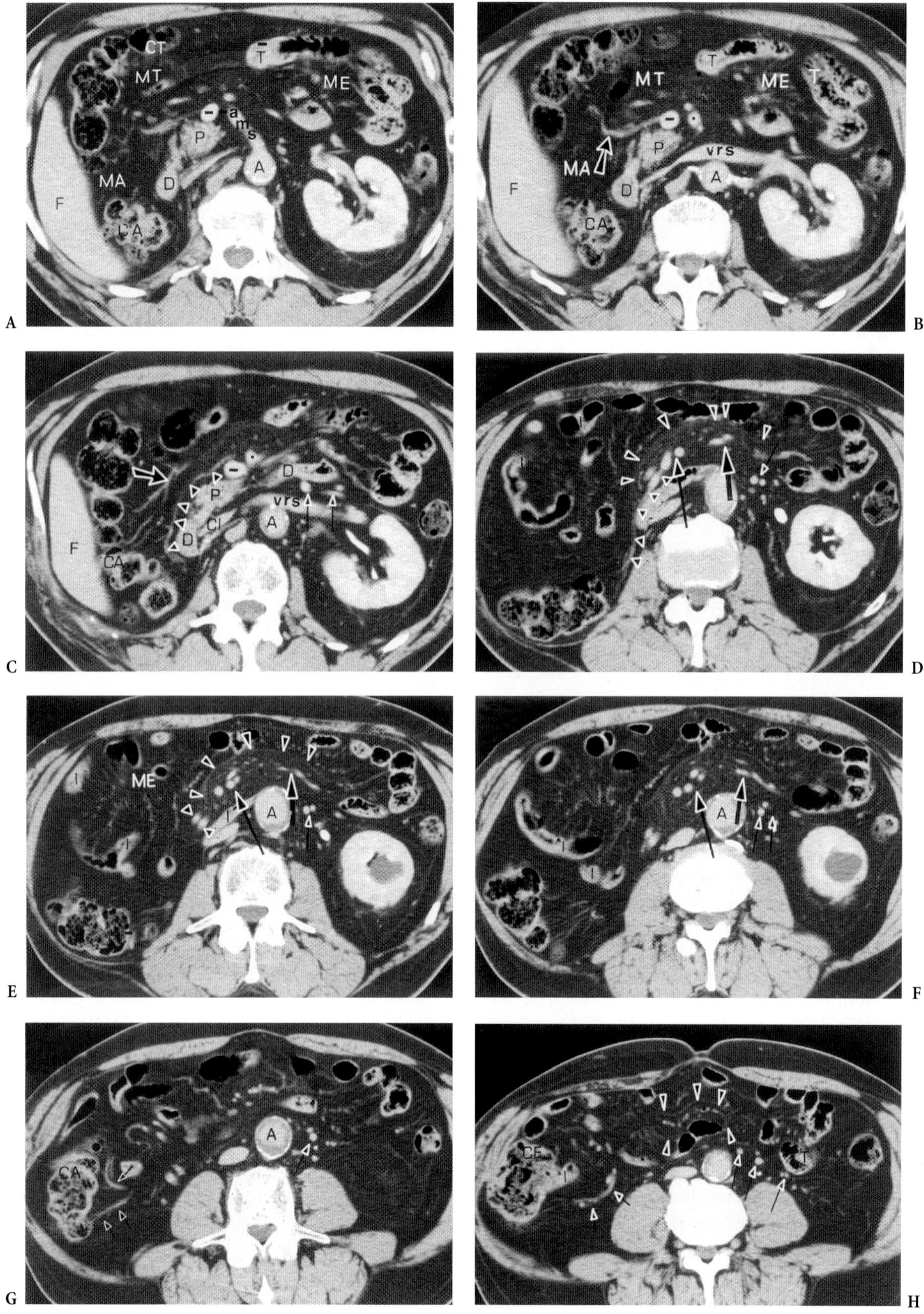
CT
T
MT
ME
a
m
s
P
A
MA
D
F
CA
A
T
MT
ME
T
P
vrs
MA
A
D
F
CA
B
D
P
vrs
Cl
A
D
F
CA
C
D
I
ME
A
I
E
A
F
A
CA
G
CE
T
H

It is sometimes also possible to recognize the right colic branches, which are in pairs or in groups of three and have a tubular appearance, extending downward and obliquely on the right up to the mesocolic side of the cecum and of the descending colon, where the right marginal colic artery comes out (Fig. 4.52); this artery can be recognized for its punctiform aspect.

It is not rare to observe the terminal ileal branch; after extending along the right psoas, this ramification penetrates the mesentery surrounding the cecum from behind and from the left; it then subdivides into thin vessels around the bowel (Fig. 4.54).

4.2.1.1.3
Inferior Mesenteric Artery

The inferior mesenteric artery (Figs. 4.52, 4.64, 4.66, 4.72) originates 4–5 cm under the superior mesenteric artery, coming out from the anterior aortic wall just on the left of the middle line, with the aspect of a small spur. Thereafter, it continues downwards and slightly backwards with a punctiform appearance, progressively moving away from the aorta and getting close to the bigger punctiform image of the homonymous vein, which is less dense and is located more laterally. The inferior mesenteric artery extends in retroperitoneal planes, between the posterior parietal peritoneum and the anterior renal fascia.

At hypogastric levels, it is possible to recognize its three main collateral branches: the left colic artery, the sigmoidal artery and the superior hemorrhoidal artery.

The *left colic artery* is the first branch coming out from the main trunk; it extends on the left side. Its aspect depends on its variable paths: if the vessel extends upwards or downwards, it is punctiform, whereas if the artery is horizontal, it appears as a thin curvilinear line, moving progressively away from the trunk of the inferior mesenteric artery up to the descending colon.The *left marginal colic artery* can be recognized by its punctiform aspect along all the medial border of the descending colon (Figs. 4.52, 4.59).

The *sigmoidal artery* (Figs. 4.17, 4.52, 4.64) has variable aspects and orientations according to the position and sinuosity of the sigmoid. Its most frequent position within the sigmoid mesocolonic adipose areolar tissue is above or on the posteromedial border of the bowel, which the artery follows along the total extension from the left to the right, as a thin sinuous line or a series of small dense points.

The *superior hemorrhoidal artery* (Figs. 4.52, 4.64, 4.66) is frequently visible in the upper tract as a thin line extending obliquely and backward from the inferior mesenteric artery toward the median line up to the front of the promontory. Farther on it subdivides into the right and left pararectal branches, which extend downward on the sides of the rectum with a punctiform aspect.

4.2.1.2
Pelvic and Genital Arteries

The main trunks of the pelvic arteries (common, external and internal iliac arteries) are clearly visible, whereas it is difficult to recognize the secondary branches.

The *common iliac arteries* appear round and extend in front of the first sacral vertebrae at a high level, opening apart and diverging from their aortic origin up to the pelvic aperture, where they subdivide into the *external iliac arteries* (Figs. 4.99, 4.104) anteriorly and the *internal iliac* or *hypogastric arteries* (Figs. 4.32, 4.104) posteriorly; they have a round appearance and are located in the laterorectal spaces on both sides of the pelvis.

The *inferior epigastric arteries* (Figs. 4.5, 4.6, 4.8, 4.9, 4.32, 4.99), which originate from the external iliac artery, appear punctiform and coupled with the homonymous veins in the preperitoneal space in a lateral position. Ascending from the pelvis, they tend

Fig. 4.52A–H. Submesocolic vessels. **A–C** Superior mesenteric artery (*dot*) and vein (*small line*), with **D–F** relative junctions with the ileocolic trunks (*long arrow*) on the *right* and jejunoileal (*long thick arrow*) on the left. Some horizontal branches originate at different levels. We recognize: the right middle colic vein (*curved arrow*) within the transverse mesocolon (**B**), the right colic vessels (*triangles*) (**C, D, E**) and the terminal branches of the ileocolic vessels (*short arrows*), which continue in the marginal colic vessels at the confluence of the mesentery with the mesocecum and the ascending mesocolon (**G, H**). Most of the secondary vessels emptying into the small intestine extend in a craniocaudal direction with a punctiform (**E–H**) or bead-like aspect within the mesentery The adipose areolar tissue around the trunks of the superior mesenteric vessels and of their main branches (**D–F, H**) is denser than that located in the mesenteries and in the retroperitoneum, from which it is separated by a very thin lamina (*small arrowhead*) (**C–H**) On the *left*, we can follow the inferior mesenteric vessels (*long thin arrows*) up to their subdivisions in sigmoidal vessels inside and superior hemorrhoidal vessels outside (**H**). On the internal side of the descending colon, we recognize the punctiform images of the marginal vessels extending vertically within the root of its mesentery

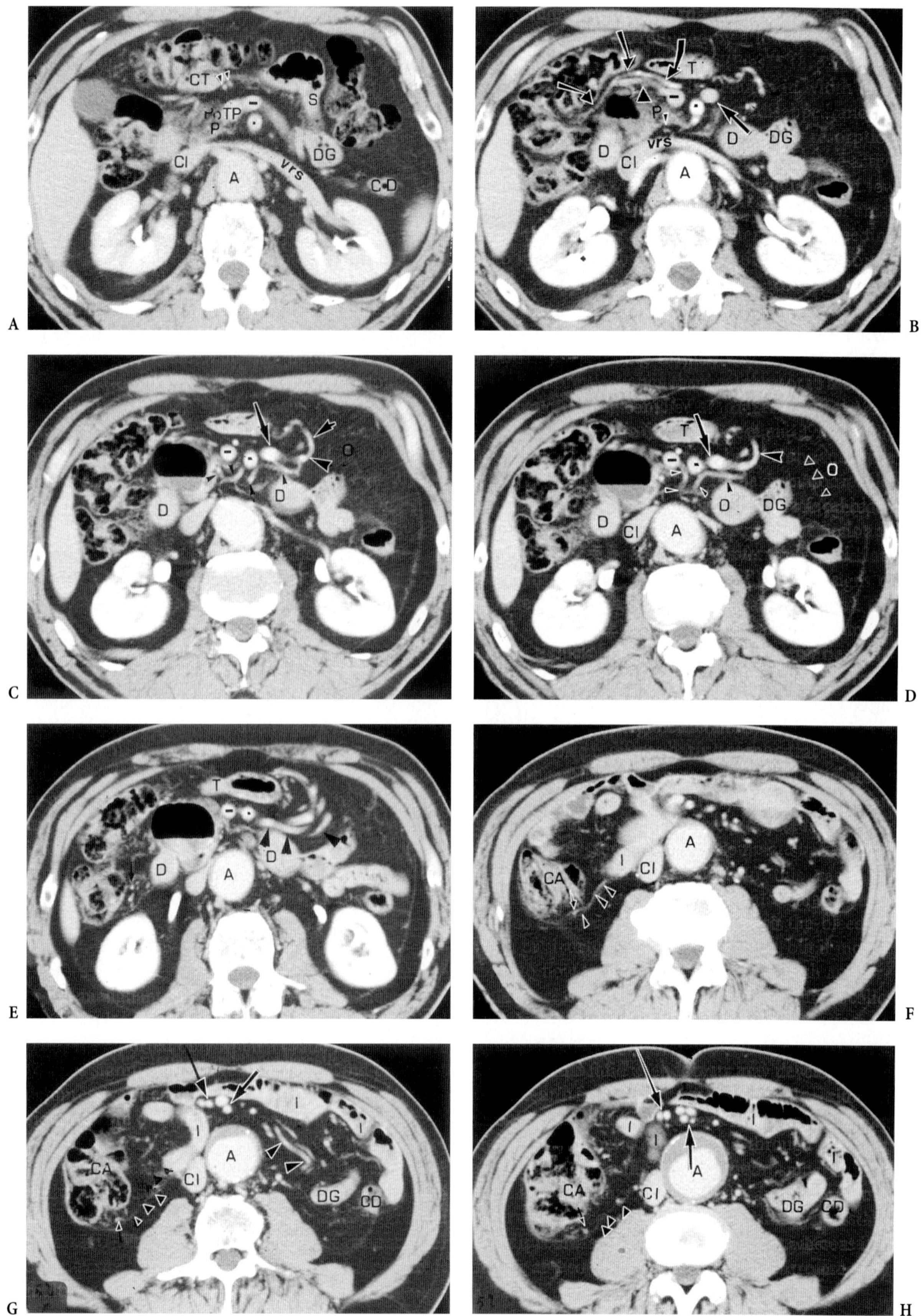
A
CT
S
P TP
P
CI
A
vrs
DG
C D
B
T
P
D
D
CI
vrs
A
DG
C
O
D
D
D
T
O
D
DG
D
CI
A
E
T
D
D
A
F
A
CA
I
CI
G
I
I
I
A
CA
CI
DG
CD
H
I
I
I
A
CA
CI
DG
CD
I

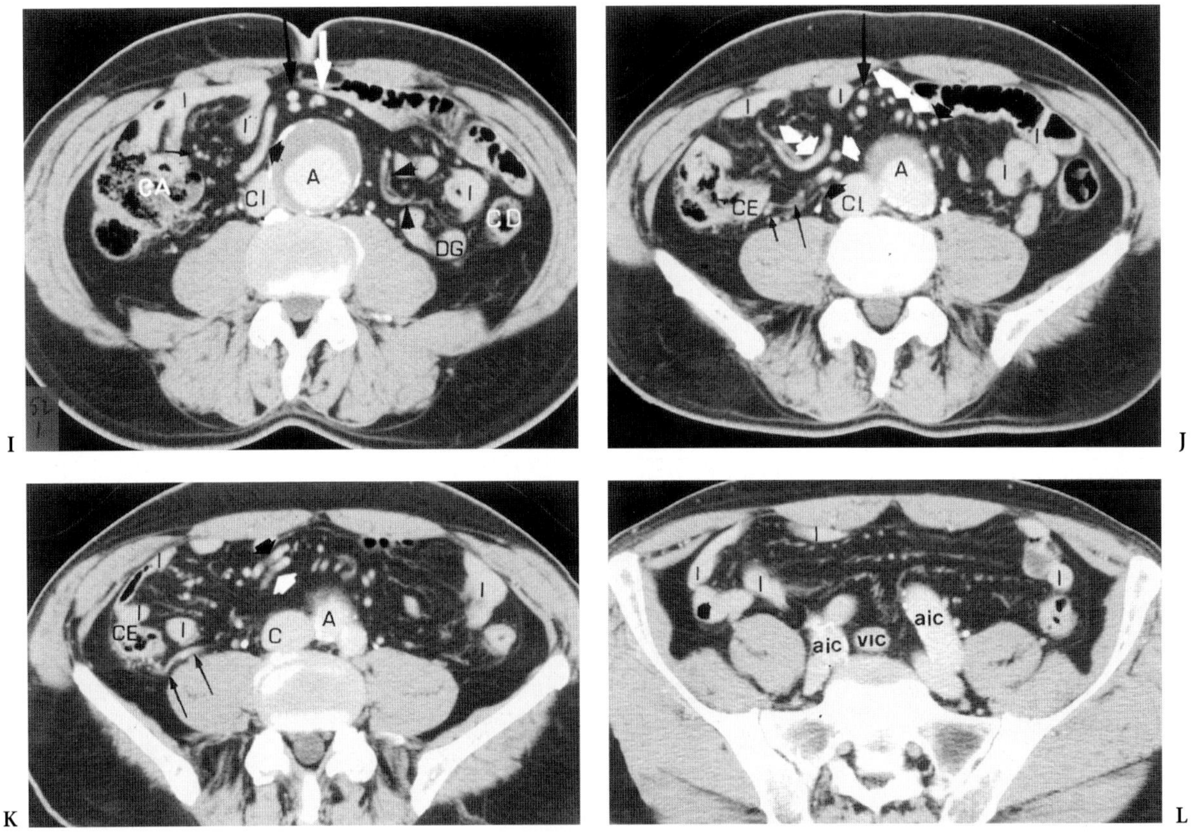

I J

K L

Fig. 4.53A–L. Submesocolic vessels. Superior mesenteric vessels and secondary branches. The trunks of the superior mesenteric artery (*point*) and vein (*small line*) extend together in a craniocaudal direction with a roundish aspect (from **A–E**) They subdivide (**B–D**, **G–I**) into jejunoileal branches (*arrow*) on the left and ileocolic (**G–J**) (*long arrow*) branches on the right. Before the subdivision, the superior mesenteric trunks generate the right (**B**) middle colic artery (*curved arrows*) and vein (*triangle*), and the inferior pancreatoduodenal arteries (*small arrowhead*), which extend from below upwards (**B–D**). The secondary ramifications (*large arrowhead*), extending upward and on the left side for the jejunum (**C–E**) and downwards for the ileum (**G, I**) originate from the jejunoileal branches. The ileal vessels (*stubby white arrows*) extending downwards (I, L, M), the middle (*small arrowhead*) (**F**) and inferior (*triangles*) (**G, H**) colic vessels for the ascending colon and the cecal vessels (*long thin arrows*) (**J, K**) originate from the ileocolic branches. On the medial side of the ascending colon (**E–J**), we observe the punctiform images of the marginal colic vessels (*small arrows*). The peripheral ileal vessels extend along three transverse parallel lines with a bead-like aspect (**L**). All these vessels represent important markers for recognizing the mesocolon, mesentery and retroperitoneum; in particular, the superior mesenteric vessels for the mesenteric root, the middle colic vessels for the transverse mesocolon, the jejunal and ileal vessels for the mesentery, the right paracolic branches for the ascending mesocolon The right colic branches are located within the retroperitoneum between the posterior parietal peritoneum and the anterior renal fascia

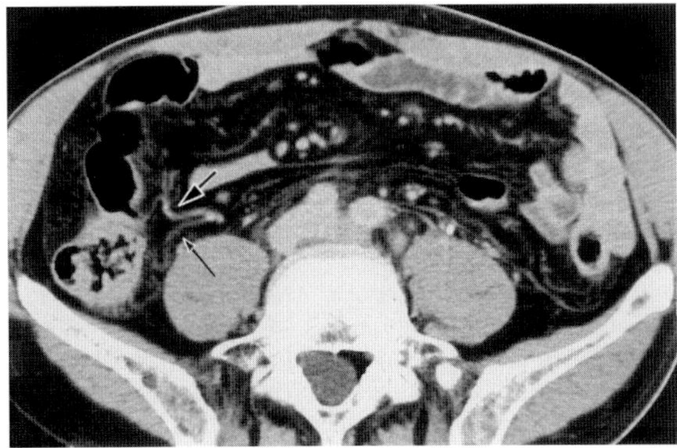

Fig. 4.54. Submesocolic arteries. Subdivision of the terminal branches of the ileocolic artery

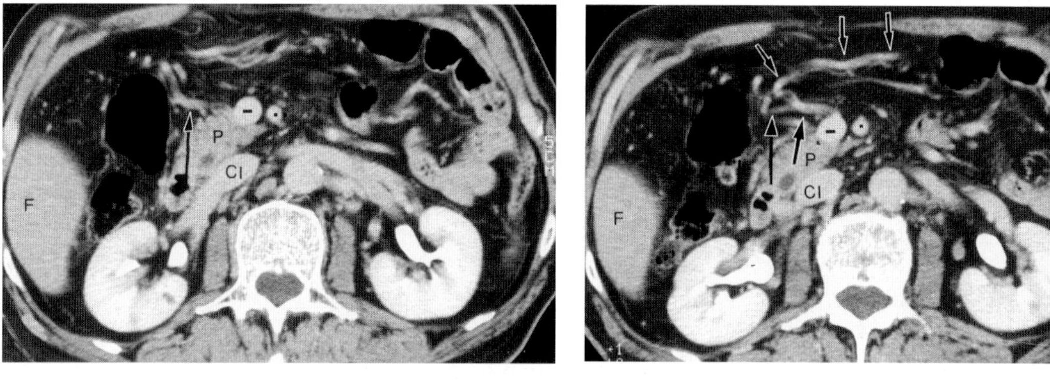

Fig. 4.55A, B. Supra- and inframesocolic veins. Gastrocolic venous trunk (*thick arrow*) (**B**), emptying into the superior mesenteric vein (*small line*), and affluent veins: right gastroepiploic (*arrows*) and right middle colic (*long arrow*) veins

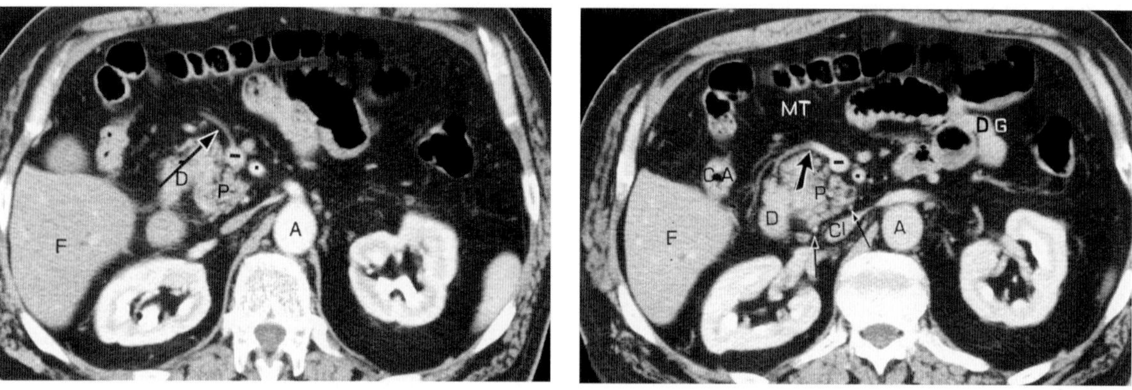

Fig. 4.56A, B. Mesocolic vessels. **A** Right middle colic (*long arrow*) and **B** right colic (*curved arrow*) veins. Posteroinferior pancreatoduodenal arteries (*small arrows*)

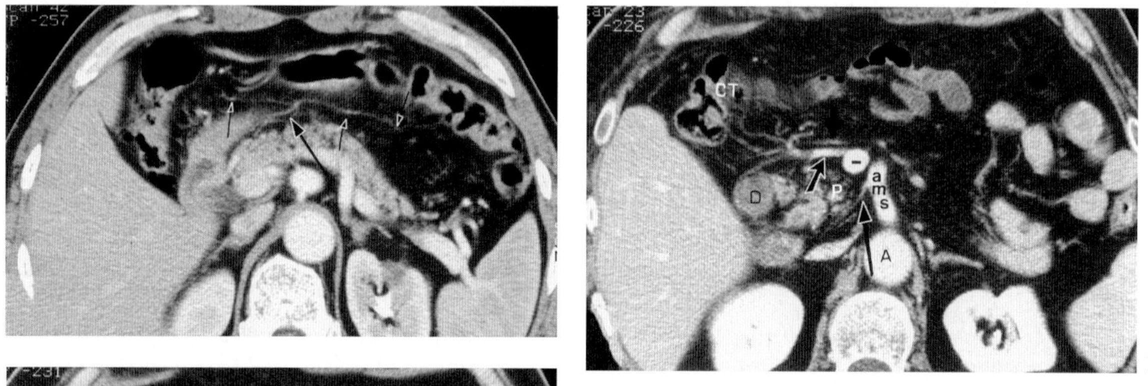

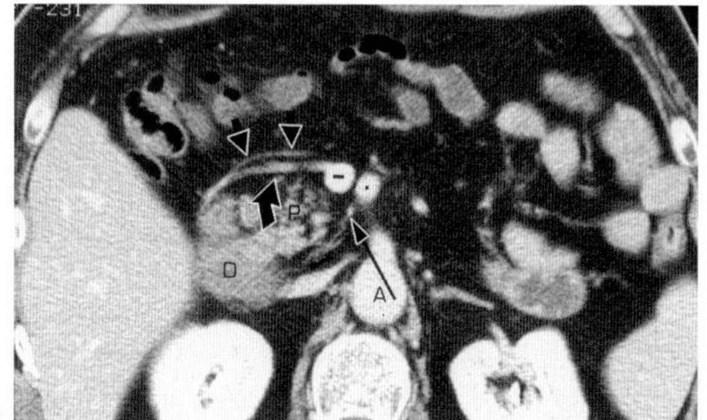

Fig. 4.57A–C. Mesocolic vessels. **A** Middle colic artery (*long arrow*) and its marginal branches for the transverse colon. **B C** Right colic artery (*stubby arrows*) and vein (*curved arrows*) for the hepatic flexure of the transverse colon and the ascending colon. Inferior pancreatoduodenal artery (*long arrow*)

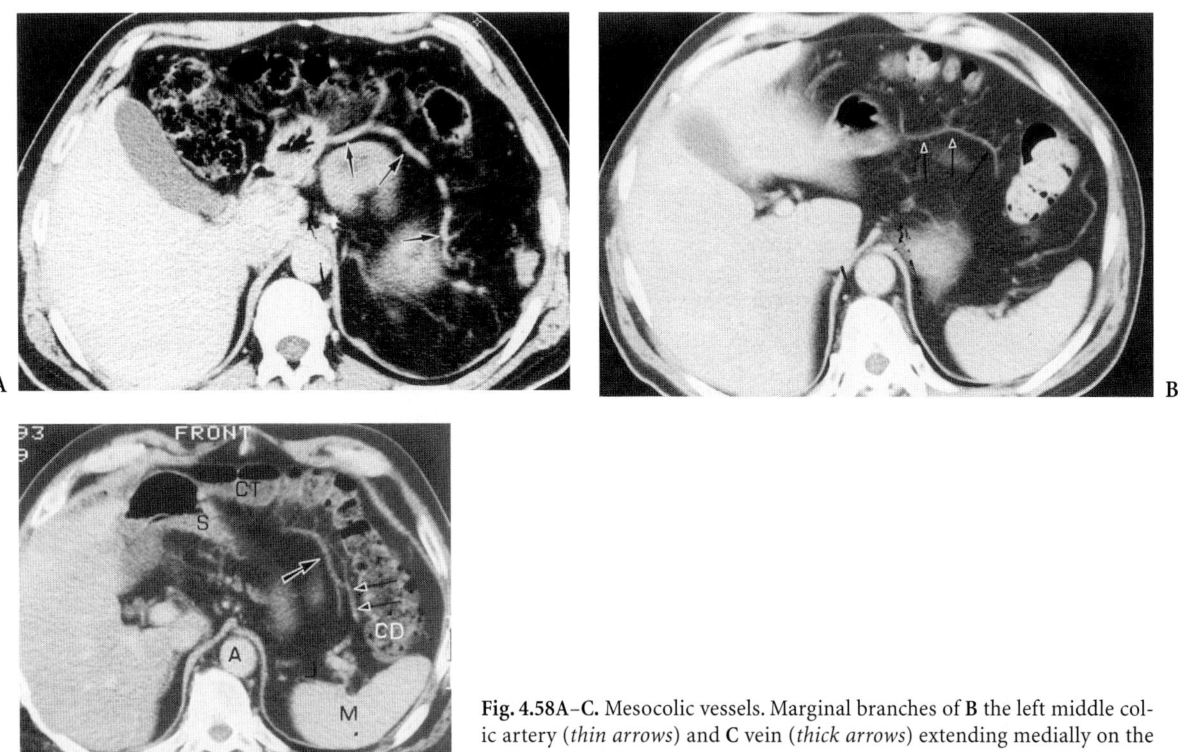

Fig. 4.58A–C. Mesocolic vessels. Marginal branches of **B** the left middle colic artery (*thin arrows*) and **C** vein (*thick arrows*) extending medially on the mesocolic side along the splenic flexure of the colon

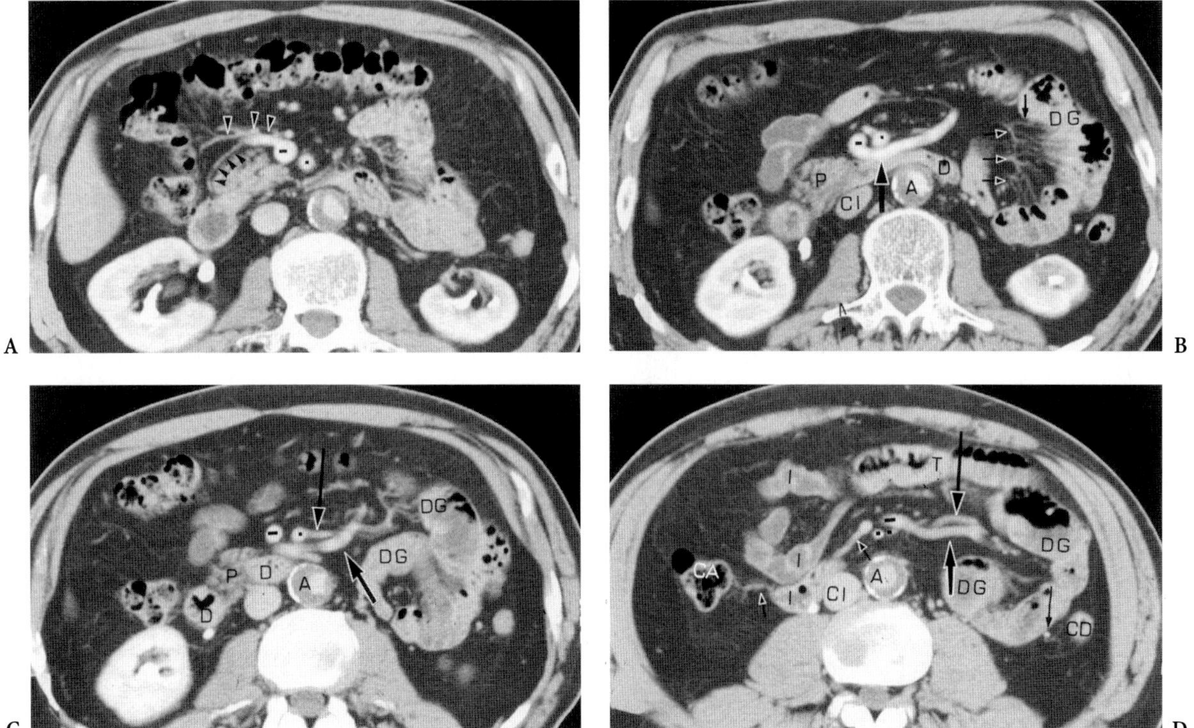

Fig. 4.59A–D. Superior mesenteric vessels: proximal branches. **A** Right superior colic vein (*large arrowhead*) and right ileal veins (*small arrowhead*). **B** Jejunal veins: main trunk (*large arrow*) and peripheral branches (*thin arrows*) in the mesentery. **C** Jejunal artery (*long arrow*) and vein (*thick arrow*). **D** Right ileocolic vein (*thin arrow*), jejunal artery (*long arrow*) and vein (*thick arrow*) Left marginal colic artery (*long thin arrow*) from the inferior mesenteric artery

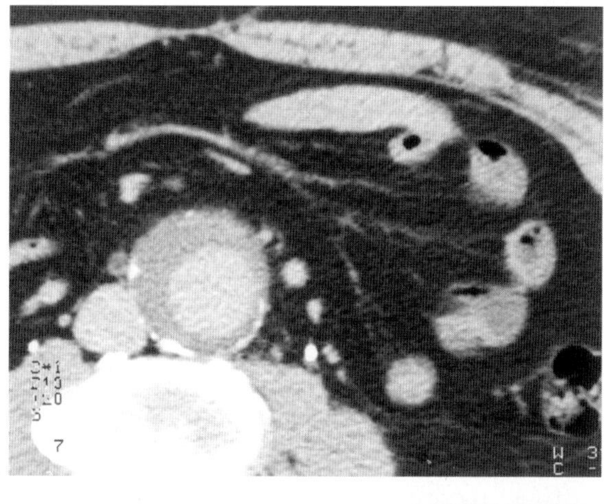

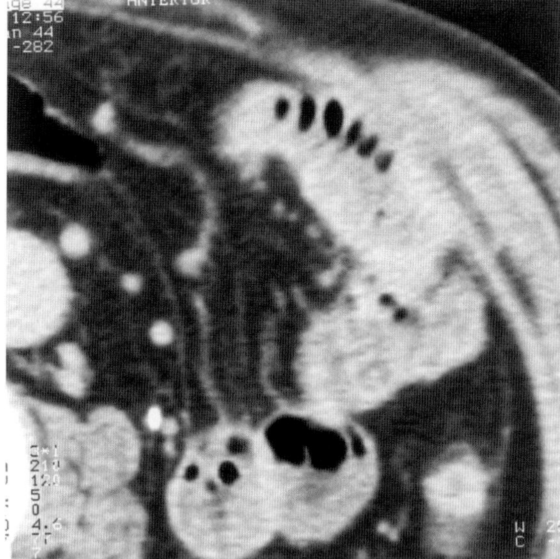

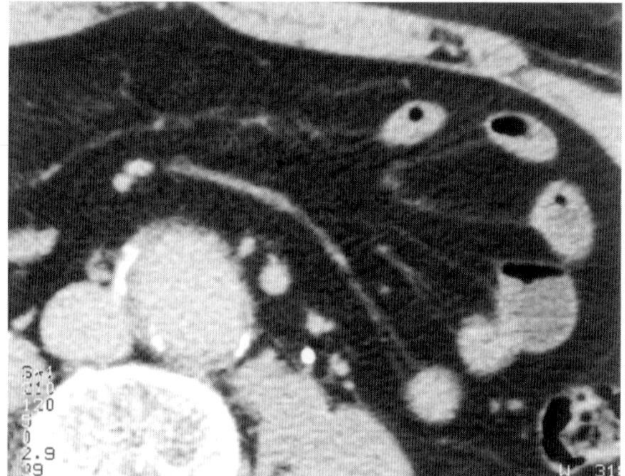

Fig. 4.60A–C. Submesocolic vessels. Terminal jejunoileal branches

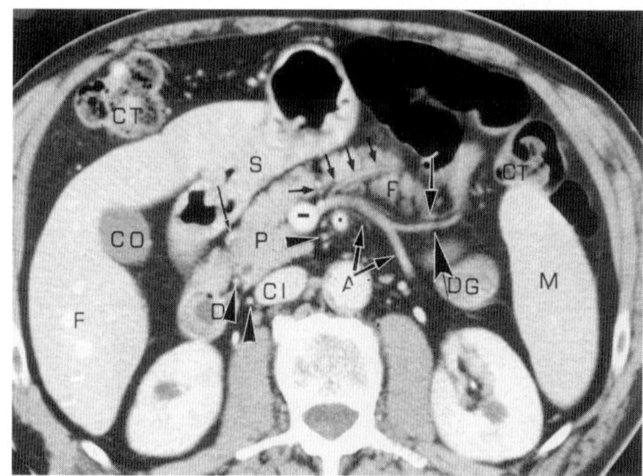

Fig. 4.61. Inferior mesenteric vessels. Inferior mesenteric vein (*thick arrows*) at the confluence with the superior mesenteric vein (*small hyphen*), next to the splenomesenteric confluent Left superior colic vein (*spearhead*) coming from the splenic flexure of the colon The homonymous artery (*medium-sized arrows*) extends parallel to the vein, but it is very thin. Other structures observed are: inferior pancreatic venous branches

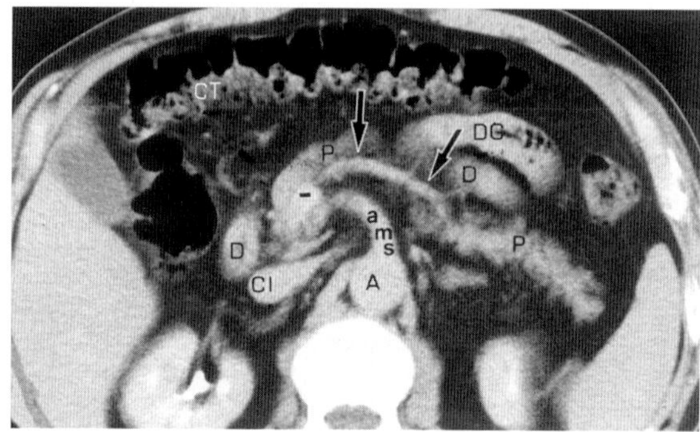

Fig. 4.62. Inferior mesenteric vein. Confluence of the inferior mesenteric vein (*thick arrow*) with the superior mesenteric vein (-) The inferior mesenteric vein extends between the duodenojejunal flexure (*D*, *G*) and the corpus and cauda pancreatis, within the left paraduodenal space

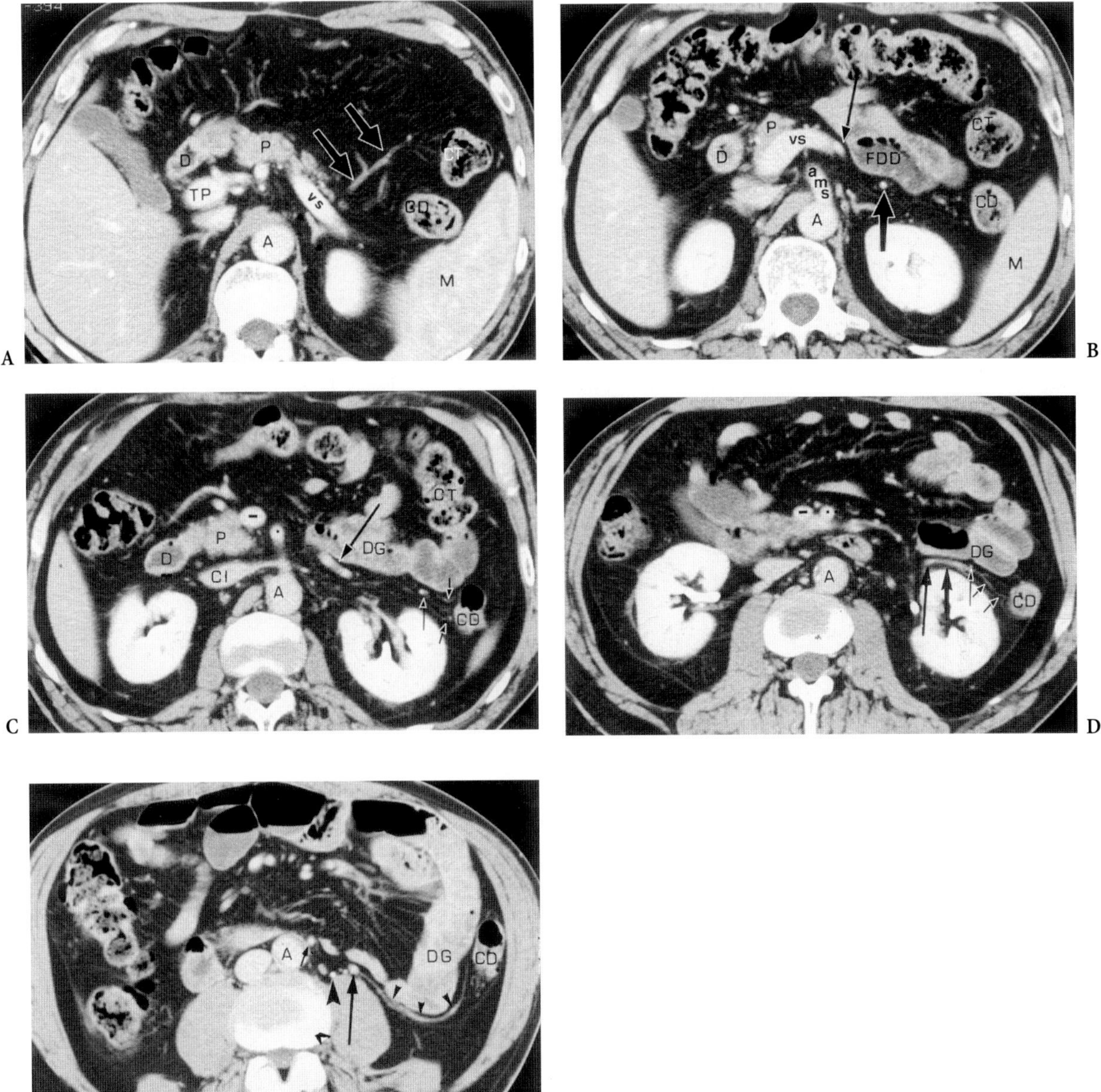

Fig. 4.63A–E. Inferior mesenteric vein: secondary branches. **A** The left superior colic vein (*large arrows*), coming from the splenic flexure of the colon, extends oblique backwards, downward and inward to reach the inferior mesenteric vein. It penetrates between the cauda pancreatis and the duodenojejunal flexure (*F, D, D*); behind this structure it joins the inferior mesenteric vein. **B** Confluence of the inferior mesenteric vein (*thick arrow*) with the splenic vein. Left superior colic branch (*large arrow*) behind the duodenojejunal flexure. **C** Superior tract of the inferior mesenteric vein (*long arrow*) from the jejunum to the anterior renal fascia. Left colic (*thin arrow*) and paracolic (*short thin arrow*) branches within the descending mesocolon, medially to the colon. **D** Intermediate left colic vein (*thick arrow*) and its paracolic branches (*thin arrows*). **E** Intermediate left colic vein (*small arrowhead*), between descending colon and inferior mesenteric vein (*long arrow*), located between the jejunal loops and the anterior renal fascia. Origin of the inferior mesenteric artery (*thin arrow*) from the aorta. *Large arrowheasd* indicate left ureter

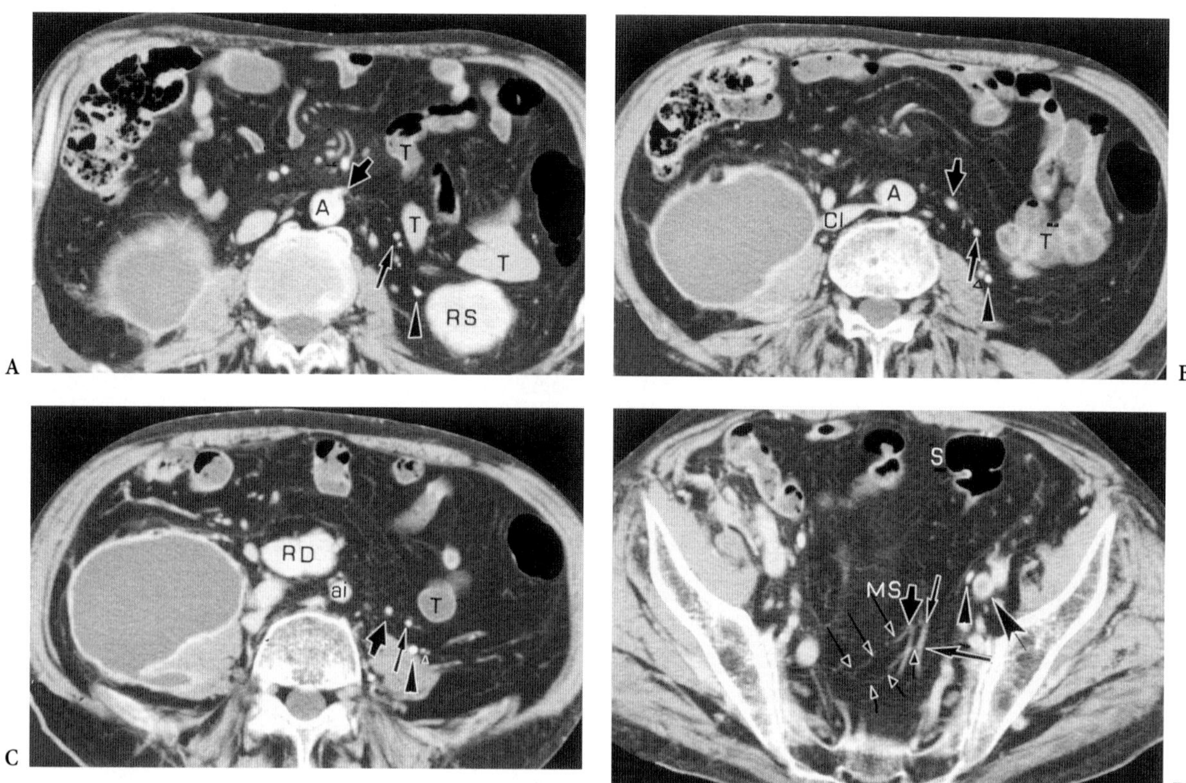

Fig. 4.64A–D. The inferior mesenteric artery (*short thick arrows*) originates from the anterior aortic wall (**A**) and extends, with a punctiform aspect, outwards and toward the left side up to the vicinity of the homonymous vein (*arrow*). Here, it is located on the medial side of the vein in retroperitoneal planes, in front of the anterior renal fascia, which separates it from the ureter (*arrowhead*) and from the ureteral and spermatic vessels (*open small triangles*) (**B, C**). Inferior tract of the inferior mesenteric vessels, which continue in the superior hemorrhoidal vessels (artery on the right and vein) is seen on the *left* (**D**). The sigmoidal artery (*long thin arrows*) and vein (*short thin arrows*) originate from the right side and extend on the superior part of the sigmoid mesocolon (**D**). Patient with an abscess located inside the right psoas fascia and a thrombosis of the left femoral and external iliac veins (*spearhead*)

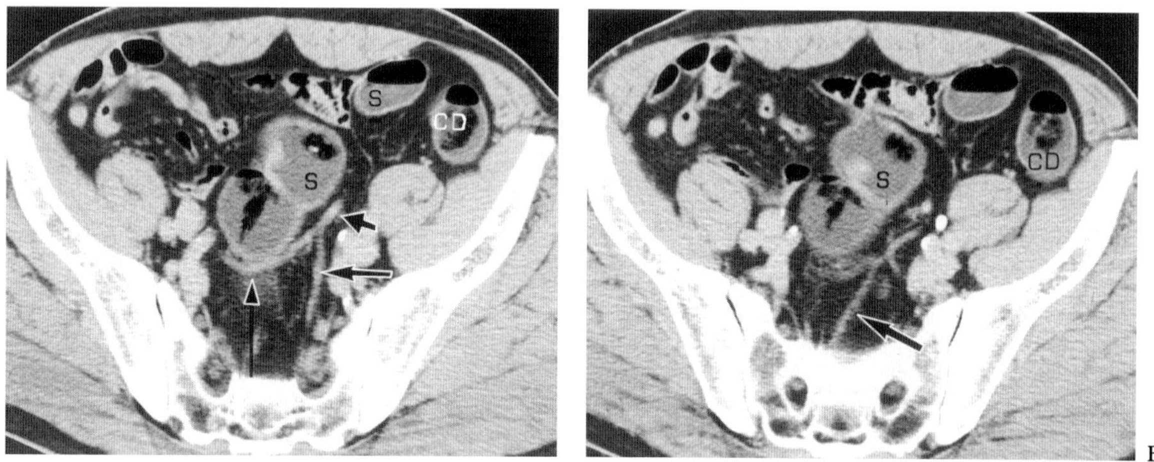

Fig. 4.65. Inferior mesenteric (*short thick arrow*), sigmoidal (*long thin arrow*) and **A** left and **B** right superior hemorrhoidal (*long thick arrow*) veins

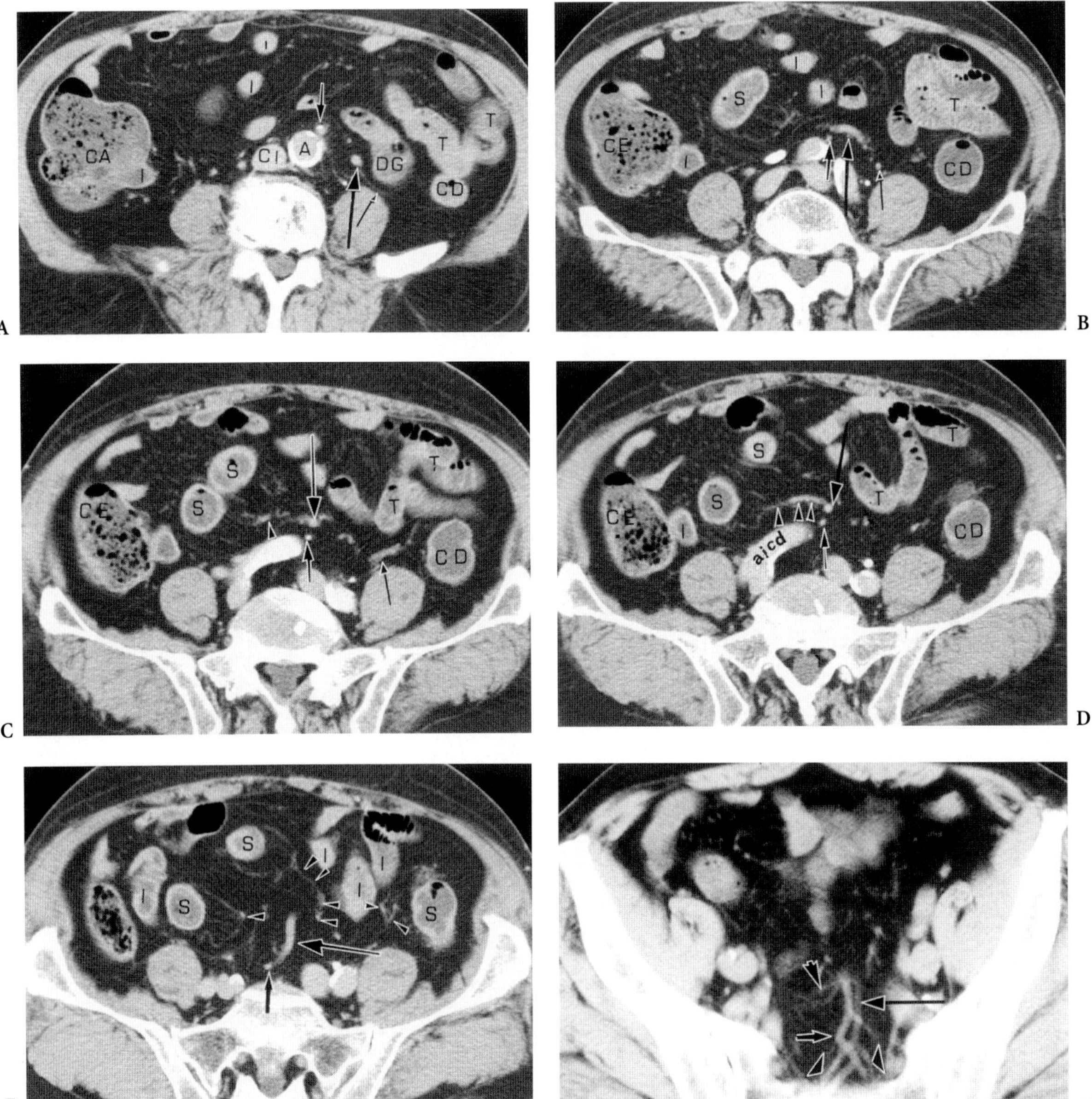

Fig. 4.66A–F. Inferior mesenteric artery and vein. **A** The inferior mesenteric artery (*arrow*) originates from the left anterolateral wall of the aorta and extends downward, with a punctiform aspect, along the median line up to the front of the promontory (**A–E**). Under this structure, it subdivides (**F**) into the superior hemorrhoidal branches (*triangles*). **B** The inferior mesenteric vein (*long arrow*) extends along the left paramedian line in front of the psoas (**A**), then veers inward (**B**) and becomes parallel to the homonymous artery (**C–E**). It collects two left colic branches (**A, B, C** *thin arrows*) from outside and the sigmoidal vein (*arrow points*) (**D, E**) from inside. Under the promontory (**F**), the two superior right and left hemorrhoidal branches (*triangles*) converge in the inferior mesenteric vein

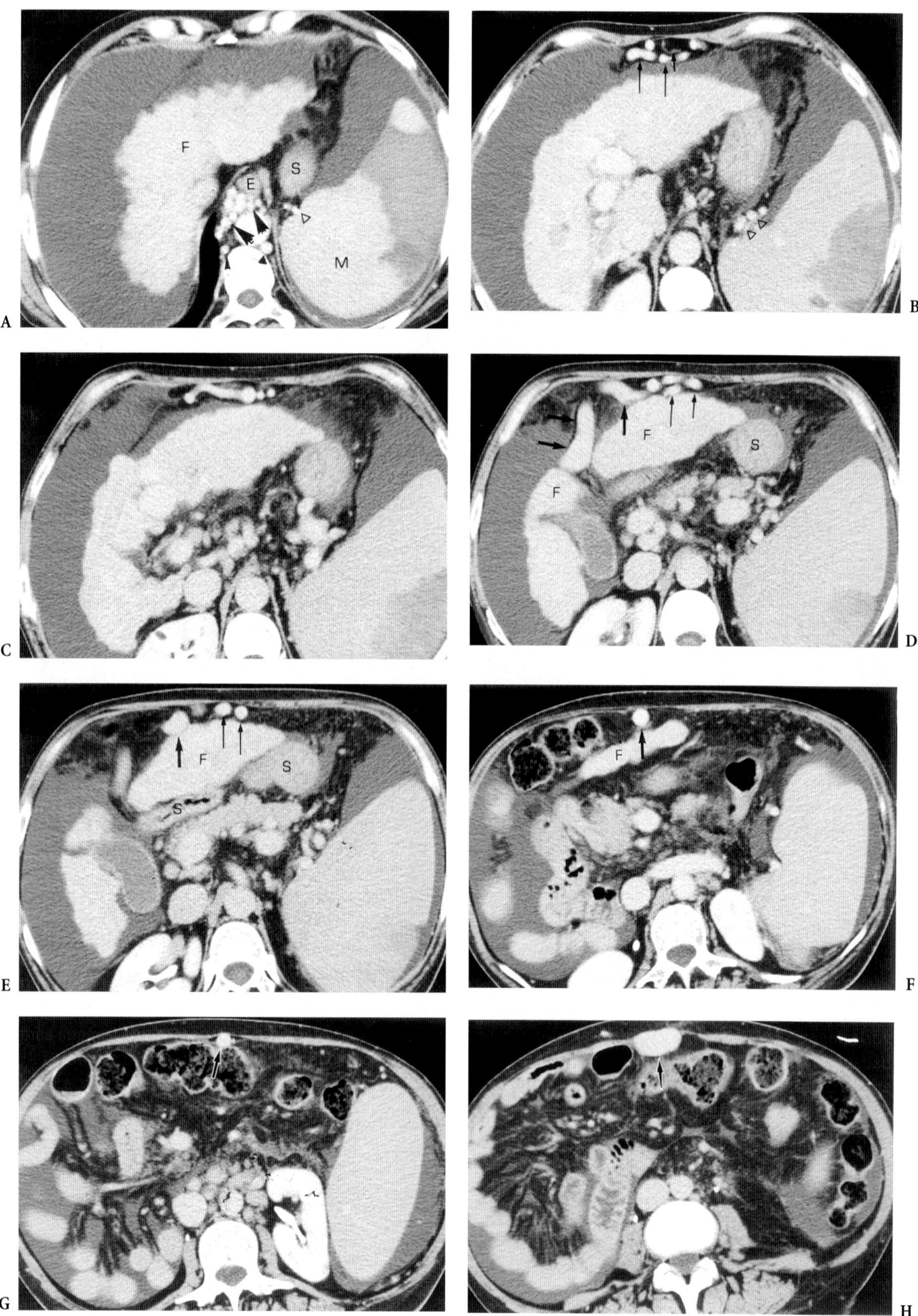
F
E
S
M
A
B
F
S
F
C
D
F
S
S
E
F
F
G
H

to extend toward the median line behind the anterior abdominal wall with unchanged punctiform aspect and a progressively reducing diameter.

Concerning the branches of the hypogastric artery, we here describe those extending to the intra- or juxtaperitoneal organs and structures: the *superior* (Fig. 4.101) and *inferior vesical*, the *middle hemorrhoidal* and the *genital arteries*. Except for the genital vessels, it is difficult to identify these arteries because they are confused with the pelvic ligaments. In elderly women, the *uterine arteries* may become visible because of the presence of calcified atheromatous plaques along their extension on both sides of the uterus and at the base of the broad ligaments. In men, the *spermatic arteries* are recognizable because of their linear aspect and their characteristic pathway from behind forward and outward toward the inguinal foramen, on the sides of the pelvis.

The *genital arteries* (Figs. 4.9, 4.64) are frequently visible in the retroperitoneal tract, in a pre- or paravertebral position, from their origin from the aorta or the renal arteries up to the pelvis, coupled with the homonymous veins; these vessels are recognizable because of the double punctiform appearance: the vein is bigger and is located outside, the artery is smaller, denser and in a medial position. These vessels are closely linked with the ureters, extending in front of them higher up and to the side lower down.

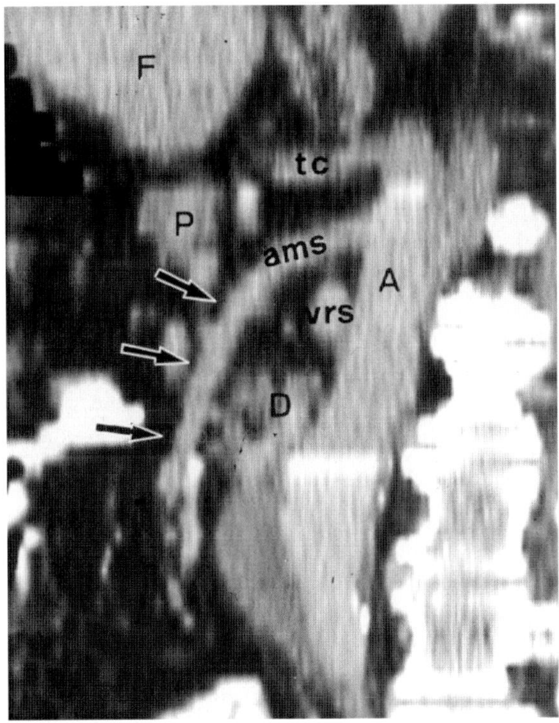

Fig. 4.68. Sagittal reconstruction of the celiac trunk and superior mesenteric artery. The two vessels originate from the anterior aortic wall. The superior mesenteric artery extends downwards behind the pancreas and in front of the left renal vein and of the third portion of the duodenum

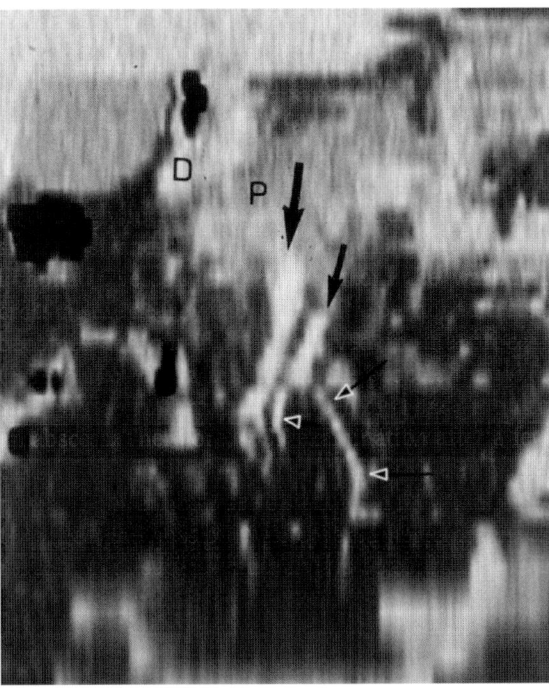

Fig. 4.69. Coronal reconstruction of the superior mesenteric artery and vein. Vertical extension of the two vessels, the vein being wider on the right side (*large arrow*) and the artery (*arrows*) thinner. Bifurcation of the artery in the ileocolic branch (*thin arrow*) on the *right* and in the jejunoileal branch (*long thin arrows*) on the *left*

Fig. 4.67A–H. Umbilical vein, superior epigastric artery, and esophageal veins in a patient with cancer that has given rise to cirrhosis, ascites, portal hypertension and splenic infarct. The umbilical vein (*arrows*), filled and expanded, participates in the outflow of the portal overload. The vessel is made opaque by the contrast medium and is visible along its entire path from the origin at the umbilical level (*H*) up to the junction with the left branch of the portal vein (*D*). In the middle tract, the umbilical vein communicates with the superior epigastric vein (*thin arrows*) (**B–E**). Within the sinuosity of the latter vein, it is possible to distinguish the thread-like image of the superior epigastric artery (**B** *thin arrow*). The esophageal veins (**A** *large arrowhead*) and the short gastric veins (**A, B** *open triangles*) are easily visible

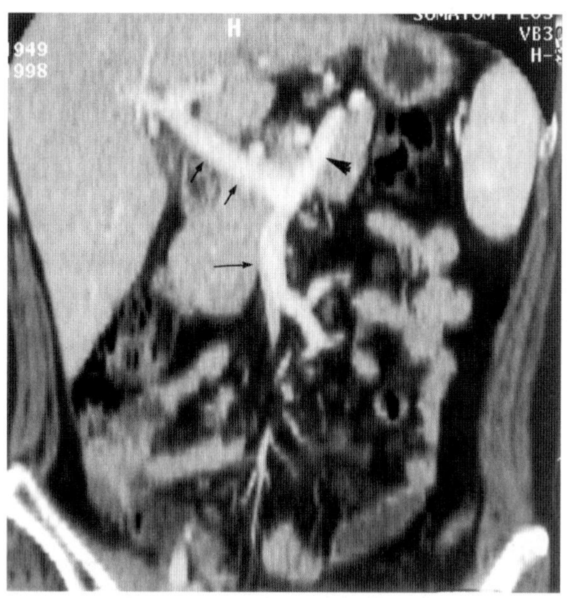

Fig. 4.70. Coronal reconstruction of the portal system. Superior mesenteric vein (*long arrow*), splenic vein (*arrowhead*) and portal trunk (*thin arrows*)

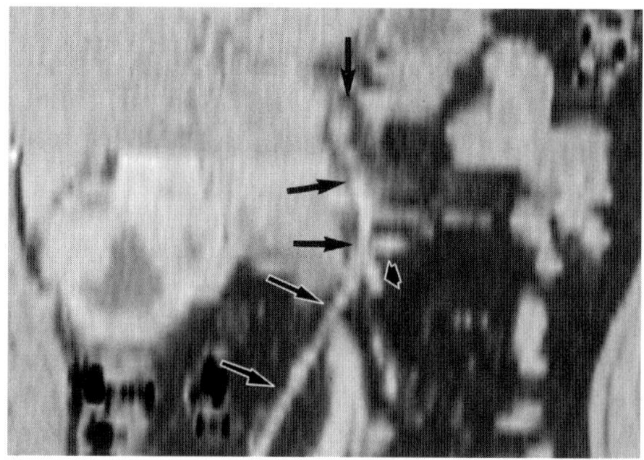

Fig. 4.71. Coronal reconstruction of the superior mesenteric vein. Besides the vessel trunk (*arrow*), we recognize its tributary ramifications: the ileocolic branch on the right (*long arrows*) and the jejunoileal branch (*stubby arrow*)

A

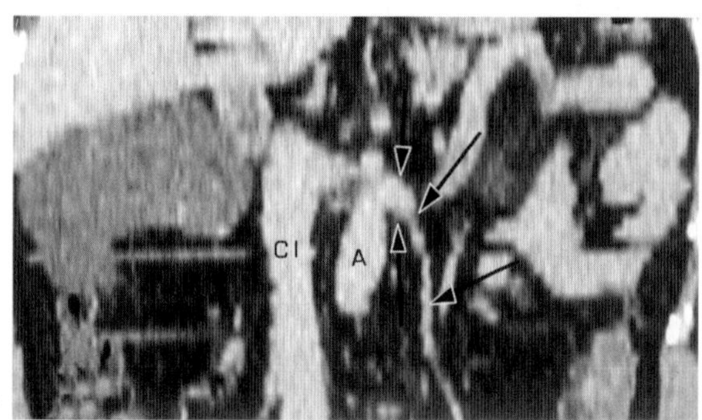

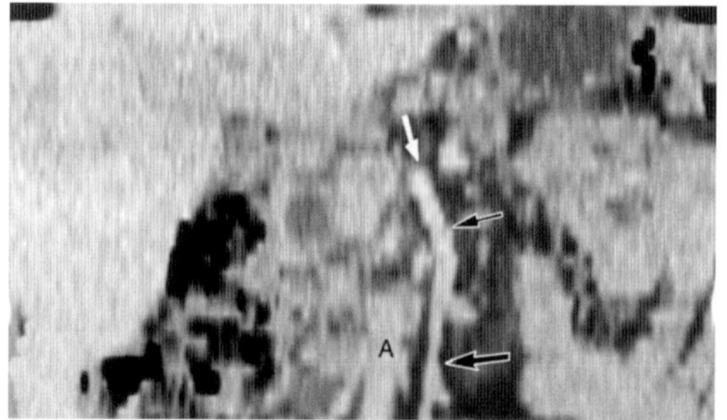

B

Fig. 4.72. Coronal reconstruction of the inferior mesenteric vessels. **A** Inferior mesenteric artery (*long arrows*) and **B** vein (*arrows*)

The inferior mesenteric vessels (the artery inside and the vein outside) are on the left side, in front of the genital vessels and the ureter.

In the presacral space the *median sacral artery* (Fig. 4.101) can be seen, extending along the homonymous vein with a punctiform appearance.

4.2.2 Veins

Mostly, veins and arteries have parallel pathways. Like arteries, veins assume tubular or punctiform aspects; however, they can be distinguished by the greater caliber and the lower density after contrast medium injection (Figs. 4.9, 4.10, 4.38, 4.45–4.47, 4.51–4.53, 4.57–4.59, 4.66).

Our analytical description will be limited to the veins that differ from arteries in orientation, path, and relationships with various peritoneal structures.

a) The *portal trunk* (Figs. 4.15, 4.42, 4.43, 4.70) can be recognized in the initial tract at the confluence of the superior mesenteric vein with the splenic vein, from its ovoid apearance on the side of the upper part of the pancreatic head. Extending upward, it passes progressively toward the right side up to the front of the inferior vena cava, from which it remains separated by Winslow's foramen, and maintains its ovoid aspect up to the transverse fissure of the liver. After its

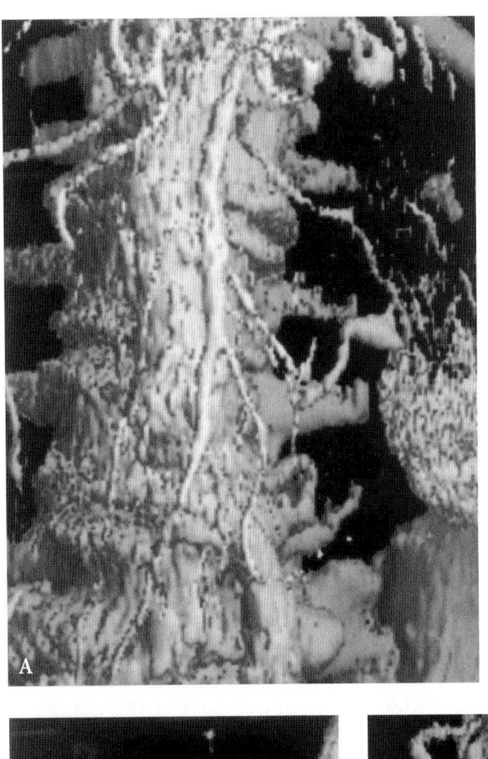

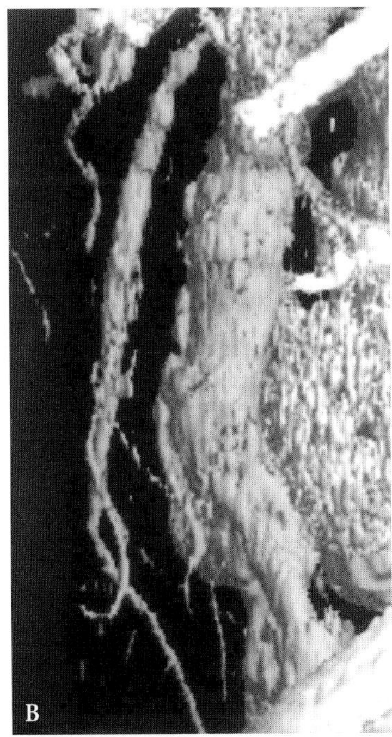

Fig. 4.73A–E. 3D reconstruction of the superior mesenteric artery. **A** Coronal, **B**, **C** sagittal, **D** right oblique and **E** left oblique views

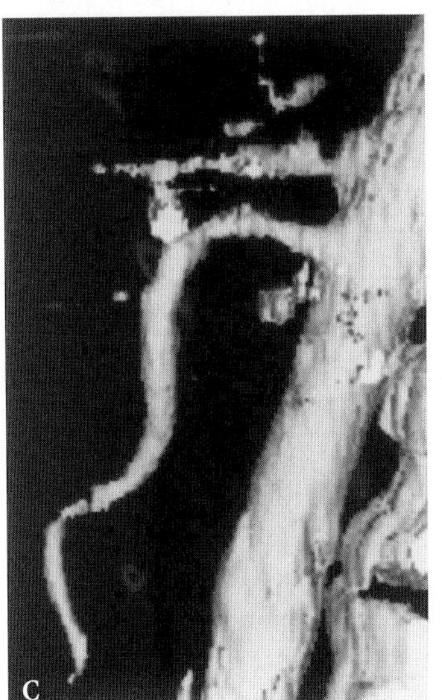

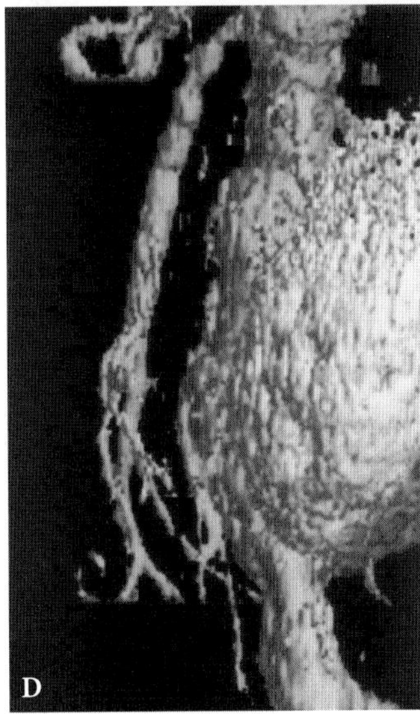

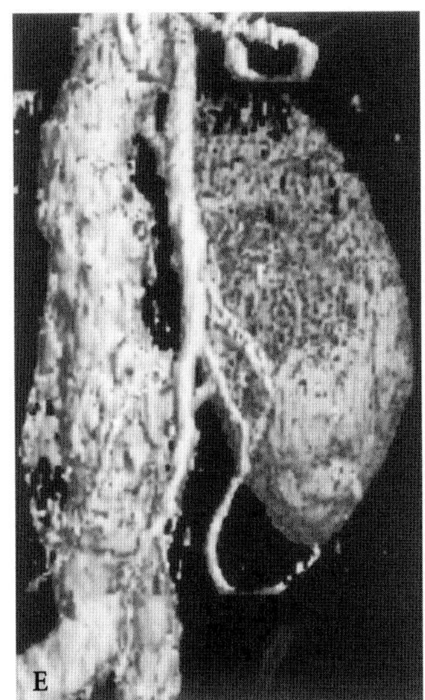

penetration through the porta hepatis, it shows an oblique linear extension within the transverse fissure, in front of the caudate lobe and behind the hepatic duct and artery.

- The *umbilical vein* (Fig. 4.67) becomes visible in the case of portal hypertension, when it is expanded again and forms a collateral circulation with inverse flux. Initially, it follows the path of the round ligament, with a round or ovoid aspect in the vertical ascending tract within the umbilical canal; it is first located anteriorly on the median line, then extends progressively toward the right side and inward, coming close to the supraumbilical fascia and to the peritoneum. When it is close to the longitudinal fissure of the liver it extends with a sinuous tubular aspect on the right side, between the inferior prolongations of the peritoneal leaves of the falciform ligament. Maintaining a tubular appearance, it penetrates the fissure from the front backward, up to its termination in the left branch of the portal vein.

b) The *splenic vein* (Figs. 4.46, 4.47, 4.49, 4.50) extends transversely, with a linear and slightly arcuate aspect, on the superoposterior border of the pancreas, from the splenic hilum to the portal trunk.

c) The *superior mesenteric vein* (Fig. 4.15, 4.47, 4.48, 4.50, 4.52, 4.53, 4.69, 4.70, 4.71) has a round aspect in the upper tract; in contrast with the artery, the vein is located in front of rather than behind the uncinate process of the pancreas, before its confluence with the splenic vein into the portal trunk. Under the superior mesenteric vein, it comes close to the homonymous artery, which it follows on the right side along all its ramifications and subdivisions. Veins and arteries have similar aspects, but the veins have a wider caliber.

The *posteroinferior pancreatoduodenal vein* (Fig. 4.48) is the first confluent branch of the superior mesenteric vein. It shows a punctiform or linear aspect posteriorly or posterolaterally to the pancreatic head; it is close to the homonymous artery at high levels, whereas it is located in more anterior planes with respect to the artery at low level, according to the different position of the two mesenteric vessels at this level, the posteroinferior pancreatoduodenal vessels being connected with the mesenteric vessels.

A variation of the direct confluence of the right gastroepiploic, subpyloric, right superior colic and anterosuperior pancreatoduodenal veins into the superior mesenteric vein is represented by the presence of a *common gastrocolic trunk*, constituted by these veins before flowing into the superior mesenteric vein. This gastrocolic trunk (Figs. 4.17, 4.47, 4.55) is visible in about 90% of cases in front of the uncinate process of the pancreas, where it extends obliquely from the front backward with a tubular aspect and reaches the right anterolateral wall of the superior mesenteric vein. The vein that is most constantly confluent is the *right gastroepiploic vein* (Figs. 4.47, 4.55). After extending along the greater curvature of the stomach, in front of and under this structure, the vein reaches the right side of the gastric antrum and of the pylorus with a sinuous extension; from there it curves backward up to the junction with the gastrocolic trunk. In contiguous planes, it is possible to follow the arch that constitutes the terminal tract of the right gastroepiploic vein and its confluence in the gastrocolic trunk. The *right superior colic vein* (Fig. 4.59) may also merge into the gastrocolic trunk. After having crossed the root of the right half of the mesocolon transversely, with a sinous tubular aspect, this vein extends from behind forward with a slightly arcuate path, and inserts into the gastrocolic trunk. The *anterosuperior pancreatoduodenal vein* (Fig. 4.48) flows into the gastrocolic trunk in front of the upper border of the pancreatic head. Because of its ascending path, it always has a punctiform appeance.

Sometimes, it is possible to observe the gastrocolic trunk and the right gastroepiploic and middle colic veins, whose appearance resembles a Y, in a single plane.

Recognition of the gastrocolic trunk is an important vascular finding, because it indicates the point of confluence of the transverse mesocolic and mesenteric roots.

d) The *inferior mesenteric vein* (Figs. 4.22, 4.52, 4.61–4.66, 4.72) shows a constant punctiform aspect from its pelvic origin up to its termination into the splenic vein, near the confluence of this latter vein with the superior mesenteric vein. The inferior mesenteric vein originates from the confluence of the *superior hemorrhoidal veins* (Figs. 4.64–4.66) (with a tubular or punctiform aspect, at the sides of the rectum-sigmoid) with the *sigmoidal veins* (Figs. 4.64–4.66) in the upper part of the pelvis, on the left paramedian line, in front of the iliac and gonadal vessels, the left ureter and outside the homonymous artery. At the abdominal level, it progressively extends toward the median line in front of the renal fascia, on the left side of the aorta, ureter, and left gonadal and ureteral vessels; thereafter, it progressively moves away from the homonymous artery, extending forward up to the posterior and external side of the duodenojejunal loop. After crossing over this structure, it bends medially up to its termination in the splenic vein (Fig. 4.63) or the superior mesenteric vein (Figs. 4.61, 4.62). In the last tract, it may maintain its punctiform aspect, or assume a linear arcuate form, with posterior concavity and a left-to-right direction.

In the intermediate tract, it receives the *left colic vein* (Fig. 4.63), which often follows a transverse path and has a linear, slightly arcuate aspect, and may be followed along its retroperitoneal extension from the descending mesocolon up to its termination into the inferior mesenteric vein. Afterwards, above the duodenojejunal flexure, the inferior mesenteric vein receives the colic branch from above, collecting the blood flowing from the splenic flexure (Figs. 4.58, 4.61). This latter branch has a tubular or a punctiform appearance and extends backwards and downwards from the flexure to the left paraduodenal space, where it penetrates between the cauda pancreatis and the duodenojejunal flexure and joins the inferior mesenteric vein.

4.3 Lymphatic System

In normal conditions, lymph nodes are not usually recognizable on CT because of their size, which is below the resolution power of the scanners presently in use.

They become visible, with a round or ovoid apearance, only when their density increases in the case of calcification, as a consequence of inflammatory processes, or thickening because of previous or active pathologies of a reactive inflammatory or tumoral nature.

Particularly, lymph nodes can be identified in the transparent subperitoneal adipose areolar tissue of ligaments and mesenteries, where they are located along the arterial paths.

It may be difficult to identify even thickening lymph nodes when adipose tissue of ligaments and mesenteries is scarce: in this case, organs and vessels must be well delineated by contrast media, able to expand and evidence the alimentary canal and make vessels intensely opaque. In addition, the increase in vascular opacity facilitates the distinction of round images that might be interpreted as vessels or lymph nodes. On the other hand, the increased opacity of the walls of the intestinal loops provides the possibility to discriminate parasite images of intestinal loops full of food or liquids, which sometimes simulate thickening lymph nodes.

The *celiac lymph nodes* (Figs. 4.78, 4.79) are located in the retroperitoneum, around the celiac trunk and in front of its bifurcation; they are the last filter before the intestinal duct for the lymph flowing from stomach, duodenum, pancreas, liver and biliary tract. The lymph coming from these organs flows preferentially into the lymph nodes located on the right side of the trunk. Furthermore, there are close connections between celiac and mesenteric lymph nodes.

The *hepatic lymph nodes* are located along the total extension of the homonymous artery; there are *deep* (Fig. 4.76) and *superficial* (Figs. 4.76, 4.77, 4.79) lymph nodes. The former lymph nodes are situated in the deepest part of the transverse hepatic incisure at the level of the subdivision of vessels and ducts. In contrast, the superficial lymph nodes have a close relationship with the hepatic artery, the portal trunk, the hepatic duct and the duodenum; they represent an important lymph nodal connection among lymphatic vessels coming from the liver, gallbladder, stomach, duodenum and pancreas, whether directly or, more frequently, with the interposition of the primary lymph nodes of the various organs. They are subdivided into *cystic* and *choledochal lymph nodes* (Fig. 4.79) in the hepatoduodenal ligament, on the right side of the pancreatic head, next to the punctiform image of the gastroduodenal artery, and in *inferior superficial lymph nodes* (Fig. 4.76–4.78); these latter lymph nodes are located in the retroperitoneum, where the hepatic artery shows a linear appearance and extends horizontally from left to right, forming the last filter before the celiac lymph nodes. In pathologic conditions, it is possible to individuate all the hepatic

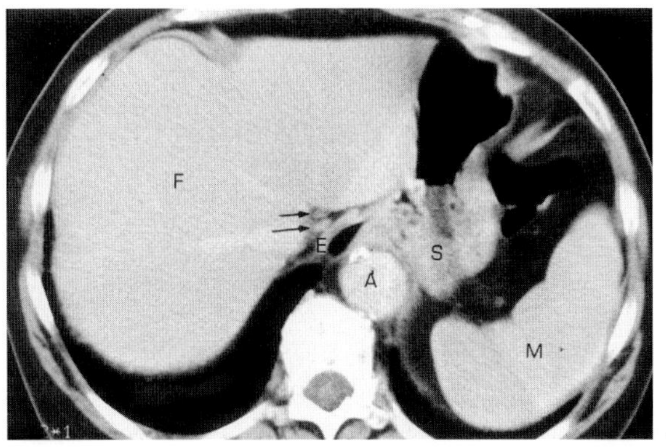

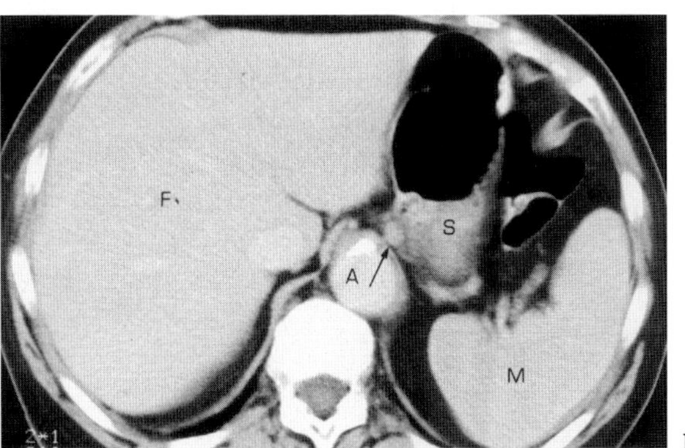

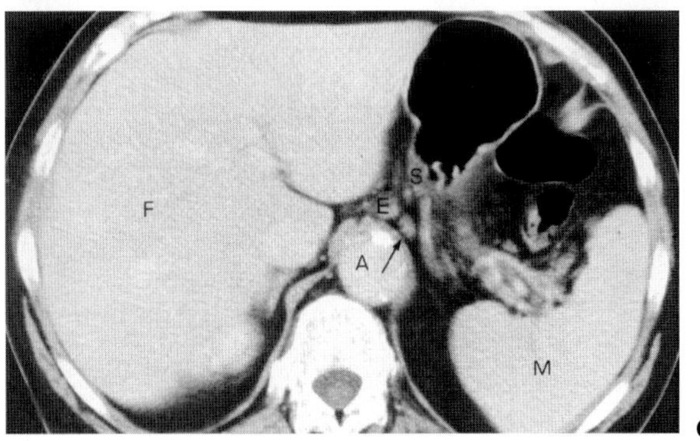

Fig. 4.74A–C. Supramesocolic lymph nodes. **A**, **B** Paraesophageal lymph nodes (*arrows*), located **A** in front of and **B** under the terminal tract of the esophagus. **C** Subcardial lymph nodes

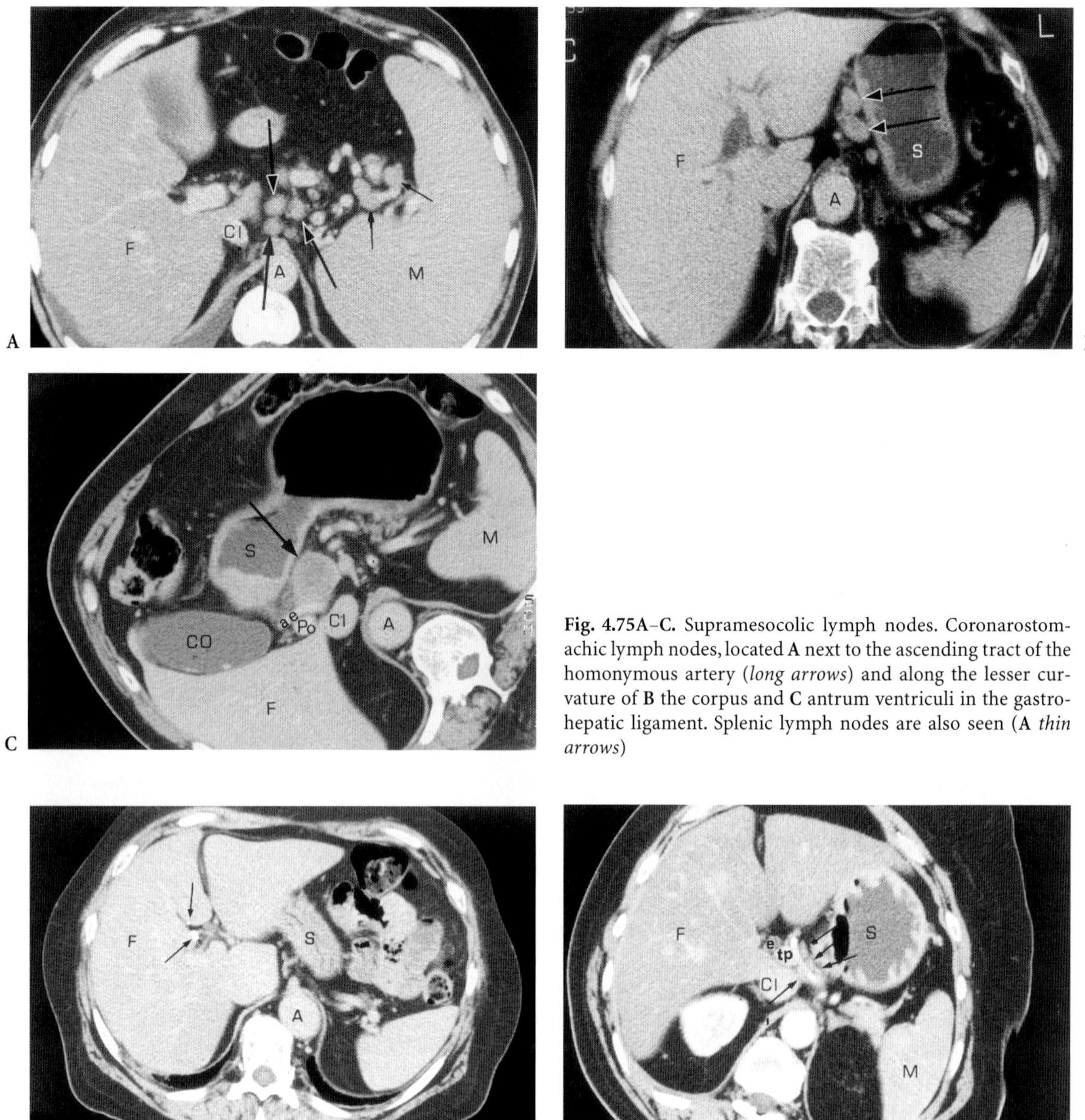

Fig. 4.75A–C. Supramesocolic lymph nodes. Coronarostomachic lymph nodes, located **A** next to the ascending tract of the homonymous artery (*long arrows*) and along the lesser curvature of **B** the corpus and **C** antrum ventriculi in the gastrohepatic ligament. Splenic lymph nodes are also seen (**A** *thin arrows*)

Fig. 4.76A, B. Supramesocolic lymph nodes. **A** Calcified deep hepatic lymph nodes (*arrows*). **B** Superficial hepatic lymph nodes (*arrows*) located on both sides of the common hepatic artery in the hepatoduodenal ligament

lymph nodes from the hepatic hilum to the celiac trunk.

The *lymph nodes of the left gastric chain* (Fig. 4.75) are situated in different planes along the lesser curvature of the stomach together with the right and the left gastric arteries within the transparency of the gastrohepatic ligament. We observe the *supra-* and *subcardial paraesophageal lymph nodes* (Fig. 4.74) in superior planes in front of the aorta and of the diaphragmatic crura; then, in underlying planes, the *lymph nodes* located posteriorly along the *ascending proximal tract of the left gastric artery*, and finally, in front of these latter, the lymph nodes filtering the lymph flowing from the corpus and antrum ventriculi along the lesser curvature.

The *lymph nodes of Winslow's hiatus* (Figs. 4.77, 4.82) are located in the space between the portal trunk and the inferior vena cava within the hepatoduodenal ligament.

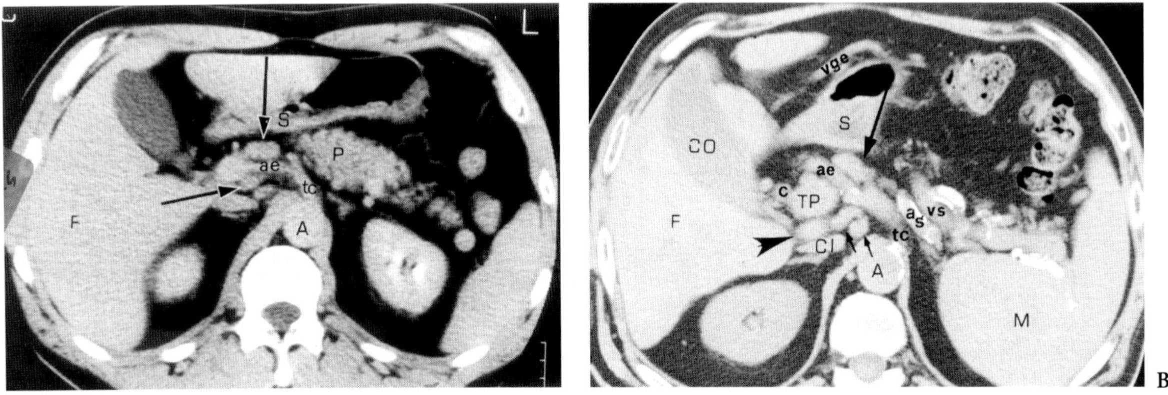

Fig. 4.77A, B. Supramesocolic lymph nodes. Superficial hepatic lymph nodes (*long arrows*) in the hepatoduodenal ligament, on both sides of the common hepatic artery, behind the portal trunk and at the level of Winslow's hiatus (*spearhead*)

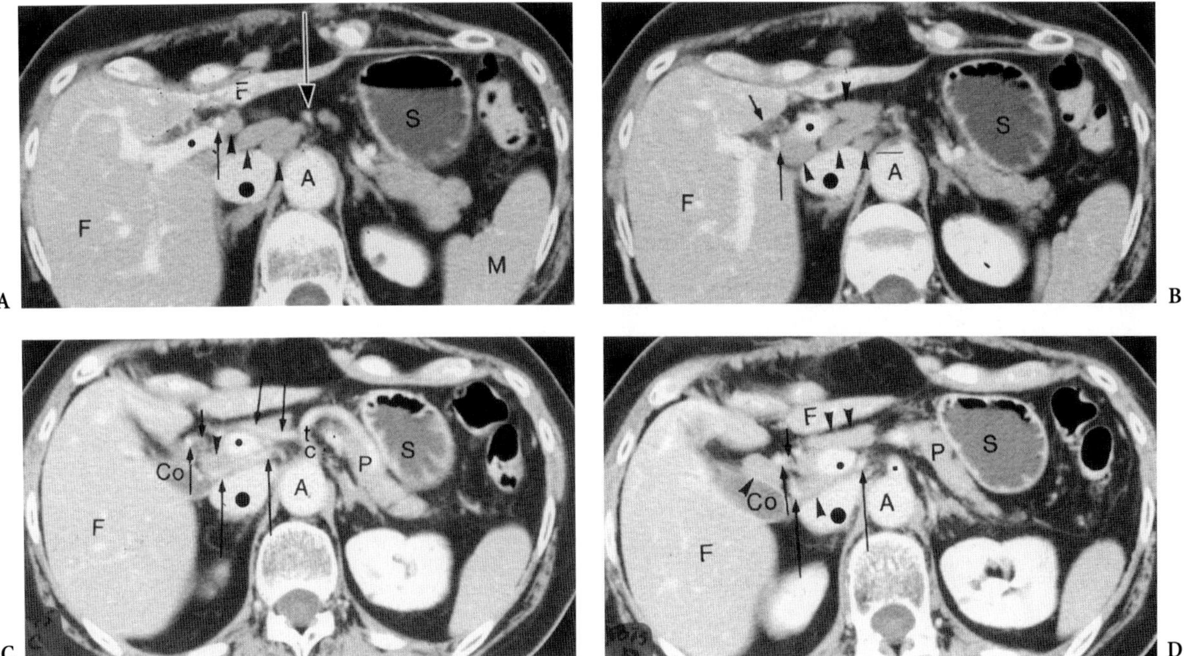

Fig. 4.78A–D. Supramesocolic lymph nodes. Lymph nodes of the hepatoduodenal ligament (*arrowhead*) and their relationships with the biliary ducts and vessels. Biliary ducts (*thin arrows*), common and left hepatic artery (*arrows*), right hepatic artery (*long arrows*) between portal vein and vena cava, coronarostomachic artery (*long thick arrows*), portal vein (*small spheres*), inferior vena cava (*large spheres*), superior mesenteric artery (*small square*)

The *gastroepiploic lymph nodes* (Figs. 4.80, 4.81) are placed along the gastroepiploic arch (constituted by the homonymous right and left arteries), in the transparency of the gastrosplenic and gastrocolic ligaments, and electively receive the lymph from the greater curvature of the stomach.

From above downward, in axial tomograms, we first observe the left gastroepiploic lymph nodes along the extension from behind forward of the relative artery within the gastrosplenic ligament. Thereafter, following the greater curvature of the stomach from the left to the right and/or from above downward, we distinguish the left and then the right gastroepiploic lymph nodes in front or under the stomach, or in an intermediate position, according to the transverse or vertical disposition of the stomach.

The *lymph nodes* of the *gastrosplenic chain* (Fig. 4.75) receive lymph electively from the fundus ventriculi and are located within the homonymous

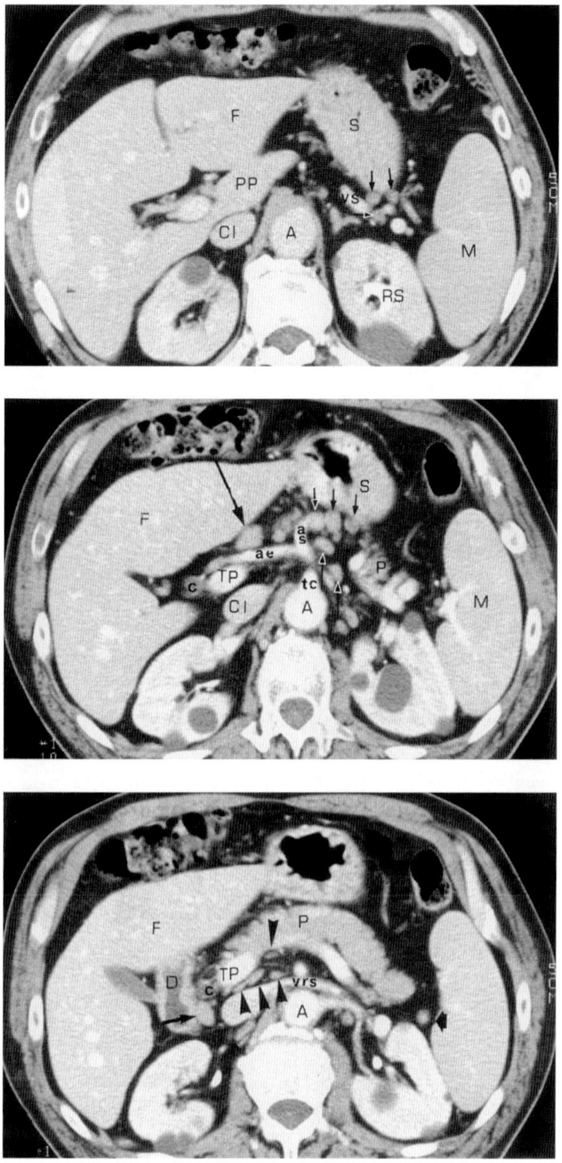

Fig. 4.79A–C. Supramesocolic lymph nodes. **A, B** Superior splenopancreatic lymph nodes (*thin arrows*) along the extension of the splenic vessels; celiac lymph nodes (*thin arrows*) on the left side of the trunk; superficial hepatic lymph nodes (*long arrow*) in front of the common hepatic artery. **C** Choledochal lymph nodes (*arrow*) between duodenum and inferior vena cava, behind the choledochus; posterior pancreatoduodenal lymph nodes (*arrowhead*) between pancreas, left renal vein and inferior vena cava, on the right side of the superior mesenteric artery. Lymph node of the splenic hilum (*stubby arrow*)

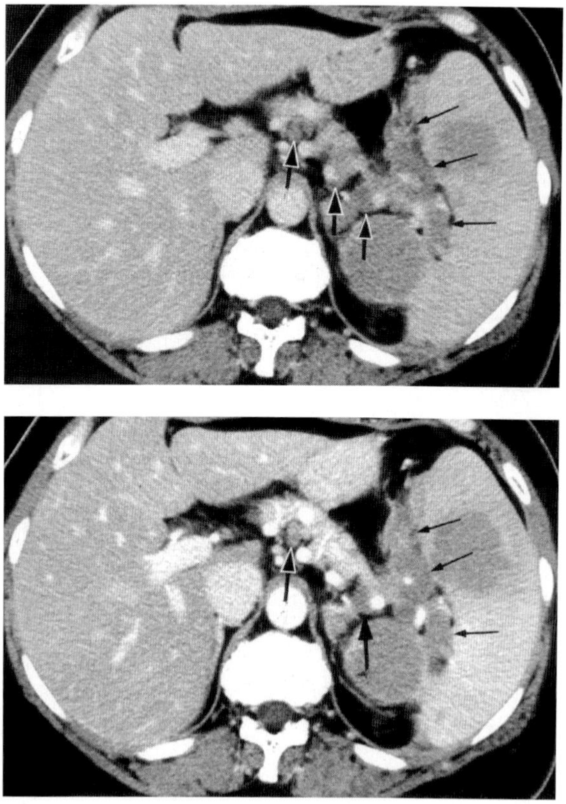

Fig. 4.80A, B. Supramesocolic lymph nodes. Splenopancreatic lymph nodes (*thick arrows*) located along the extension of the splenic artery (transversely sectioned at several points and enhancing with contrast agent) on the superior border of the corpus and cauda pancreatis. Lymph nodes of the splenic hilum (*thin arrows*) and of the proximal tract of the left gastroepiploic artery

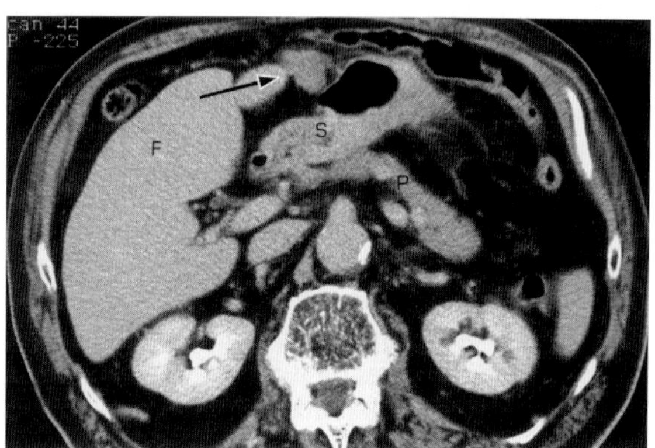

Fig. 4.81. Supramesocolic lymph nodes. Right gastroepiploic bundle of lymph nodes (*arrow*) located along the greater curvature of the corpus ventriculi in the gastrocolic ligament

ligament along the extension of the short gastric vessels, just outside and behind the fundus ventriculi and between this structure and the splenic hilum 1 or 2 cm above the left gastroepiploic lymph nodes that are situated within the same ligament.

The *splenopancreatic lymph nodes* (Figs. 4.79, 4.80) are located in the homonymous ligament within the transparency of the splenic hilum, along the extension of the lienal artery on the upper border of the pancreas. They receive the lymphatic collectors coming from the spleen and from the corpus and cauda pancreatis.

The *pancreatoduodenal lymph nodes* (Figs. 4.79, 4.82) are placed in the retroperitoneum at the level of the pancreatic head, under the hepatic artery, and represent an important connection, which receives the lymphatic vessels coming from the supramesocolic organs before terminating into the celiac trunk.

The *superior mesenteric lymph nodes* (Fig. 4.82) are situated within the mesentery along the extension of the homonymous artery, from its aortic origin at the abdominal level up to the most peripheral ramifications. From above downwards, we can identify:

a) The lymph nodes surrounding the initial tract of the artery, in front of the aorta and the anterior renal fascia, still in the retroperitoneum. They collect the lymph flowing from duodenum, pancreatic head, jejunum, ileum, right colon and transverse colon.These lymph nodes have close connections with the celiac lymph nodes located above; it is not rare in pathologic conditions for both groups of lymph nodes to appear to be affected.
b) The lymph nodes located along the mesenteric vascular axis, subdivided into two groups, anterior and posterior.
c) The intermediate jejunoileal lymph nodes (Figs. 4.82–4.84) and the ileocolic lymph nodes in the transparency of the mesenteric adipose areolar tissue along the extension of the collateral branches of the superior mesenteric artery, without typical localizations because of the high variety in the path and subdivision of these ramifications.
d) The peripheral lymph nodes, next to the right jejunoileal and colic loops, that represent the primary stations of lymph filtration.

The *ileocecal lymph nodes* (Fig. 4.82) are divided into primary and secondary. The primary lymph nodes are recognizable on the internal and posterior side of the cecum, within the pericecal areolar tissue, whereas the secondary lymph nodes are recognizable within the transparency of the base of the mesenteric root next to the ileocolic vessels, which extend obliquely toward the median line and upward, in front of the ureter, the right gonadal vessels and the inferior vena cava.

The *lymph nodes of the ascending mesocolon* or *right paracolic lymph nodes* (Figs. 4.82, 4.84) are located on the medial side of the colon, in the transparency of the mesocolon, next to the right colic vessels.

The *lymph nodes of the transverse mesocolon* or *middle colic lymph nodes* (Fig. 4.82) are placed in the transparency of the areolar tissue extending from the inferior border of the pancreas and of the second duodenal portion forward, up to the transverse colon. They are divided into marginal and secondary. The former are located behind the transverse colon, next to the peripheral branches of the middle colic vessels; according to the situation of the colon, they can be situated above, if the colon is in a low position, or under the bowel, if the colon is in a high position. The intermediate lymph nodes extend along the middle colic vessel trunks, with a transverse path.

The *lymph nodes of the descending mesocolon* or *left paracolic lymph nodes* (Figs. 4.82, 4.84–4.86) are visible on the internal side of the descending colon, next to the marginal branches of the left colic vessels. The relative intermediate lymph nodes are located medially within the areolar tissue of the descending mesocolon, along the path of the left colic vessels extending to the inferior mesenteric vessels, in front of the gonadal vessels and the left ureter.

The sigmoidal lymph nodes (Figs. 4.86–4.88) are recognizable in the transparency of the reative mesentery. The primary lymph nodes next to the peripheral sigmoidal vessels can be visible above the sigmoid or on its posterior side, according to the position, length and sinuosity of the mesentery. The intermediate lymph nodes extend along the path of the sigmoidal vessels toward the inferior mesenteric vessels inside and in front of the ureter and the left gonadal vessels. At the level of the rectosigmoid junction, they are located on the sides of the bowel, mainly on the left side, next to the hemorrhoidal vessels (Fig. 4.87).

The *inferior mesenteric lymph nodes* (Figs. 4.84, 4.86) must be searched for along the extension of the homonymous vessels in deep retroperitoneal planes in front of the iliac vessels, the ureter and the left gonadal vessels, in front and slightly on the left of the aorta.

Pararectal or *superior hemorrhoidal lymph nodes* (Figs. 4.87, 4.88) located on the sides of the rectum, along the extension of the homonymous vessels.

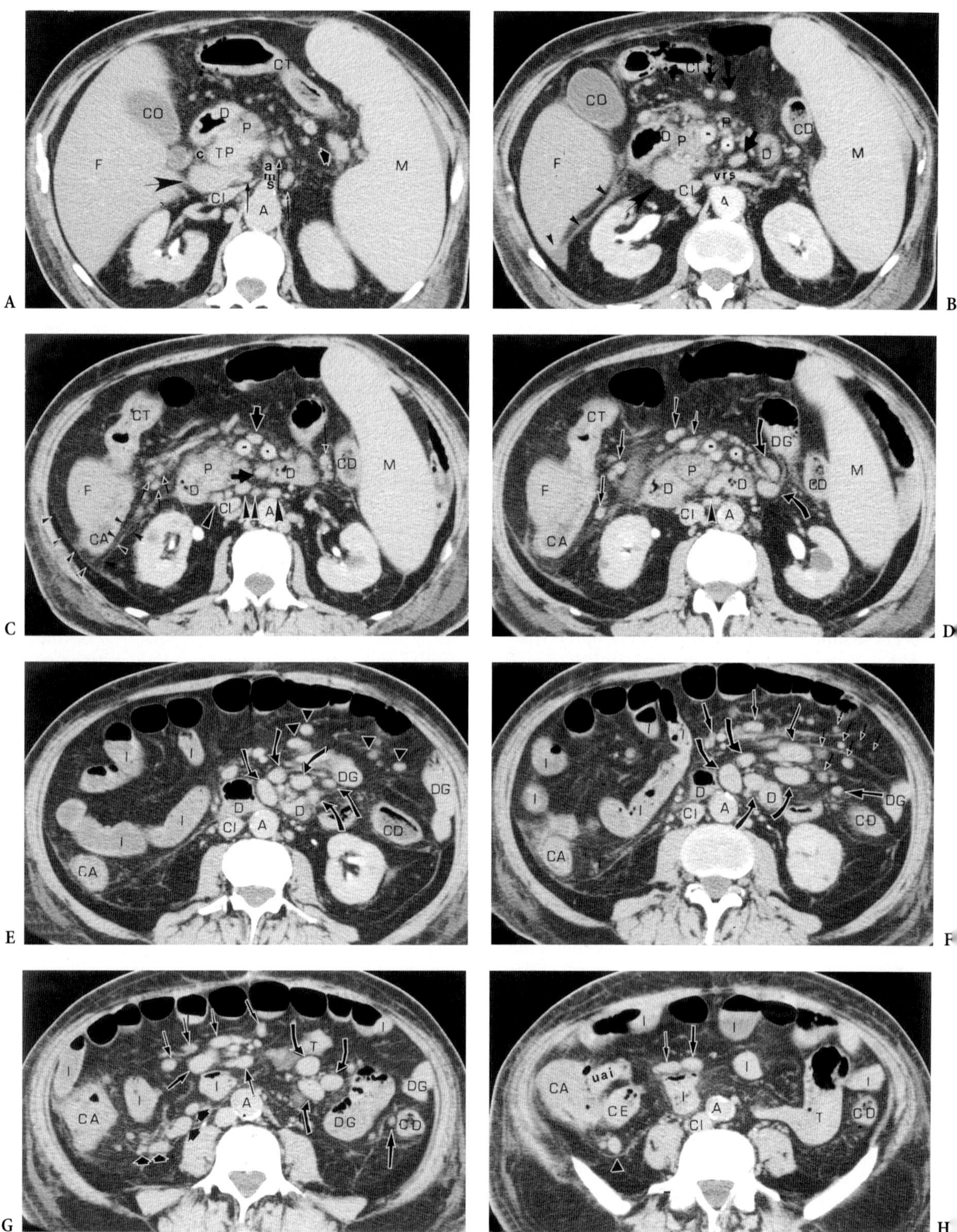
A
CT
CO
D
P
c
TP
F
M
a
m
s
CI
A
B
CT
CD
D
P
F
M
vrs
CI
A
C
CT
P
F
D
CD
M
CI
A
CA
D
CT
P
DG
F
D
CD
M
CI
A
CA
E
I
DG
D
CI
A
CD
CA
F
I
D
A
DG
CI
CD
CA
G
I
T
A
DG
CA
CD
H
I
CA
uai
CE
A
CI
T
CD

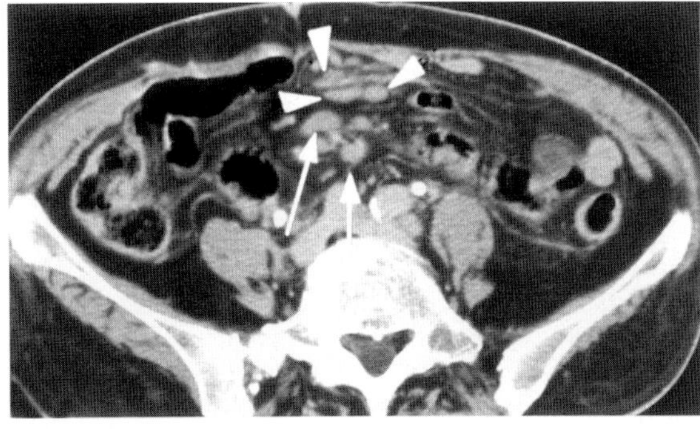

Fig. 4.83. Submesocolic lymph nodes. Jejunoileal lymph nodes (*white arrowhead*) in an anterior plane, and ileocolic lymph nodes (*long white arrows*) in a posterior plane along the extension of the homonymous vessels

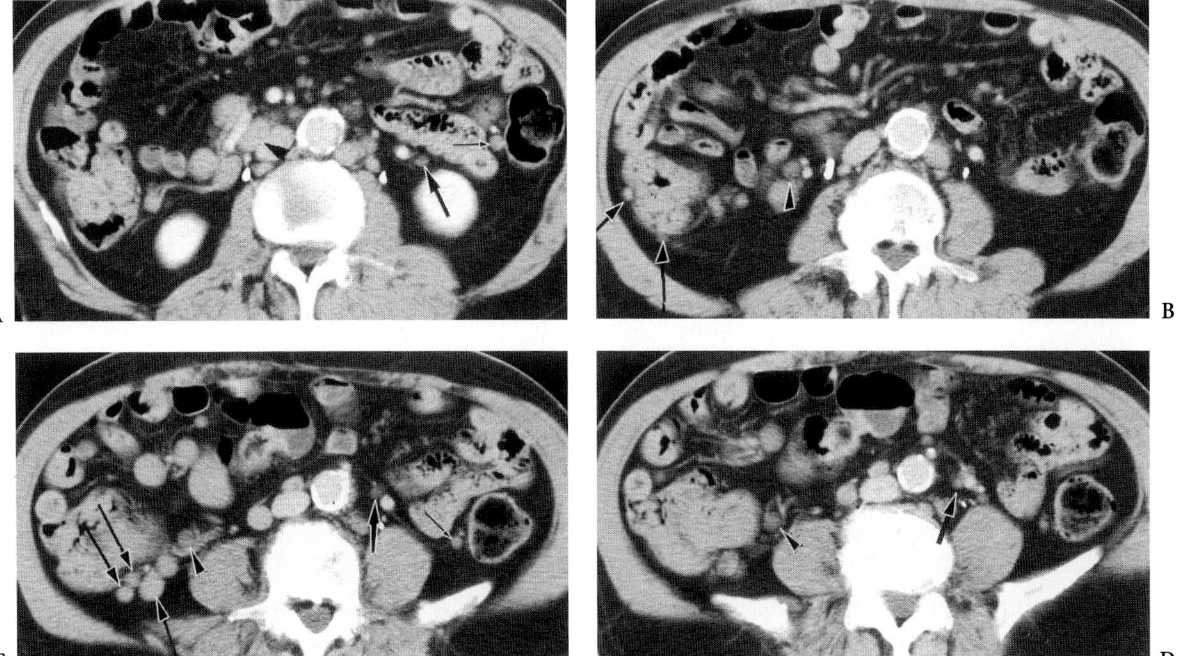

Fig. 4.84A–D. Submesocolic lymph nodes. Right paracolic (**B**, **C** *long arrows*) and left paracolic (**A** *thin arrow*), ileocolic (*arrowhead*) and inferior mesenteric (**A**, **C**, **D** *large thick arrows*) lymph nodes

Fig. 4.82A–H. Abdominal lymph nodes, peritoneum, and lateroconal and renal fasciae on the right side in a patient with non-Hodgkin lymphoma. Diffuse shading of the mesentery and mesocolon. Thickening of the lateroconal and renal fasciae (*small arrowhead*) on the right. A small amount of liquid is present in the anterior pararenal space and in the right paracolic gutter. **A** Superior mesenteric lymph nodes (*long thin arrows*) on the sides of the homonymous artery. Lymph node in Winslow's hiatus (*spearhead*) between portal trunk and inferior vena cava; lymph nodes of the splenic hilum (*stubby arrow*). **B** Lymph node of Winslow's foramen (*spearhead*); superior mesenteric lymph nodes (*short thick arrow*); middle colic lymph nodes (*curved arrow*) in the transverse mesocolon. **C** Posteroinferior pancreatoduodenal lymph nodes (*large arrowhead*); right middle colic lymph nodes (*small thin arrows*). Left paracolic lymph nodes (*thin arrow*); superior mesenteric lymph nodes (*short thick arrows*). **D** Right paracolic lymph nodes (*long thin arrows*); distal ileal lymph nodes (*arrows*), jejunal lymph nodes (*curved arrows*); posteroinferior pancreatoduodenal lymph nodes (*arrowhead*). **E** Left middle colic lymph nodes in the transverse mesocolon (*triangles*); proximal jejunal lymph nodes compressing the third portion of the duodenum (*curved arrows*). **F** Superior mesenteric lymph nodes along the extension of the jejunoileal vessels on the right: primary (*small arrows*), intermediate (*curved arrows*) and distal (*arrows*); left paracolic lymph nodes (*large arrow*). **G** Jejunoileal lymph nodes (*curved arrows*) and ileocolic lymph nodes (*arrows*) on the sides of the homonymous vessels; distal ileal lymph nodes (*short stubby arrows*); left paracolic lymph nodes (*large arrow*). **H** Ileocecal lymph nodes (*triangle*); ileocolic lymph nodes (*arrows*)

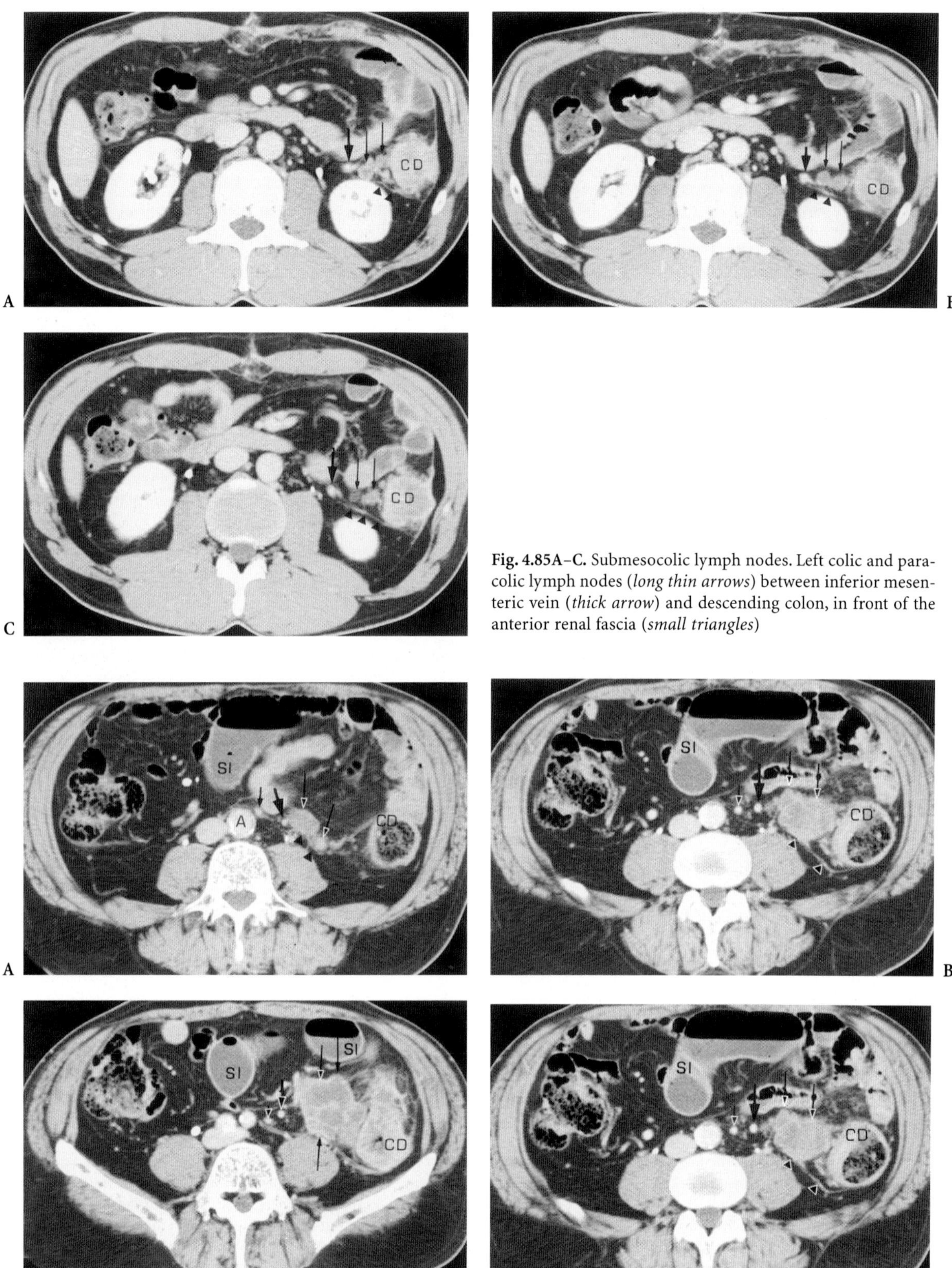

Fig. 4.85A–C. Submesocolic lymph nodes. Left colic and paracolic lymph nodes (*long thin arrows*) between inferior mesenteric vein (*thick arrow*) and descending colon, in front of the anterior renal fascia (*small triangles*)

Fig. 4.86A–D. Submesocolic lymph nodes. **A** Inferior mesenteric, **B, C** left inferior colic and paracolic, and **D** sigmoidal lymph nodes (*long thin arrows*) located among the inferior mesenteric artery (*small arrows*) and vein (*thick arrows*) medially, the descending colon outside and the anterior renal fascia (*triangles*) posteriorly

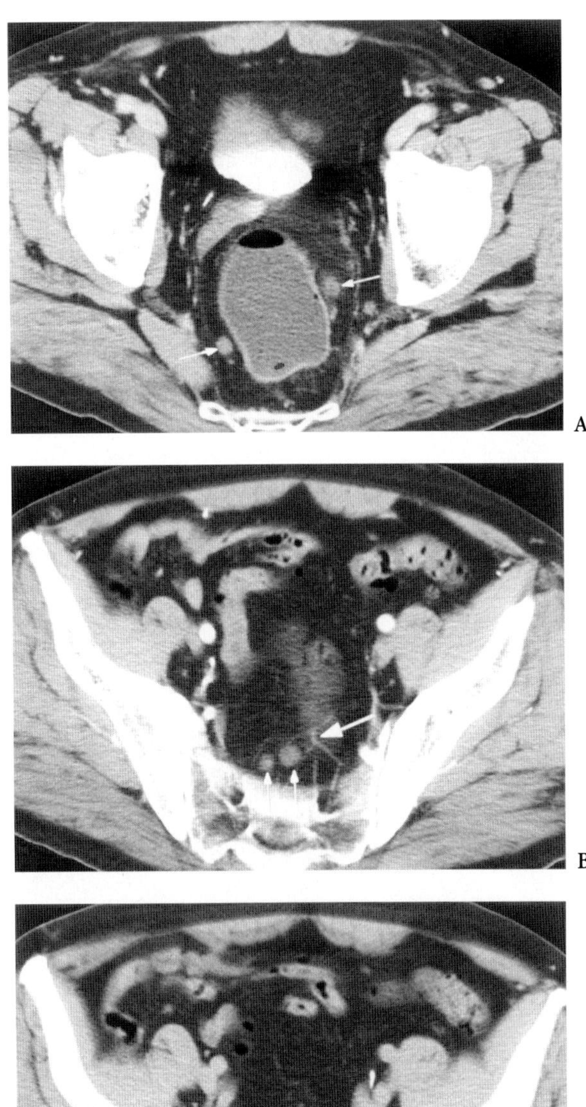

A

B

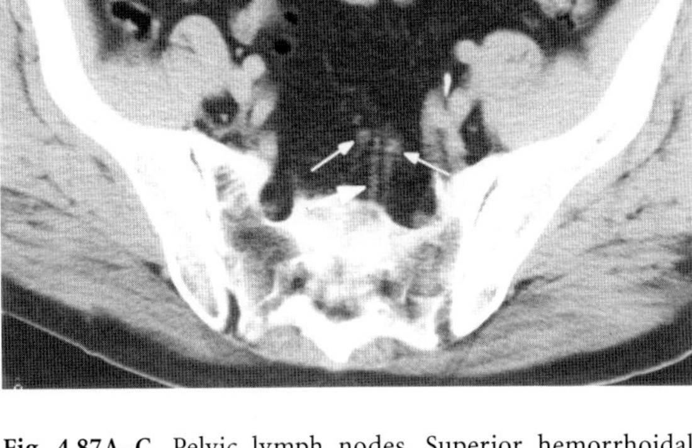

C

Fig. 4.87A–C. Pelvic lymph nodes. Superior hemorrhoidal lymph nodes (*thin arrows*) from below upward: **A** pararectal, **B** at the rectosigmoidal junction, at the sides of the superior hemorrhoidal vessels (*large arrows*), **C** at the confluence of the hemorrhoidal vessels with the inferior mesenteric vessels

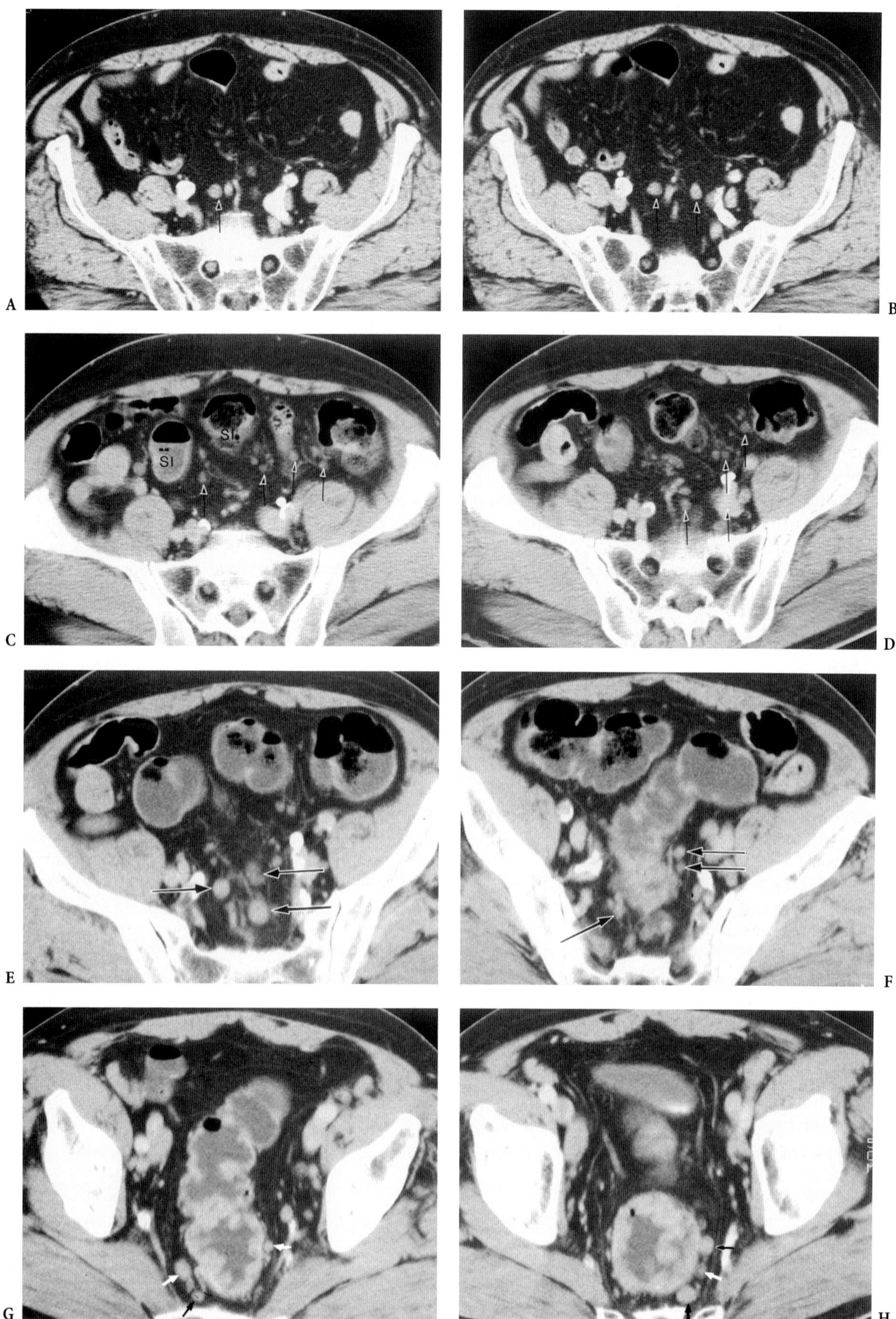

Fig. 4.88A–H. Sigmoidal lymph nodes. Distal sigmoidal lymph nodes (*thin arrows*) located **A–D** along the extension of the homonymous vessels, and **E**, **F** in marginal positions (*thick arrows*) above and on the sides of the sigmoid. **G**, **H** Pararectal and superior hemorrhoidal lymph nodes on the sides of the rectum (*arrows*)

4.4 Nervous System

In normal subjects, identification of the abdominopelvic nerves is almost impossible. Occasionally, the sciatic nerve is an exception.

In order to obtain an almost complete topographical map of the lumbar and sacrococcygeal spinal nerves, the abdominal sympathetic nerves and their ramifications, we utilized the images obtained from a patient affected by neurofibromatosis.

The description reported here is based only on our interpretation of the CT scans, because we did not find any significant reference about this matter in the literature.

In this description, we will first analyze the nervous structures in the upper abdominal planes, where the sympathetic nervous system, with the celiac-mesenteric plexus, and its ramifications are located; then, we will examine the nervous structures situated in lower planes, which are constituted by the lumbar and the sacrococcygeal plexus of the spinal nerves, spreading to the abdominopelvic wall and the lumboaortic and sacral sympathetic plexuses, which innervate the pelvic organs.

4.4.1 Sympathetic System

Going from above downward, we can successively distinguish:

- The *greater* and *lesser splanchnic nerves* (Fig. 4.89A) in the retrocrural space, on the sides of the aorta and medially to the azygos veins on the right and the hemiazygos veins on the left, with a round aspect.
- The *coronarostomachic plexus* (Fig. 4.89A), extending along the ascending proximal tract of the homonymous artery, with a round aspect, in a median prevertebral position in the upper part of the gastrohepatic ligament.
- The *celiac plexus* (Fig. 4.89B–D) on the median line in front and on the sides of the big vessels, with a tubular aspect on the sides of the celiac trunk.
- The hepatic plexus (Fig. 4.89B, C) in the same plane as the celiac plexus, on both sides of the homonymous artery with its pyloric, gastroduodenal, gastroepiploic and pancreatic branches (Fig. 4.89D).
- The *splenic plexus* (Fig. 4.89A–C), also located in the same plane as the previously described plexus, first in a posterior position and then on the sides of the splenic artery.
- On both sides of the aorta in a posterolateral position, we can distinguish the two *adrenal plexus* with an arcuate tubular appearance and, in a lower position, the two *renal plexuses* extending along the homonymous arteries (Fig. 4.89B–E).
- The *superior mesenteric plexus* (Fig. 4.89D, E) is placed in the same plane around the superior mesenteric artery trunk and in front of the aorta; this plexus continues the celiac plexus downwards without interruption. The superior mesenteric plexus (Fig. 4.89F, G, I, J) can be followed on the side of the homonymous artery from the origin up to its terminal tract. The main trunk is parallel to the vessel, has a round form and decreases progressively in diameter during its extension downward and toward the periphery; along its extension, it generates collateral branches. Some of these have a horizontal path and a linear aspect (*middle colic plexus*, some *ileal branches*); other ramifications show a circular aspect (*ascending* and *descending colic plexus*) (Fig. 4.89G, I, J). Mostly, the *peripheral paracolic* and *terminal ileal branches* appear circular and adjacent to the corresponding segment within the mesocolon and the mesentery (Fig. 4.89G, I, J).
- The *inferior mesenteric plexus* (Fig. 4.89I, K) has a circular aspect and can be followed along the side and the total path of the homonymous artery and its subdivisions in *left colic* (Fig. 4.89I), *sigmoidal* (Fig. 4.89L–O) and *superior hemorrhoidal* (Fig. 4.89L, M) *branches*, next to the homonymous arteries. The sigmoidal plexus extends in a horseshoe shape with anterior concavity above the vesica. <At the pelvic level, it is possible to distinguish the hypogastric, middle hemorrhoidal and vesical plexus on the right side.
- The *hypogastric plexus* (Fig. 4.89N) is widely expanded and has a posterolateral location around the homonymous vessels, adjacent to the musculoskeletal wall.
- The *vesical plexus* (Fig. 4.89O, P) has a bead-like aspect and extends along the homonymous artery horizontally and forward on the sides of prostate and urinary bladder.
- The *middle hemorrhoidal plexus* (Fig. 4.89O) is characterized by round and serpiginous images outside the rectum.

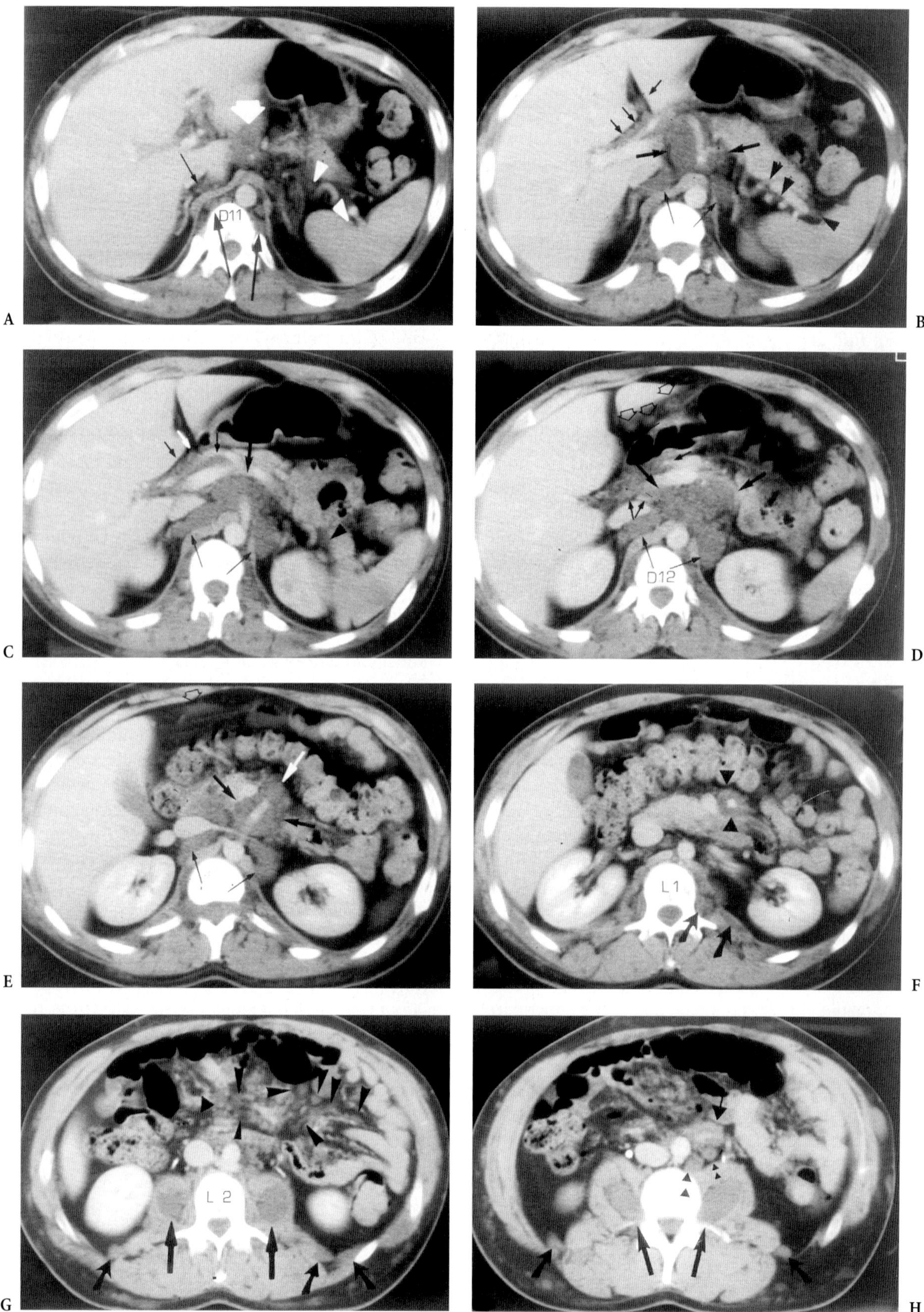
A
D11
B
C
D
D12
E
F
L1
G
L 2
H

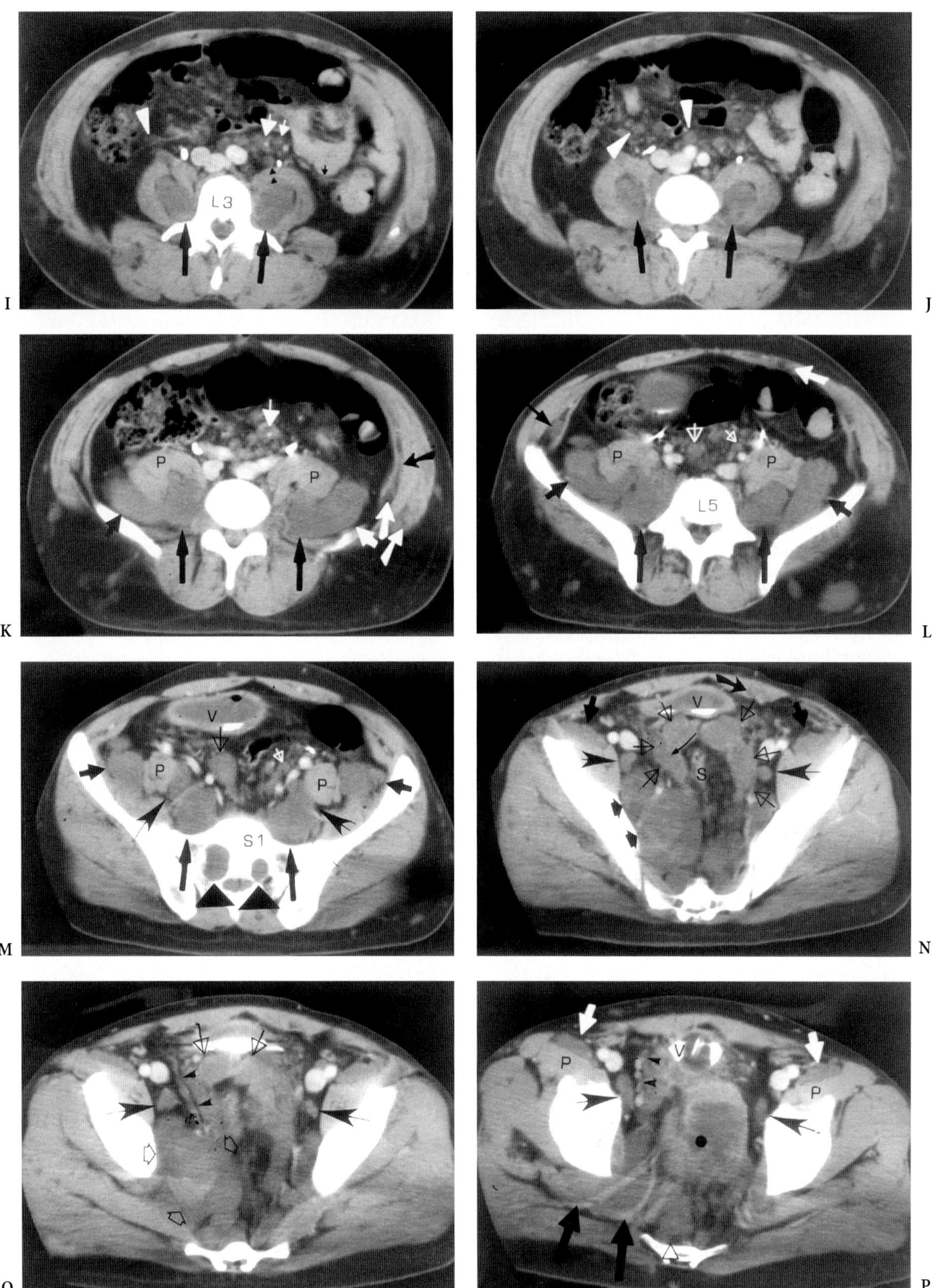

Fig. 4.89A–R →

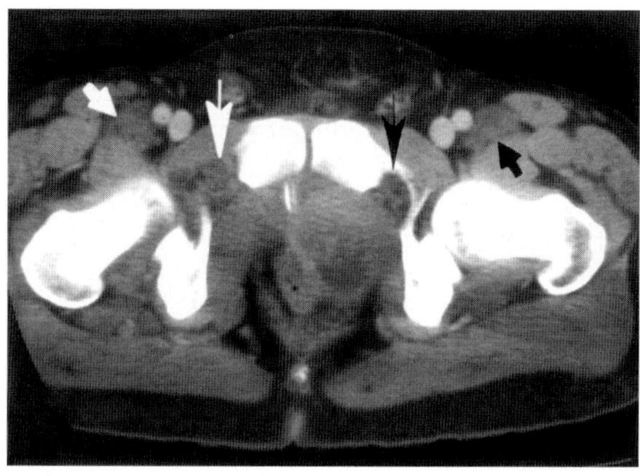

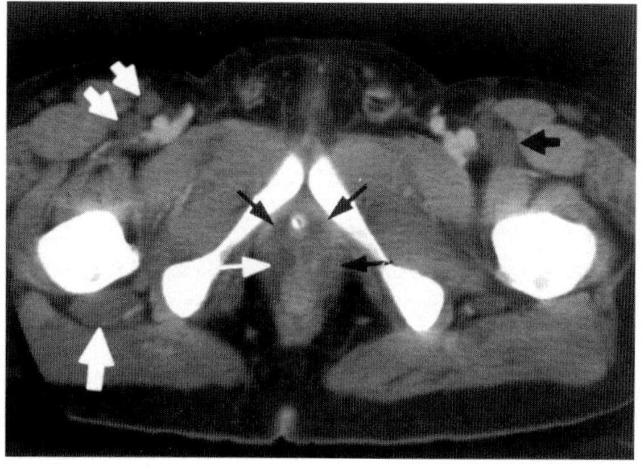

Fig. 4.89A–R. Nervous system. Patient with plexiform neurofibromatosis. Abdominal sympathetic system.

1) Greater and lesser splanchnic nerves (*long arrows*) (**A**) behind the diaphragmatic crura outside the azygos and hemiazygos veins, respectively.
2) Celiac plexus (thick arrows) (**B, C, D**) in front of the diaphragmatic crura and around the celiac trunk.
3) Coronarostomachic plexus (*short thick arrow*) (**A**); it has a round aspect and is located around the ascending tract of the homonymous artery.
4) Hepatic plexus (**B, C** *short thin white arrows*) in the transverse fissure and in the hepatoduodenal ligament; pyloric and pancreatic branches (**D**).
5) Splenic plexus (**A–C** *arrowheads*); only a few tracts are visible.
6) Right gastroepiploic plexus (**D** *open stubby arrows*) between the left lobe of the liver and the gastric antrum.
7) Paramedian renal and adrenal plexus (**B–E** *thin arrows*) in front of the diaphragmatic crura.
8) Superior mesenteric plexus; it continues downwards the celiac plexus (**D, E** *thick arrow*) around the origin of the superior mesenteric artery.
9) Superior mesenteric plexus: trunk (**F** *triangles*) around the homonymous artery and secondary branches extending horizontally and vertically (**G, I, J** *arrowhead*).
10) Inferior mesenteric plexus (**H** *double large triangle*) around the origin of the homonymous artery from the aorta and along its extension on the left side in the retroperitoneum (**I, K**).
11) Left colic plexus (**I** *thin arrow*) outside the inferior mesenteric nerve.
12) Sigmoidal plexus (**L, M** *large open arrows*) and its ramifications on the sides of the sigmoid (**N, O**).
13) Superior hemorrhoidal plexus (**L, M** *small open arrow*).
14) Left spermatic plexus (**H, I** *small double triangles*) extending medially along the ureter.

System of the spinal nerves.

- Lumbar plexus (**G–K** *large arrows*) within the thickness of the psoas muscles and between the insertions of these muscles on the transverse processes and the vertebral bodies.
- Abdominogenital nerves (**F–H, K** *curved black or white arrows*). The left nerve is more easily visible from its origin at L-1 level (**F**) up to the anterior musculus rectus (**N**), and then, between the psoas and the transverse muscle fascia (**F, G**), between the transverse and internal oblique muscle (**K**) (at the level of the iliac crest), between the internal and external oblique muscles (**K**), and finally within the thickness of the rectus muscle (**L, N**) anteriorly.
- Femoral (or crural or lumboinguinal) nerve (*short thick black* or *white arrow*) (**K–N, P–R**): from the lumbar region up to the femoral ring and Scarpa's triangle, at a high level behind the psoas, then on the side and finally in front of the psoas. At the inguinal level (**Q, R**), it is located outside the femoral vessels.
- Obturator nerve (*black* or *white spearhead*) (**M–P**), recognizable because of its extension behind the external iliac vessels on the medial side of the ileopsoas (**M–P**) up to inside the obturator canal (**Q**).
- Sacrococcygeal plexus (**K–M** *large arrows*); it extends the lumbar plexus downward, behind the psoas and the iliac vessels, extending in front of the sacrum on the two sides of the median line.
- Median sacral nerve (**P** *open triangle*) on the median line in front of the sacrum.
- Right superior and inferior gluteal nerves (**P** *large thick arrows*): they continue the sacrococcygeal plexus downward and outward, extending between the muscular fasciae of the greater and lesser gluteus.
- Nerves of the levator ani on the two sides of this muscle and of the urethra (*short thick arrows*) (**R**).
- Pelvic visceral plexus of the sympathetic system.
- Right hypogastric plexus (**N** *short stubby arrow*) on the posterolateral side of the pelvic cavity.
- Median hemorrhoidal plexus (*open stubby arrows*); these nerves are more evident on the right side (**O**).
- Vesical plexus (**O, P** *arrowhead*); they extend along the path of the homonymous arteries.

Neurosarcoma (**P** *circle*)

4.4.2 Lumbosacral Plexus of the Spinal Nerves

4.4.2.1 *Lumbar Plexus*

The lumbar plexus (Fig. 4.89G–K) is recognizable by its posterior position among the psoas insertions on the lumbar transverse apophyses and the vertebral bodies.

Among the branches of the lumbar plexus, we can distinguish the abdominogenital, femoral and obturator nerves, according to their relationships with the iliac vessels and the ileopsoas muscles.

- The *abdominogenital nerves* (Fig. 4.89F–H, K, L, N) come out from the lumbar plexus at L-1 level; first, they extend on the side between the psoas and the trasverse muscle fascia up to the level of the iliac crest; thereafter they turn forward between the transverse and oblique internal muscles, and finally penetrate medially the anterior rectum muscle.
- The *femoral nerves* (Fig. 4.89K–R) can be followed from the lumbar region to the groin; they are recognizable by their relationships with the psoas: extending from above downward first behind, then on the side, and finally, in the femoral ring and in the inguinal region, in the front of the psoas, outside the femoral vessels.
- The *obturator nerves* (Fig. 4.89M–P) are located behind the external iliac vessels on the internal side of the psoas. At a lower level, in the pelvic cavity, they penetrate the obturator canal (Fig. 4.89Q).

4.4.2.2 *Sacrococcygeal Plexus*

The sacrococcygeal plexus (Fig. 4.89K–M) continues downward and without interruptionfrom the lumbar plexus on the paramedian line on both sides, in front of the sacrum and behind the psoas and the iliac vessels, with a multinodular aspect and a very sharp anterior profile owing to the transverse fascia. In front of it, the transparency of the retroperitoneal adipose tissue which separates the fascia from the rectum stands out.

Along the median presacral line, the round image of the middle sacral nerve comes out (Fig. 4.89P).

The bundle of the posterior branches of the sacrococcygeal plexus (*internal obturator nerve, superior* and *inferior gluteus, superior* and *inferior gemellus, quadratus femoris, pyramidalis, levator ani*) (Fig. 4.89M–P), that converges in the greater ischiatic incisure and through this structures comes out of the pelvis, is well recognizable as a unit, but not as single components. Outside the pelvis, some nerves can be followed along a more or less extended tract. In

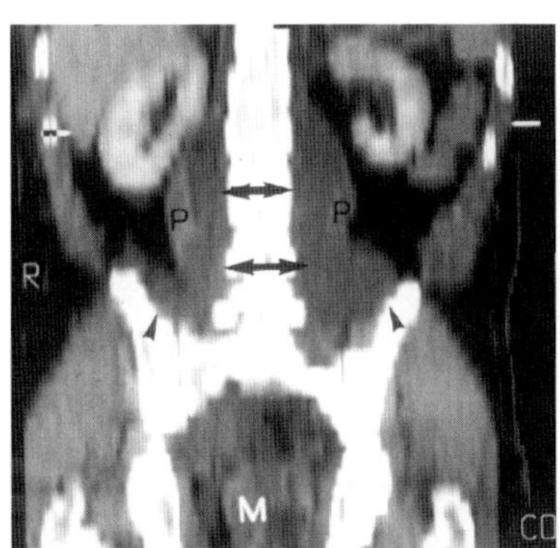

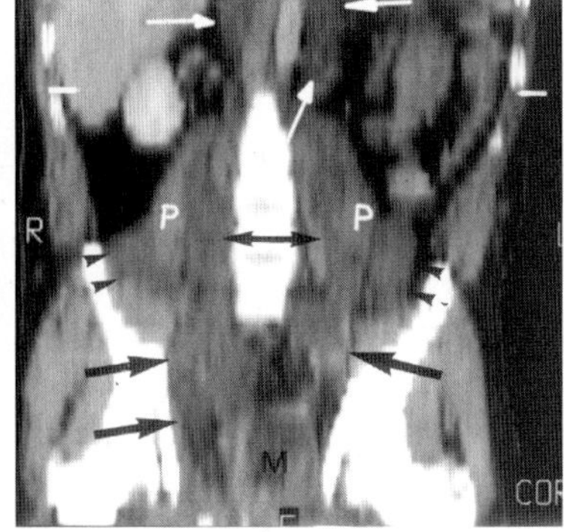

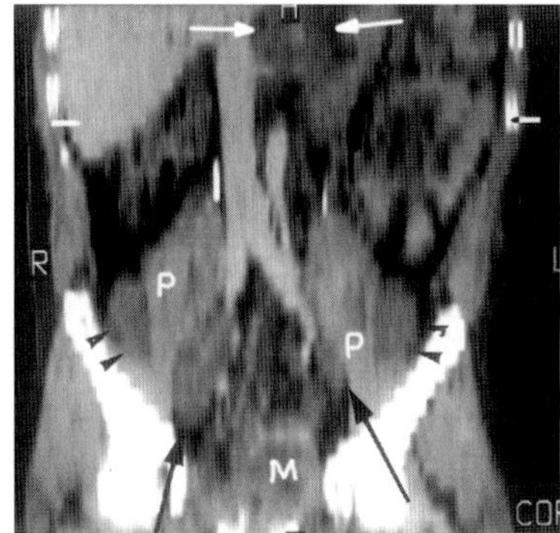

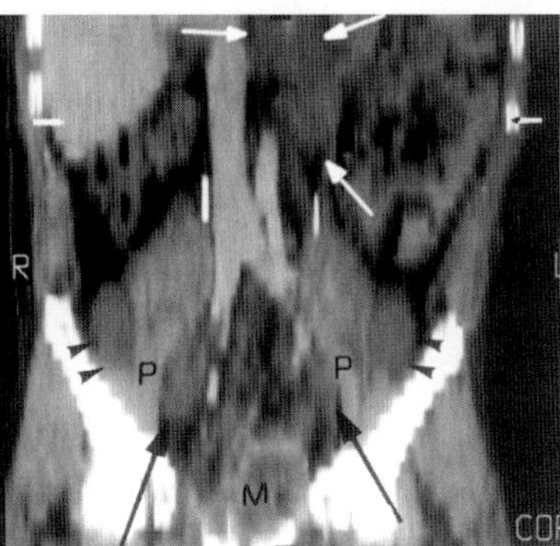

Fig. 4.90A–D. Nerves. Coronal reconstructions from behind forwards. **A, B** The lumbar plexus (*short thick arrows*) between psoas and spinal column and its continuation in the sacral plexus (*long thick arrow*). The celiac-mesenteric plexus (*thin white arrow*) is visible at a high level at the sides of the aorta. Obturator nerves (*arrowhead*) are seen at the sides of the psoas inside the alae ossis ilii. **C, D** The celiac plexus is visible in front of the aorta at a high level At a low level, the obturator nerves (*long arrows*) can be distinguished inside the psoas and behind the external iliac vessels The lumbar plexus extends at the sides of the psoas and between these muscles and the alae ossis ilii, it continuing downward in the femoral nerves (*arrowhead*)

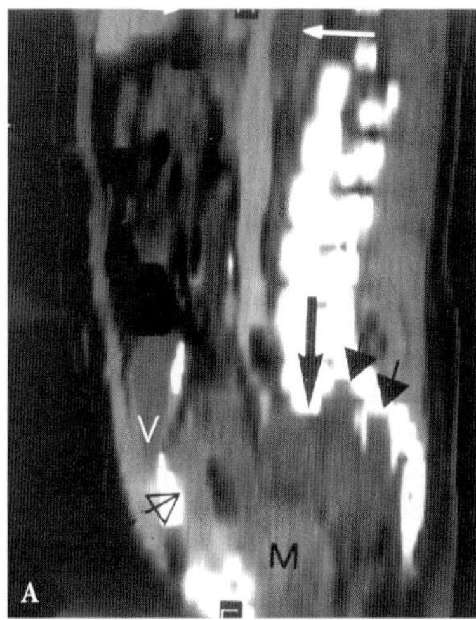

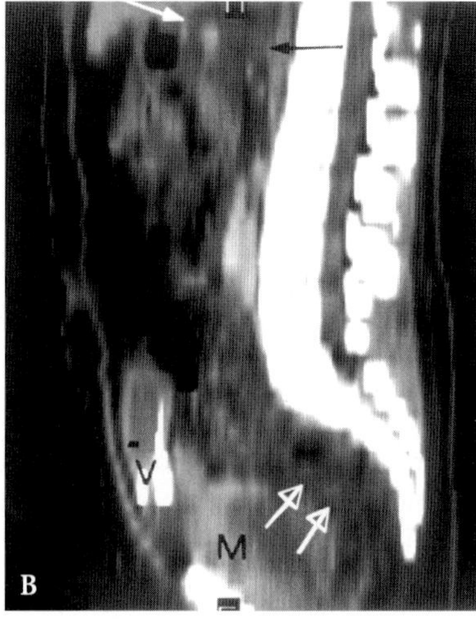

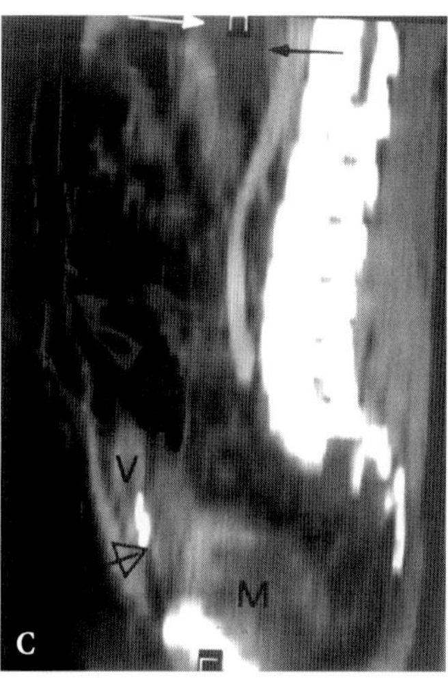

Fig. 4.91A–C. Nerves. Sagittal reconstruction from right to left. **A** Right paramedian section (caval plane): at a high level, the celiac plexus (*long thin white arrow*) is visible behind the inferior vena cava and in front of the aorta; the hepatic plexus (*short thin white arrow*) is visible in the front of the inferior vena cava. At a low level and posteriorly, the sacral plexus (*long thick arrow*) and the right S1 and S2 spinal nerves (*stubby arrows*) enlarging the conjugation foramina. The urinary bladder is pushed upward and is compressed against the abdominal wall by the nervous tumor (*M*); at a higher level, the sigmoidal plexus (*large open arrow*) is seen. **B** Medial section: at a high level and in front of the spinal column, the celiac mesenteric plexus (*long thin arrows*). **C** Left paramedian section (aortic plane): at a high level, the celiac-mesenteric plexus in front of the aorta (*thin white arrow*). The left renal plexus is visible in median planes behind the aorta (*long white arrow*). At a low level, the sacral plexus and the S1 and S2 spinal nerves are observed making an impression in the conjugation foramina (*long thick arrow*). In front of the plexus, the middle hemorrhoidal vessels and plexus are seen. The tumoral mass pushing up the urinary bladder and the sigmoidal vessels and plexus (*open arrow*) is located in the anterior planes

particular, the *gluteal nerves* (Fig. 4.89P) along the path extending among the muscular bundles and the *nerves innervating the levatores ani* (Fig. 4.89R) are recognizable from the close relationship that they establish with these muscles around the anal canal (Fig. 4.89R).

The utilization of *coronal, sagittal* and *oblique* reconstructions gives a complete and detailed spatial representation of the *celiac-mesenteric plexus* and of the spinal branches.

In the median and left paramedian sagittal sections and in the coronal sections, the celiac-mesenteric plexus is located in front of the first two lumbar vertebrae and of the aorta, and behind the inferior vena cava (Figs. 4.90, 4.91).

In the oblique reconstructions, the *lumbar plexus* (Fig. 4.92) appears to be located posteromedial to the psoas throughout its length; in the coronal reconstructions it extends between the psoas and the lumbar spinal column (Fig. 4.90).

In the paramedian and oblique sagittal reconstructions, the *sacrococcygeal plexus* (Figs. 4.91, 4.92) is easily recognizable in front of the last lumbar vertebrae and the sacrum, as a lumpy mass with smooth anterior profile; anteriorly, the transparency of the retroperitoneal adipose tissue stands out.

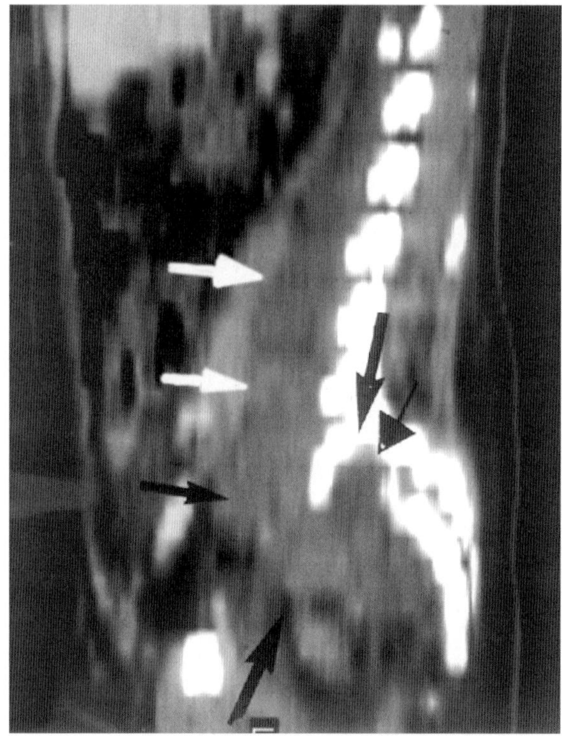

Fig. 4.92. Nerves. Lumbar and sacrococcygeal plexuses (*arrows*) and first right spinal nerve (*stubby arrow*). Left anterior oblique reconstruction

4.5 Extraperitoneal Structures Connected with the Peritoneum

There are some extraperitoneal structures that deserve particular attention because of their close relationships with the peritoneum: – the preperitoneal space of the upper abdomen: the supraumbilical fascia and the umbilical canal; – the subumbilical preperitoneal space; – Tte subperitoneal pelvic space; – the anterior renal and lateroconal fasciae and the anterior pararenal space, and – the transverse fascia.

4.5.1 Preperitoneal Space of the Superior Abdomen: Supraumbilical Fascia and Umbilical Canal

The *umbilical canal* (Figs. 4.17B–E, 4.19F, 4.93–4.95, 5.11, 6.4) appears as a biconvex lens-like structure, with a larger transverse diameter between the abdominal wall and the dense line of the anterior parietal peritoneum, reinforced by the *supraumbilical fascia.*This canal is located between the ensiform apophysis and the umbilicus and is occupied by adipose tissue with a density which is generally lower in comparison with peritoneal fat. Within its context, the punctiform images of the superior epigastric vessels in the upper part, and of the round ligament (Fig. 4.93) or the umbilical vein in the lower part stand out. It is possible to follow his total path from the umbilicus to the longitudinal fissure of the liver (Figs. 4.67, 4.93).

In the sagittal reconstructions (Fig. 4.95) the umbilical canal appears as a low-density band extending from above downwards between the ensiform apophysis and the umbilico and between the anterior abdominal wall and the peritoneum, which is easily recognizable in the median vertebral plane (Fig. 4.19F). In contrast, it becomes shorter and less thick in the paramedian planes (Fig. 4.19E, G), disappearing more laterally (Fig. 4.19D, H).

In the coronal reconstructions (Fig. 4.94), in the point of maximal expansion and depth on the median line in the anterior planes, it appears as an ovoid flat area with adipose density.

4.5.2 Subumbilical Preperitoneal Space

The subumbilical preperitoneal space is located between the posterior aponeuroses of the musculus rectus abdominis and the musculus obliquus abdominis and the peritoneum; it comprises: – the transversalis fascia, – the umbilicoprevesical space, – the umbilicovesical fascia, – the preperitoneal or umbilicoperivesical space, and – the peritoneum.

In normal conditions, the *transversalis fascia* is not usually visible, because it constitutes a unique linear image with the muscular aponeuroses. However, in particularly favorable conditions, it can be observed in the suprapubic region as a thin horizontal line in front of the urachus and the umbilicovesical ligaments, between the transparency of the adipose areolar tissue of the *retromuscular space* and that of the *preperitoneal space.*

In the abdominal tract, the *umbilicovesical fascia* cannot be distinguished from the transversalis fascia, because the two fasciae are divided only by the very thin interstice containing the adipose tissue of the *umbilicoprevesical space.*

The *umbilicoperivesical* or *preperitoneal space* (Figs. 4.5, 4.6, 4.8–4.10, 4.19) is usually well defined in subjects with sufficient amount of adipose tissue as a thin transparent transverse interstice between the anterior abdominal wall and the thin dense line of the parietal peritoneum; in this space, the punctiform images of the *median umbilicovesical ligament* (*urachus*) on the median line, of the *inferior epigastric vessels* on the sides, and occasionally, of the *lateral umbilicovesical ligaments* in an intermediate position, are identifiable.

The *median umbilicovesical ligament* (urachus) (Figs. 4.6, 4.10, 4.11, 4.33, 4.100) shows a fairly elevated density and is identifiable in the recess of the anterior abdominal wall, which is located behind the linea alba between the expansions of the bundles of the abdominal rectus muscles, where the adipose tissue is usually abundant.

The *lateral umbilicovesical ligaments* are very small and are not easily recognizable in the superior part at paraumbilical level on both sides of the median line; they become more and more evident as they move away, extending downwards and backwards up to the two sides of the urinary bladder. When liquid is present in the peritoneal cavity, they appear as two symmetrical paramedian incisures imprinting the peritoneum (Figs. 4.32, 4.33).

Outside these ligaments, in the triangular space of the *inguinocrural fossae*, we observe the *lower epigastric vessels* (Figs. 4.5–4.10, 4.32, 4.99), which show a punctiform aspect in pairs or in a group of three. They can be followed along their total extension from the external iliac vessels up to the highly located point, where they cross the transversalis fascia to penetrate the rectus muscle. Here, they produce a small inflexion in the covering peritoneum, but this

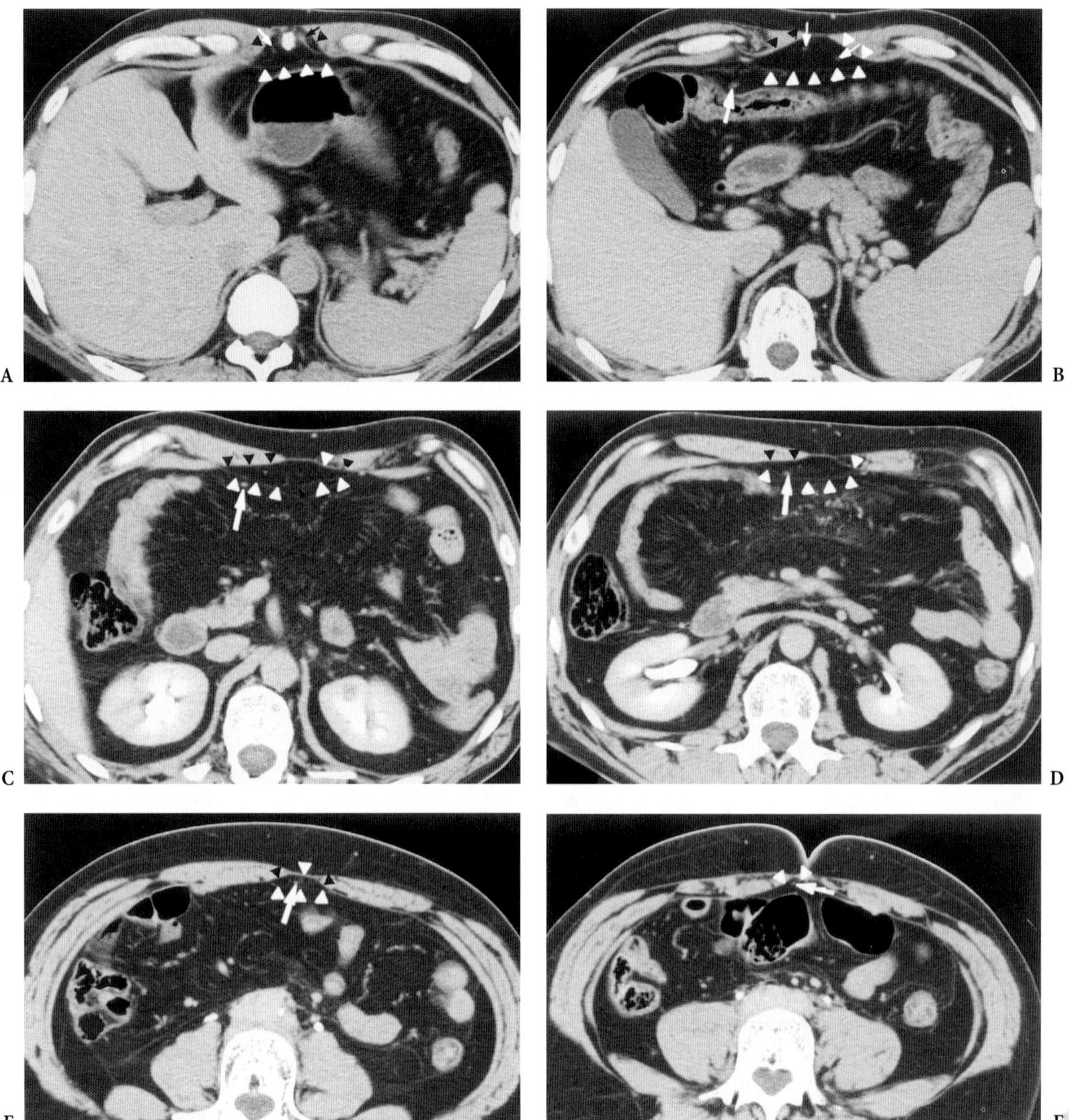

Fig. 4.93A–F. Umbilical canal, supraumbilical fascia and round ligament. The umbilical canal (*white triangles*) is located behind the linea alba, among the inflexion of the rectus abdominis muscle, the ensiform apophysis (**A**) and the umbilicus (**F**). It is limited posteriorly by the dense line of the parietal peritoneum thickened by the supraumbilical fascia; it has the aspect of a biconvex lens with a major transverse diameter and is occupied by adipose tissue. At a high level inside, the dense punctiform images of the superior epigastric vessels can be distinguished (**A–C** *short thin arrows*). The dense punctiform image of the round ligament (**B–D** *white arrow*) is visible along its total extrahepatic extension, surrounded by a thin fascia (**B, C** continuation of the falciform ligament) up to the umbilical canal (**D**) and to the umbilicus (**E, F**)

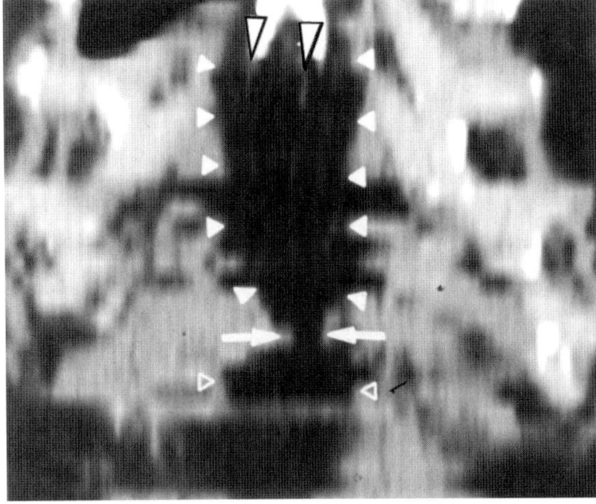

Fig. 4.94. Umbilical canal. Coronal reconstruction. Vertically extended median disposition of the umbilical canal (*triangles*). At the umbilical level (*arrows*), the canal narrows to a cuneiform stricture, expanding again in the umbilicovesical space (*open triangles*). At a high level, the superior epigastric vessels are seen (*arrowheads*)

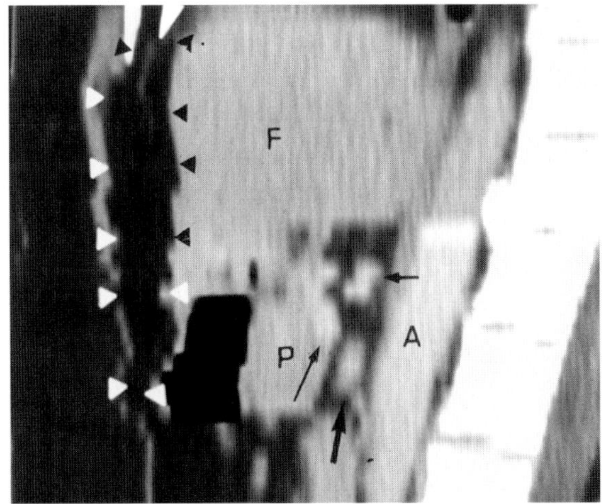

Fig. 4.95. Umbilical canal. Median sagittal reconstruction. The umbilical canal (*triangles*) is visible between the ensiform apophysis and the umbilico, behind the linea alba and in front of the liver and the stomach. At a high level, we observe the superior epigastric vessels (*arrowhead*)

A

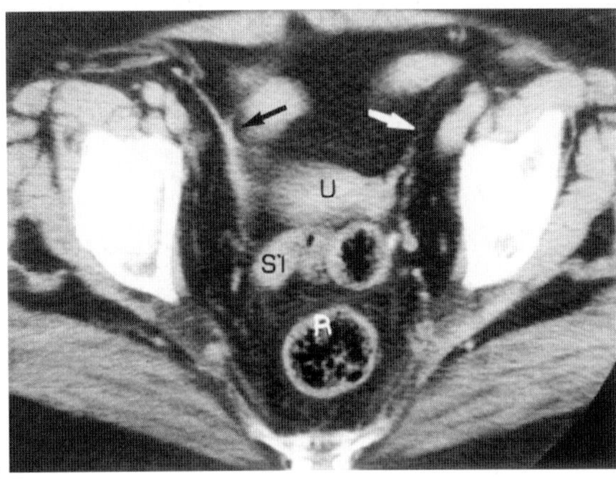

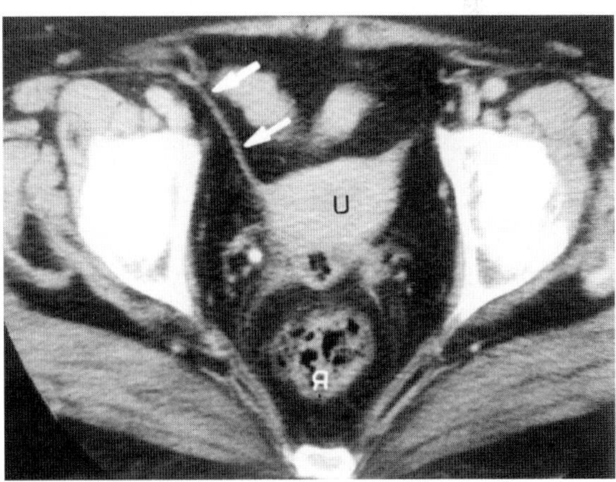

B

Fig. 4.96. Subperitoneal pelvic spaces, fasciae and ligaments (woman). Round ligaments (*arrows*) extending forward and outward from the lateral cornua of the fundus uteri toward the inguinal canals

inflexion is visible only when the intraperitoneal liquid is abundant (Fig. 4.32).

The *parietal peritoneum* (Figs. 4.5–4.11) appears as a thin dense linear image that extends along the abdominal wall both anteriorly and on the sides and is located between the transparencies of the pre- and intraperitoneal adipose tissue.

4.5.3 Subperitoneal Pelvic Space

The subperitoneal pelvic space corresponds to the transparency of the adipose tissue located on the sides of the pelvic organs (urinary bladder, uterus or seminal vesicles, prostate, rectum) and confined outside by the transversalis fascia covering the musculoskeletal structures of the pelvic wall.

In favorable conditions, we can recognize the crossing fasciae, ligaments and vessels, and the subdivision spaces that make it up.

In normal conditions its upper limits are always indefinite and only the presence of liquid in the peritoneal recesses (supra-, para- and retrovesical, retrouterine and pararectal) clearly delineates its contours.

In the transparenct image of the subperitoneal adipose areolar tissue, at the sides of the pelvic

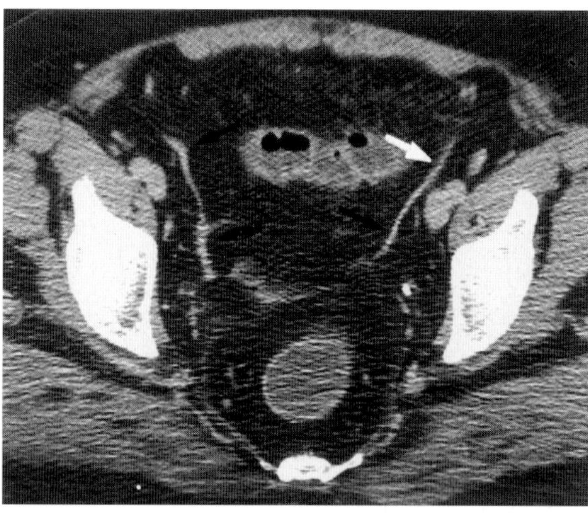

Fig. 4.97. Pelvic ligaments (woman). The round ligaments (*arrows*) located symmetrically on both sides of the pelvis

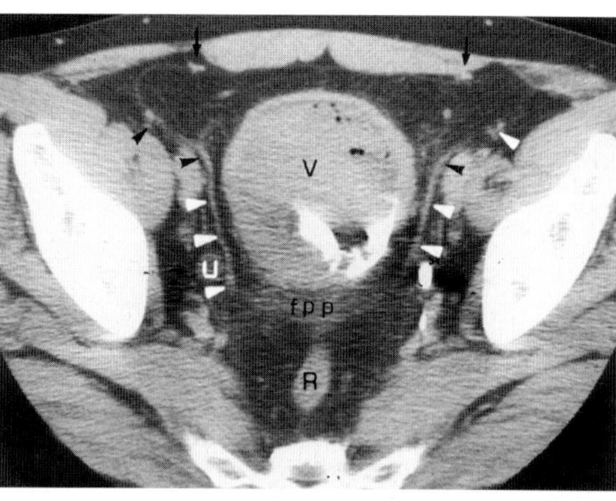

Fig. 4.99. Pelvic structures (man). Deferent structures (*arrowhead*): characteristic extension of the seminal vesicles toward the inguinal canal along the lateral border of the peritoneum, medially to the external iliac vessels and to the ureter. Inferior epigastric vessels are seen (*arrows*) anteriorly, in front of the dense linear image of the peritoneum

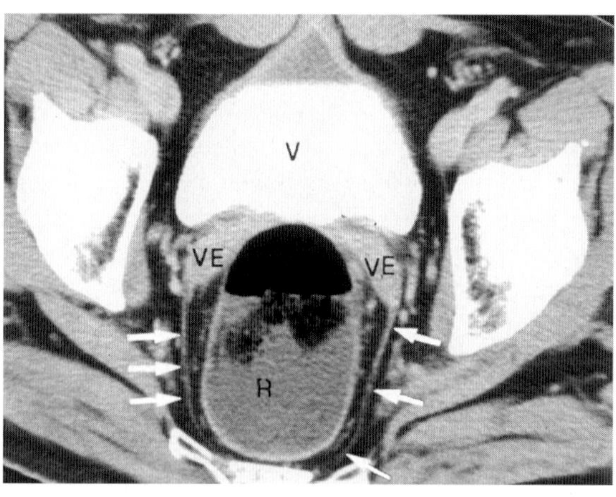

Fig. 4.98. Pelvic fasciae and ligaments (man). Denonvilliers' fascia surrounding the seminal vesicles (*VE*). The vesicosacral ligaments (*arrows*) extend from the lateral border of the seminal vesicles to the sacrum, merging with the sacro-recto-genito-pubic fascia

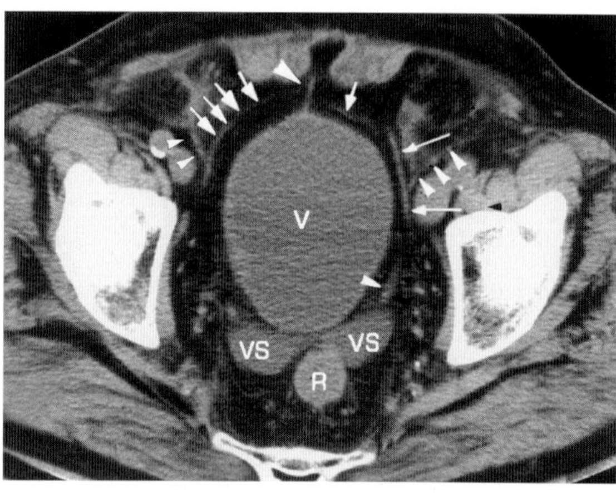

Fig. 4.100. Pelvic structures (man). Median umbilicovesical ligament (urachus) at the insertion point on the vesical cupula (*large arrowhead*). The umbilicovesical fascia (*small arrows*) shows a semicircular disposition in front of the urinary bladder, dividing the prevesical space (anteriorly) from the perivesical space (posteriorly). The left lateral umbilicovesical ligament (*long thin arrows*) extends along the left vesical wall. *Left*: deferent structures (*small arrowhead*) from the seminal vesicles to the inguinal canal

organs, it is subdivided into secondary spaces by the linear images of the fibrovascular laminae.

These laminae comprise: – the sacro-recto-genito-pubic ligaments or internal fascia; – the umbilicovesical fascia; – the lateral umbilicovesical ligaments; – the genital ligaments in women: (a) the broad and round ligaments, (b) the vesicogenital ligaments, (c) the cardinal or transverse cervical ligaments, (d) the uterosacral and uterolumbar ligaments; and – the genital ligaments in men: (a) the prostatoperitoneal fascia of Denonvilliers, (b) the vesicosacral ligaments; and the lateral ligaments of the rectum.

The *sacro-recto-genito-pubic ligaments* or *internal fascia* (Figs. 4.98, 4.101–4.103) appear as two dense sagittal bands between sacrum and pubis separating

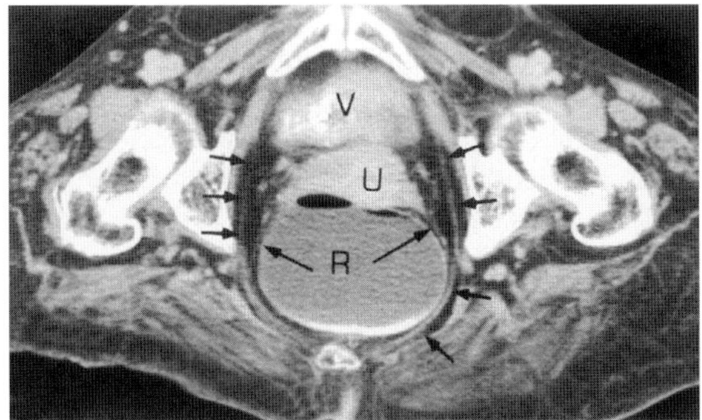

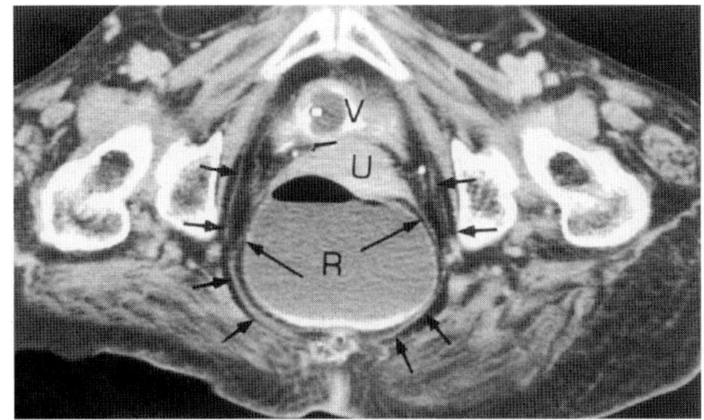

Fig. 4.101. Pelvic fasciae and spaces (woman). The sacro-recto-genito-pubic fasciae (*short arrows*) are located symmetrically on both sides and are separated from the musculoskeletal wall by the transparency of the laterorectal space. On the median line: urinary bladder, uterus and rectum. Among fasciae and pelvic organs, on both sides the superior vesical vessels can be recognized anteriorly and the uterosacral ligaments (*long arrows*) are seen extending from the external margins of the uterus backward and outward and then merging with the sacro-recto-genito-pubic fasciae on the side of the rectum. The umbilicoprevesical space is located inside the sacro-recto-genito-pubic fasciae, between these and the umbilicovesical fascia surrounding the urinary bladder on three sides and extending backward up to the rectum The pre- and retrorectal spaces are located around the rectum inside the uterosacral ligaments and the sacro-recto-genito-pubic fasciae Between rectum and coccyx a thin transverse lamella can be observed separating the retrorectal space from the presacral space, where the median sacral vessels are located

the lateral subperitoneal (or laterorectal) pelvic adipose spaces, where vessels, lymph nodes and external iliac and hypogastric nerves stand out from the medial adipose spaces surrounding the pelvic organs.The sacro-recto-genito-pubic ligaments are more easily visible in the posterior half of the pelvis, where they merge with the vesicosacral ligaments in men and the uterosacral and vaginosacral ligaments in women.

The *umbilicovesical fascia* (Figs. 4.33, 4.100–4.102) is not visible in the abdominal tract because it adheres to the transversalis fascia. In contrast, in the prevesical tract, where it moves away and extends posteriorly, it appears as a thin semicircular line with a posterior concavity, which is limited anteriorly by the transparency of the adipose tissue of the prevesical space and inside by the perivesical fat (Fig. 4.100). This linear image may be strengthened by the parietal peritoneum, which descends in front of the urinary bladder with both sides raised by the umbilicovesical ligaments. In this case, the punctiform images of the omental vessels are recognizable within the adipose tissue located behind the fascia.

Its posterior continuation along the lateral face of the cervix of the uterus (or of the seminal vesicles and prostate in men) and of the rectum is only occasionally visible in normal subjects, whereas it becomes easily visible as the medial limit in the extraperitoneal urinary collections.

The *lateral umbilicovesical ligaments* (Figs. 4.32, 4.33, 4.100) are not visible in the abdominal tract, whereas they are recognizable in the pelvis as thin, slightly arcuate linear images with internal concavity, which extend from the anterior pelvic wall to the hypogastric arteries along the lateral wall of the urinary bladder. The presence of liquid in the peritoneal cavity gives a better separation of these ligaments as two symmetrical paramedian incisures on the anterior profile of the peritoneum, which in lower planes subdivide the paravesical peritoneal cavity into medial and lateral inguinal fossae. Between these ligaments and the lateral pelvic wall there is subperitoneal areolar tissue, which continues downwards in the laterorectal space where vessels, lymph nodes, and external iliac nerves are located.

The *broad* and *round ligaments* (Figs. 4.32, 4.34, 4.96, 4.97) appear as two bilateral and symmetrical linear images, which are slightly concave toward the internal side: they extend from the extremity of the corpus uteri forward and slightly outward toward the inguinal canal, along the pelvic wall, medially to the iliac vessels and to the ureters.

The *vesicogenital ligaments* appear as thin, slightly arcuate, laminae located on the two sides between the posterolateral vesical wall and the uterus, within the transparent image of the subperitoneal adipose areolar tissue.

The *cardinal* or *transverse cervical ligaments* are visible only in very favorable conditions. In planes underlying the broad ligaments, they are visible as two thin bands extending laterally from the uterine cervix up to their junction with the sacro-recto-genito-pubic ligaments

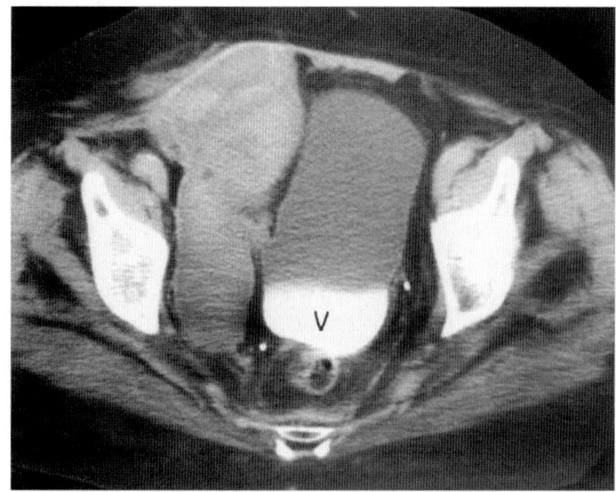

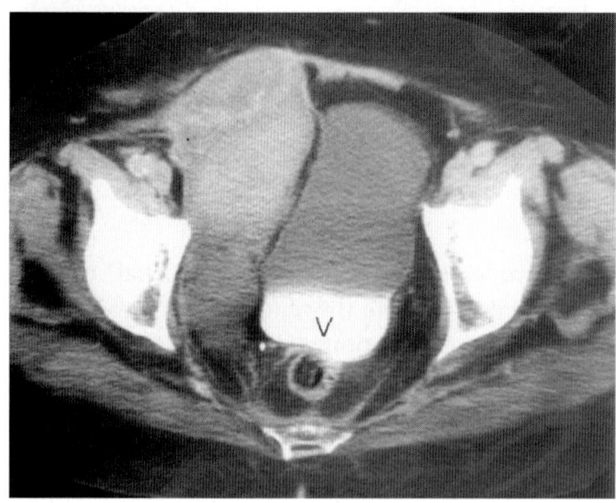

Fig. 4.102. Subperitoneal spaces. The right prevesical space is occupied by a recent posttraumatic hematoma, seen extending along the vesical wall, between the sacro-recto-genito-pubic ligament outside and the umbilicovesical fascia inside, and closed posteriorly by the fusion of these two laminae The prevesical space shows a cuneiform penetration between the transparencies of the laterorectal space outside and the perivesical space inside

The *uterosacral ligaments* (Fig. 4.101) have the aspect of an arcuate band; extending obliquely, outward and backward, they connect the uterine cervix to the sagittal laminae of the sacro-recto-genito-pubic ligaments.

The *prostatoperitoneal fascia of Denonvilliers* (Figs. 4.98, 4.99) appears as a thick transverse band, which is located in the median part of the pelvic cavity and separates the retrovesical subperitoneal space from the prerectal space. It is wider at a high level, where it surrounds the seminal vescicles, and extends posterolaterally on the two sides (becoming thinner with a mouse-tail-like aspect and surrounding the vesicodeferential vessels) up to its junction with the sacro-recto-genito-pubic ligaments

The *vesicosacral ligaments* (Fig. 4.98) appear as two thin arcuate laminae on the two sides between the posterolateral vesical wall and the sacrum, which they reach after joining with the sacro-recto-genito-pubic ligament.

The *lateral ligaments* or *alae of the rectum* (Fig. 4.103) appear as short bands located transversely between the sides of the bowel and the sacro-recto-genito-pubic ligaments. Within their thickness the middle hemorrhoidal vessels are recognizable. In men the observation of the *deferential ducts* and *vessels* is frequent; they are covered by the parietal peritoneum (Fig. 4.99) and appear as slightly arcuate linear images extending forward from the two sides of Denonvilliers' fascia, along the lateral vesical wall, up to the internal orifice of the inguinal canal and medially to the lower epigastric vessels.

The fasciae and ligaments described above subdivide the subperitoneal space into secondary spaces, which can be recognized separately only when they are occupied by adipose tissue or by liquid or when they are limited by thickening fasciae: (a) the laterorectal spaces, (b) the prevesical space, (c) the perivesical space, and (d) the perirectal space.

The *laterorectal spaces* (Figs. 4.101, 4.102, 4.104) are easily recognizable, not only from the constant presence of adipose tissue inside them, the sagittal disposition and the arcuate lateral position between

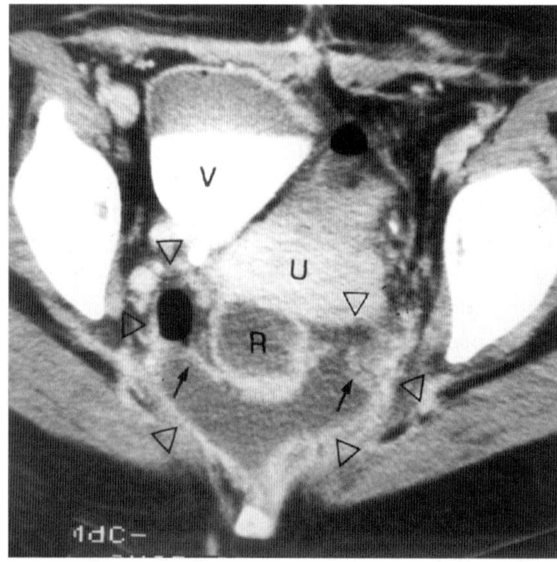

Fig. 4.103. Pelvic structures (woman). The perirectal space is occupied by an abscess surrounding the rectum and is limited anteriorly by the base of the uterus and the broad ligaments, and laterally by the umbilicovesical fascia, which is blended with the sacro-recto-genito-pubic ligament. The pre- and retrorectal spaces (*open triangles*) are separated by the thin transverse laminae of the alae recti (*small arrows*)

the osteomuscular wall outside and the laminae of the sacro-recto-genito-pubic ligaments inside, but also because they are crossed by the external iliac vessels.

The other subperitoneal spaces are located inside the sacro-recto-genito-pubic ligaments and the adipose tissue of the laterorectal space and have a transverse or predominantly transverse orientation.

The *prevescical space* (Figs. 4.11, 4.37, 4.100–4.102, 5.17) is located between the transversalis and the umbilical fasciae and is limited laterally by the sacro-recto-genito-pubic ligament. In normal subjects it is not easily recognizable, because it is very thin and is occupied by a very small amount of adipose tissue. It becomes visible when it contains liquid, with a molar tooth-like aspect (Auh et al. 1986a, b), with the crown located as an arch in front of the urinary bladder and the roots on the vesical sides.

Between the urinary bladder and the prevesical space, there is an interstice of low attenuation owing to the adipose tissue of the perivesical space. When only a half of the prevesical space contains liquid, the interstice becomes conical, with a posterior apex (Fig. 4.102).

The *perivesical space* (Figs. 4.11, 4.100, 4.102) appears as a thin interstice of low attenuation owing to the adipose tissue that is located on the sides of the urinary bladder, the internal genital organs and the rectum; it is limited anteriorly by the thin dense arcuate line of the umbilicovesical fascia, in the back of which the punctiform image of the median umbilicovesical ligament (urachus) stands out. Posteriorly, the perivesical space is limited medially by the sagittal linear images of the vesicosacral ligaments in men and uterosacral ligaments in women, which separate this space from the pelvic viscera, and externally by the curved line of the lateral umbilicovesical ligament and the umbilicovesical fascia, which separate the perivesical from the prevesical space. Inside the perivesical space, we can individuate the linear or punctiform images of the arteries and the visceral pelvic venous plexus. As a whole, the space has an arcuate aspect with anterior median convexity.

The *perirectal space* (Figs. 4.101, 4.103) is well visible because it is occupied by more or less abundant adipose tissue. Its lateral contours are constituted by the linear images of the posterior prolongation of the sacro-recto-genito-pubic ligaments, strengthened by the sacrogenital ligaments, and are always clearly visible. Similarly, the punctiform or sinuous images of the hemorrhoidal vessels and of the perirectal venous plexus are frequently recognizable within its context. The subdivision of the perirectal space in

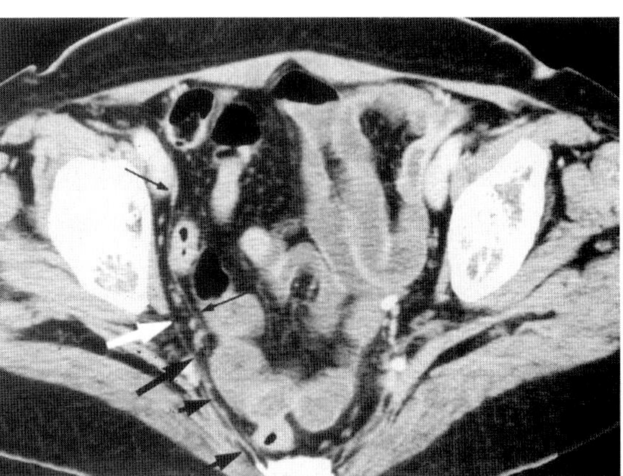

Fig. 4.104. Pelvic structures. The pelvic peritoneum (*thin arrows*) and the right transverse fascia (*thick arrows*) become thicker and merge posteriorly (*arrowhead*). Between these structures, the laterorectal extraperitoneal space is occupied by adipose tissue and by the external iliac vessels anteriorly, and by the branches of the hypogastric vessels posteriorly

pre- and *retrorectal* is visible only in the presence of liquid (or gas) inside. In this case, the laterorectal ligaments or alae recti can be recognized between the bowel and the sacro-recto-genito-pubic fascia (Fig. 4.103).

Behind the retrorectal space, a thin dense transverse band is sometimes visible in front of the sacrum; it is separated from the sacrum by an interstice of adipose tissue (*presacral space*), where, occasionally, the punctiform images of the middle sacral vessels are visibile (Fig. 4.101).

4.5.4 Anterior Renal and Lateroconal Fasciae and Anterior Pararenal Space

The *anterior renal fascia* (Figs. 4.105–4.107) is easily visible on CT because of its transverse and vertical orientation and because of the constant presence of adipose tissue on both sides.

It appears as a thin opaque line (1–2 mm thick), slightly concave posteriorly, which crosses the abdomen from one side to the other in front of the kidneys, adrenal glands, inferior vena cava and aorta and behind the ascending and descending colon, pancreas, third duodenal portion and mesenteric vessels.

It is more obviously visible and slightly thicker on the left side, where it is strengthened laterally by the lateroconal fascia and medially by the retroduo-

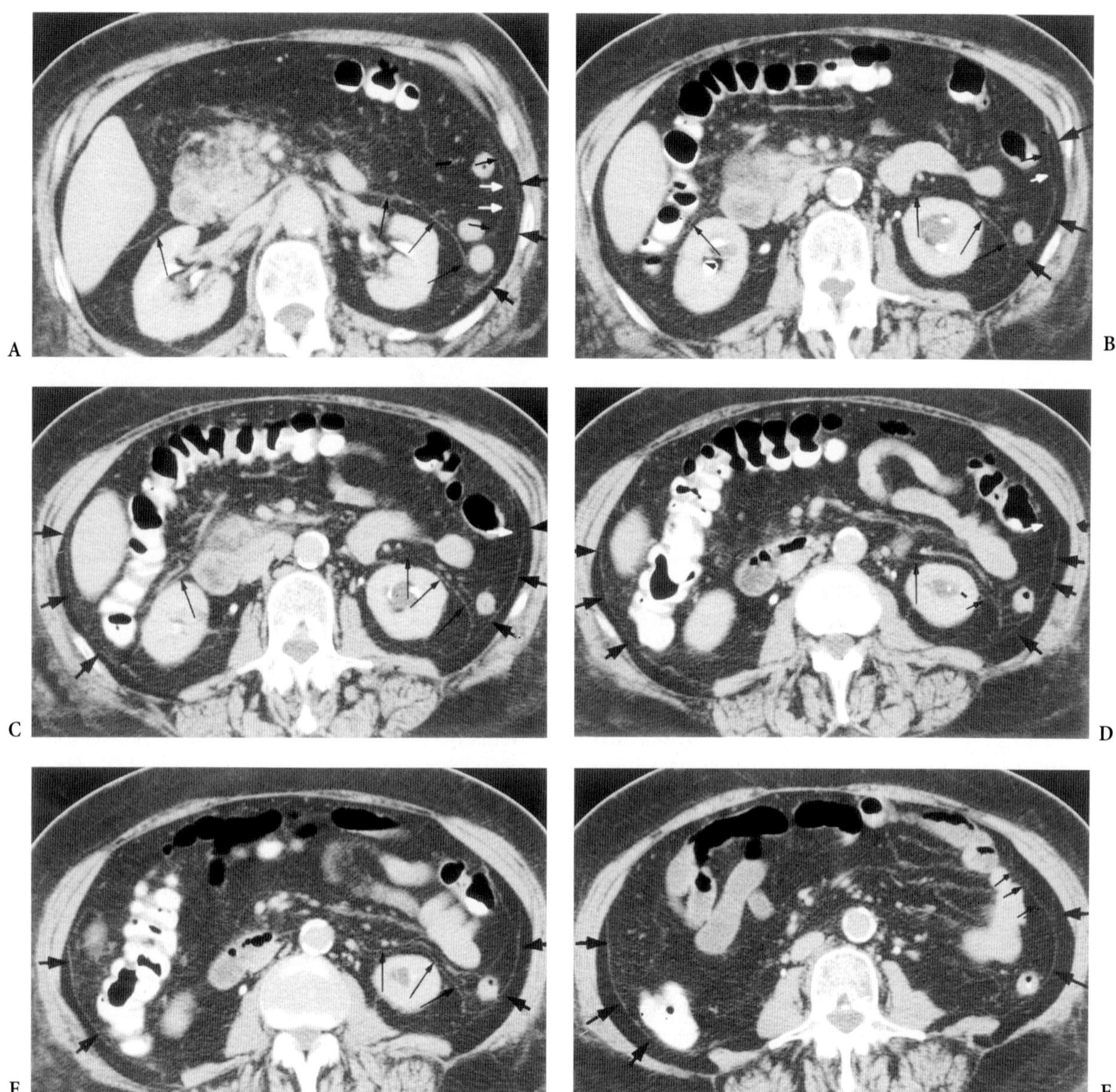

Fig. 4.105. Anterior and lateroconal renal fasciae and left lateroconal compartment in a patient recovering from acute necrotic hemorrhagic pancreatitis. Slight thickening makes fasciae and peritoneum easily visible. On the *left*, the anterior renal (*long thin arrows*) and lateroconal (*short thick arrows*) fasciae are recognizable along their entire length up to the left iliac fossa. On the same side the peritoneum (*short thin arrows*) can also be distinguished because of the presence of adipose tissue in the anterior pararenal space between the peritoneum itself and the lateroconal fascia. The lateroconal compartment, with the descending colon, is visible as a triangle limited by the peritoneum and the anterior pararenal and the lateroconal fasciae.On the *right*, the total extension of the lateroconal fascia is visible, whereas the anterior renal fascia can be recognized only in the superior planes as a *very thin line* extending in front of the kidney

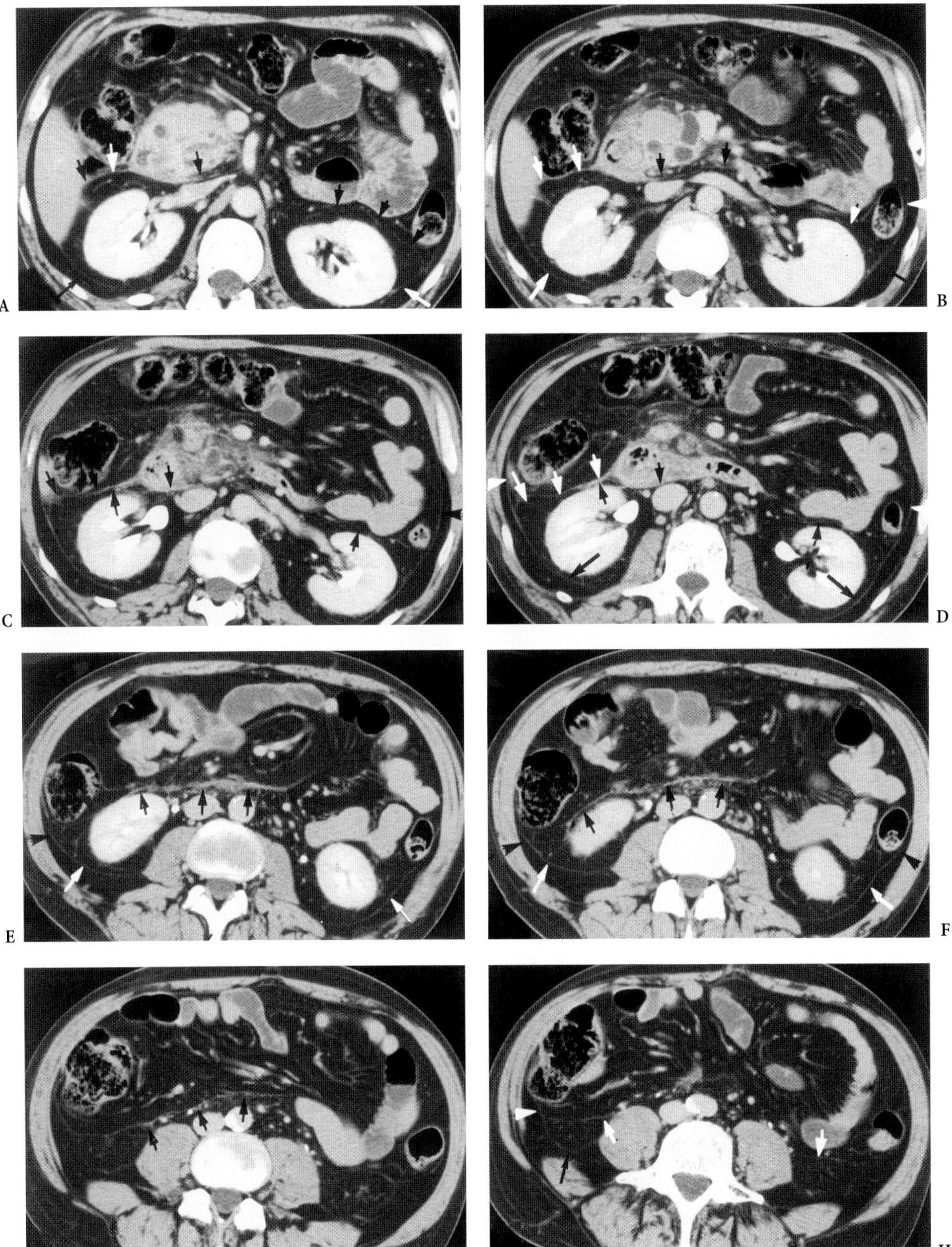

Fig. 4.106. Anterior renal fascia, lateroconal fascia, and anterior pararenal space in a patient with acute pancreatitis of the pancreatic head. The anterior renal fascia (*short arrows*) is thicker on the median line and on the right side; its total transverse and vertical extension is visible as an arcuate line passing among the anterior pararenal space, the renal compartment and the prevertebral space. At the sides, it continues backwards in the posterior renal fascia (*long arrows*). On the *left*, the dense sagittal line of the lateroconal fascia (*arrowhead*) joins the renal fascia and the peritoneum

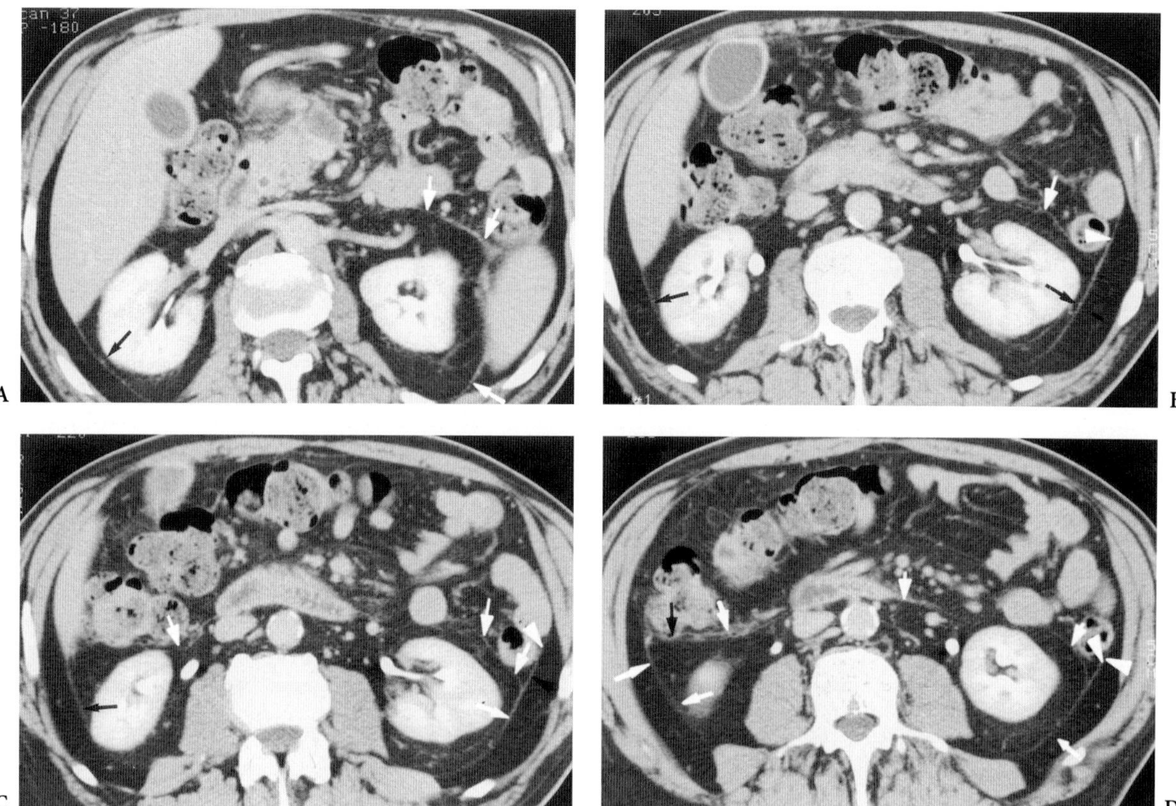

Fig. 4.107. Anterior renal fascia, left lateroconal fascia and space in a patient with acute pancreatitis. The anterior renal fascia is thicker (*short arrows*) in front of the renal compartments and the prevertebral space and behind the anterior pararenal space. On the *left*, it joins the lateroconal fascia (*arrowhead*); together, these fasciae limit the lateroconal space, where the descending colon stands out. The two fasciae join and continue backward in the posterior renal fascia (*arrows*)

denopancreatic fascia of Treitz and the retropancreatic fascia of Toldt, and in the points where it adheres to the posterior peritoneum.

The *lateroconal fasciae* (Figs. 4.82, 4.105–4.107) are visible outside the ascending and descending colon as thin lamellae with an anteroposterior extension, connecting the renal fascia with the lateral parietal peritoneum, with which they merge.

The *anterior pararenal space* (Figs. 4.19, 4.22, 4.105–4.107, 5.10) is located between the posterior parietal peritoneum and the anterior renal fascia and is confined on the sides by the lateroconal fasciae. Its thickness varies according to the presence or absence of organs inside. Its posterior limits are well defined by the arcuate line of the renal fascia, whereas the anterior limits cannot usually be recognized in normal conditions. In fact, in the suprapancreatic planes, the pararenal space is virtual because of the adhesion of the renal fascia to the posterior peritoneum, and blends with the posterior profile of the intraperitoneal organs.

In the underlying planes, the median and left paramedian expansions of the pancreatic compartment and the lateral expansions of the *right* and *left lateroconal compartments* are clearly visible in the anterior pararenal space.

In the subpancreatic planes, the anterior pararenal space expands at the level of the mesocolic and mesenteric roots; the transparency of the pararenal adipose tissue continues into that of the mesocolic and mesenteric fat without interruption. In contrast, in the intermediate tracts between mesentery and mesocolon, the anterior pararenal space is identifiable in the curved line formed by the renal fascia and by the posterior peritoneum. Only when the two laminae are detached by an effusion, as often happens during acute pancreatitis, does the space become recognizable.

Sagittal reconstruction yields extensive representation of this space from the diaphragm to the pelvis, between the parietal peritoneum and the anterior renal fascia, in front of the renal compartment (Figs. 4.19, 4.22).

Furthermore, the presence of intraperitoneal fluid, which delineates the anterior profile of the space, makes it possible to evaluate its differing thickness at various levels: this is greater on the median line, where the transparency of the retroperitoneal adipose tissue continues into the mesenteric transparency, whereas it is minimal in the intermediate tracts, where peritoneum and anterior renal fascia adhere.

4.5.5 Abdominal Transversalis Fascia

The abdominal transversalis fascia is not visible in normal conditions, because of its close adhesion with the aponeuroses of the abdominal wall muscles and the spinal column; it becomes visible between the fascia itself and the adjacent parietal structures when fluid collections are present (Fig. 4.104).

Bibliography

Peritoneum, Ligaments, Mesenteries, Peritoneal Cavity and Extraperitoneal Structures

Ahn CY, Ahn HK, Han KS (1983) Superior aspect of the perirenal space: anatomy and pathological correlation Clin Radiol 39:368–372

Auh YH, Rubenstein WA, Markisz JA, Zirinsky K, Whalen JP, Kazam E (1986) Intraperitoneal paravescical spaces: CT delineation with US correlation. Radiology 159:311–317

Auh YH, Rubenstein WA, Schneider M, Reckler JM Whalen JP, Kazam E (1986) Extraperitoneal paravescical spaces, CT delineation with US correlation. Radiology 159:319–332

Baert AL, Wackenheim A, Jeanmart L (1980) Abdominal computer tomography. (Atlas of pathological computer tomography, vol 2) Springer, Berlin Heidelberg New York

Balfe DM (1988) Upper abdominal peritoneal spaces and ligaments. In: Fishman EK, Jones B, et al (eds) Computed tomography of the gastrointestinal tract. Churchill Livingstone, New York

Balfe DM, Peterson RR, Lee JKT (1983) Normal abdominal anatomy. In: Lee JKT, Sagel SS, Stanley RJ, et al (eds) Computed body tomography. Raven Press, New York

Balfe DM, Mauro MA, Koehler RE, Lee JKT, Weiman PJ, Picus D, Paterson RR (1984) Gastrohepatic ligament: normal and pathologic CT anatomy. Radiology 150:485–490

Buy JN, Moss AA, Singler RC (1982) CT guided celiac plexus and splanchnic nerve neurolysis. J Comput Assist Tomogr 6:315–319

Callen PW, Filly RA, Korobkin M (1978) Ascitic fluid in the anterior paravesical fossa: misleading appearance on CT scans AJR Am J Roentgenol 130:1176–1177

Camerini E, Busoni F, Vignali C, Sbragia P (1988) Moderne acquisizioni tomodensitometriche sugli spazi para e perirenali in condizioni normali e patologiche. Radiol Med 76:284–288

Charnsangavej C, DuBrow RA, Varma DGK, Herron DH, Robinson TJ, Whitley NO (1993) CT of the mesocolon. 1. Anatomic considerations. Radiographics 13:1035

Chou C K, Liu G C, Chen L T, Jaw T S (1993} MRI Demonstration of peritoneal ligaments and mesenteries Abdom Imaging 18:126–130

Coppolino F, Fischietti SG, Priolo GD, Chiarenza R, Loreto C (1990) Anatomia TC ed imaging anatomico integrato: pelvi maschile. In: del Vecchio E, Loreto C (eds) TC imaging integrato pelvi e bacino. Idelson, Naples

Dalla Palma Ludovico (1989) Il retroperitoneo diagnostica per immagini. LINT, Trieste

DeMeo JH, Fulcher AS, Austin RF (1995) Anatomic CT demonstration of peritoneal spaces, ligaments, and mesenteries: normal and pathologic processes. Radiographics 15:755–770

Dodds WJ, Foley WD, Lawson TL, Stewart ET, Taylor A (1985) Anatomy and imaging of the lesser peritoneal sac. AJR Am J Roentgenol 144:567–575

Dunnick NR, Jones RB, Doppman JL, Speyes SI, Myers CE (1979) Intraperitoneal contrast infusion for assessment of intraperitoneal fluid dynamics. AJR Am J Roentgenol 133:221–223

Feldberg MA (1983) Computed tomography of the retroperitoneum: an anatomical and pathological atlas with emphasis on the fascial planes. Martinus Nijhoff, The Hague

Feldberg MA, van-Leeuwen MS (1990) The properitoneal fat pad associated with the falciform ligament. Imaging of extent and clinical relevance. Surg Radiol Anat 12:193–202

Fosbager MR, Walsh JW (1994) CT of the female pelvis: a second look. Radiographics 14:51–66

Frezza F, Pozzi Mucelli RS (1992)Valutazione anatomica delle fascie renali nel soggetto normale mediante impiego di apparecchiatura per tomografia computerizzata con tecnologia avanzata. Radiol Med 84:274–282

Goldberg HI, Gould RC, Feuerstein IM, e al (1989) Evaluation of ultrafast CT scanning of the adult abdomen. Invest Radiol 24:537

Goodman P, Raval B (1990) CT of the abdominal wall. AJR Am J Roentgenol 154:1207

Goodman P, Balachandran S (1992) CT evaluation of the abdominal wall. Crit Rev Diagn Imaging 33:461–493

Gossios KJ, Tsianos EV, Kontogiannis DS, et al (1992)Water as contrast medium for computed tomography study of colonic wall lesions. Gastrointest Radiol 17:125

Grassi R, Rotondo A, Smaltino F (1991) Valutazione TC dei meso e dei recessi peritoneali. Proceedings of the Meeting of the Gastroenterology Section of SIRM, Rome

Haaga JR (1984) Improved technique for CT – guided celiac ganglia block. AJR Am J Roentgenol 42:1201–1204

Heiken JP (1989) Abdominal wall and peritoneal cavity. In: Lee J, Sagel S, Stanley R, et al (eds) Computed body tomography with MRI correlation. Raven Press, New York

Hureau J, Pradel J (1988) Tomodensitometrie du tronc. Piccin, Padua

Hureau J, Agossou-Voyeme AK, Germain M, Pradel J (1991) The posterior interparietoperitoneal spaces or retroperitoneal spaces. 1. Normal topographic anatomy. J Radiol 72:101–116

Innocenti P, Dal Pozzo G (1990) Anatomia TC ed immagine integrato: pelvi femminile. In: Del Vecchio E, Loreto C (eds) TC imaging integrato pelvi e bacino. Idelson, Naples

Jeffrey RB, Federle MP, Goodman PC (1981) Computed Tomography of the lesser peritoneal sac. Radiology 141:117–122

Jeffrey RB, Federle MP, Goodman PC (1985) Computed tomography of the lesser peritoneal sac AJR Am J Roentgenol 144:567–575
Jeffrey RB (1983) Computed tomography of the peritoneal cavity and mesentery. In: Moss AA, Gamsu G, Genant HK, et al (eds) Computed tomography of the body. Saunders, Philadelphia
Jeffrey RB Jr (1991) Imaging of the peritoneal cavity Curr Opin Radiol 3:471–473
Kazam E, Whalen JP (1983) Anatomy. In: Margulis AR, Burhenne HJ (eds) Alimentary tract radiology, 3rd edn. Mosby, St Louis, pp 292–342
Kazam E, Auh YH, Rubenstein WA, Whalen JP (1986) Cross-sectional anatomy of the abdomen. In: Taveras JM, Ferrucci JT, et al (eds) Radiology: diagnosis – imaging – intervention. Lippincott, Philadelphia
Kazam E, Auh YH, Rubenstein WA (1988) Normal TC antomy of the pelvis with ultrasound MRI correlations. In: Putnam CE, Ravin C (eds) Textbook of diagnostic imaging. Saunders, Philadelphia, pp 380–390
Kazam E, Rubenstein WA, Markise JA, Whalen JP, Zirinsky HJ, et al (1989) Alimentary tract radiology, 4th edn. Mosby-YearBook, St Louis
Kazam E, Auh YH, Rubenstein WA (1990) Computed tomography of the lower urinary tract and pelvis. In: Pollack HM (ed) Clinical urography. Saunders, Philadelphia, pp 407–432
Levitt RG (1983) Abdominal wall and peritoneal cavity In: Lee JKT, Sagel SS, Stanley RJ, et al (eds) Computed body tomography. Raven Press, New York
Lim JH, Auh YH, Suh SJ e Kim KW (1990) Right perirenal space: CT evidence of communication between the bare area of the liver. Clin Imaging 14:239–244
Louis O, Bollaert A, Osteaux M, Grivegnee A (1983) CT of peritoneal effusions and their anatomic topography. J Belge Radiol 66:107–112
Love L, Meyers MA, Chruchill RJ, et al (1981) Pictorial essay: Computed tomography of extraperitoneal spaces. AJR Am J Roentgenol 136:781–789
Marano P (1992) Diagnostica per immagini, vol I. CEA, Milan
Matsumoto M (1983) CT diagnosis of total body: CT diagnosis of abdomen, lymph node. Asakurashoten, Tokyo
Merine D, Fishman EK, Jones B (1989) CT of the small bowel and mesentery. Radiol Clin North Am 27:707–715
Meyers MA (1973) Peritoneography: normal and pathologic anatomy AJR Am J Roentgenol 117:353–365
Meyers MA (1986) Computed tomography of the gastrointestinal tract. Springer, New York Berlin Heidelberg
Meyers MA (1988) Dynamic radiology of the abdomen: normal and pathologic anatomy, 3rd edn. Springer, New York Berlin Heidelberg
Meyers MA (1992) Radiologia dinamica dell'addome. Verduci, Rome
Meyers MA, Oliphant M, Berne AS, Feldberg MAM (1987) The peritoneal ligaments and mesenteries: pathways of intraabdominal spread of disease. Radiology 163:593–604
Min P Q, Yang Z G, Lei Q F, Gao X H, Long W S, Jiang S M, Zhou D M (1992) Peritoneal reflections of left perihepatic region: radiologic-anatomic study. Radiology 182:553–557
Naidich DP, Megibow AJ, Hilton S, et al (1983) Computed tomography of the diaphragm: peridiaphragmatic fluid collection. J Comput Assist Tomogr 7:641–649
Oldfield AL, Wilbur AC (1993) Retrogastric colon: CT demonstration of anatomic variations. Radiology 186:557
Oliphant M, Berne AS (1982) Computer tomography of subperitoneal space: demonstration of direct spaces of intrabdominal diseases. J Comput Assist Tomogr 6:1127–1137
Osborne TM (1990) CT peritoneography in peritoneal dialysis patients. Australas Radiol 34:204
Osteaux M, Louis O, Dieirickx K, Darras T, Jeanmart L (1985) La cavité péritonéale. In: Vasile N (ed) Tomodensitométrie corps entier. Vigot, Paris
Pistolesi GF, Procacci C, Tonegutti M, D'Attoma N, Della Sala S, Bicego E, Dompieri P, Residori E (1990)Analyse des différents espaces des régions extra-péritonéales. Radiol J CEPUR 10:195–204
Pozzi Mucelli RS, Cova M, Magnaldi S (1991) Anatomia della pelvi maschile in TC e RM. In: Dalla Palma L (ed) Radiourologia. Lint, Trieste, pp 191–209
Pozzi Mucelli RS, Shariat Razavi I (1994) Aspetti anatomici delle fasce e dei legamenti pelvici in tomografia computerizzata. Radiol Med 88:458–464
Pozzi Mucelli RS, Shariat Razavi I (1994) Le fasce, i legamenti e gli spazi pelvici nella patologia neoplastica in tomografia computerizzata Radiol Med 88:465–471
Pozzi Mucelli RS, Sponza M (1996) Peritoneo. In: Pozzi Mucelli RS (ed) Trattato italiano di tomografia computerizzata. Gnocchi, Naples
Radier C, Baumelou A, Bousquet JC, Bellin MF, Grellet J (1989) X-ray computed tomographic aspects of medium-sized free peritoneal effusions (supramesocolic level). J Radiol 70:95–102
Rotondo A, Grassi R, Contino A, Smaltino F (1991) Spazi peritoneali In: Dal Pozzo M (ed) Compendio di tomografia computerizzata. UTET, USES, Verona
Roub LW, Drayer BP, Orr DP, Oh KS (1979) Computed tomographic positive contrast peritoneography Radiology 131:699–704
Rubenstein WA, Auh YH, Whalen JP, Kazam E (1983) The perihepatic spaces: computed tomographic and ultrasound imaging. Radiology 149:231–239
Rubenstein WA, Auh YH, Zirinsky K, Kneeland B, Whalen IP, Kazam E (1985) Posterior peritoneal recesses: assessment using CT. Radiology 156:461–468
Rubenstein WA, Whalen JP (1986) Extraperitoneal spaces. AJR Am J Roentgenol 147:1162–1164
Silverman PM, Kelvin FM, Korobkin M, Dunnick NR (1984) CT of the normal mesentery. AJR Am J Roentgenol 143:953–957
Solomon A, Rubinstein Z (1984) Importance of the falciform ligament, ligamentum teres, and splenic hilus in the spread of malignancy as demonstrated by computed tomography. Gastrointest Radiol 9:53–56
Takahashi N, Itoh K, Haba H, Ishii Y (1989) Anatomy of hepatoduodenal ligament on MR imaging. Rinsho-Hoshasen 34:1585–1589
Vincent LM, Mauro MA, Mittelstaedt CA (1984) The lesser sac and gastrohepatic recess: sonographic appearance and differentiation of fluid collections. Radiology 150:515–519
Vishakar SO, Bellon EM (1984) The bare area of the spleen: a constant CT feature of the ascitic abdomen. AJR Am J Roentgenol 141:953–955
Watrin J, Rohmer P e Weill F (1985) Etude scanographique des ligaments et mésos péritonéaux. J Radiol 67:775–781
Wegener OH (1992) Whole body computed tomography, 2nd edn. Blackwell Scientific, Oxford
Weill F, Watrin J, Rohmer P (1986) Ultrasound and CT of peri-

toneal recesses and ligaments: a pictorial assay Ultrasound Med Biol 12:977–989
Weinstein JB, Heiken JP, Lee JKT, et al (1986) High resolution CT of the porta hepatis and hepato-duodenal ligament. Radiographics 6:55–73
Whiteley VC, Walsh JW, Wheelock JB, et al (1984) CT of the normal and abnormal parametria in cervical cancer AJR Am J Roentgenol 142:507–603
Wojtowicz J, Rzymski K, Czarnecki R A (1982) CT evaluation of the intraperitoneal fluid distribution Fortschr Rontgenstr 137:95–99

Arteries and Veins

Abu-Yousef MM (1990) Is it calcification of the ductus venosus or calcification of the ligamentum teres? Radiology 176:291
Alexander MS, Blake RA, Gelman R (1991) Visualization of a recanalized umbilical vein on hepatobiliary imaging with CT correlation. Clin Nucl Med 16:517
Baum PA, Matsumoto AH, Teitelbaum GP, Zuurbier RA, Barth KH (1989) Anatomic relationship between the common femoral artery and vein: CT evaluation and clinical significance. Radiology 173:775
Carrington BM, Martin DF (1987) Position of the superior mesenteric artery on computed tomography and its relationship to retroperitoneal disease. Br J Radiol 60:997–999
Coin CG, Chan YS (1977) Computed tomographic arteriography J Comput Assist Tomogr 1:165–168
Hricak H, Amparo E, Fisher MR, et al (1985) Abdominal venous system: assessment using MR. Radiology 156:415–422
Ishikawa T, Tsukune Y, Okyama Y, Fujikawa M, Sakuyama K, Kujii M (1980) Venous abnormalities in portal hypertension demonstrated by CT AJR Am J Roentgenol 134:271–276
Korobkin M, Kressel HY, Moss A (1978) Computed tomographic angiography of the body. Radiology 126:807–811
Kuhns LR, Borlaza G (1980) Normal Roentgen variant: aberrant right hepatic artery on computed tomography. Radiology 135:391–396
Lafortune M (1990) Is it calcification of the ductus venosus or calcification of the umbilical vein? Radiology 176:290
Maramonti M, Gallini C, Giuliano A (1992) Studio del tripode celiaco: reperti normali e varianti anatomiche. XXXV Congress of SIRM, Genua 1992. Radiol Med 84 [Suppl 1]:198
Marn CS, Glazer GM, Williams DM, Francis IR (1990) CT-angiographic correlation of collateral venous pathways in isolated splenic vein occlusion: new observations. Radiology 175:375–380
Moncada R, Reynes C Churchill R, Love L (1979) Normal vascular anatomy of the abdomen on computed tomography. Radiol Clin North Am 17:25–37
Moody AR, Poon PY (1992) Gastroepiploic veins: CT appearance in pancreatic disease AJR Am J Roentgenol 158:779
Mori H, Miyake H, Aikawa H, et al (1991) Dilated posterior superior pancreatico-duodenal vein: recognition with CT and clinical significance in patients with pancreaticobiliary carcinomas Radiology 181:793–800
Mori H, McGrath FP, Malone DE, Stevenson GW (1992) The gastrocolic trunk and its tributaries: CT evaluation. Radiology 182:871–877
Morin C, Lafortune M, Pomier G, Robin M, Breton G (1992) Patent paraumbilical vein: anatomic and hemodynamic variants and their clinical importance. Radiology 185:253
Reuter SR, Redman HC, Cho KJ (1986) Gastrointestinal angiography, 3rd edn. Saunders, Philadelphia
Rizzo AJ, Haller JO, Mulvihill DM, Cohen HL, Da Silva MG (1989) Calcification of the ductus venosus: a cause of right upper quadrant calcification in the newborn Radiology 173:89
Rizzo AJ, Haller JO (1990) Is it calcification of the ductus venosus or calcification of the ligamentum teres?: reply. Radiology 176:291
Rubin GD, Dake MD, Napel SA, McDonnel CH, Jeffrey RB Jr (1993) Three-dimensional spiral CT angiography of the abdomen: initial clinical experience. Radiology 186:147
Shapir J, Rubin J (1984) CT appearance of the inferior mesenteric vein. J Comput Assist Tomogr 8:877–880
Silverman PM, Patt RH, Garra BS, et al (1991) MR imaging of the portal venous system: value of gradient-echo imaging as an adjunct to spin-echo MR. AJR Am J Roentgenol 157:297–301
Sponza M, Pozzi Mucelli RS, Pozzi Mucelli F (1993) Anatomia arteriosa del tripode celiaco e dell'arteria mesenterica superiore con tomografia computerizzata. Radiol Med 86:260–267
Weinstein JB, Heiken JP, Joseph KT, et al (1986) High resolution CT of the porta hepatis and hepato-duodenal ligament. Radiographics 6:55–73
Winter TC III, Freeny PC, Nghiem HV, et al (1995) Hepatic arterial anatomy in transplantation candidates: evaluation with three-dimensional CT arteriography. Radiology 195:363–370
Winter TC, Nghiem HV, Freeny PC, Hommeyer SC, Mack LA (1995) Hepatic arterial anatomy: demonstration of normal supply and vascular variants with three dimensional CT angiography. Radiographics 15:771–780
Zerin JM, DiPietro MA (1991) Mesenteric vascular anatomy at CT: normal and abnormal appearances. Radiology 179:739
Zirinsky K, Auh YH, Rubenstein WA, Kneeland JB, Whalen JP, Kazam E (1985) The portocaval space: CT with MR correlation. Radiology 156:453–460

Lymphatic System

Ritcher E, Feyerabend T (1990)Normal lymph node topography.CT atlas. Springer, Berlin Heidelberg New York

Section 2

Primary and Secondary Pathology of the Peritoneum

5 Fluid Collections

CONTENTS

5.1 General Considerations

Fluid collections in the peritoneal cavity and in subperitoneal spaces are usually a consequence of pathologic processes affecting intraperitoneal organs; occasionally, they may represent the extension of collections from extra- or retroperitoneal compartments. Fluids can be constituted by transudate, exudate, blood, pus, bile, lymph, urine, pancreatic fluid, mucin or food, and are produced by a variety of processes: inflammatory, vascular, traumatic, neoplastic (primary or secondary), metabolic or consequent to hepatic, renal, cardiac failure or surgery (Table 5.1).

In the peritoneal cavity, fluid collections may be confined in the recess where they have been generated, blocked by active peritoneal reactions (Figs. 5.7, 5.8), or may spread over the whole peritoneal cavity (Figs. 5.1–5.3) according to the mechanisms described in the chapter 2 (Physiology and Physiopathology of the Peritoneum). On the other hand, subperitoneal collections spread into tissues sur-

Table 5.1. Causes of peritoneal collection

Transudative ascites
Portal hypertension
Morgagni-Laennec atrophic cirrhosis
Congestive heart failure
Constrictive pericarditis
Inferior vena cava obstruction
Hepatic vein occlusion (Budd-Chiari syndrome)
Portal vein obstruction
Hypoalbuminemia
Nephrotic syndrome
Malabsorption syndrome
Exudative ascites
Peritoneal carcinomatosis (due to ovarian, colic, gastric, hepatic, pancreatic, pulmonary or mammary tumors or to melanomas)
Mesothelioma
Infections
Tuberculosis
AIDS and related syndromes
Chronic renal failure
Chylous ascites
Obstruction or discontinuity of lymphatic flow: congenital, tumoral, traumatic, surgery-induced, tubercular or due to filariasis
Hematic collections
Traumas
Surgical operation
Anticoagulant therapy / hemorrhagic diathesis
Spontaneous rupture of tumors rich in vessels
Spontaneous rupture of hemorrhagic and endometriotic cyst or of ectopic gestation
Bile collections
Rupture of the biliary tree due to: surgical operation, biliary drainage, transcutaneous or endoscopic cholangiography, traumas, intraluminal hypertension
Urine collections
Traumas
Instrumental procedures
Intraluminal hypertension
Derivative surgical procedures
Seromas
Surgical operations
Pancreatic collections
Acute pancreatitis
Endoscopic cholangiopancreatography
Surgical operations
Purulent collections[a]
Extension of visceral inflammations
Intestinal perforations
Surgical operations

[a] see Chap. 6

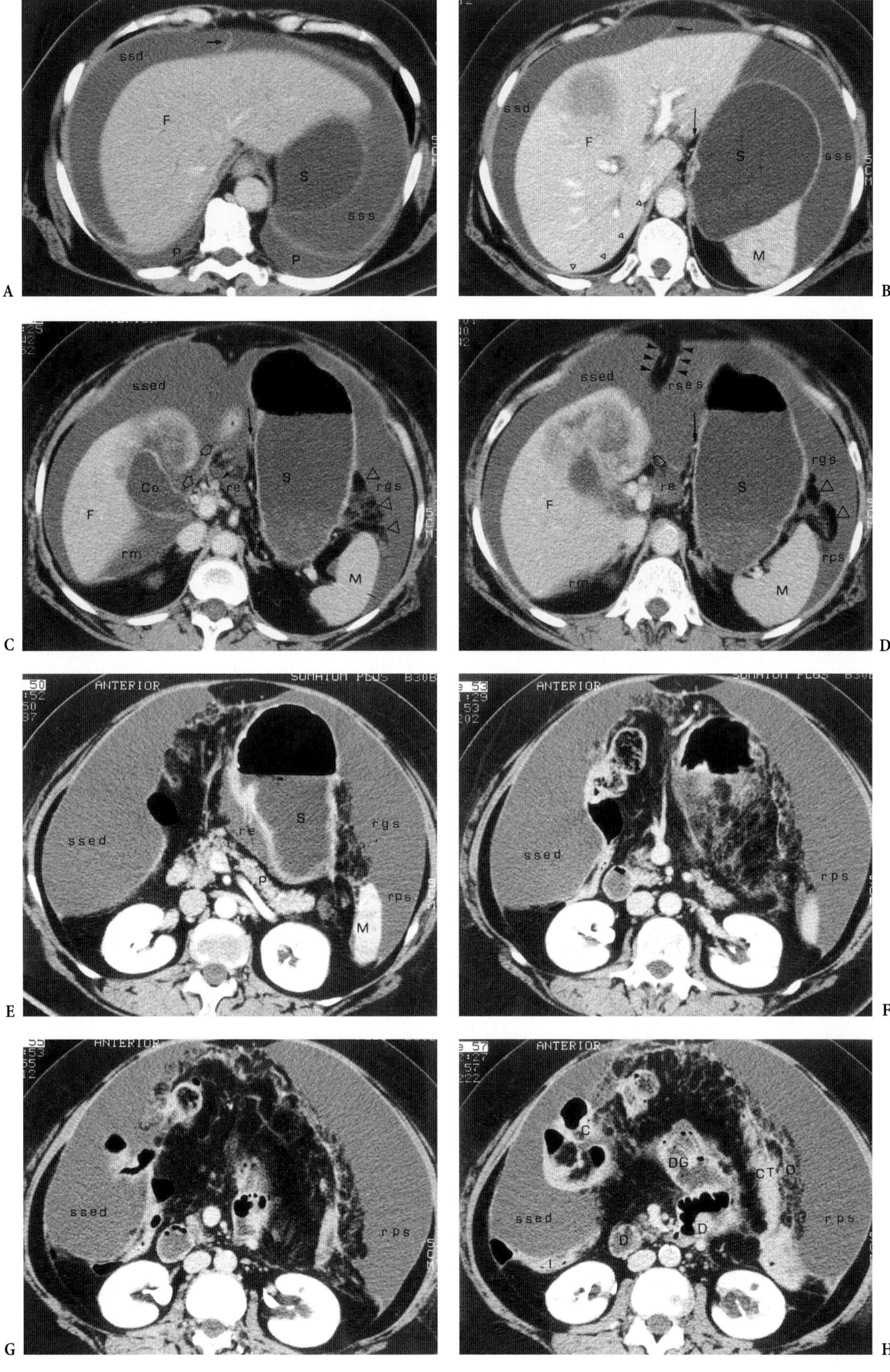

A
ssd
F
S
sss
P
B
ssd
F
S
sss
M
C
ANTERIOR
ssed
Co
re
S
rgs
F
rm
M
D
ssed
rses
re
S
rgs
F
rps
rm
M
E
ANTERIOR
SOMATOM PLUS
ssed
re
S
rgs
P
rps
M
F
ANTERIOR
ssed
rps
G
ANTERIOR
ssed
rps
H
ANTERIOR
C
DG
CT
O
ssed
rps
D
D
I

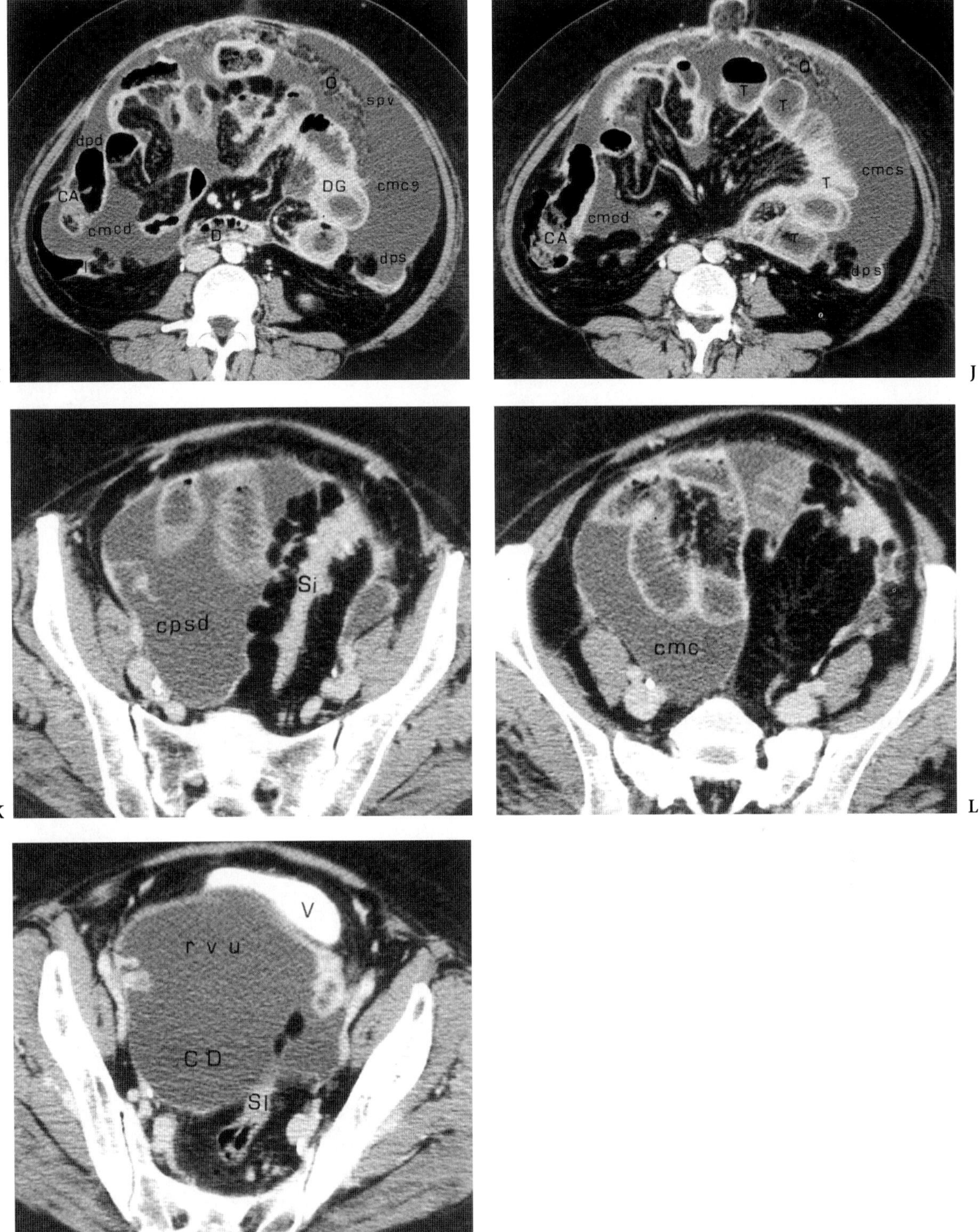

Fig. 5.1A–M. Peritoneal and pleural collections. Exudative ascites in patients with ovarian carcinomatosis. The ascites occupies the whole peritoneal cavity. All signs of malignant ascites are present: peritoneal collection, diffuse thickening of the supra and submesocolic and pelvic peritoneum, omental and mesenteric infiltration. Bilateral pleural collection. All the signs that differentiate ascites from pleural fluid are present : the pleural fluid (*P*) has a crescent shape behind the bare area of the liver and displaces the diaphragmatic crura (Dwyer's sign) medially. In the right subphrenic space the fluid cannot reach the posteromedial border of the liver, being blocked by the coronary ligament (*small open triangles*). In the left subphrenic space, the reflection of the splenopancreatic ligament (bare area of the spleen) prevents the posteromedial wall of the spleen from being surrounded by the fluid. The interface between the liver, the spleen and the pleural fluid is poorly defined, whereas it is sharp in the peritoneal collection (Teplick interface sign)

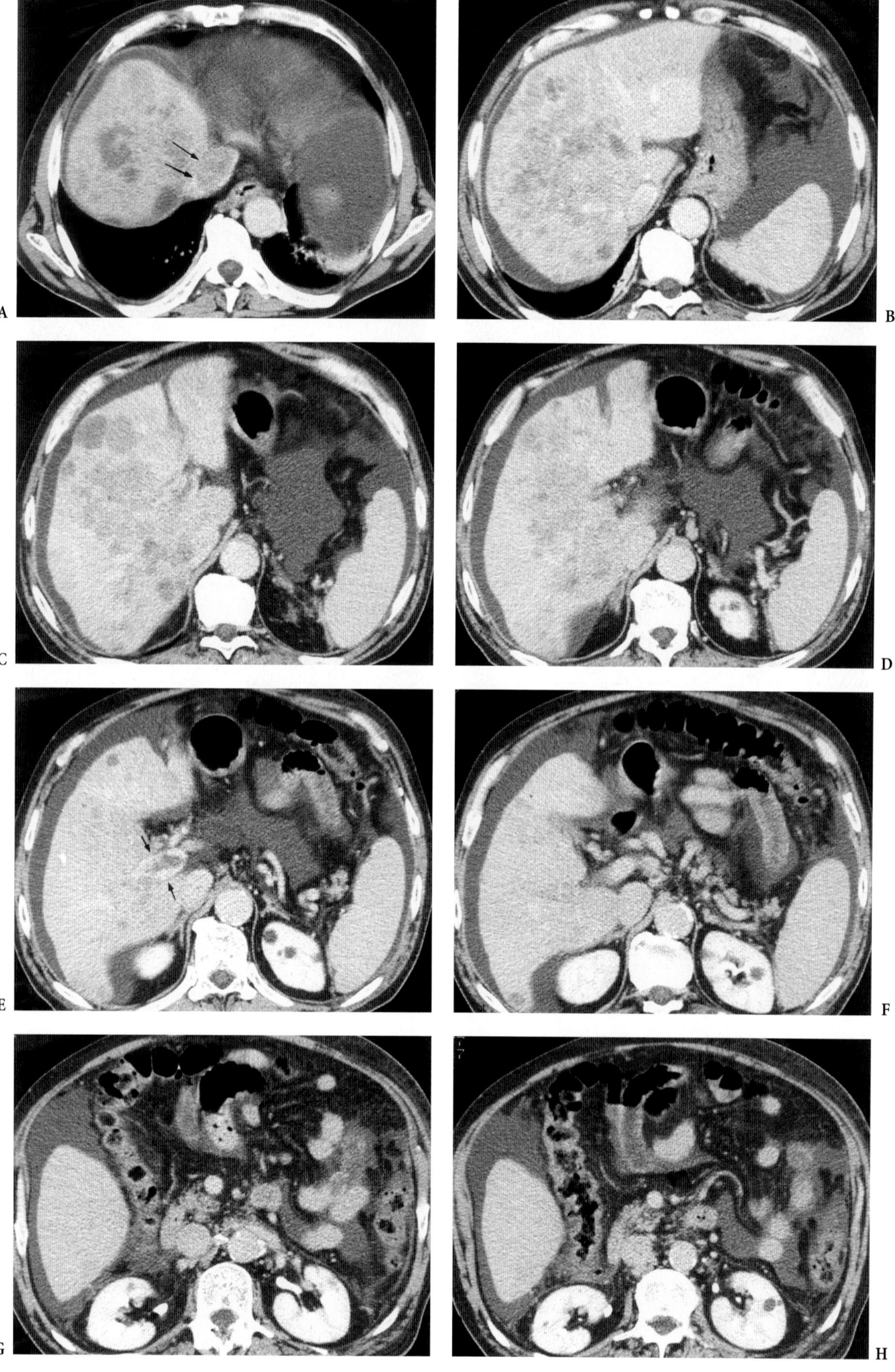
A
B
C
D
E
F
G
H

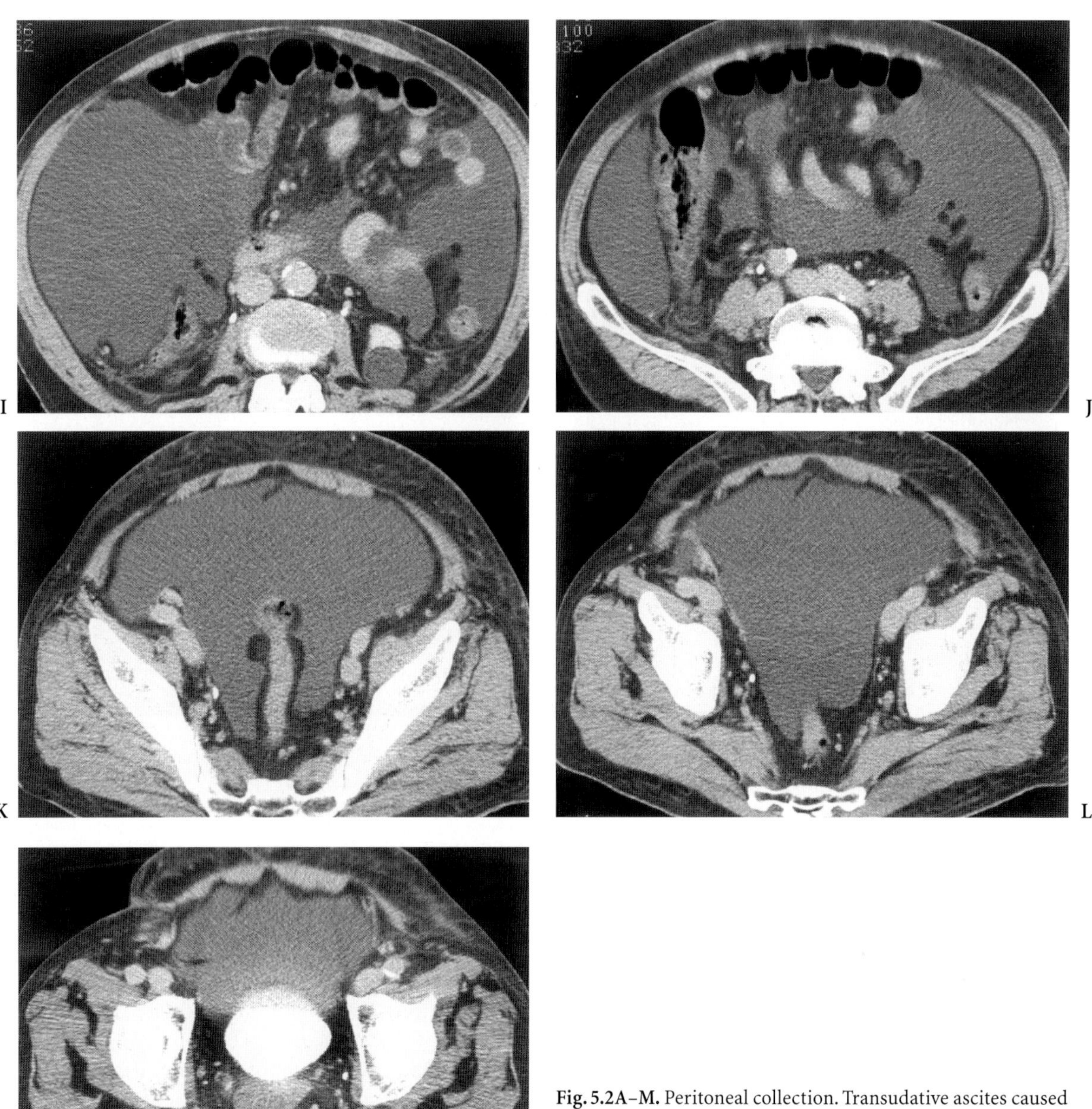

Fig. 5.2A–M. Peritoneal collection. Transudative ascites caused by caval (*long arrows*) and portal (*small arrows*) thrombosis in cancer cirrhosis. Massive fluid collection in the entire peritoneal cavity. Dilatation of the splenic, superior and inferior mesenteric veins with their affluents

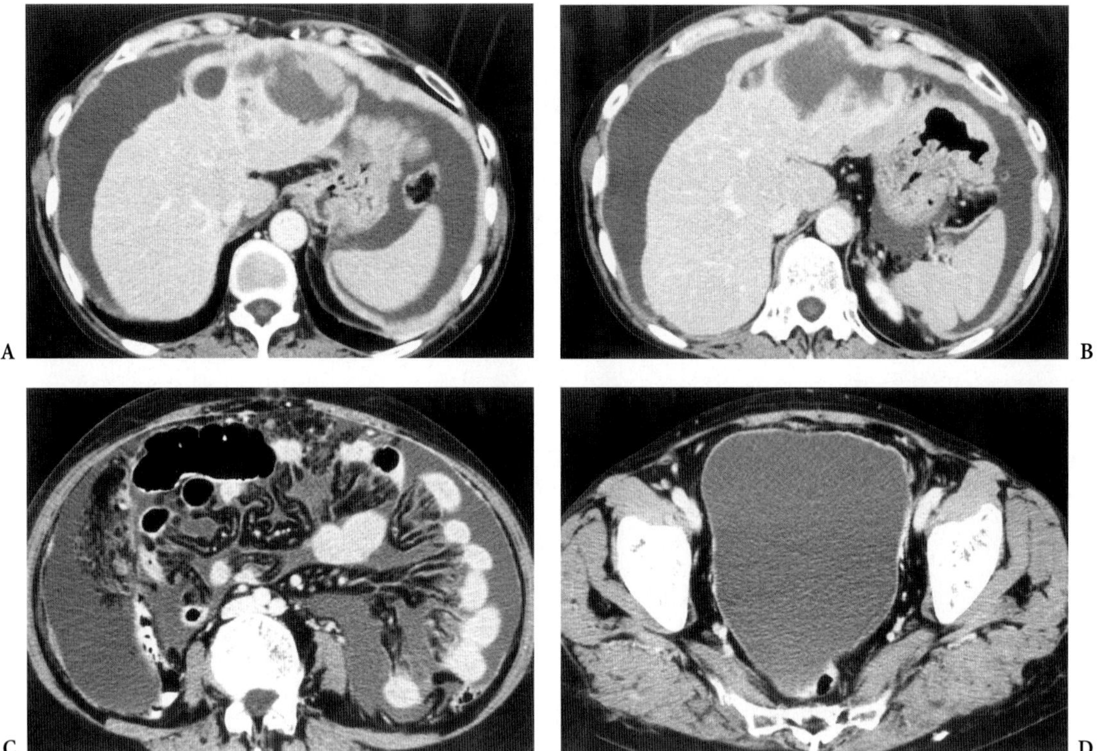

Fig. 5.3A–D. Peritoneal collection. Massive hemorrhagic and exudative ascites caused by rupture of a hepatocarcinoma .Diffuse thickening of the parietal peritoneum as a result of carcinomatous seeding

rounding the organ where they have been generated. After detachment of the perivascular fat, they spread along ligaments and may reach the retroperitoneum.

Position, nature, composition and consistency of collections represent determinant conditions for diffusion. Therefore, exudates and transudates, which are more fluid and produce a lower stimulation of the peritoneal reactivity, reach the lowest recesses and spaces in the peritoneal cavity more quickly, in contrast to pus, blood, bile and urine collections. The peritoneum tries to construct a protective barrier around these latter accumulations.

Usually, it is not difficult to localize intraperitoneal fluid effusions and collections, because of their shape and disposition and their positions relative to the abdominal organs. However, there are specific CT appearances that can raise differential diagnostic problems between

1. Pleural and subphrenic fluid
2. Subcapsular hepatic and splenic collections, and perihepatic and perisplenic peritoneal collections
3. Collections in the anterior pararenal space and in the posterior peritoneal recesses
4. Collections in the paracolic gutters, in the laterconal compartments and in the perirenal compartment
5. Collections in the peritoneal cavity and in the subperitoneal spaces
6. Intra- and extraperitoneal and extrafascial pelvic collections

5.1.1 Pleural and Subphrenic Fluid (Figs. 5.l, 5.4–5.6)

In scans of the upper abdomen, small fluid collections in the pleural costophrenic spaces and in the subphrenic recesses show the same semicircular or crescent shape between the liver or the spleen and the abdominal wall. Some signs are useful to distinguish supra- from subdiaphragmatic collections: the pleural fluid (Fig. 5.1, 5.4–5.6) lies posterior to the bare area of the liver and displaces the diaphragmatic crus from the spine (Dwyer's sign) (Dwyer 1978).The right subphrenic fluid (Figs. 5.1, 5.6) is seen only lateral to the liver, being blocked dorsally

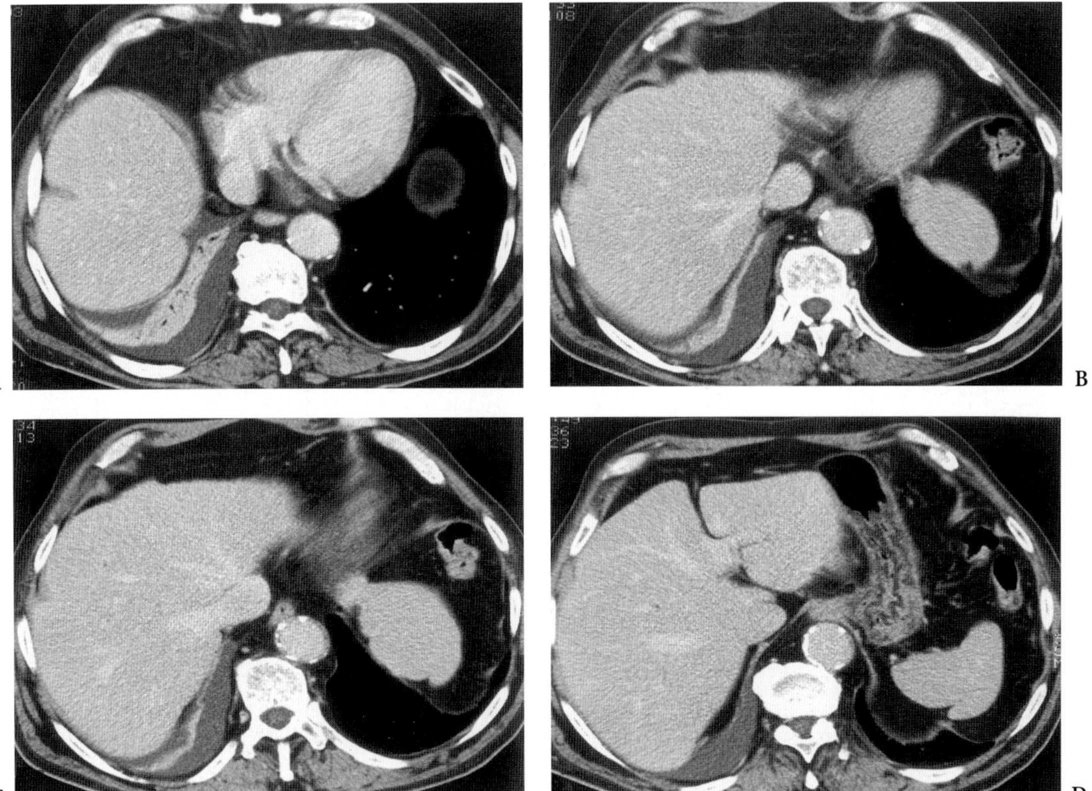

Fig. 5.4A–D. Right pleural collection. Semicircular collection in the costophrenic sulcus, extending posteromedially to the liver up to the back of the diaphragmatic crus, which is pushed anteriorly and laterally (Dwyer's sign). The collection causes collapse of the basal segments of the lung. The interface with the collapsed lung is sharp, and that with liver is ill defined (Teplick's interface sign)

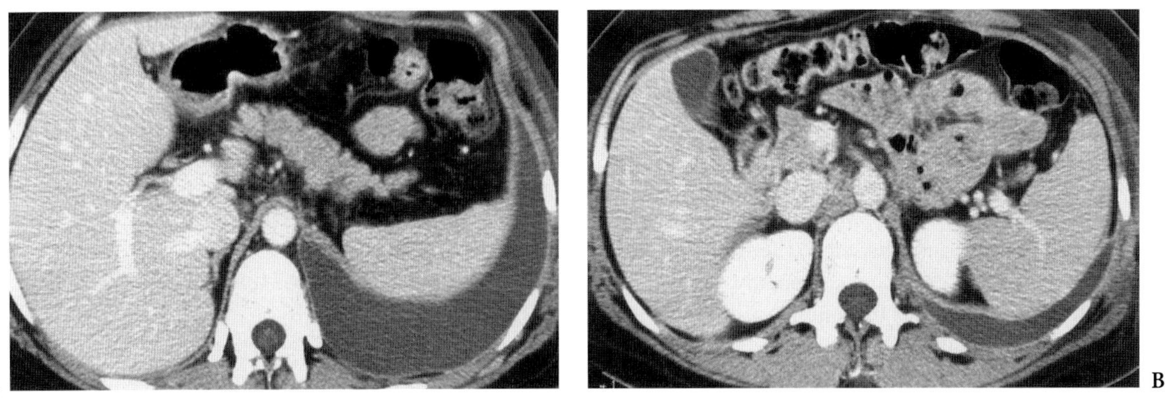

Fig. 5.5A, B. Left pleural collection. Semicircular collection in the posterior costophrenic sulcus displacing the diaphragmatic crus medially (Dwyer's sign). Its width decreases downward. The interface between the fluid and the spleen is ill defined (Teplick's interface sign)

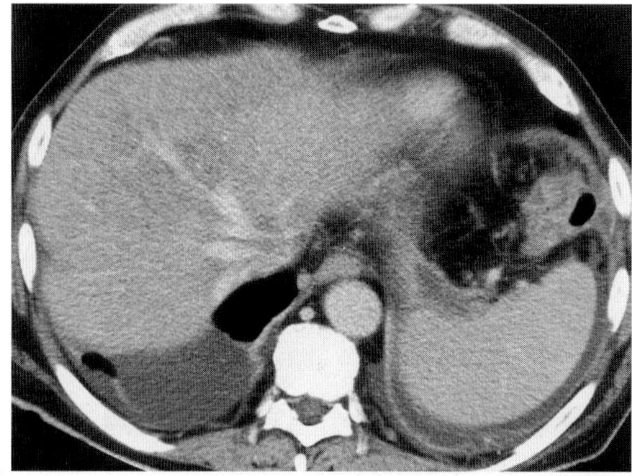
A

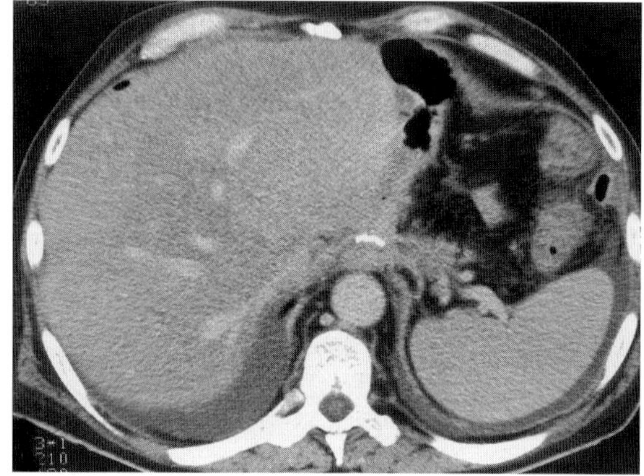
B

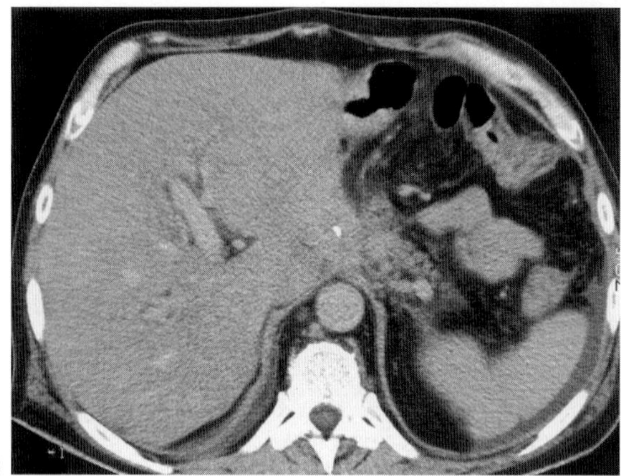
C

Fig. 5.6A–C. Bilateral pleural and perisplenic collections. Pleural effusions diffusing in a semicircular shape behind the liver and the spleen, and spreading medially up the back of the crura of the diaphragm, which they are pushing away from the spine (Dwyer's sign). On the left a slightly thickening diaphragm is easily visible, with the pleural collection outside and the subphrenic collection inside (sign of the diaphragm). The subphrenic collection surrounds the spleen, except at the hilum, owing to the presence of the splenopancreatic ligament (splenic bare area). Ill-defined interface between the pleural fluid, the liver and the spleen; sharp interface between the peritoneal collection and the spleen (Teplick's interface sign)

by the coronary ligament (bare area) (Fig. 5.1). On the left, the collection is seen around the spleen; it does not penetrate to the medial side of the organ, because it is blocked by the reflection of the splenopancreatic ligament (Fig. 5.1).

- The interface between the liver and spleen (Figs. 5.4–5.6) is very sharp when the fluid is subphrenic, and ill defined in the presence of pleural fluid (Teplick's interface sign) (Teplick et al. 1982).
- The pleural fluid is situated outside the diaphragm, whereas the subphrenic fluid is located inside (diaphragm sign) (Figs. 5.1, 5.6).
- When the fluid is conspicuous, the pleural collections spread upwards (Fig. 5.1), becoming progressively thicker and causes collapse of the lung; in contrast, the shape and disposition of the subphrenic collections conform to that of every single peritoneal cavity.
- When doubts about the location of fluid persist, further scans with the patient in a recumbent position and/or sagittal or coronal reconstructions may be needed (Griffin et al. 1984).

5.1.2 Subcapsular Hepatic and Splenic Collections and Perihepatic and Perisplenic Peritoneal Collections (Figs. 5.7, 5.8, 6.7, 6.8)

Subcapsular hepatic and splenic collections differ from perihepatic and perisplenic peritoneal collections in some significant features:

a) Subcapsular collections are round, whereas periton-eal collections are fusiform with cuspidate extremities.
b) Peritoneal collections are confined by ligaments, whereas intraparenchymal accumulations spread in front of the hepatic and splenic bare area.
c) In contrast to subcapsular accumulations, peritoneal collections show a "step" (Figs. 5.5, 5.7, 5.8, 6.8), or a short lucent space, at their extremities between fluid and visceral profile.
d) The poorly defined contours indicate an intraparenchymal collection.

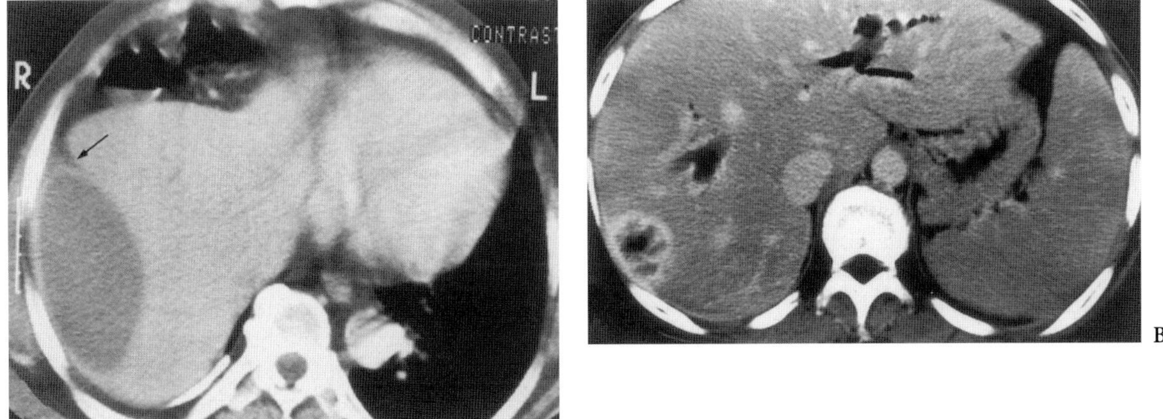

Fig. 5.7A, B. Subphrenic and intrahepatic collections. **A** Abscess in the right subphrenic recess. "Step" between the abscess and the hepatic border (*arrow*). **B** Round peripheral intrahepatic abscessed collection with thick enhanced wall and multiloculated cavity

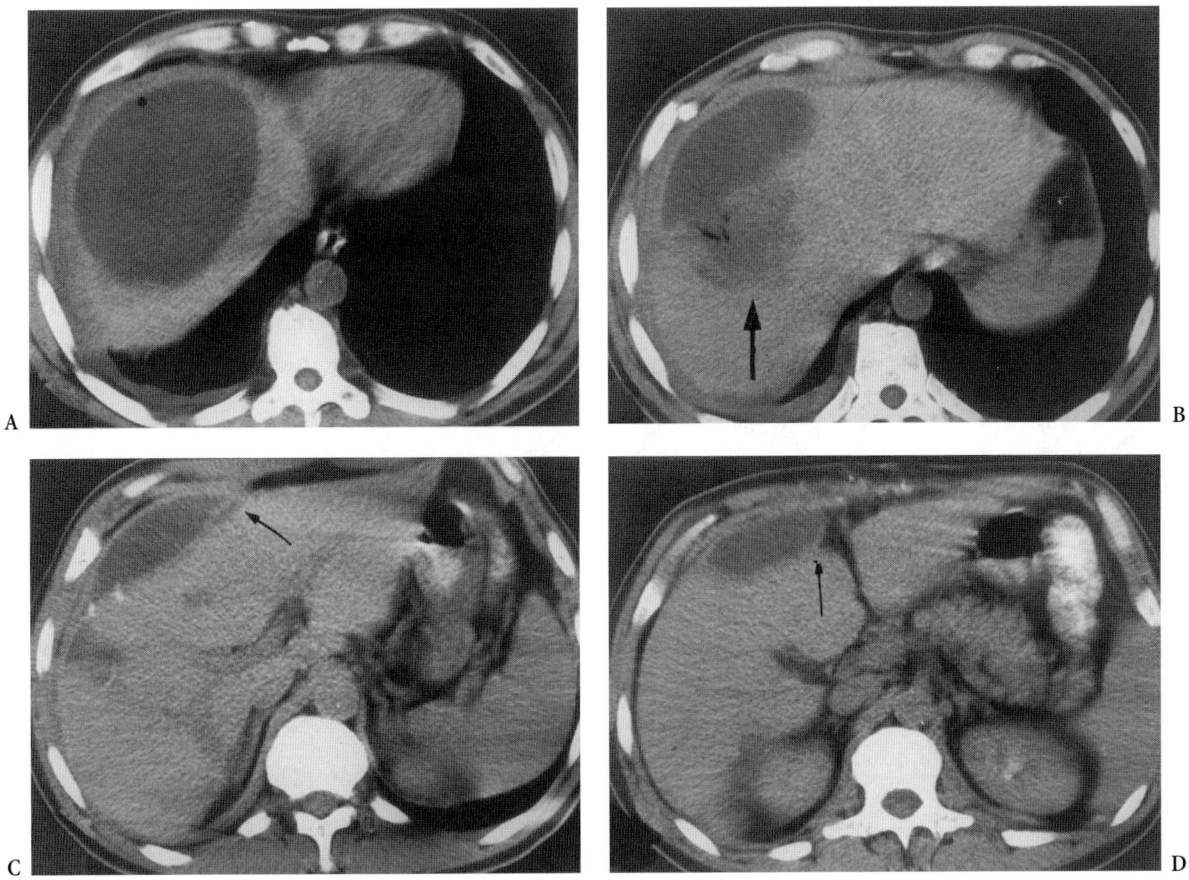

Fig. 5.8A–D. Subphrenic and intrahepatic abscesses. **A,C,D** The subphrenic abscesses are characterized by a sharp profile and a round disposition between the cupula of the liver and the diaphragm and a cuspidate fusiform shape at the side, with step and block at the level of the falciform ligament (*small arrow*). **B** In contrast, the hepatic abscess (*thick arrow*) has an indistinct curled profile

5.1.3 Collections in the Anterior Pararenal Space and in the Posterior Peritoneal Recesses (Figs. 5.9–5.11)

Fluid collections in the anterior pararenal space are usually secondary to necrotic-hemorrhagic pancreatitis; they can easily be distinguished from collections in the lesser sac, in Morrison's recess and in the splenopancreatic recess, because of their different shape, orientation, limits and expansion. However, since the retroperitoneal collections frequently spread over the peritoneal cavity during necrotic-hemorrhagic pancreatitis, evaluation of any possible peritoneal involvement and accurate detection of the cavities involved are often needed before the therapeutic program can be selected. These evaluations are easily performed in the presence of a wide peritoneal involvement, with fluid collections in cavities far distant from the concomitant peripancreatic accumulation, whereas they are difficult, or even impossible, when the peritoneal involvement is limited to the cavities located near the pancreatic compartment, such as the lesser sac and the splenopancreatic recess. In this connection, it can also be difficult to specify the exact intra- and/or retroperitoneal localization of fluid collections during surgery, because it is difficult to make out the peritoneum; only the persistence of the retrogastric lucent transversal line makes it possible to say definitively that retroperitoneal collections have not diffused into the bursa omentalis (Rubenstein et al. 1983).

Even a minimal amount of fluid in the posterior peritoneal spaces can be confused with thickening of the anterior renal fascia; however, when the thin transversal line of the fascia is followed at the sides, where it does not make close contact with the peritoneum, this is sufficient to allow recognition of thickening of the fascia resulting from the presence of peritoneal fluid.

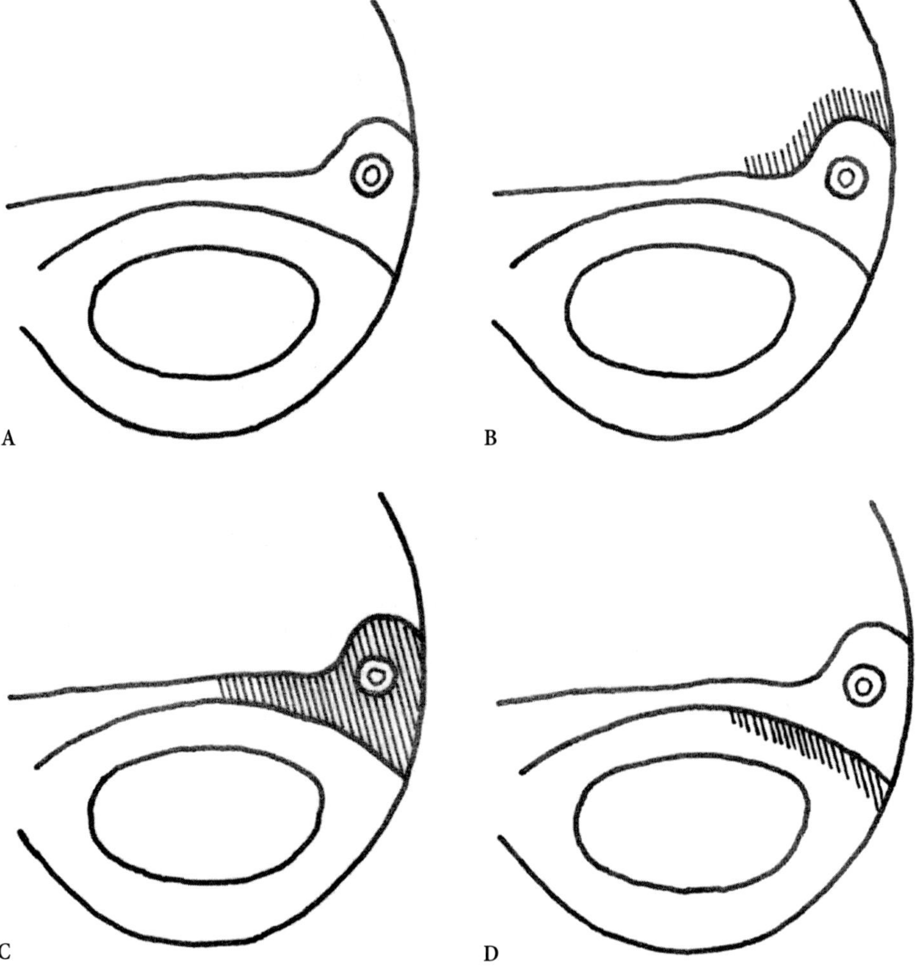

Fig. 5.9. A Diagram of sites of fluid collections: B paracolic gutter; C lateroconal compartment; D perirenal compartment

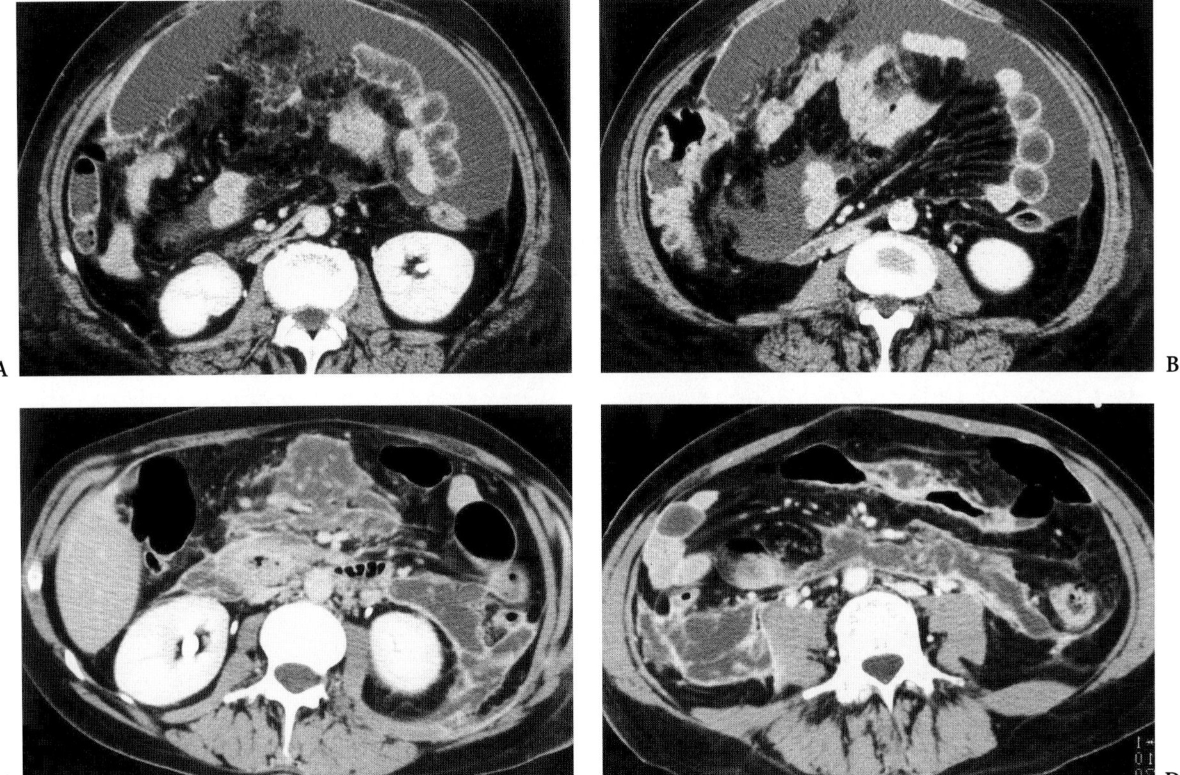

Fig. 5.10A–D. Collections in the posterior peritoneal recesses and in the anterior pararenal space. **A, B** Malignant ascites expanding the inframesocolic cavities and the left paracolic gutter. **C, D** Collection in the anterior pararenal space extending forward to the mesentery in a patient with necrotic pancreatitis. The difference in the collections, their profiles, and position relative to vessels, peritoneum and fasciae is very clear. The intraperitoneal collection shows a sharp profile all around; it diffuses in front and at the sides of the clear spaces representing the mesenteries and the retroperitoneum, and in front of both the ascending and the descending colon, in the respective lateroconal compartments (**A, B**). The collection in the anterior pararenal space is clearly limited on the posterior side by the anterior renal fascia and penetrates the lateroconal compartments laterally, behind both ascending and descending colon (**C, D**). The subperitoneal collection in the mesentery is recognizable by its position in front of the mesenteric vessels (*C*)

5.1.4 Collections in Paracolic Gutters, in Lateroconal Compartments and in the Anterior Pararenal Compartment (Figs. 5.9, 5.10)

Fluid collections in the paracolic gutters are located in front of the ascending or descending colon and in front of the adipose tissue of the corresponding mesentery, sinking to varying depths at their sides (Jeffrey 1983; Jolles and Coulam 1960). Even though the peritoneal cavity sometimes seems to surround the colon completely, it is always possible to recognize the thin lucent line of the mesentery connecting colon and retroperitoneum.

Collections in the lateroconal compartments are usually seen along the anterior renal fascia, where this blends with the lateroconal fascia. When small amounts of fluid are present, only a thickening of the fascia is observed; in contrast, more conspicuous collections spread around and particularly behind the ascending and descending colon (Fig. 5.31).

Fluid collections in the anterior pararenal compartment are limited anteriorly by the arcuate line of the anterior renal fascia, which often becomes thicker and separates the fluid from the lucent adipose tissue located in the lateroconal compartments and from the ascending and descending colon.

5.1.5 Collections in the Peritoneal Cavity and Subperitoneal Spaces

When peritoneal fluid (Figs. 5.10, 5.11A, 5.12) spreads over recesses and cavities, it adopts the characteristic shapes and dispositions described in the

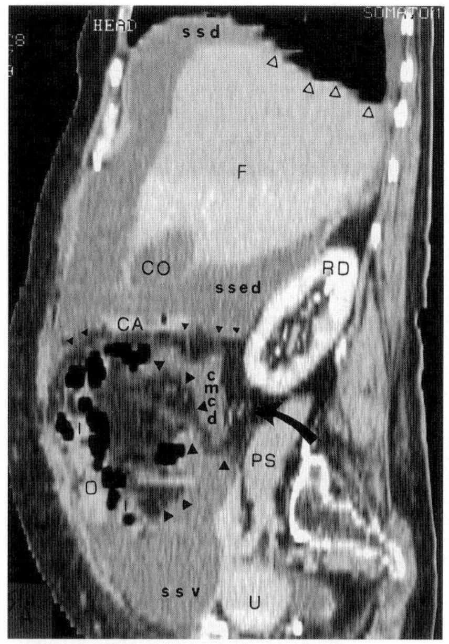

A

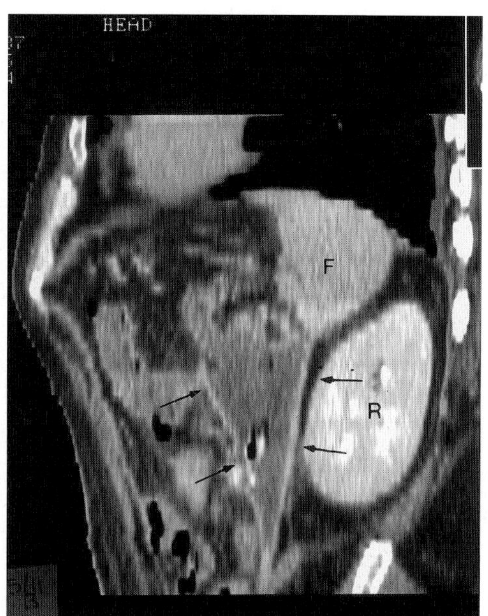

B

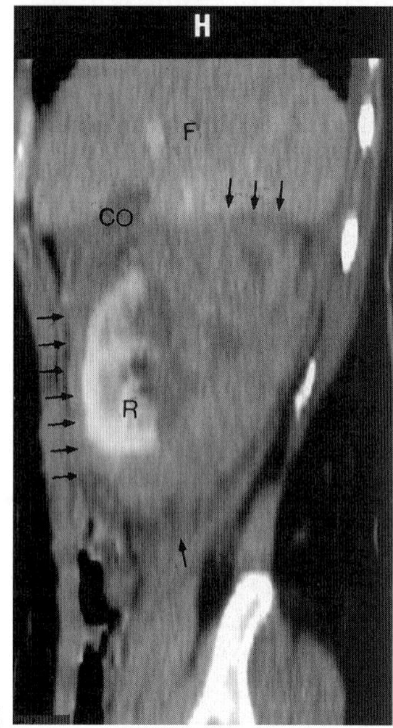

C

Fig. 5.11. Disposition of fluid collections in **A** the peritoneal cavity, and in **B** the anterior pararenal and **C** the perirenal spaces. Utility of the sagittal reconstructions. **A** Ascites. **B** Acute necrotic pancreatitis. **C** Hematoma caused by traumatic rupture of the kidney. Utility of sagittal reconstruction for easy location of the collections: the ascites well limited by peritoneum, the pancreatic collection between the peritoneum and the renal fascia, and the blood effusion in the perirenal space

CT anatomy section. These collections show a sharp peritoneal boundary with preservation of the adjacent subperitoneal fat. When the patient moves to a changed lying position the collections modify their shape only slightly and the fluid does not flow out of the recess where it is contained.

In contrast, the subperitoneal collections (Figs. 5.10, 5.14, 5.15) follow the orientation of ligaments and mesenteries; their profile is sharp only on the peritoneal side, whereas it is indefinite and shaded on the side of the areolar tissue, where they are held.

With changes in the lying position, the fluid moves in dependence on the ligaments that are containing it, and may diffuse into the retroperitoneum.

5.1.6 Intra- and Extraperitoneal and Extrafascial Pelvic Collections (Figs. 5.13–5.18)

It is usually easy to perform a correct set of images of the intra- or subperitoneal pelvic collections, in view of their different shapes, dispositions, and pro-

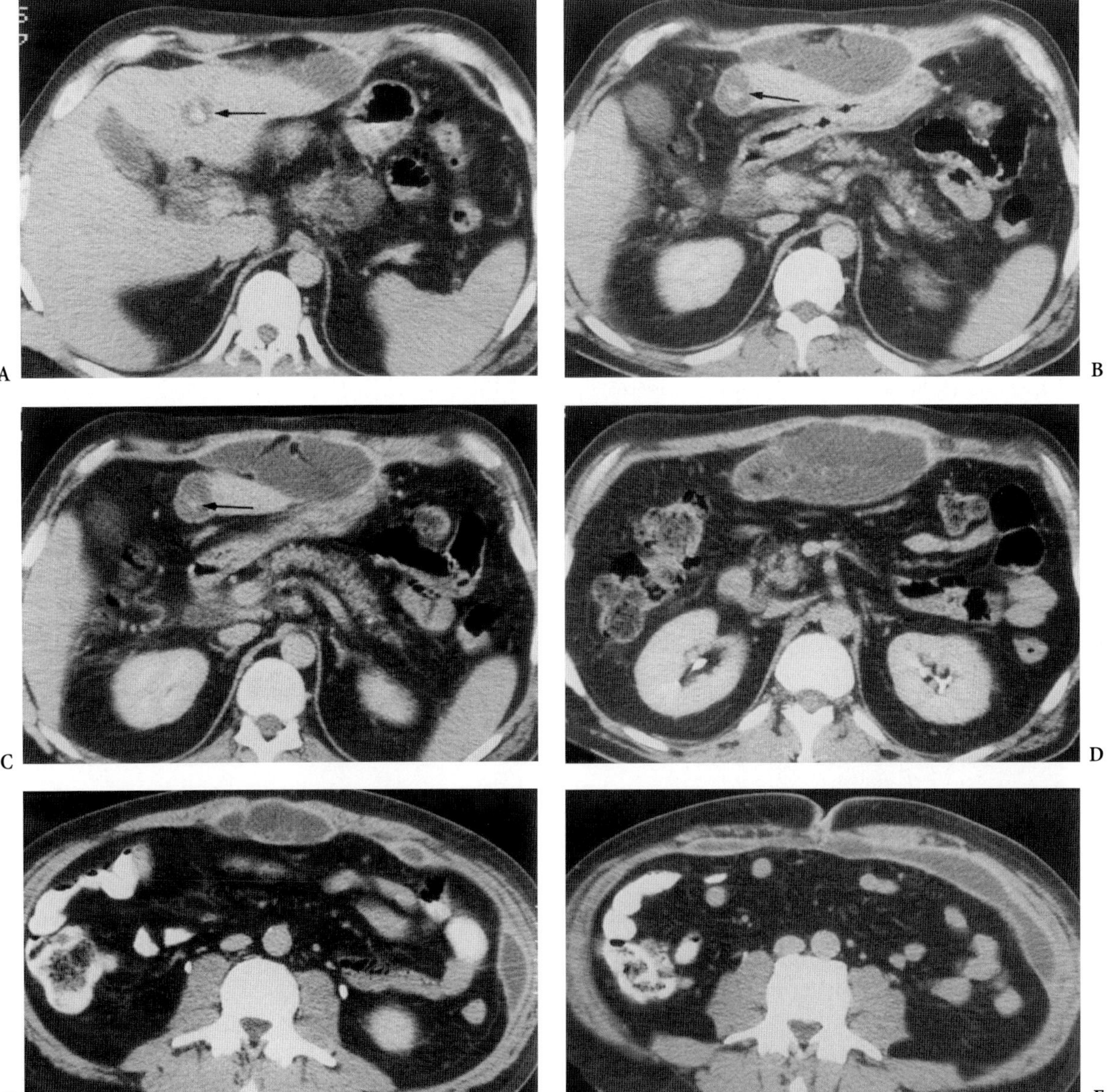

Fig. 5.12A, B. Inflammatory collection in the anterior preperitoneal spaces. The collection occupies the umbilical canal, which appears widened with thickened and contrast-enhancing walls. Higher up, the fluid diffuses toward the right, surrounding the umbilical vein up to the longitudinal fissure of the liver in the space between the leaves of the falciform ligaments. The umbilical vein (*arrow*) is surrounded by the fluid; the vein is made opaque by the contrast medium and is easily recognized in the intrahepatic tract. In the median tract of the umbilical canal only the negative punctiform image of the teres ligament is visible. At the level of the umbilicus the fluid spreads laterally into the preperitoneal space between the peritoneum and the transversalis fascia

files, and their expansion, extension and mobility in adapting to different lying positions, their positions relative to vessels and organs, and the possible concomitant fluid collections in other peritoneal spaces and their different pathologic causes (Figs. 4.32–4.37, 4.102, 4.103).

Furthermore, the pelvic peritoneal recesses filled with fluid have a specific appearance owing to the prominence of vessels, ligaments and organs pushing up the lower peritoneum, which are symmetrically arranged whether they are located on the median line or sited at the sides (Figs. 4.32–4.35).

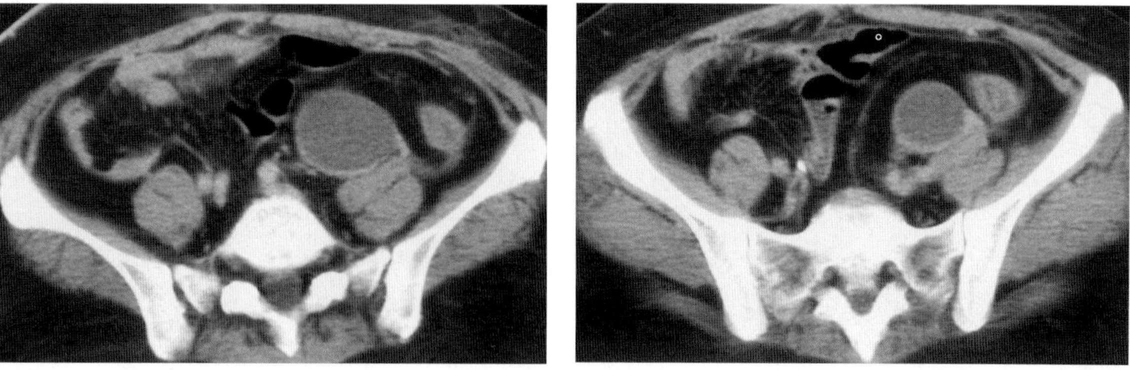

Fig. 5.13A, B. Intraperitoneal pelvic collection. Postsurgical saccate collection with sharp borders in the left parasigmoidal space, limited medially by the clarity of the sigmoid mesocolon with the sigmoid vessels and laterally by fat of the lateral extraperitoneal spaces

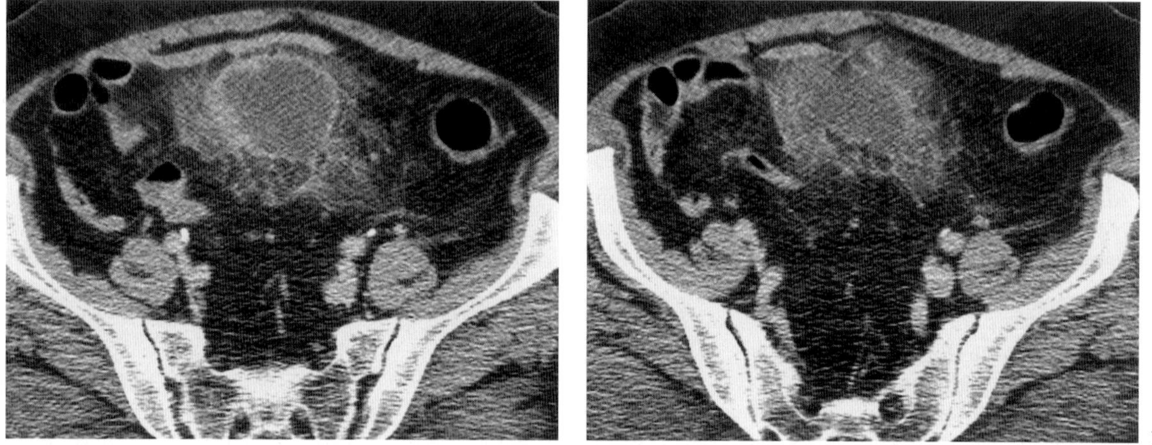

Fig. 5.14A, B. Pelvic subperitoneal collection. Abscess into the pelvic mesentery. In contrast with the previous collections showing very sharp peritoneal borders, the subperitoneal collection shows ill-defined limits

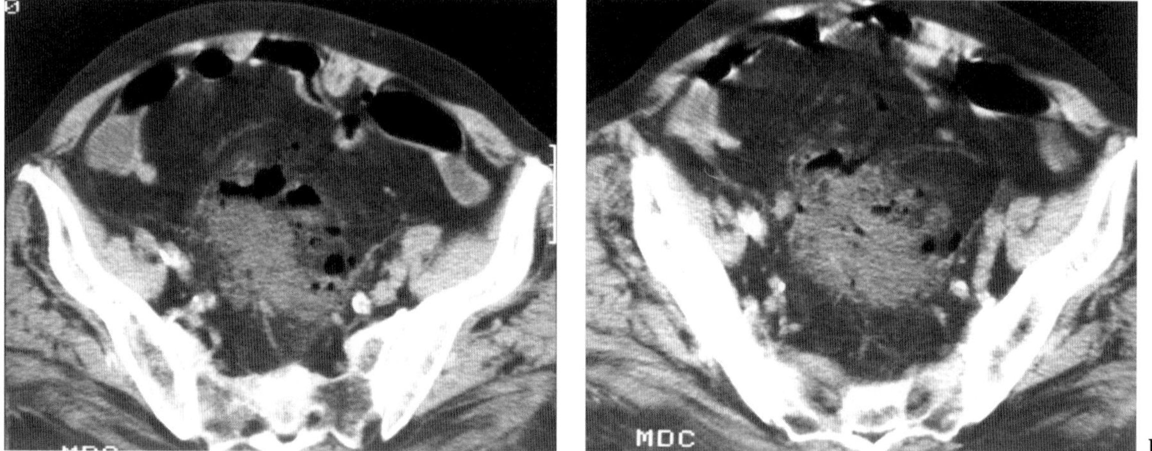

Fig. 5.15A, B. Pelvic sub- and retroperitoneal collection. Poorly defined fluid collection in the sigmoid mesocolon extending into the retroperitoneal space owing to rupture of a sigmoidal diverticulum

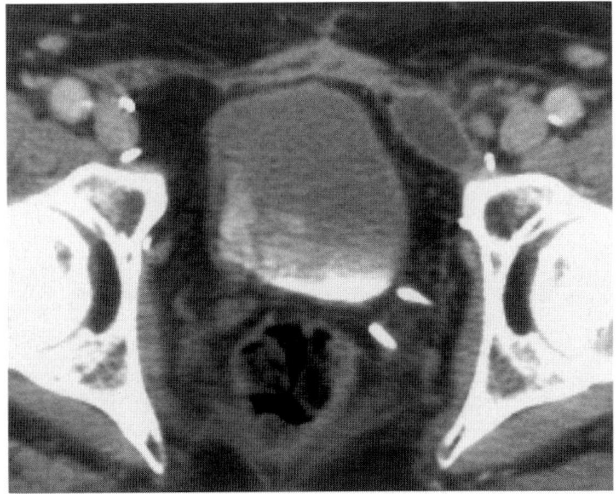
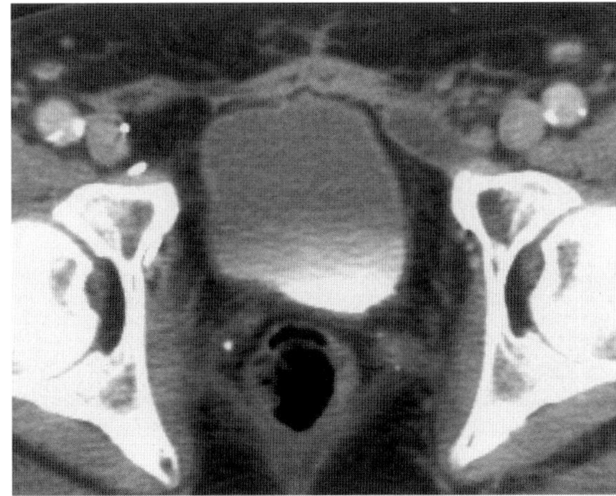

Fig. 5.16A, B. Anterior extrafascial pelvic collection. Serous postsurgical collection outside the transversalis fascia

In contrast to peritoneal collections, which are usually caused by liver cirrhosis or tumors, subperitoneal fluid generally has traumatic or iatrogenic causes; that is to say it is usually the consequence of vesical or prostatic biopsies or pelvic surgery. These collections also have a shape that is peculiarly their own, which is correlated to the arrangement of fasciae and spaces (Figs. 4.102, 4.103, 5.29–5.31).

A characteristic "molariform" shape is adopted by fluids in the perivesical space: a wider expansion in the anteromedial pre- and subvesical space corresponds to the crown, and a cuneiform posterior process extends at the sides of the urinary bladder (AUH et al. 1986a, b) (Fig. 5.17).

Furthermore, the intrafascial lateral subperitoneal collections can be distinguished from the extrafascial fluids located between the transversal pelvic fascia and the muscular aponeuroses by two elements: the shape and the position of the collection compared with the adipose tissue contained in the laterorectal space. The intrafascial subperitoneal collections show a medial convexity and diffuse into the areolar tissue in the laterorectal space, around the iliac vessels (Figs. 5.27, 5.29–5.31); in contrast, the extrafascial collections (Figs. 5.16, 5.18, 5.28) are fusiform, elongated in the anterior-posterior direction along the pelvic fascia, and they push the subperitoneal lateral fat and the internal and external iliac vessels medially. The thickening of the transversalis fascia that is almost always present provides further information that can be useful in the distinction between these types of collections and others.

5.2 Ascites

Ascites is an accumulation of transudate, exudate or chyle in the peritoneal cavity. It may be caused by various pathologies and is usually seen as a complication of a pathologic condition that is already known (Table 5.1).

Transudative ascites results from abnormally slow removal of peritoneal fluid caused by portal hypertension resulting from an intrahepatic (cirrhosis), prehepatic (portal thrombosis) or posthepatic (Budd-Chiari syndrome, thrombosis of the inferior vena cava, constrictive pericarditis, congestive heart failure) obstruction of flow. Transudative ascites can also be due to hypoalbuminemia, which favors the accumulation of fluid in the peritoneum through alterations to the mechanisms for fluid and solute exchange through serous and vascular membranes.

Exudative ascites is caused by an irritant stimulation of the peritoneal serosa with more rapid fluid production. The most frequent causes are the peritoneal neoplastic spread of abdominal tumors, prevalently ovarian and intestinal (carcinomatosis), and infections (peritonitis). Less commonly, it may be caused by a mesothelioma or by tuberculosis, and occasionally by chronic renal failure or myxedema.

Chylous ascites is an accumulation of chyle in the peritoneal cavity, caused by slowed or interrupted lymph flow through lymph nodes as a result of inflammatory, lymphomatous or metastatic adenopathies, or by traumatic or surgical obstruc-

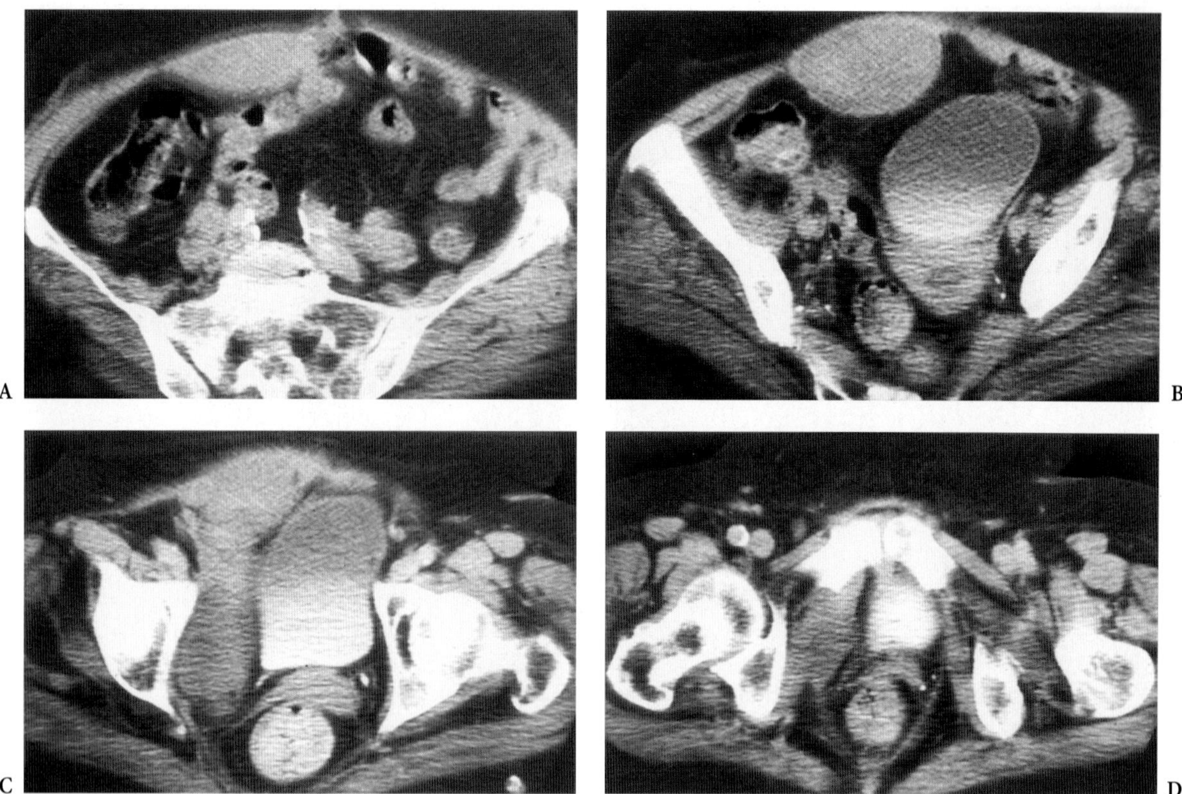

Fig. 5.17A–D. Extraperitoneal pelvic collection. Recent traumatic high-density hemorrhage in the right rectus abdominis muscle extending below the semicircular line of Douglas in the umbilico-prevesical space, between the transversalis fascia and the peritoneum, and in the pelvis between the umbilico-vesical fascia (located medially) and the pubic-genito-recto-sacral fascia (situated laterally). Here the collection shows a characteristic cuneiform shape, with posterior apex and very sharp borders

tion of the main lymphatic trunks (intestinal duct, cisterna chyli, thoracic duct) and less commonly by congenital abnormalities (atresia, stenosis, lymphangiectasia) or filariosis. Accumulation of chylous ascites also occurs when a large number of collectors are involved without adequate lymphatic flow through collateral pathways.

The ascitic fluid may occupy the whole of the peritoneal cavity (Figs. 5.1–5.3) or may be collected in one or more recesses, or finally, it may be confined to the pocket where it was generated, limited by peritoneal reactive adhesions.

When the ascitic fluid occupies the entire peritoneal cavity it delineates the various recesses, which can each be distinguished by its configuration, situation, position relative to organs and surrounding structures and by the thin dense line dividing it from the restraining peritoneum (Figs. 5.1–5.3).

The ascitic fluid is usually homogeneous, with low attenuation values (0–20 HU), with no differences that might help to establish its nature and etiology. However, a higher density suggests a tubercular, purulent or hematic nature of the collection (Bydder and Kreel 1980; Federle and Jeffrey 1983), while very low or negative attenuation values are indicative of a chylous fluid. Plaques and nodules of different thickness dotting the internal surface of the peritoneum and associated with ascites are usually signs of carcinomatosis (Figs. 4.17, 4.20, 5.1, 5.3).

5.3 Hematic Collections

Intraperitoneal (hemoperitoneum) (Fig. 5.3) and subperitoneal hematic collections occur as the consequence of hepatic, splenic or mesenteric trauma, biopsy or postsurgical bleeding attributable to incomplete hemostasis, with spontaneous rupture of a vascular neoplasm (chiefly a hepatic adenoma, hepatocarcinoma, cavernous angioma, or angiosar-

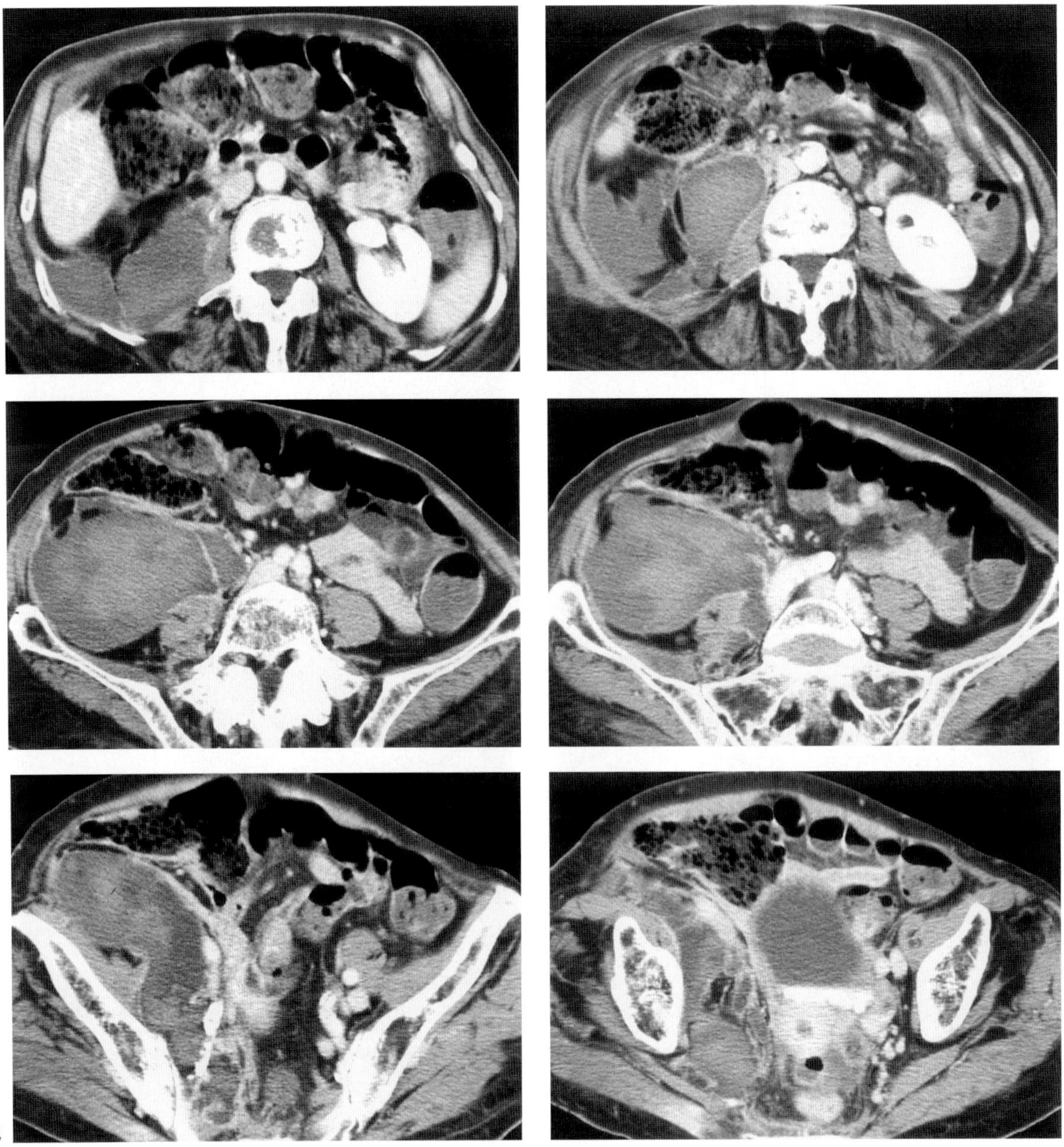

A B C D E F

Fig. 5.18A–F. Extrafascial abdominopelvic collection. Recent nonhomogeneous hemorrhagic collection, after biopsy of the right iliac crest, in the extrafascial space, pressing on the transversalis fascia and the extraperitoneal spaces

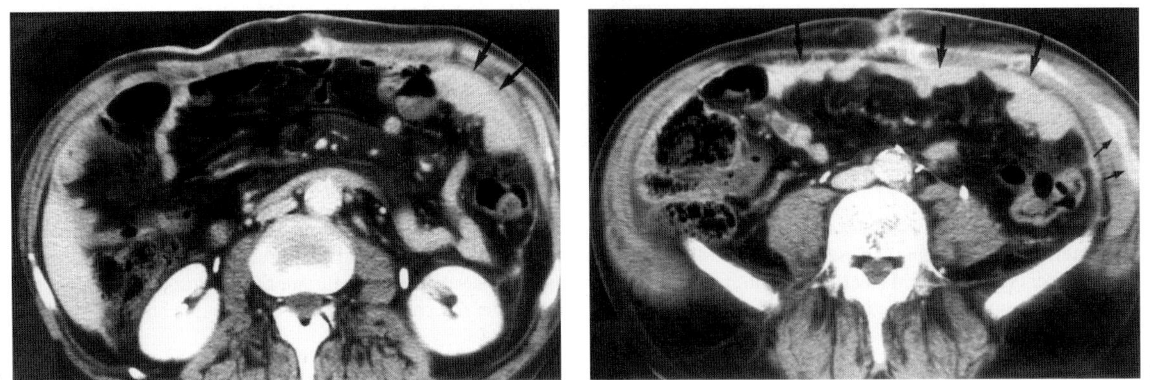

Fig. 5.19A, B. Hematic collections. Spontaneous hemorrhage of the omentum and of the abdominal wall. The recent hyperdense hemorrhage adopts a semicircular shape in the anterior part of the abdominal cavity and penetrates between the ileal loops (*thick arrows*) and the left abdominal transverse muscle bundles (*thin arrows*)

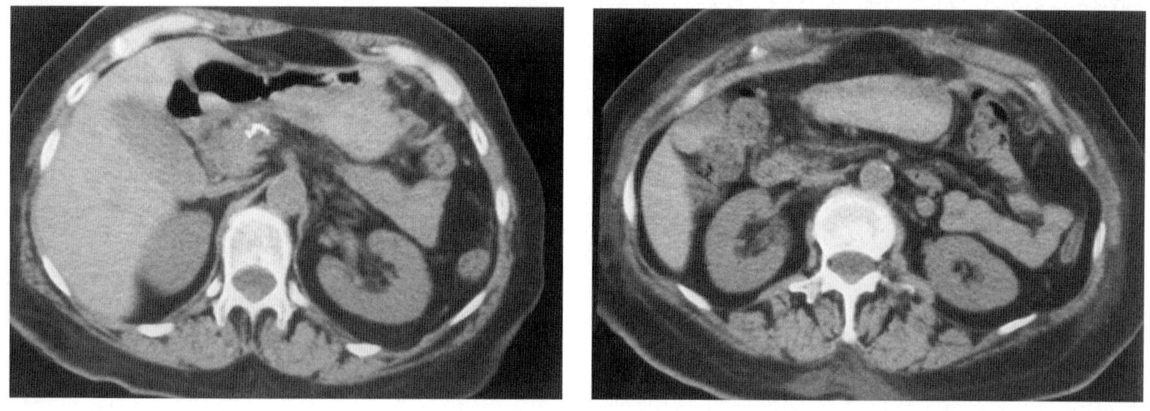

Fig. 5.20A, B. Intraperitoneal hematic collection. Postsurgical (splenectomy and resection of the corpus and cauda pancreatis) collection in the left inferior recesses of the lesser sac. Peculiar hyperdensity of the recent hemorrhage without contrast medium. Transverse orientation of the collection just behind the stomach; the fluid continues downward as far as the conjunction of the smaller omentum with the transverse mesocolon

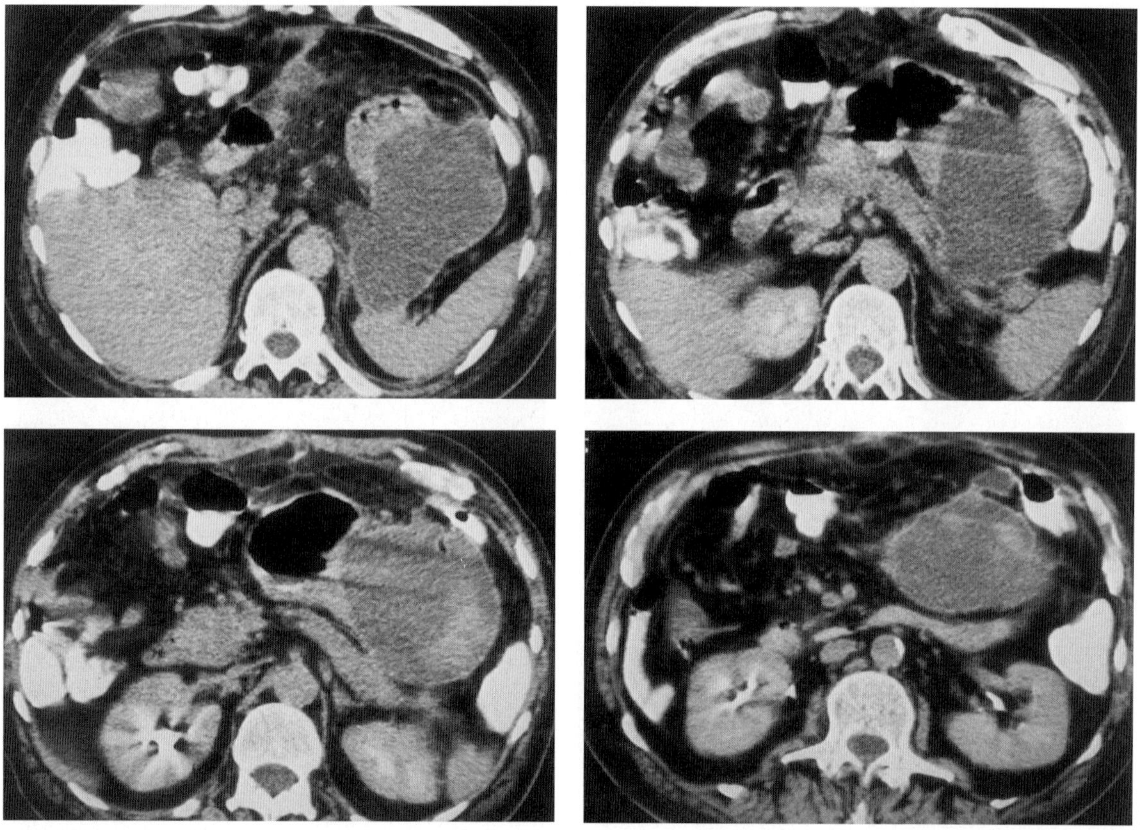

Fig. 5.21A–D. Hematic intraperitoneal collection. Wide collection in the left recesses of the lesser sac after gastro-esophageal resection. The collection is in close contact with the posterior wall of the gastric stump and is separated from the pancreas, spleen and jejunal loops by a thin clear fissure; in the lower part it stops at the level of the junction of the smaller omentum with the transverse mesocolon. There is a high-attenuation area within the low-density collection where hemolysis is not yet complete

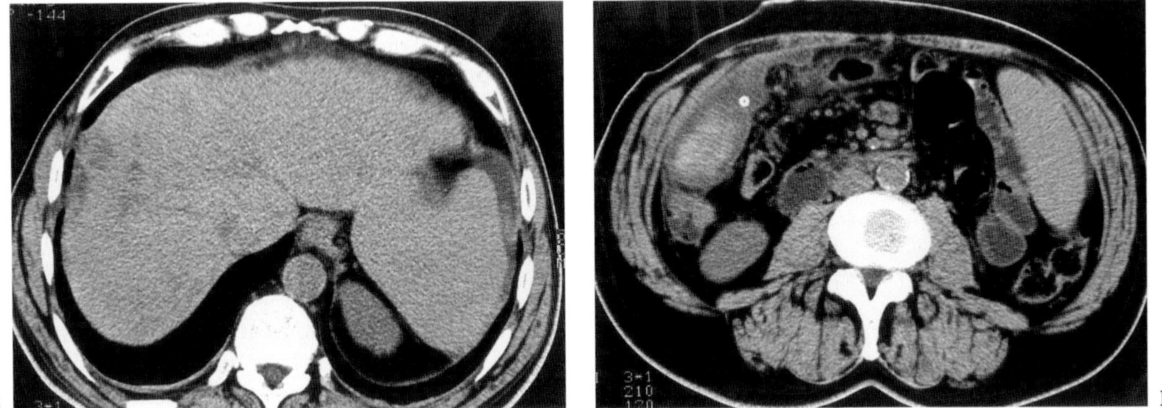

Fig. 5.22A, B. Intraperitoneal hematic collections. Subhepatic and perisplenic hemorrhage following biopsy. Initial peripheral hemolysis

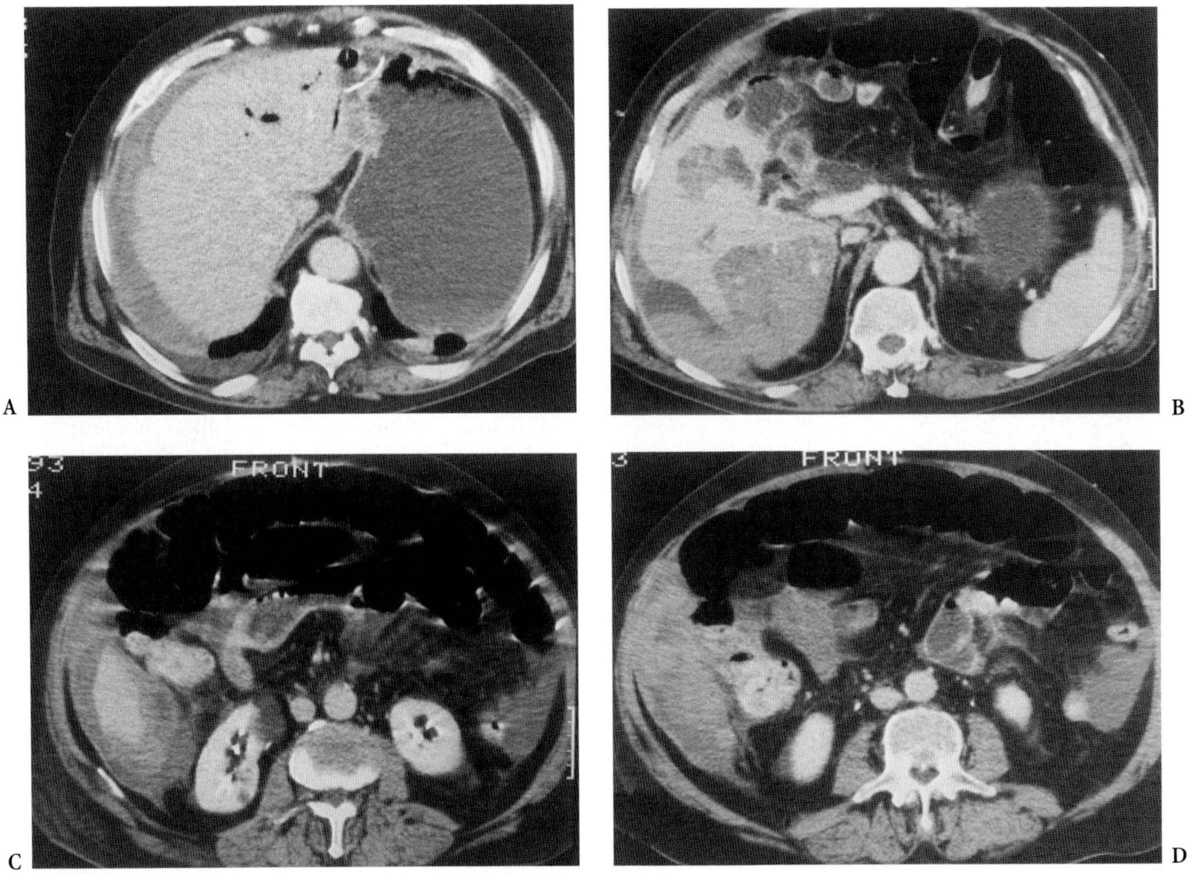

Fig. 5.23A–D. Intraperitoneal hematic collection. Postsurgical (gastro-duodeno-cephalo-pancreatectomy) hemorrhage. High-attenuation nonhomogeneous areas surrounded by low-density fluid in the **A**, **B** subphrenic and **C**, **D** right subhepatic spaces. Swollen gastric stump owing to stenosis of the gastro-jejunostomy; ischemia of the VI hepatic segment

coma), spontaneous rupture of hemorrhagic, luteinic or endometriotic cysts, ectopic pregnancy, excessive use of anticoagulants or bleeding diatheses.

CT findings (Federle and Jeffrey 1983; Haaga 1988; Heiken 1989; Jeffrey et al. 1991) in hemorrhagic collections vary according to the age of the bleeding and to the degree of peritoneal absorption. Initially, the attenuation of the collection is the same as that of the circulating blood and soft structures (Fig. 8.9); then, within a few hours, it increases and

A
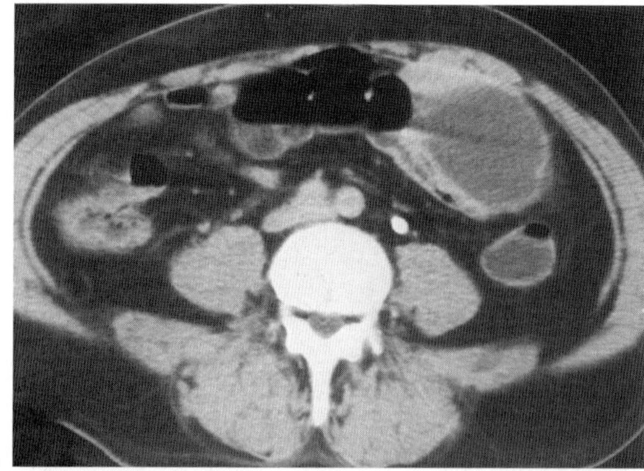
B
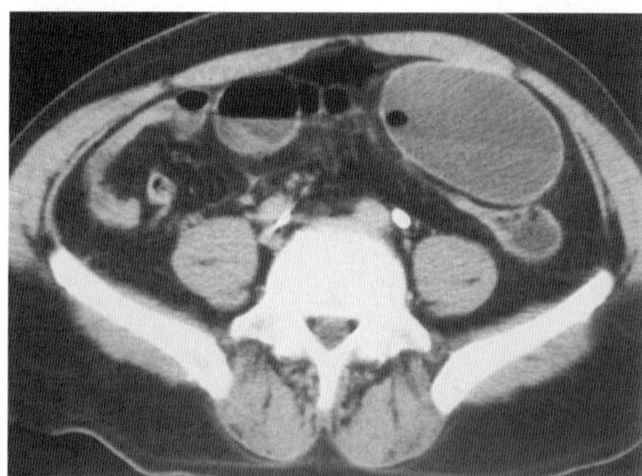
C
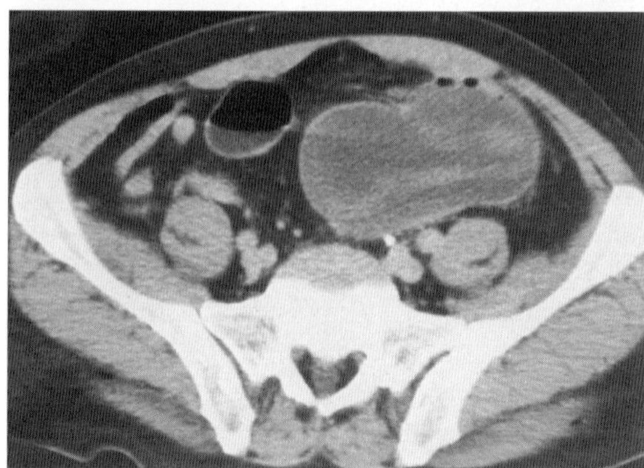

Fig. 5.24A–C. Intraperitoneal hematic collection. Intraperitoneal hemorrhage owing to rupture of the intestinal wall secondary to lithotripsy. Within the fluid, there are small air bubbles – indices of rupture – and dense hematic areas

reaches high values (greater than 50 HU), a change that is connected with clotting and with the concentration of hemoglobin (Figs. 4.102, 5.17, 5.19, 5.20, 8.4, 8.9, 8.11, 8.12). Finally, it is followed by a gradual decrease (until the values for water are reached) because of the remarkable thrombolytic activity of the peritoneum. The attenuation usually decreases from the periphery toward the center and shows a hyperdense area surrounded by a low-density halo, widening as the lysis increases (Figs. 5.18, 5.21–5.24, 8.9).The collection gradually reduces in width until it is totally resorbed with complete disappearance or fibrous residuals. In the peritoneal cavity resorption of serous fluid is rapid because of the intense activity of the serosa. Alternate concentric layers of low and high density or persistent linear strands or areas of high attenuation are due to intermittent bleeding or to irregular reabsorption of clot (Wolwerson et al. 1983). Sometimes a layer of serous fluid over denser clotted blood is caused by erythrocyte sedimentation (hematocrit effect).

An active bleeding may be revealed by contrast medium extravasation in the mesentery or in the peritoneal cavity on dynamic CT scan (Jeffrey et al. 1991; Mirvis 1989; Shanmuganathan et al. 1993, 1995).

Old hematomas appear to be surrounded by a thick dense fibroplastic and vascular pseudocapsule.

In patients with abdominal trauma, a focal high-density area attributable to the localized clotted blood with high hemoglobin content (sentinel clot) is a significant marker of the bleeding source.

According to the organ and structure where the lesion occurred, the hemorrhage may spread into the areolar tissue of the ligaments or mesenteries, into the omentum (Fig. 5.19) or within the peritoneal cavity (Figs. 5.20–5.24).

When the subperitoneum and the omentum are involved, besides diffuse hazing of the adipose tissue, bleeding may appear in an early phase as a small high-density mass displacing or compressing an intestinal loop that progressively reduces the attenuation values and size until complete resorption, with or without fibrotic residue.

In the peritoneal cavity, the hemorrhagic fluid may be localized in a recess next to the bleeding organ or structure where it originated, but it mostly tends to flow toward the lowest parts, such as Morrison's recess, when the bleeding is supramesocolic, and the pelvis when it is submesocolic. Therefore, to determine the extent of posttraumatic bleeding, a complete scan of the abdomen and pelvis may be suggested; in fact, it is possible that after splenic ruptures the hemorrhagic fluid moves from the left to the right subhepatic recesses and through the right paracolic gutter to the pelvic cavity.

The hemorrhagic nature of a peritoneal fluid observed after a recent trauma cannot be established according to CT density unless it contains diffuse areas with attenuation values greater than 30 HU.

5.4 Bilomas

Bile collections(bilomas) are due to rupture of the biliary tree or of the gallbladder induced by trauma or biliary surgery, drainage, percutaneous biopsy, cholangiography or are spontaneous, resulting from a sudden increase of the intraluminal pressure caused by choledochal obstructions.

Bilomas originate in leakage from the gallbladder. Initially, they are located in the peritoneal pericholecystic space, then expanding up into the gastrohepatic and subhepatic recesses to occupy most of the width of the supramesocolic space, displacing the duodenum and the gastric antrum medially and the hepatic flexure of the colon downward. After trauma or invasive diagnostic procedures, they may collect in the peritoneal recess, but they are usually confined by a quick plastic-inflammatory response of the peritoneum, which forms a thin capsule around them.

On CT, bilomas appear as a low-density (0–20 HU) cyst-like structure with a thin, but always well-defined wall (Figs. 5.25, 5.26).

A biloma must be suspected when a sub- or perihepatic fluid collection forms just after surgery, trauma or invasive diagnostic procedures involving the biliary tract.

CT i.v. cholangiography with exaiodate contrast medium (Endocistobil, Biligrafin etc.) or PIPIDA scintigraphy showing opaque contrast or radionuclide extravasation may be helpful in determining whether an active bile leak is present, and if so in identifying the site of the leakage (Sty et al. 1982;

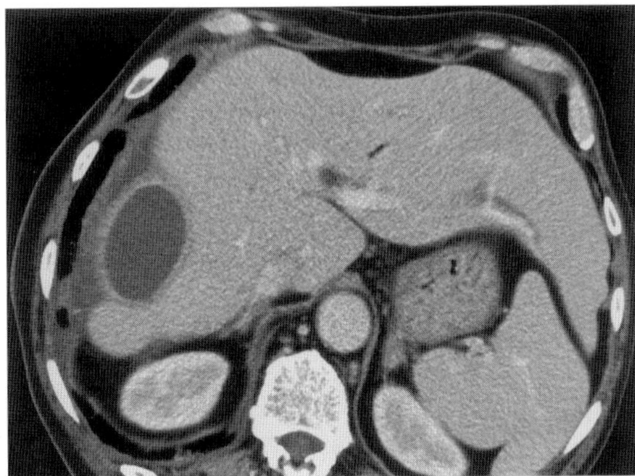

Fig. 5.25. Bile collections. Intra- and extraperitoneal and pleural iatrogenic biloma (transhepatic cholangiography). The intraperitoneal fluid is limited by a thick, dense reactive capsule

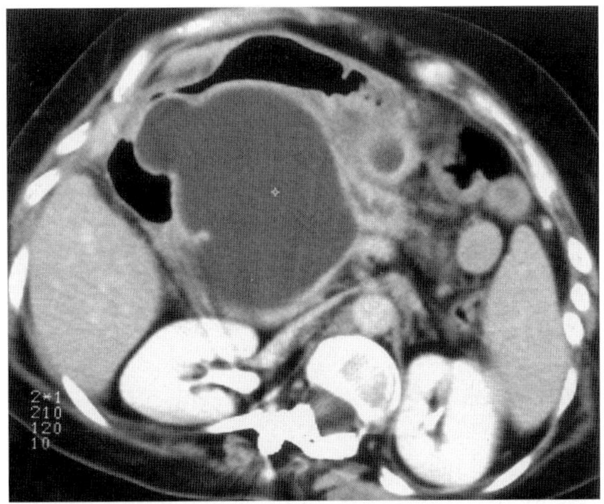

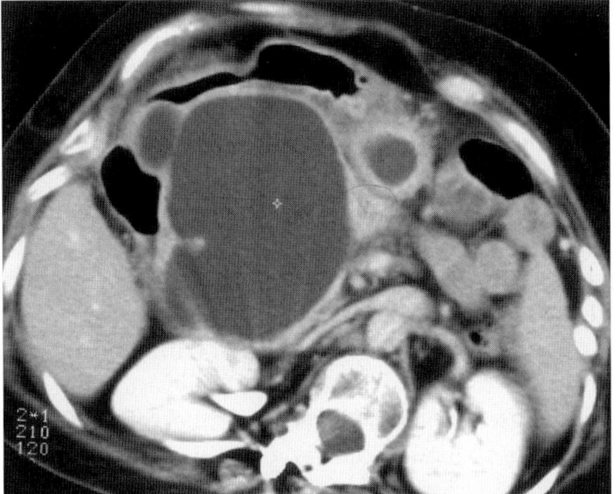

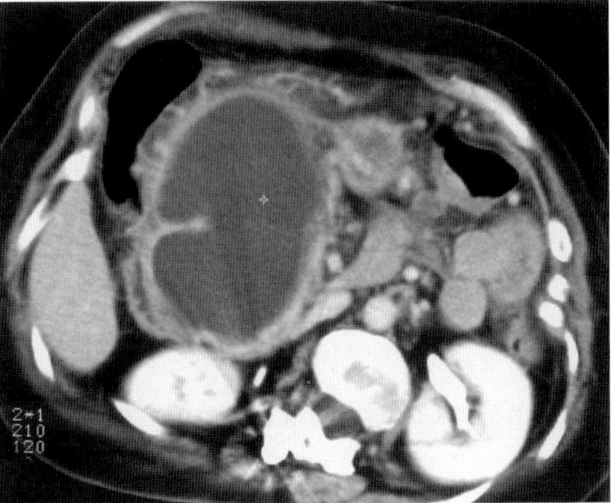

Fig. 5.26A–C. Bile collection. Biloma caused by leaking from the cystic duct after laparoscopic cholecystectomy. The fluid collection occupies the hepatoduodenal ligament, and spreads over the pancreatic compartment surrounded by the gastric antrum anteriorly, the second duodenal portion (on the right side and posteriorly), the pancreas (on the left side and above), and the superior mesenteric vessels (*below*)

Weissmann et al. 1979).In most cases it cannot be identified. More conveniently, a percutaneous aspiration through a thin needle can allow a correct diagnosis of bile collections even after bile extravasation has ceased, and at the same time it also allows the placement of an external drainage system, which often makes surgery unnecessary.

5.5 Urinomas

Abdominal urine collections (urinomas) are usually due to the extravasation of urine into retroperitoneal spaces after ruptures of the urinary tract, which can result, for example, from traumatic instrumental procedures or sudden increases in intraluminal pressure. In the subperitoneal spaces urine collections occur only as secondary events, because of diffusion through the direct communication with the retroperitoneal spaces at the mesenteric or the mesocolic level. Peritoneal involvement is usually due to complications of surgical shunt operations (total cystectomy with uretero-cutaneous or sigmoidal stoma, or ileal neovesica), to relaxation of a ureteral anastomosis, or to traumatic rupture of the vesical dome.

CT after i.v. contrast medium injection with late scanograms or after retrograde cystography showing the extravasation of opaque contrast is essential for diagnosis and management of urinomas, because it can establish the presence of an active urine leakage, identify the site of the leakage, which is sometimes far distant from the urinoma, and disclose the pathway followed by the urine (Sivit et al. 1995).

On unenhanced CT scans the urine collections (Figs. 5.27, 5.28) have water-attenuation values similar to those of other collections.

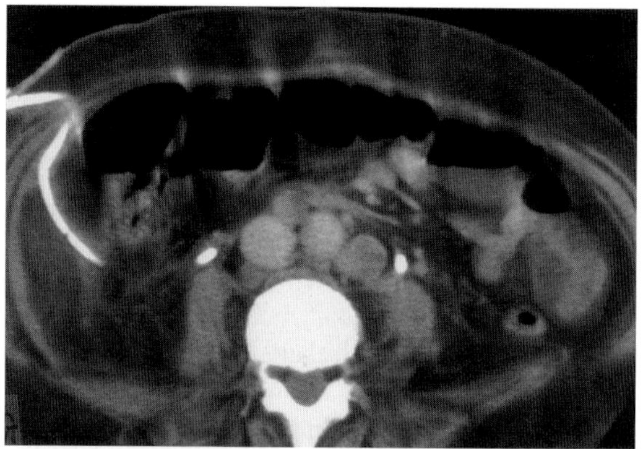

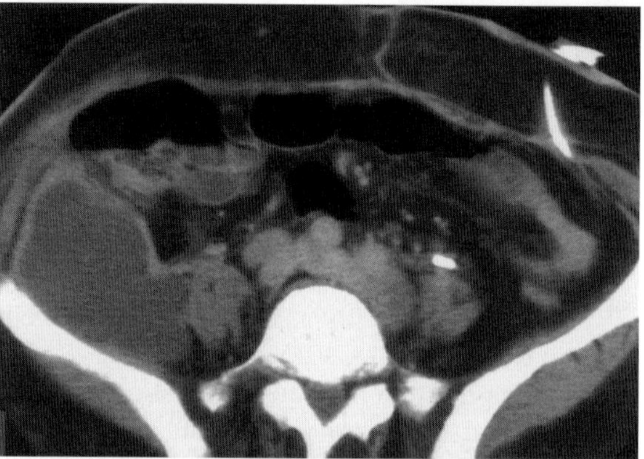

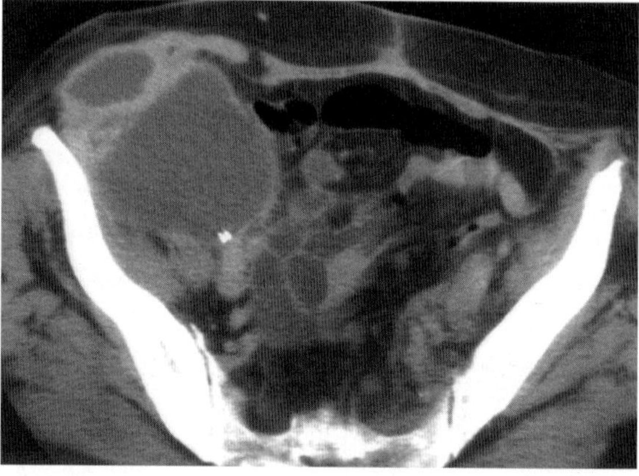

Fig. 5.27A–C. Extraperitoneal urine collection. Patient had undergone total cystectomy and bilateral uretero-cutaneostomy. The collection was generated by urine dripping on the sides of the cutaneous insertion of the right ureter into the lateral extraperitoneal space, in front of the psoas and of the internal iliac muscles and inside the transversalis fascia; it pushes the ascending colon and the ileal loops medially

5.6 Lymphatic Collections (Lymphoceles)

Lymphoceles are cystic collections of lymph resulting from section of lymphatic collectors during lymphadenectomy, renal transplantations or abdominal and pelvic surgery.

On CT scans, the lymphoceles are identifiable as cyst-like structures that are round, ovoid or irregular in shape; they are characterized by a fluid content with a density lower than 10 HU. Their wall is extremely thin, but always detectable, and it gives

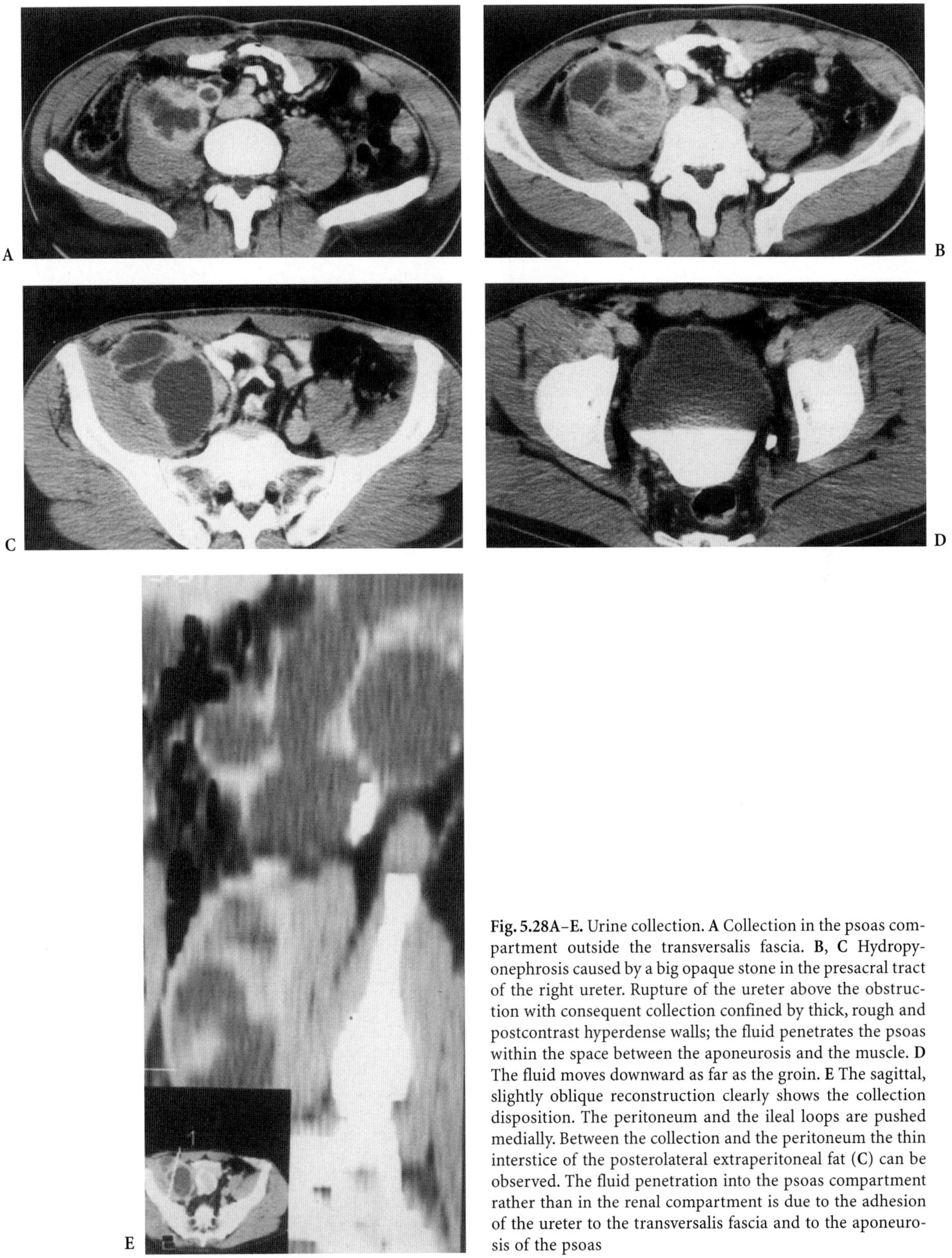

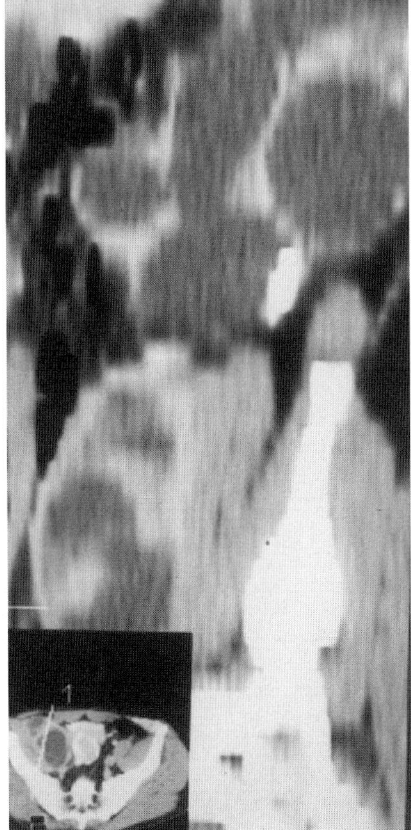

Fig. 5.28A–E. Urine collection. **A** Collection in the psoas compartment outside the transversalis fascia. **B, C** Hydropyonephrosis caused by a big opaque stone in the presacral tract of the right ureter. Rupture of the ureter above the obstruction with consequent collection confined by thick, rough and postcontrast hyperdense walls; the fluid penetrates the psoas within the space between the aponeurosis and the muscle. **D** The fluid moves downward as far as the groin. **E** The sagittal, slightly oblique reconstruction clearly shows the collection disposition. The peritoneum and the ileal loops are pushed medially. Between the collection and the peritoneum the thin interstice of the posterolateral extraperitoneal fat (**C**) can be observed. The fluid penetration into the psoas compartment rather than in the renal compartment is due to the adhesion of the ureter to the transversalis fascia and to the aponeurosis of the psoas

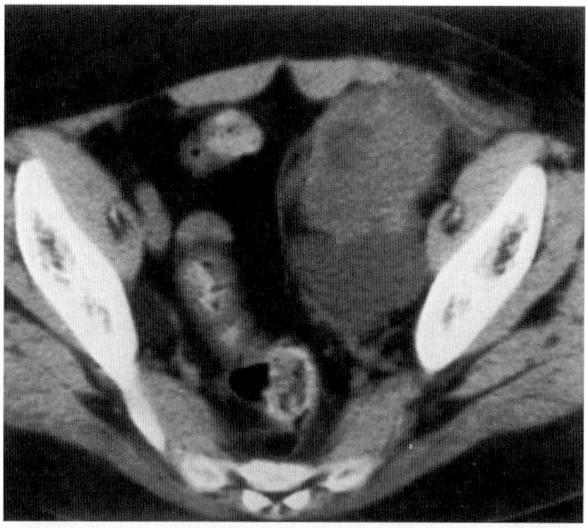

A 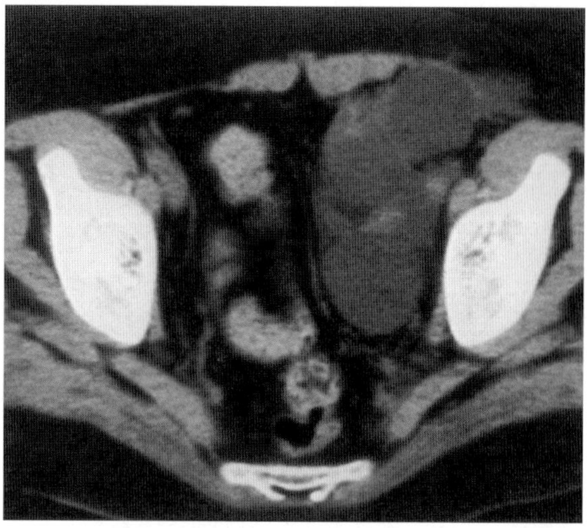 B

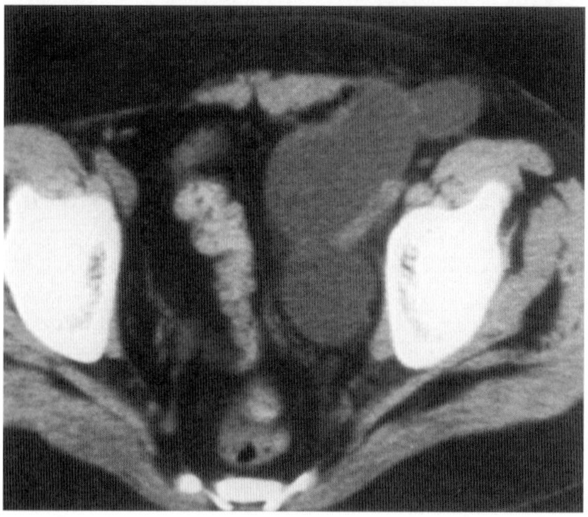

C

Fig. 5.29. Lymphatic collection (lymphocele). Patient operated on for renal transplantation. Well-delimited water-density collection in the pelvic extraperitoneal space

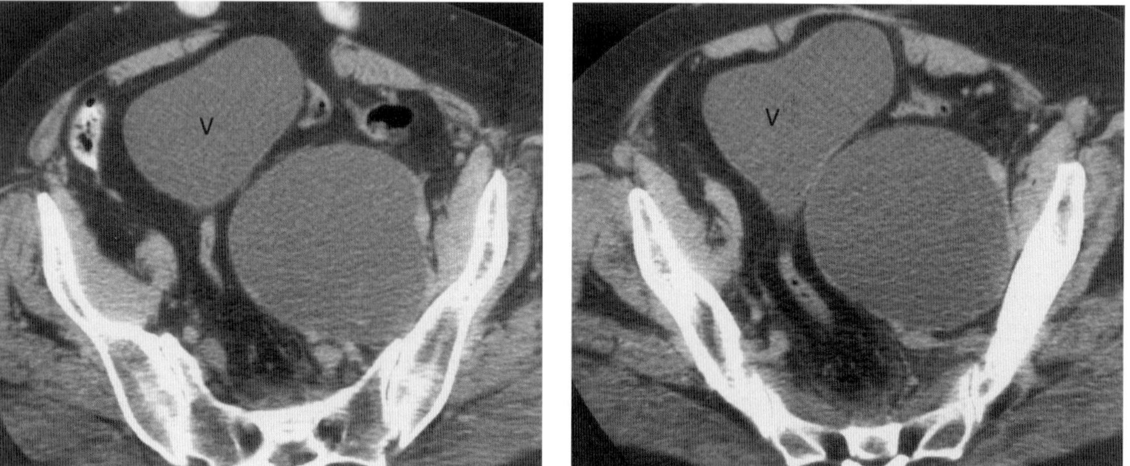

Fig. 5.30A, B. Lymphatic collection (lymphocele). Patient had undergone hystero-ovariectomy. Wide low-density homogeneous thin-walled collection in the lateral extraperitoneal space, below and medial to the iliac vessels, which are pulled apart and compressed. The urinary bladder and the sigmoid with its mesentery are displaced inward and are clearly separated from the fluid by fat

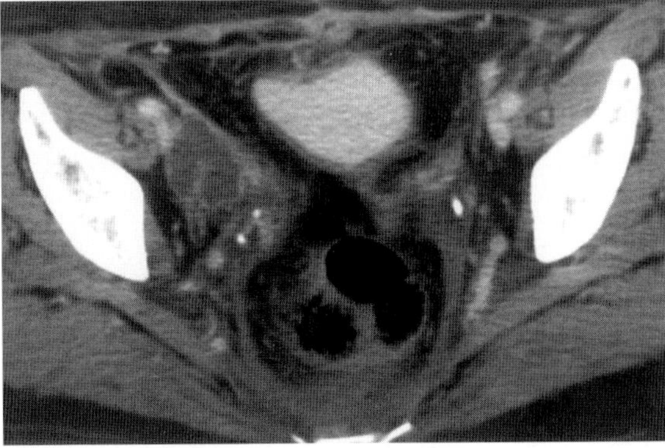

Fig. 5.31. Lymphatic collection (lymphocele). Patient had undergone hysterectomy and lymphadenectomy. Low-attenuation, homogeneous, thin walled collection in the right lateral extraperitoneal space, posterior to the external iliac vessels

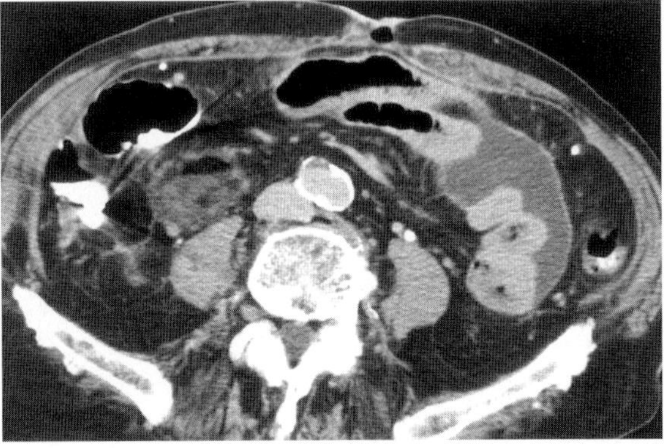

Fig. 5.32. Intraperitoneal seroma. Low-density, homogeneous serous collection surrounding the ileal loops and limited laterally by thickened peritoneum in a patient who had undergone small-bowel resection.

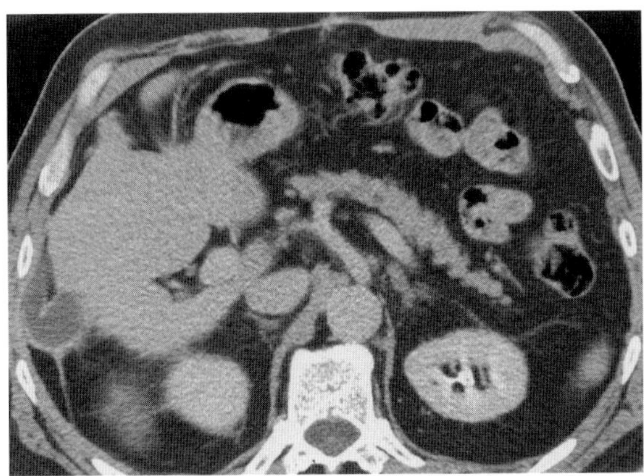

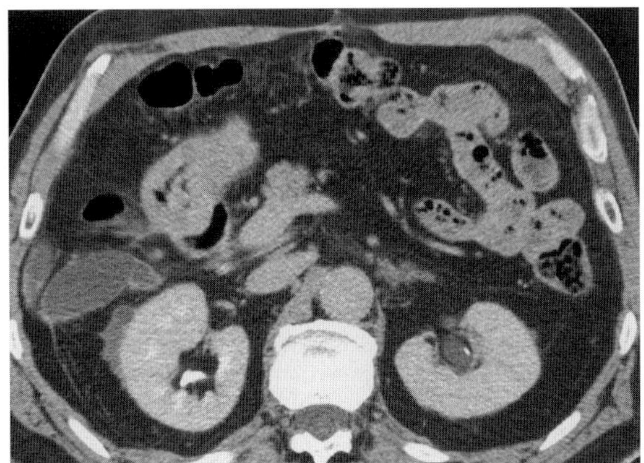

Fig. 5.33A, B. Seroma. Low-density homogeneous serous collection located among the right posterolateral peritoneum, lateroconal fascia and the anterior renal fascia in a patient who had undergone VI segmental hepatectomy

them a smooth profile. They are located in the extraperitoneal spaces along iliac or lumboaortic lymphatic pathways or next to a transplanted kidney or, occasionally, inside the peritoneum. Injection of contrast medium does not modify their characteristics (Figs. 5.29–5.31, 6.14).

The diagnosis of lymphocele is usually easy, providing account is taken of the clinical history and of the structure and location of the lesion.

5.7 Seromas (Serous Peritoneal Pseudocysts)

Seromas are peritoneal loculated collections limited by postsurgical, postinflammatory or posttraumatic adhesions. Inside the sac there is continuous secretion of peritoneal serosa without intracavitary upward flux and reabsorption by the dialytic membrane, which is more active in the subdiaphragmatic spaces. This condition causes a fluid collection, which tends to become enclosed in a cyst.

According to the same mechanism and from the same causes, analogous formations may develop at pelvic level; they contain a fluid secreted by the ovary during its normal activity in fertile women who are not taking oral contraceptives (Hoffer et al. 1988; Hedelstrom and Forsberg 1990; Kurachi et al. 1993; Mazziotti et al. 2000).

On CT scans seromas appear as round or ovoid or irregular loculated collections of the same density as water, limited by the thickened peritoneum (Figs. 5.13, 5.16, 5.32–34, 6.3).

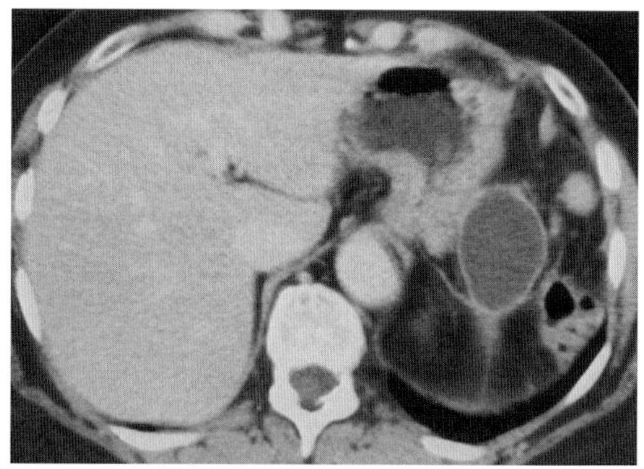

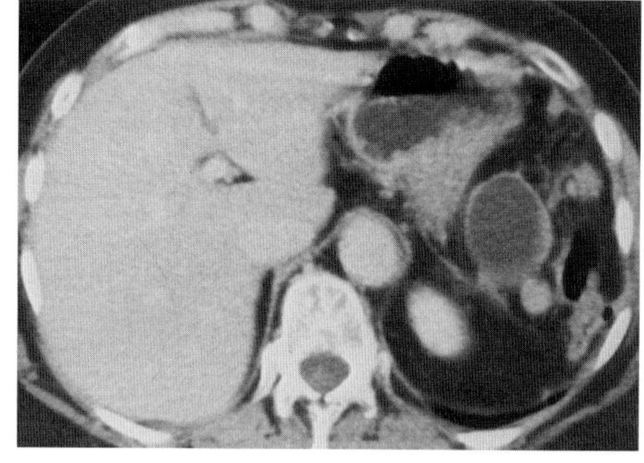

A B

Fig. 5.34A, B. Seroma. Saccate serous collection in the splenic compartment after splenectomy and resection of the corpus and the cauda pancreatis. It is possible to establish the position of this collection on the grounds of its position relative to the stomach, the anterior renal fascia and the left flexure of the colon. Two small accessory spleens have developed at the sides, outside the collection

Bibliography

General considerations

Auh YH, Rubenstein WA, Markisz JA, Zirinsky K, Whalen JP, Kazam E (1986a) Intraperitoneal paravesical spaces: CT delineation with US correlation. Radiology 159:311–317

Auh YH, Rubenstein WA, Schneider M, Reckler JM, Whalen JP, Kazam E (1986b) Extraperitoneal paravesical spaces: CT delineation with US correlation with US. Radiology 159:319–332

Baer JW (1990) Extraperitoneal mass effect by ascites under tension. Gastrointest Radiol 15:3–8

Brindicci D, Ettorre GC, Francioso G, Angone G, Grimaldi F, Monteduro M (1990) La TC nelle asciti. Radiol Med 80:889–892

Bydder GM, Kreel L (1980) Attenuation values of fluid collections within the abdomen. J Comput Assist Tomogr 4:145–150

Callen PW, Marks WM, Filly RA (1979) Computed tomography and ultrasonography in the evaluation of the retroperitoneum in patients with malignant ascites. J Comput Assist Tomogr 3:581–584

Callen PW, Filly RA, Korobkin M (1978) Ascitic fluid in the anterior paravescical fossa: misleading appearance on CT scans. AJR Am J Roentgenol 130:1176–1177

Churchill RA, Meyers MA (1986) Intraperitoneal fluid collections. In: Meyers MA (ed) Computed tomography of the gastrointestinal tract. Spinger, New York Berlin Heidelberg

Churchill RJ(1989) CT of intra-abdominal fluid collections. Radiol Clin North Am 27:653–666

Cohen JM, Weinreb JC, Maravilla KR (1985) Fluid collections in the intraperitoneal and extraperitoneal spaces: comparison of MR and CT. Radiology 155:705–708

Cooper C, Silverman PM, Davros WJ, et al (1993) Delayed contrast enhancement of ascitic fluid on CT: frequency and significance. AJR Am J Roentgenol 161:787

Di Giandomenico E, Storto ML, Dimarzo G, Delli Pizzi C, Pirronti T, Ciccotosto C, Filippone A, Bonomo L (1988) La tac nello studio delle raccolte addominali. Incontri di Radiologia 6:33–41

Dwyer A (1978) The displaced crus: a sign for distinguishing between pleural fluid and ascites on CT. J Comput Assist Tomogr 2:598–599

Federle MP, Jeffrey RB (1983) Hemoperitoneum studied by computed tomography. Radiology 148:187–192

Gore RM, Callen PW, Filly RA (1982) Lesser sac fluid in predicting the etiology of ascites. CT findings. AJR Am J Roentgenol 139: 71–74

Griffin DJ, Gross BH, McCracken S, Glazer GM (1984) Observation on CT differentiation of pleural and peritoneal fluid. J Comput Assist Tomogr 8:24–28

Haaga JR (1988) The peritoneum and mesentery. In: Haaga JR, Alfidi RJ (eds) Computed tomography of the whole body, 2nd edn). Mosby, St Louis, pp 1137–1199

Halvorsen RA, Fedyshin PJ, Korobkin M, et al (1986) Ascites or pleural effusion? CT differentiation: four useful criteria. Radiographics 6:135–149

Hammerman AM, Oberle PA, Susman N (1990) Opacification of ascitic fluid on delayed contrast computed tomography scans. Clin Imaging 14:222–224

Heiken JP (1989) Abdominal wall and peritoneal cavity. In: Lee JKT, Sagel SS, Stanley RJ (eds) Computed body tomography with MRI correlation, 2nd edn). Raven Press, New York, pp 675–705

Krauetz GW, Cho KC, Baker SR (1988) Radiologic evaluation of pancreatic ascites. Gastrointest Radiol 13:163–166

Jeffrey RB (1980) CT demonstration of peritoneal implants. AJR Am J Roentgenol 135:323–326

Jeffrey RB (1983) Computed tomography of the peritoneal cavity and mesentery. In: Mossa AA, Gamsu G, Genant HK (eds) Computed tomography in the body. Saunders, Philadephia

Jeffrey RB, Federle MP, Goodman PC (1981) Computed tomography of the lesser peritoneal sac. Radiology 141:117–122

Jolles H, Coulam CM (1980) CT of ascites: differential diagnosis. AJR Am J Roentgenol 135:315–322

Levi C, Gray JE, McCullough EC, Hattery RR (1982) The unreliability of CT numbers as absolute values. AJR Am J Roentgenol 139:443–447

Louis O, Bollaert A, Osteaux M, Grivegnee A (1983) CT of peritoneal effusion and their anatomic topography. J Belge Radiol 66:107–112

Meyers MA (1988) Dynamic radiology of the abdomen. Normal and pathologic anatomy. Springer, New York Berlin Heidelberg

Meyers MA (1992) Radiologia dinamica dell'addome. Verduci, Rome

Minutoli A, Volta S, Gaeta M (1990) Delayed enhancement of ascites following high dose contrast CT for liver metastases. J Comput Assist Tomogr 13:916–917

Naidich DP, Megibow AJ, Ross CR, et al (1983) Computed tomography of the diaphragm: peridiaphragmatic fluid localization. J Comput Assist Tomogr 7:663–640

Osteaux M, Louis O, Darras T, et al (1985) La cavité péritonéale. In: Vasile N (ed) Tomodensitométrie corps entier. Vigot, Paris, pp 323–332

Pandolfo I, Gaeta M, Scrivano E, et al (1989) Mediastinal pseudotumor due to passage of ascites through the esophageal hiatus. Gastrointest Radiol 14:209–211

Parienty RA, Pradel J, Picard JD, et al (1981) Visibility and thickening of the renal fascia on computed tomograms. Radiology 139:119–124

Proto AV, Lane EJ, Marangola JP (1976) A new concept of ascitic fluid distribution. AJR Am J Roentgenol 126:974–980

Rabal B, Hall JT, Jackson H (1985) CT diagnosis of fluid on lesser sac mimicking thrombosis of inferior vena cava. J Comput Assist Tomogr 9:956–958

Raval B, Lakmi N (1987) CT demonstration of preferential routes of the spread of pelvic disease. Crit Rev Diagn Imaging 27:17–48

Rubenstein WA, Auh YH, Whalen JP, Kazam E (1983) The perihepatic spaces: computed tomographic and ultrasound imaging. J Radiol 149:231–239

Rust RJ, Kopecky KK, Holden RW (1984) The triangle sign: a CT sign of intraperitoneal fluid. Gastrointest Radiol 9:107–113

Seltzer SE (1987) Analysis of the tethered bowel sign on abdominal CT as a predictor of malignant ascites. Gastrointestinal Radiol 12:245–249

Teplick JG, Teplick SK, Goodman LR, Haskin ME (1982) Interface sign: a CT sign for distinguishing pleural and intraabdominal fluid. Radiology 144:359–362

Vibhakar SD, Bellon EM (1984) The bare area of the spleen: a constant CT feature of the ascitic abdomen. AJR Am J Roentgenol 142:953–955

Wojtowicz L, Rzymski K, Czarneck R (1982) A CT evaluation of intraperitoneal fluid distribution. Rofo Fortschr Geb Roentgenstr Bildgeb Verfahr 137:95–99

Hematic Collections

Alexander ES, Clark RA (1982) Computed tomography in the diagnosis of abdominal hemorrhage. JAMA 248:1104–1107

Chintapalli K, Dodds WJ, Olson DL (1988) Computed tomography characteristics of intermesenteric hematomas. Comput Tomogr 12:122–128

Federle MP, Jeffrey RB (1983) Hemoperitoneum studied by computed tomography. Radiology 148:187–192

Haaga JR (1988) The peritoneum and mesentery. In: Haaga JR, Alfidi RJ (eds) Computed tomography of the whole body, 2nd edn. Mosby, St Louis, pp 1137–1199

Heiken JP (1989) Abdominal wall and peritoneal cavity. In. lee JKT, Sagel SS, Stanley RJ (eds) Computed body tomography with MRi correlation, 2nd edn. Raven Press, New York, pp 675–705

Hidaka H, Irie H, Hirata H, Shigematsu A, Matsukuma K, Tatsuma T, Era S (1990) Mesenteric hematoma; a pediatric case. Rinsho Hoshasen 35:525–528

Jeffrey RB Jr, Cardoza JD, Olcott EW (1991) Detention of active intraabdominal arterial hemorrhage: value of dynamic contrast-enhanced CT. AJR Am J Roentgenol 156:725–729

Lewin JR, Patterson EA (1980) CT recognition of spontaneous intraperitoneal hemorrhage complicating anticoagulant therapy. AJR Am J Roentgenol 134:1271–1272

McCort J (1976) Intraperitoneal and retroperitoneal hemorrhage. Radiol Clin North Am 14:391–405

New PFJ, Aronow S (1976) Attenuation measurements of whole blood fractions in computed tomography. Radiology 121:635–640

Pombo F, Arrojo L, Perez Fonta J (1991) Haemoperitoneum secondary to spontaneous rupture of hepatoareolar tissue carcinoma: CT diagnosis. Clin Radiol 43:321

Radin DR (1991) Intramural and intraperitoneal hemorrhage due to duodenal ulcer. AJR Am J Roentgenol 157:45

Raghavendra BN, Grieco AJ, Balthazar EJ, Megibow AJ, Subramanyam BR (1982) Diagnostic utility of sonograph and computed tomography in spontaneous mesenteric hematoma. Am J Gastroenterol 77:570–573

Rubin GD, Jeffrey RB Jr, Walter JF (1991) Pancreatic microcystic adenoma presenting with acute hemoperitoneum: CT diagnosis. AJR Am J Roentgenol 156:749

Sivit CJ, Peclet M, Taylor GA (1989) Lifethreatening intraperitoneal bleeding: demonstration with CT. Radiology 171:430

Wolverson MK, Crepps LF, Sundaram M, Heiberg E, Vas WG, Shields JB (1983) Hyperdensity of recent hemorrhage at body computed tomography: incidence and morphologic variation. Radiology 148:779–784

Bilomas

Erb RE, Mirvis SE, Shanmuganathan (1994) Gallbladder injury secondary to blunt trauma: CT findings. J Comput Assist Tomogr 18:778–784

Sty JR, Starshack RJ, Hubbard AM (1982) Radionuclide hepatobiliary imaging in the detection of traumatic biliary tract disease in children. Pediatr Radiol 12: 115–118

Vasquez JL, Thorsen MK, Dodds WJ, Quiroz FA, Martinez ML, Lawson TL, Steward ET, Foley WD (1985) Evaluation and treatment of intraabdominal bilomas. AJR Am J Roentgenol 144:933–936

Weissmann HS, Chun KJ, Frank M, Koenigsberg M, Mlistein DM, Freeman LM (1979) Demonstration of traumatic bile leakage with cholescintigraphy and ultrasonography. AJR Am J Roentgenol 133:843–847

Urinary Collections

Kane NM, Francis JR, Ellis JH (1989) The value of CT in the detection of bladder and posterior urethral injuries. AJR Am J Roentgenol 153:1243–1246

Lis LE, Cohen AJ (1990) CT cystography in the evaluation of bladder trauma. J Comput Assist Tomogr 14:386–389

Lowe FC, Fishman EK, Oesterling JE, et al (1989) Computerized tomography in the diagnosis of bladder rupture. Urology 33:341–343

Mee S, McAninch J, Federle MP, et al (1987) Computerized tomography in bladder rupture: diagnostic limitations. J Urol 137: 207–209
Mirvis SE (1989) Diagnostic imaging of the urinary system following blunt trauma. Clin Imaging 13:269–280
Sandler CM, Hall JT, Rodriguez MB, et al (1986) Bladder injury in blunt pelvic trauma. Radiology 158:633–638
Sivit CJ, Cutting JP, Eichelberger MR (1995) CT diagnosis and localization of rupture of the bladder in children with blunt abdominal trauma: significance of contrast extravasation in pelvis. AJR Am J Roentgenol 164:1243–1246

Lymphatic Collections

Dodd GD, Rutledge F, Wallace S (1970) Postoperative pelvic lymphocysts. AJR Am J Roentgenol 108:312-323
Gillimand JD, Spies JB, Brown SB, et al (1989) Lymphoceles: percutaneous treatment with povidone-iodine sclerosis. Radiology 171:227-229
Kim JK, Jeong YY, Kim YH, Kim YC, Kang HK, Choi HS (1999) Postoperative pelvic lymphocele: treatment with simple percutaneous catheter drainage. Radiology 212:390-394
Meyers AM, Levine E, Myburgh JA, et al (1977) Diagnosis and management of lymphoceles after renal transplantation. Urology 10:497-502
Petru E, Tamussino K, Lahousen M, et al (1989) Pelvic and paraaortic lymphocysts after radical surgery because of cervical and ovarian cancer. Am J Obstet Gynecol 161:937-941
Sweizer R, Cho S, Kountz SL, Belzer FO (1972)Lymphoceles following renal transplantation. Arch Surg 104:42-45
Van Sonnenberg E, Mueller PR, Ferrucci JT Jr (1984) Percutaneous drainage of 250 abdominal abscesses and fluid collections: results, failures and complications. Radiology 151:337-341
Van Sonnenberg E, Wittich GR, Casola G, et al (1986) Lymphocele: imaging characteristics and percutaneous management. Radiology 161:593-596
White M, Mueller PR, Ferrucci JT, et al (1985)Percutaneous drainage of postoperative abdominal and pelvic lymphoceles. AJR Am J Roentgenol 145:1065-1069
Zuckerman DA, Yaeger TD (1997) Percutaneous ethanol sclerotherapy of postoperative lymphoceles. AJR Am J Roentgenol 169:433-437

Seromas

Hederstrom E, Forsberg L (1990) Entrapped ovarian cyst: an unusual case of persistent abdominal pain. Acta Radiol 31:285–286
Hoffer FA, Kozakewich H, Colodny A, et al (1988) Peritoneal inclusion cyst: ovarian fluid in peritoneal adhesions. Radiology 169:189–191
Kurachi H, Murakami T, Nakamura H, et al (1993) Imaging of peritoneal pseudocyst: value of MR imaging compared with sonography and CT. AJR Am J Roentgenol 160:589–591
Mazziotti S, Blandino A, Gaeta M, Scribano E, Salamone I, Pandolfo I (2000) Pseudocisti peritoneali. Radiol Med 99:109–111

6 Acute Inflammatory Diseases

CONTENTS

6.1 General Considerations

Acute inflammatory processes in the peritoneal cavity (peritonitis) and in the subperitoneal spaces are usually caused by direct or lymphatic diffusion of inflammations affecting the abdominal viscera (appendicitis, diverticulitis, cholecystitis, pancreatitis) or the consequences of postsurgical abdomino-pelvic infections or dehiscence of anastomoses or sutures. Less frequently, sub- or intraperitoneal inflammations can be caused by traumatic or pathologic (gastroduodenal ulcer, intestinal tumors) or iatrogenic (e.g. following transhepatic cholangiography or endoscopy) perforation of the intestinal wall.

Usually, such inflammatory processes are associated with high fever, abdominal pain, leukocytosis and contraction of the abdominal wall; however, sometimes they show an unspecific pattern: general malaise, light fever, asthenia and vague abdominal pain.

Subperitoneal inflammatory processes include a wide range of abnormalities, from fat congestion and edema with leukocyte accumulation in a tissue invaded by bacteria up to the development of a phlegmon, a mature abscess with a purulent central collection surrounded by a richly vascular pseudocapsule.

These processes can extend into other subperitoneal spaces, the retroperitoneum or the peritoneal cavity or they can have a favorable evolution up to complete healing or healing with residuals, such as fibrous scars or small encysted collections, which can sometimes cause a relapse of the infection.

CT scanning shows different findings in acute subperitoneal inflammatory processes:

- In the early phase the subperitoneal collection next to the altered visceral wall or in the site of the surgical operation fat has a hazy appearance with thin linear or sinuous strands owing to edematous and congestive responses and to the enlargement of blood and lymphatic vessels (Figs. 6.1, 6.23). Sometimes, this haziness is quite opaque and must be searched for with windows capable of performing an elective study of adipose tissue. The proximal intestinal wall is thick and has a shaded profile. It shows a strikingly increased postcontrast density and thin sinuous strandings, owing to the dilated blood and lymphatic vessels coming out from the wall and crossing the nearby fatty tissue. The peritoneum also becomes thicker if it is involved in the process (Figs. 6.1, 6.23). In this phase the process may still heal quickly, or it may be followed by a phlegmon or an abscess. Therefore, a CT examination after a few days of adequate therapy is always useful. In this phase, if gas bubbles are observed in the inflammatory area, the possibility of covered perforations or relaxation of sutures must always be considered.

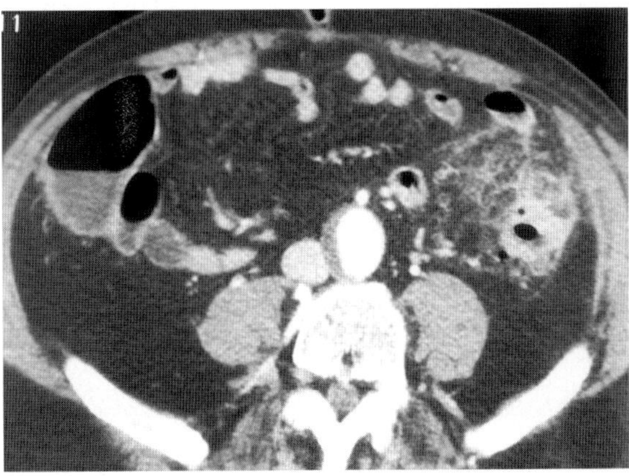

Fig. 6.1. Pericolic and peridiverticular inflammatory process with hazing and stranding of the pericolic fat. The nearby peritoneum is becoming thick

- A phlegmon (Fig. 6.24) appears as a homogeneous mass of soft tissue, increasing in density after contrast medium injection and with poorly defined margins, and surrounded by hazing fat, whose density progressively decreases with increasing distance from the phlegmon.

- The abscess (Figs. 6.3, 6.4, 6.18, 6.19, 6.25, 6.27) appears as a round, oval or more complex water-density collection limited by a more or less thick and uniform wall that increases strongly in density after i.v. contrast medium administration owing to the rich vascular content of the tissue of which they are constituted. The presence, the thickening and the degree of increment in postcontrast density of the walls indicate the level of maturity of the collections: absence of modifications at the beginning, very clear alterations after a few days, when the collections tend to be confined by a capsule.

A

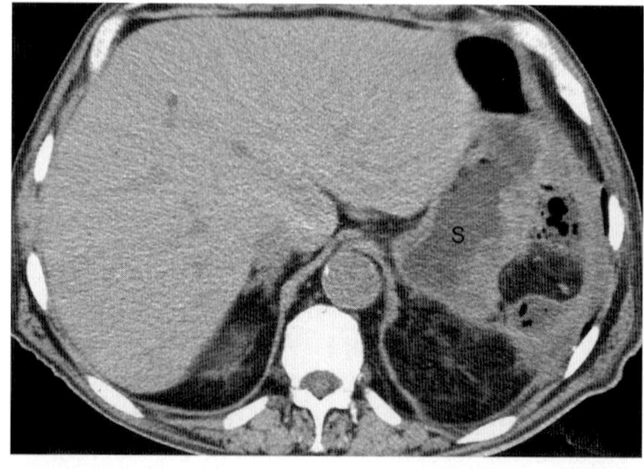

B

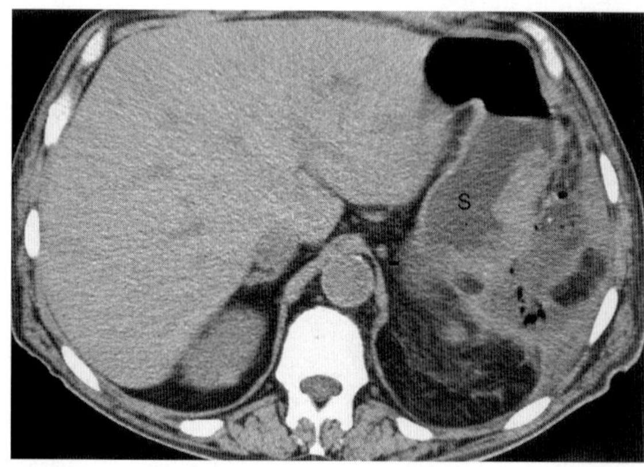

Fig. 6.2A, B. Abscess in the splenic compartment after splenectomy. Collection of same density as water or higher, with some gas bubbles inside, limited by thick, enhancing wall, in the splenic compartment between gastrocolic ligament and anterior pararenal space

- Mature abscesses (Figs. 6.3–6.6, 6.15, 6.20) have a thick and intensely enhancing wall and contain nonhomogeneous water-dense or higher density fluid, mostly associated with air bubbles or air-fluid level. The peritoneum and the adjacent fasciae are thick and dense.

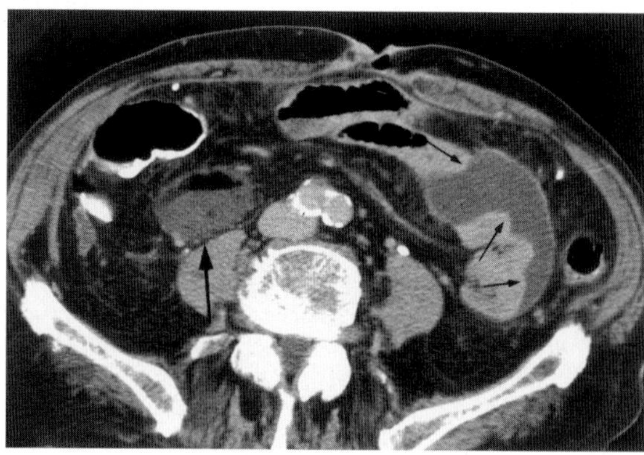

Fig. 6.3. Mesenteric abscess and peritoneal seroma. The patient had undergone ileo-ceco-colic resection and ileo-transversostomy. Abscessed collection with air-fluid level and thick nonhomogeneous wall located in the root of the mesentery *heavy arrow*) in front of the distal ileocolic vessels. Serous waterdense homogeneous collection (*small arrows*) surrounding an ileal loop and limited by thin, slightly enhancing peritoneum

Usually, when CT is considered in the clinical context, there are no problems with differential diagnosis; however, particular care is needed to avoid misinterpretation of the air-fluid levels observed inside the abscesses as dilated intestinal loops leaning on each other; conversely, abscesses can also be misinterpreted as intestinal loops. Usually, a resolving condition is recognized by the finding of a thick contrast-enhanced wall around the abscesses. If doubt persists, it is useful to change the patient's position or to give a water-soluble contrast medium orally.

After a recent surgical operation, it is necessary to establish carefully whether the gas present has always been there or has developed since surgery. Even when relaxation of anastomoses or intestinal perforation is suspected, it is advisable to give a water-soluble contrast agent orally, because this makes the intestinal loops opaque and penetrates into the collections.

Sometimes the abscesses do not differ in appearance from hematic, bile, or saccate ascitic collections or necrotic tumors. In these cases, the main differential elements are the clinical data and the patient's history: fever, pain, leukocytosis, a recent surgical operation, a known pathology (ulcer, diverticula, etc.). The absence of traumas or anticoagulant ther-

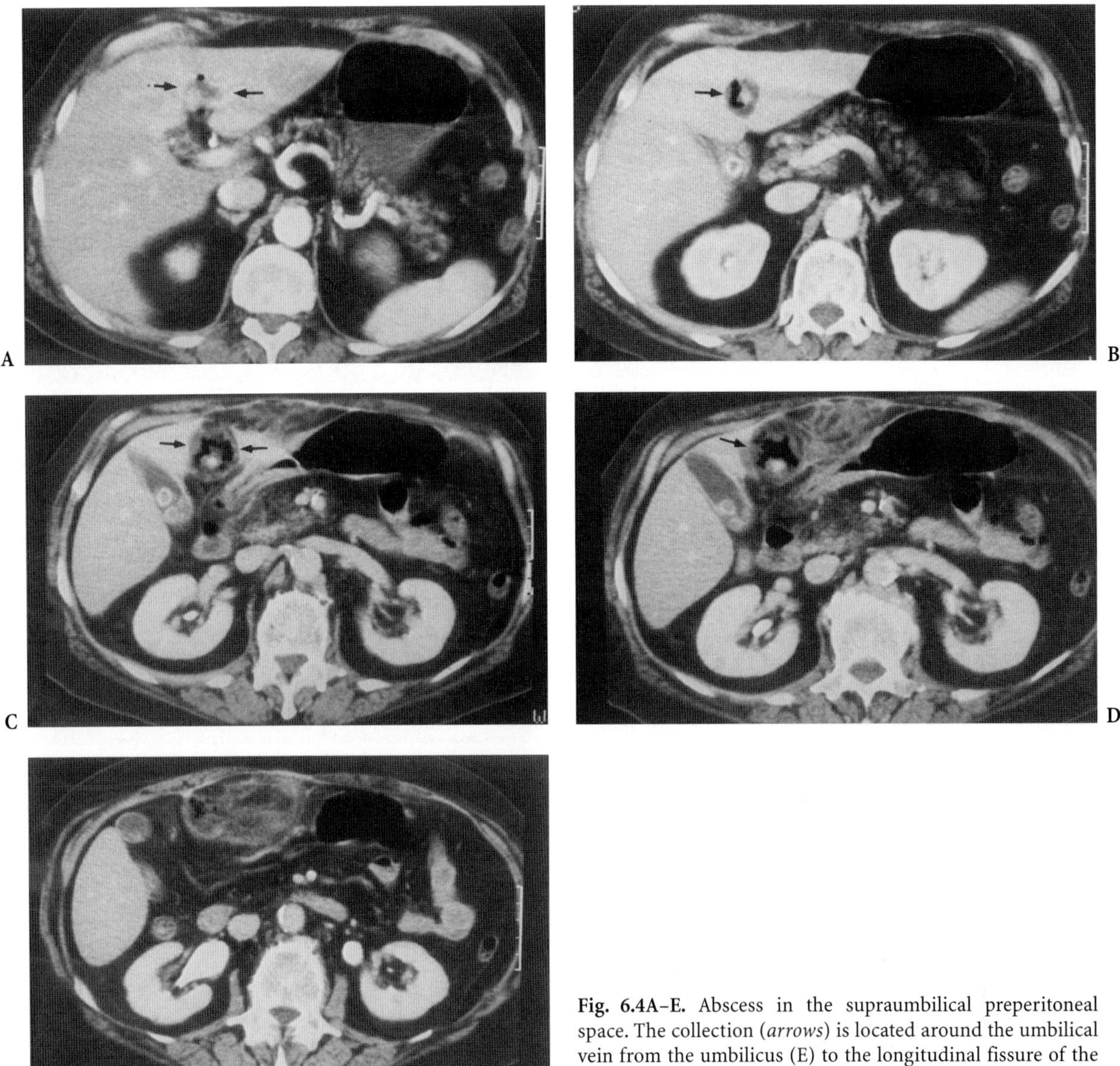

Fig. 6.4A–E. Abscess in the supraumbilical preperitoneal space. The collection (*arrows*) is located around the umbilical vein from the umbilicus (E) to the longitudinal fissure of the liver (A–B)

apies is helpful in clarifying the problem. A peripheral contrast enhancement is an important sign suggesting an inflammatory process. In order to distinguish a silent tumor infiltrating the large intestine from an inflammatory process, it is useful to supplement CT with the administration of a water enema and hypotonic drugs.

In contrast to subperitoneal abscesses, *peritoneal inflammatory collections* are always well confined by the thickening and enhancing peritoneum, which surrounds them as a dense and uniformly thick capsule. Abscesses can remain located in the site where they have developed or spread to preferential distant sites, such as the right subphrenic and subhepatic spaces (for abscesses originating above the mesocolon) and the pelvic recesses (for those located below the mesocolon).

The collections caused by diseases of the right and left upper abdomen (cholecystitis, gastric perforation, surgery of the upper abdomen) and of the right submesocolic region, spreading along the paracolic gutter (appendicitis), are preferentially located in the right subphrenic and subhepatic spaces (Figs. 5.7, 6.8, 6.7, 6.8).

Lesser sac abscesses are usually secondary to perforated ulcers of the posterior gastric wall or to expansion of an acute pancreatitis (Figs. 6.11, 6.12).

Abscesses caused by appendicitis, diverticulitis, pathologies of the uterus and adnexa uteri, surgery of the lower digestive tract or gynecological opera-

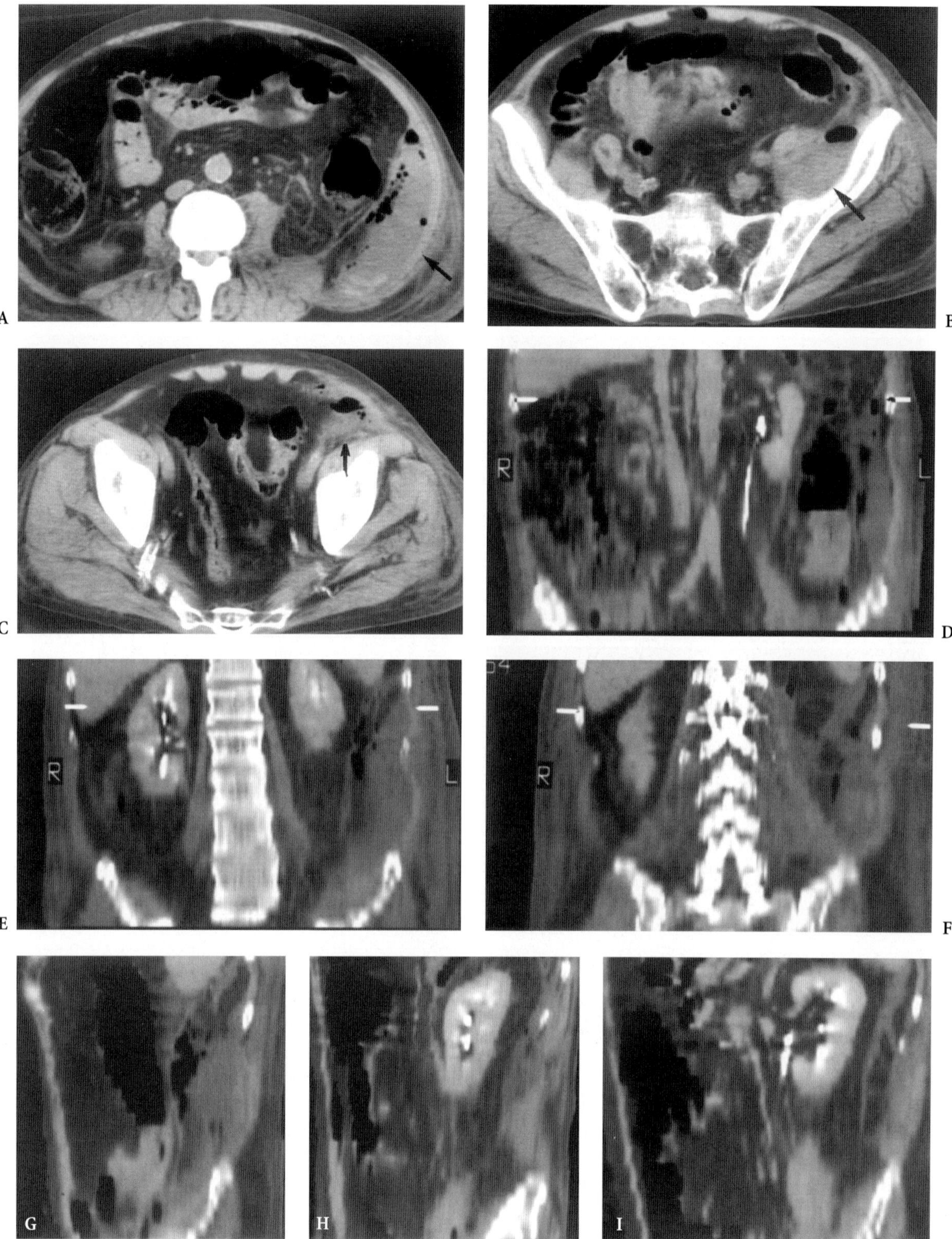

Fig. 6.5A–I. Extraperitoneal abscess. A–C Dense abdomino-pelvic collection with gas bubbles inside between the transversalis fascia outside and the lateroconal and posterior renal fasciae, extending forward in front of the peritoneum, showing the continuity of the preperitoneal with the retrorenal space. This relationship is better seen in the sagittal (D–F) and coronal (G–I) reconstructions

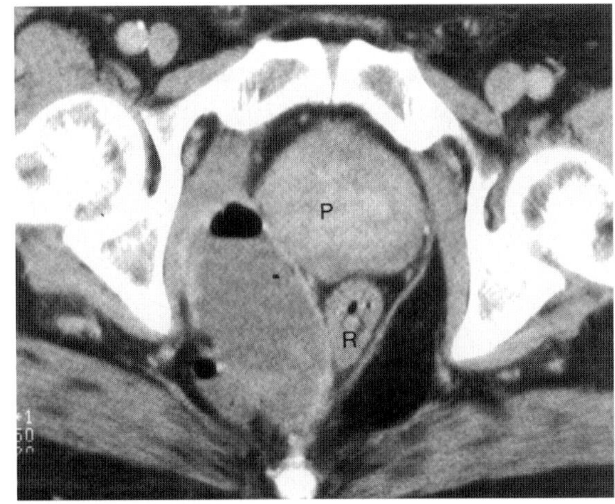

Fig. 6.6. Extrafascial abscess. Air-fluid collection in the right ischiorectal fossa limited medially by the levator ani muscle, which separates them from the perirectal and periprostatic fat

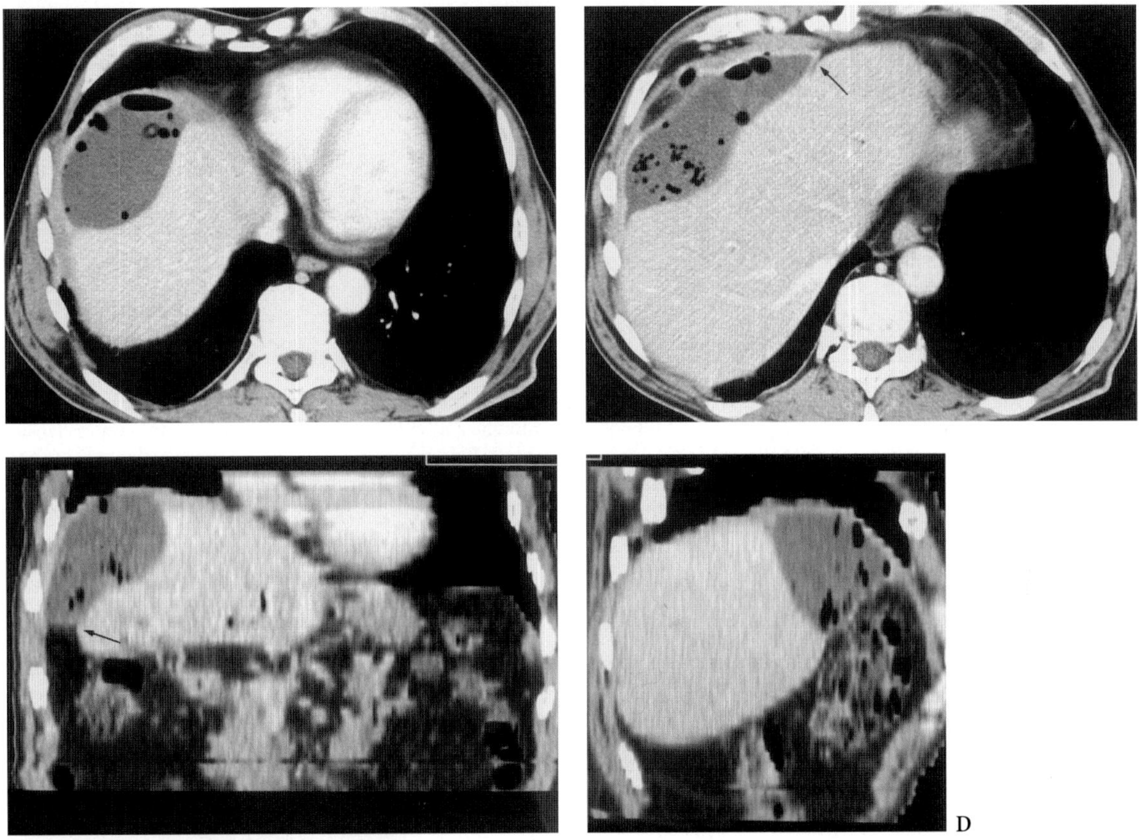

Fig. 6.7A,–E. Right subphrenic abscess. A Lateral fusiform collection, with thickening and postcontrast hyperdense wall. B The step (*arrow*) between the collection and the hepatic profile indicates that it is located outside the liver. The coronal (C), sagittal (D) and oblique (E) reconstructions provide a spatial localization of the collection

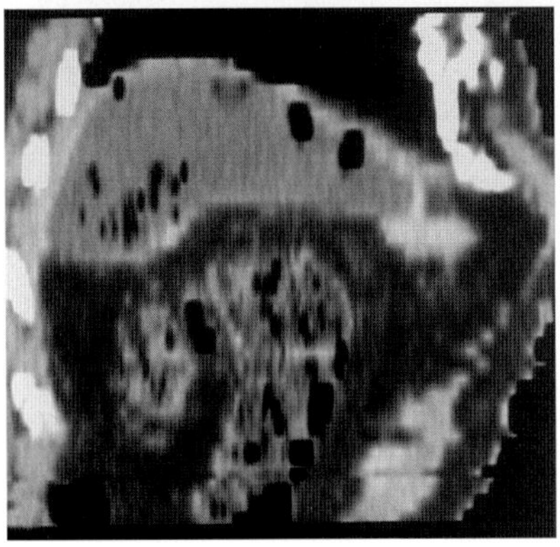

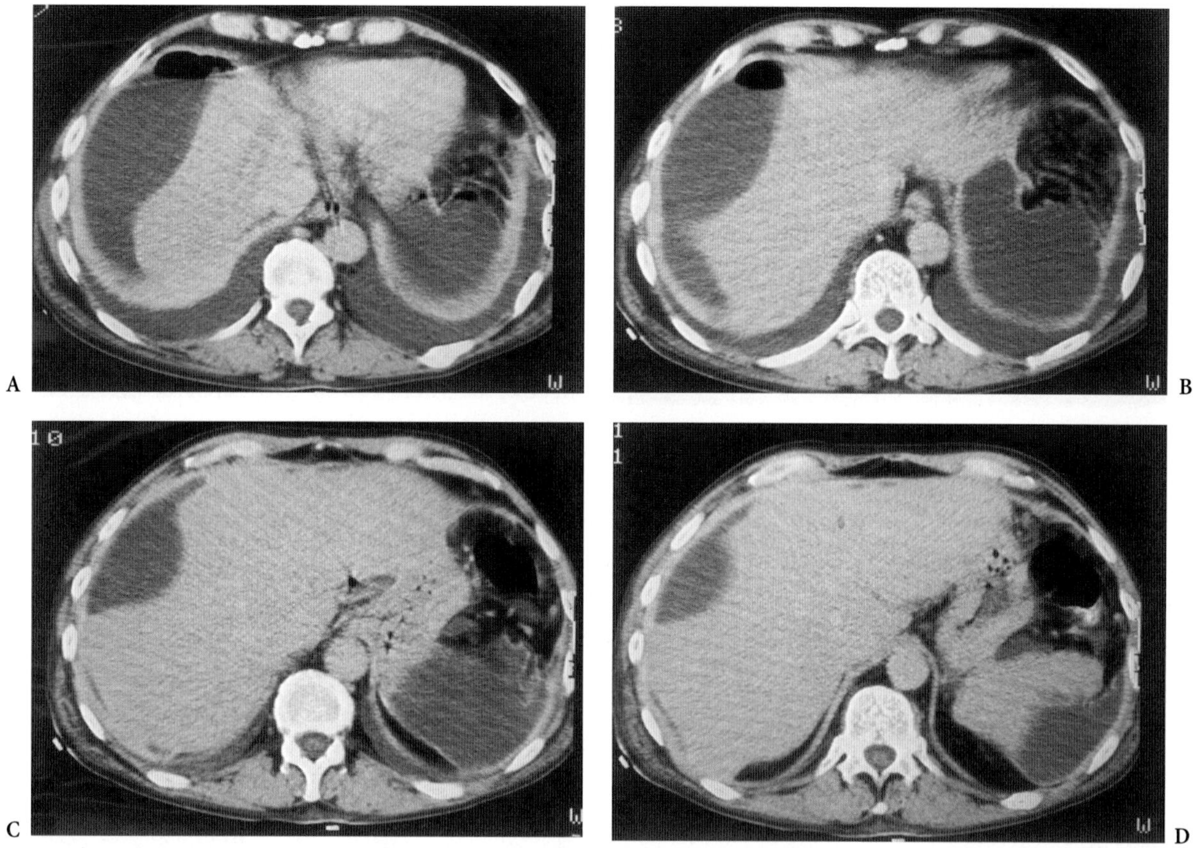

Fig. 6.8A–D. Right and left subphrenic abscesses and bilateral pleural collection. A Large right lateral subphrenic air-fluid collection limited anteriorly by the falciform ligament and posteriorly by the coronary ligament. B Left subphrenic water-density collection, displacing the stomach medially, limited behind by the posterior peritoneum pressing on the anterior renal fascia. C, D The pleural collections can be distinguished by their retrodiaphragmatic position and median continuous expansion up to the respective crura diaphragmatis, which are pushed away from the spine

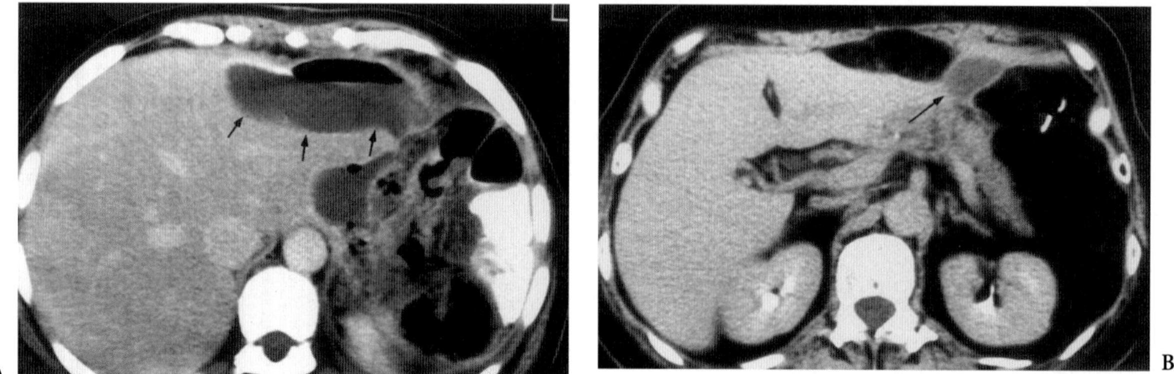

Fig. 6.9A, B. Intraperitoneal postgastrectomy abscess. Wide air-fluid collection (*arrows*) in the left subphrenic space limited medially by the falciform ligament (A). Only a small amount of fluid remains after percutaneous drainage and antibiotic treatment (B)

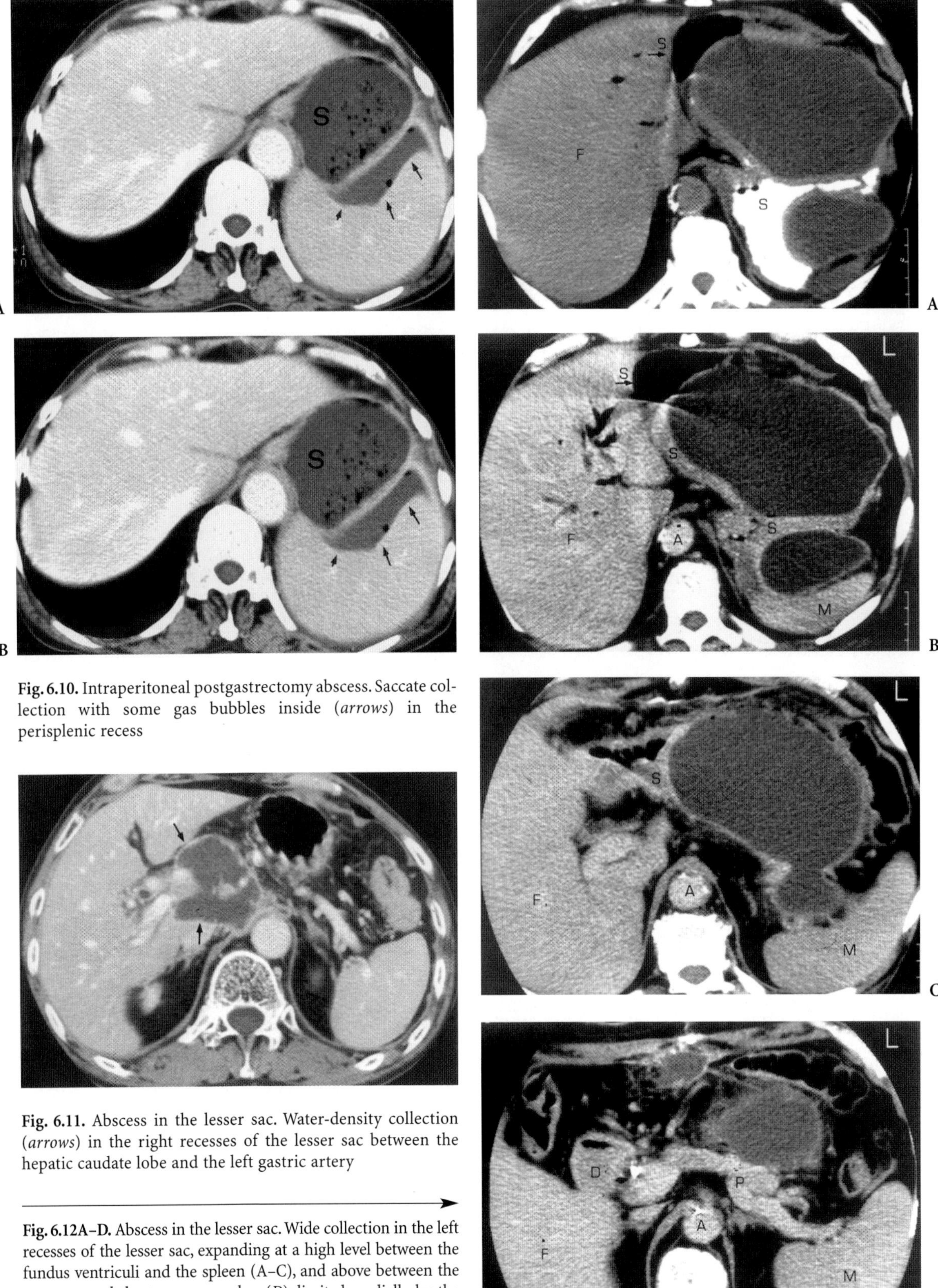

Fig. 6.10. Intraperitoneal postgastrectomy abscess. Saccate collection with some gas bubbles inside (*arrows*) in the perisplenic recess

Fig. 6.11. Abscess in the lesser sac. Water-density collection (*arrows*) in the right recesses of the lesser sac between the hepatic caudate lobe and the left gastric artery

Fig. 6.12A–D. Abscess in the lesser sac. Wide collection in the left recesses of the lesser sac, expanding at a high level between the fundus ventriculi and the spleen (A–C), and above between the pancreas and the transverse colon (*D*), limited medially by the gastrohepatic ligament and laterally by the gastrosplenic ligament (*A*). Inferiorly, it is blocked by the transverse mesocolon (C, D)

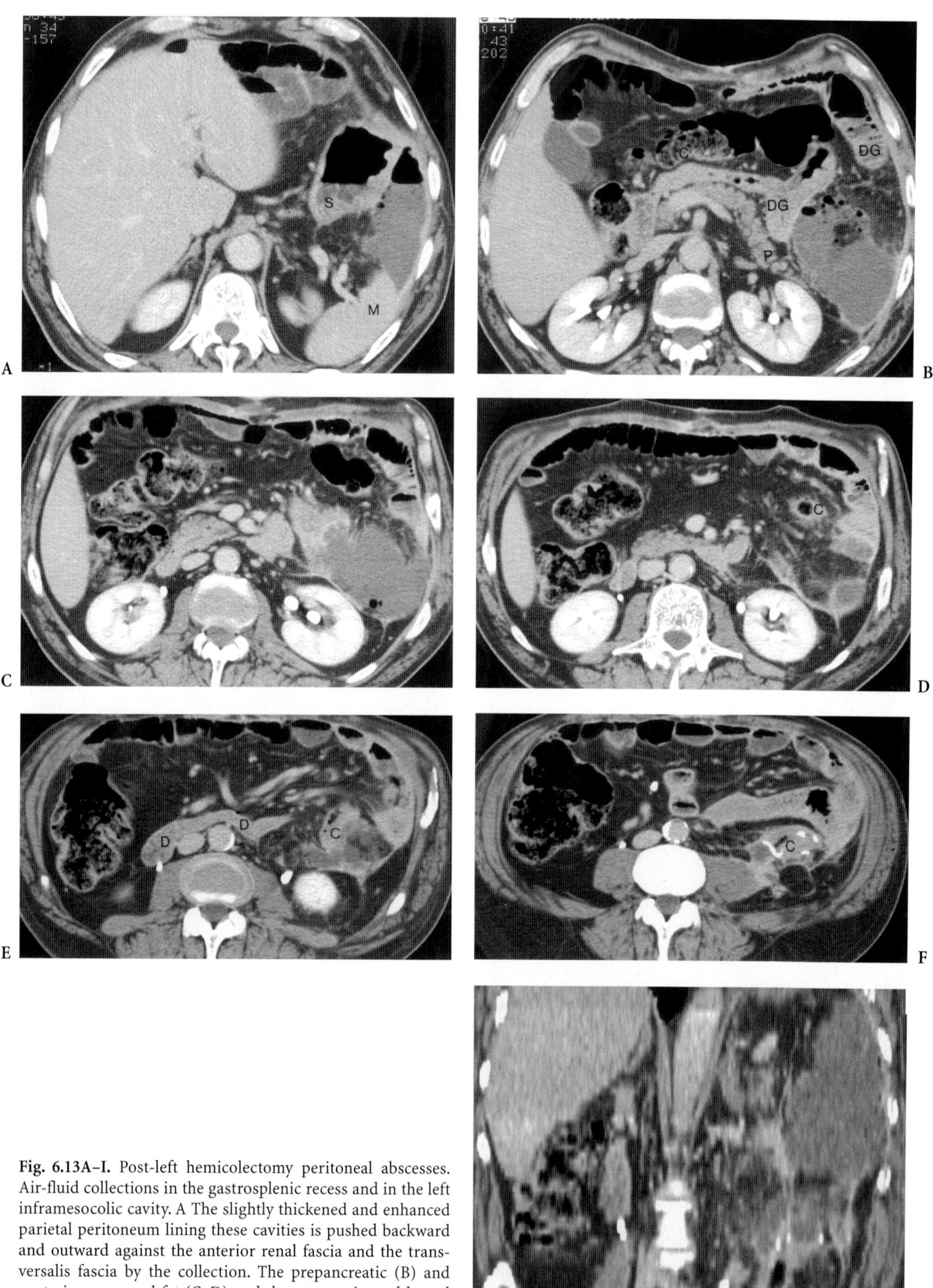

Fig. 6.13A–I. Post-left hemicolectomy peritoneal abscesses. Air-fluid collections in the gastrosplenic recess and in the left inframesocolic cavity. A The slightly thickened and enhanced parietal peritoneum lining these cavities is pushed backward and outward against the anterior renal fascia and the transversalis fascia by the collection. The prepancreatic (B) and posterior pararenal fat (C, D) and the extraperitoneal lateral adipose tissue are clear (A–C). A, F Axial scans; G, H coronal reconstructions; H sagittal reconstruction

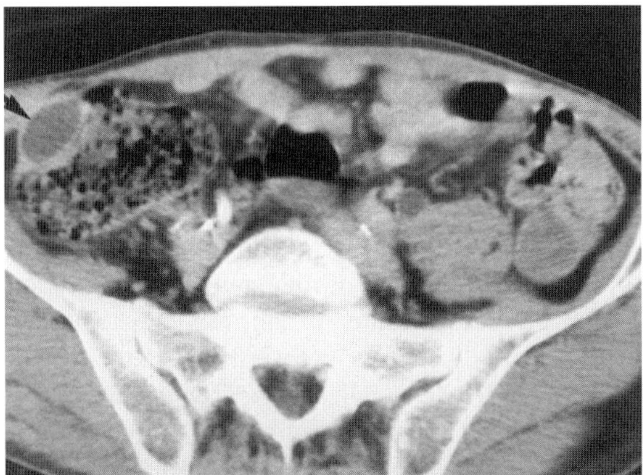
A

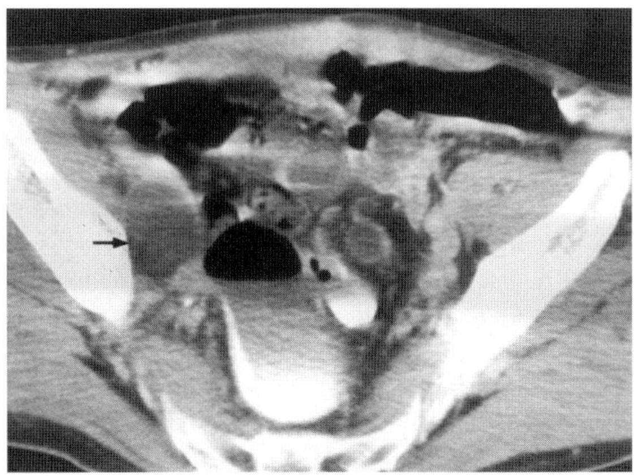
B

Fig. 6.14A, B. Paracecal abscess and iliac lymphocele. Patient had undergone total cystectomy with pelvic lymphoadenectomy and uretero-sigmoidectomy. A The abscess shows a saccate aspect within the paracecal peritoneal cavity. B The lymphocele is located in the lateral extraperitoneal space between the transversalis fascia and the sacro-recto-genito-pubic fascia, behind the external and in front of the internal iliac vessels . The wall of the lymphocele is thin and smooth and does not become opaque after contrast medium; on the other hand, the wall of the abscess is hyperdense and thickening

tions are located in the pelvic peritoneal compartments: at the sides and in front of the urinary bladder, in the pouch of Douglas and in the pararectal peritoneal recesses.

However, the width and disposition of the abscessed collections after surgery are very variable, and it is not always easy to establish their correct intra- or extraperitoneal localization because of the altered relationships among the remaining structures and the discontinuity of the peritoneum and of the ligaments (Fig. 6.13). Furthermore, it is not rare to observe multiple, saccate or communicating collections, which may occupy both subperitoneal spaces and the peritoneal cavity.

When peritoneal or subperitoneal inflammatory processes are suspected, CT makes it possible to establish their presence, site, phase (edema / congestion, phlegmon, abscess), positions relative to organs and abdominal structures, extension and diffusion. In addition, CT frequently makes it possible to specify the causes and to indicate the routes that might be used for withdrawal of pathological samples and / or for drainage, thus, providing all information necessary to decide on the most appropriate treatment.

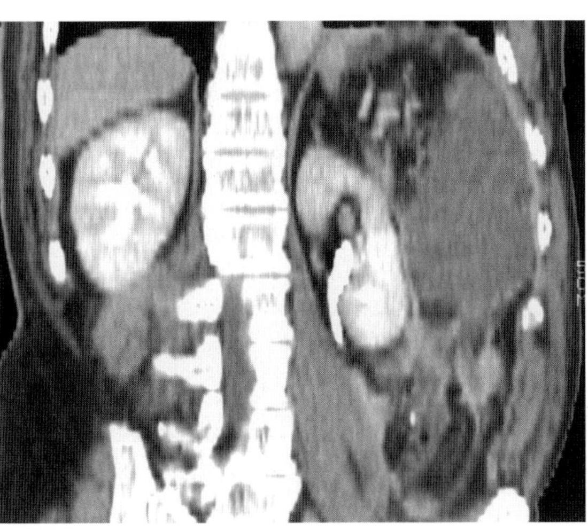
H

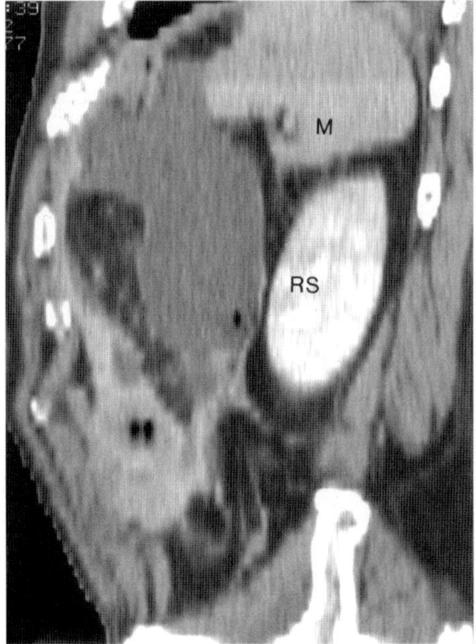

I

6.2 Acute Appendicitis

We are in complete agreement with Balthazar et al.'s (1986) statement that the use of CT in the study of acute appendicitis reduces the number of unnecessary laparotomies and, in complex cases, may suggest the use of a percutaneous drainage or indicate the most convenient surgical approach for the treatment of abscesses. This is due to the high sensitivity (96%), specificity (89%), and positive (96%) and negative (95%) predictive values of CT, which can be improved by the use of thin collimation helical scanning. The findings that may be revealed by CT in acute appendicitis are displayed in Table 6.1.

Furthermore, when the site of the appendix is atypical (subhepatic, pelvic, retro- or subumbilical or in the left quadrant) the CT allows differential diagnosis against other acute abdominal diseases (lithiasic and nonlithiasic cholecystitis, diverticulitis, pancreatitis, adnexitis, ureteral lithiasis, subphrenic abscess, terminal ileitis, etc.) that may have similar clinical signs (pain, fever, leukocytosis).

While ultrasonography is the method of choice for use in children, young people and pregnant women because of the absence of roentgen rays, low cost and good predictive value, in all other patients CT appears to be useful or even indispensable for confirmation of the localization of an inflammatory process of the appendix and evaluation of its evolutionary phase (simple inflammation, phlegmon, abscess, peritonitis). In comparison with ultrasonography, CT has the advantages of always localizing the appendix (even in the almost constant presence of intestinal meteorism or in the case of an atypical localization of the appendix) and of being more pre-

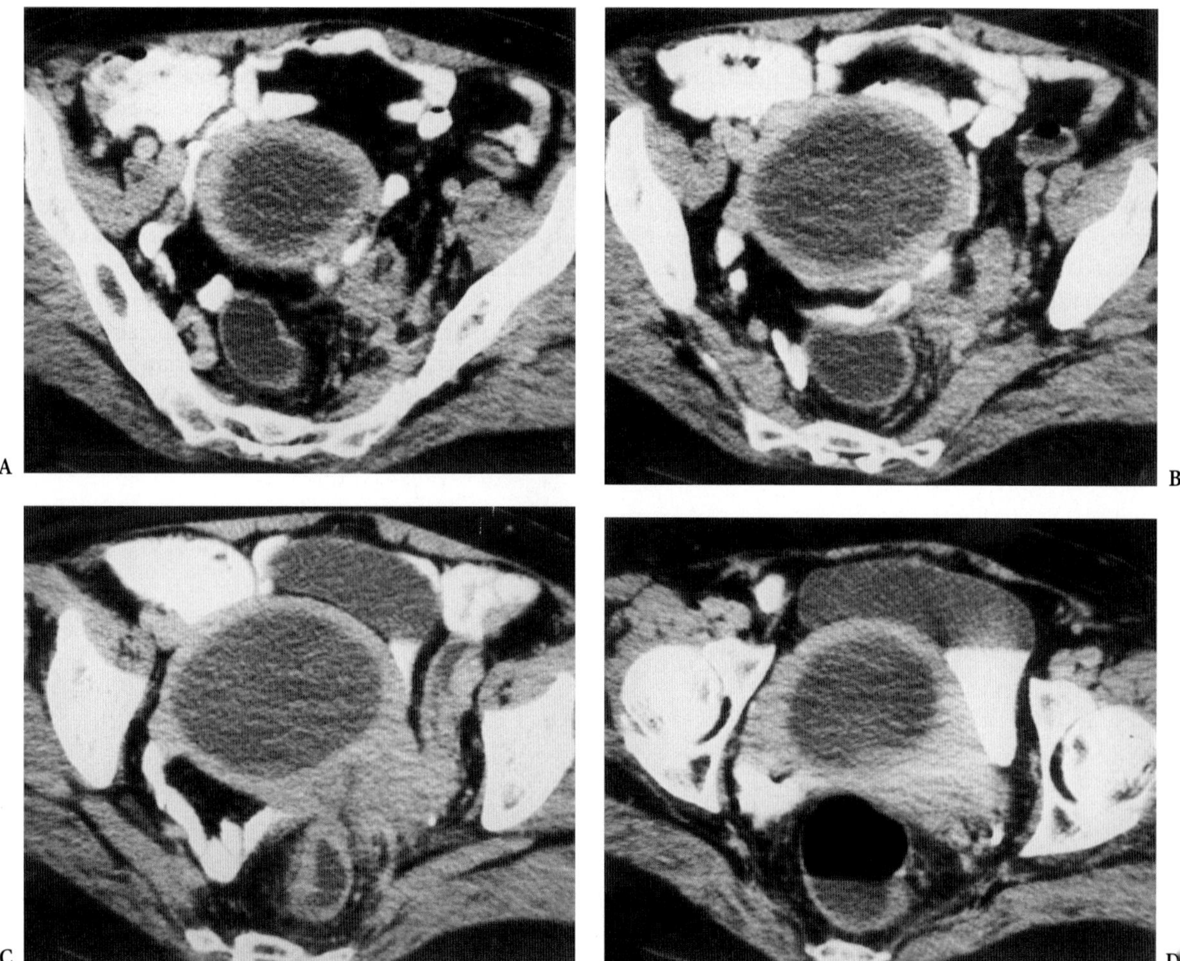

Fig. 6.15A–D. Pelvic abscess that has led to perforation of Meckel's diverticulum. Wide collection with thickening, enhancing wall involving the sigmoid, the ileal loops, the uterus and the adnexae

Table 6.1. CT findings in acute appendicitis

Pathological findings	CT findings
Inflammation limited to the appendiceal wall	Enlarged appendix (max. outer transverse dia. >6 mm) Thickened (>2–3 mm) enhancing wall Fluid and one or more apppendicoliths
Periappendiceal inflammation (edema, congestion)	Periappendicular fat hazing and stranding
Peritoneal involvement	Peritoneal thickening
Phlegmon	Small high-enhancing paracecal mass
Recent abscess	Paracecal collection into a hyperdense mass with poorly defined limits
Mature abscess	Paracecal fluid or air-fluid collection with thick enhancing capsule
Retroperitoneal diffusion of collection	Continuity of collection in the retroperitoneum
Peritonitis	Intraperitoneal fluid
Subphrenic abscess	Subphrenic gas bubbles or air-fluid level

cise in the evaluation of any concomitant subperitoneal and peritoneal alterations, which can affect the choice of treatment.

In normal subjects, CT shows the appendix in the paracecal fat as linear when it is collapsed and as tubular or annular when it contains gas, fluid, feces or barium (Fig. 6.16), with a maximum outer transverse diameter less than 6 mm. It has a thin wall (<1 mm),which increases in density after contrast injection, and a sharp profile.

Acute appendicitis is diagnosed when the appendix is dilated (with outer transverse diameter >6 mm) and the appendiceal wall is thickened all round by up to 2–3 mm and enhanced by contrast medium injection (Fig. 6.17). Fluid and one or more calcific appendicoliths are frequently seen inside (Fig. 6.18–6.20).

When there is periappendiceal diffusion of the inflammation, the fat surrounding the appendix is hazed and crossed by strands and the adjacent peritoneum is thickened.

A small, strongly enhancing, homogeneous mass with indefinitely shaded contours suggests a phlegmon.

An early abscess (Figs. 6.18, 6.19) shows attenuation values comparable to those of water or slightly higher (0/+30 HU) in a hyperdense, poorly defined mass, whereas mature abscesses (Fig. 6.20) are limited by a thick and complete capsule. Small gas bubbles or air-fluid levels inside the collection are the expression of a perforation of the appendix or of infection by an anaerobic microorganism. When collections penetrate the peritoneum, they tend to spread upward along the right paracolic gutter into the upper perihepatic spaces or downward into the pouch of Douglas, whereas gas expands under the diaphragm into the right subphrenic recess (Figs. 9.4, 9.6).

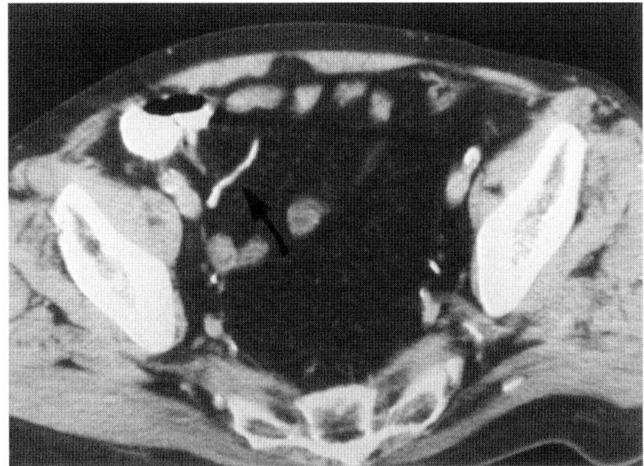

Fig. 6.16. Normal appendix. Thin tubular appendix filled with barium (*arrow*)

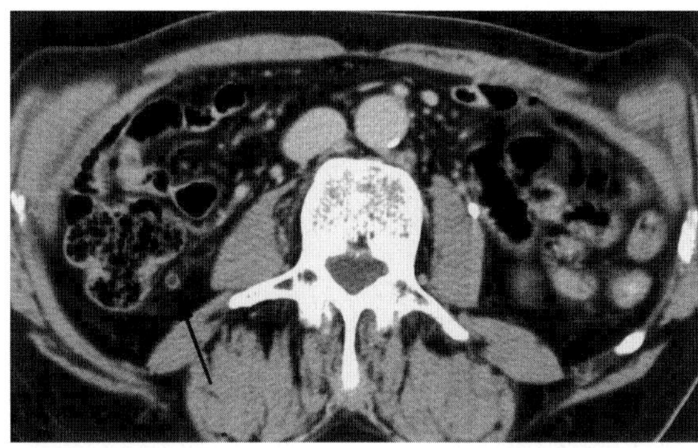

Fig. 6.17. Acute mild appendicitis. Fluid-filled appendix with annular contrast-enhancing wall in cross section

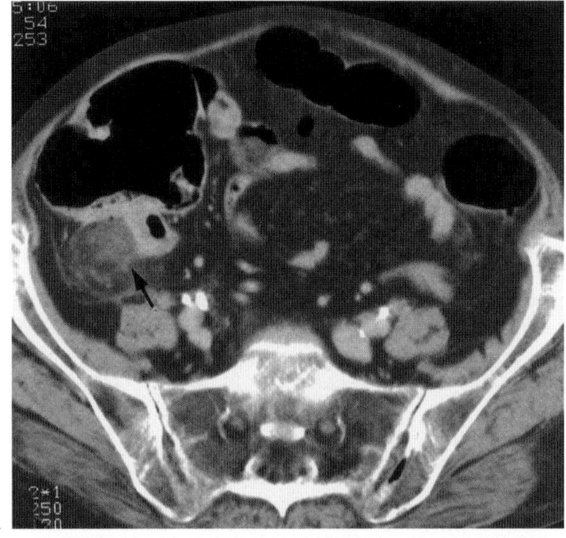

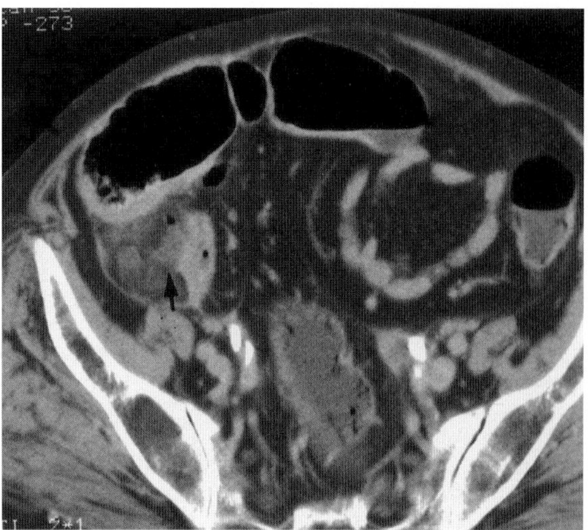

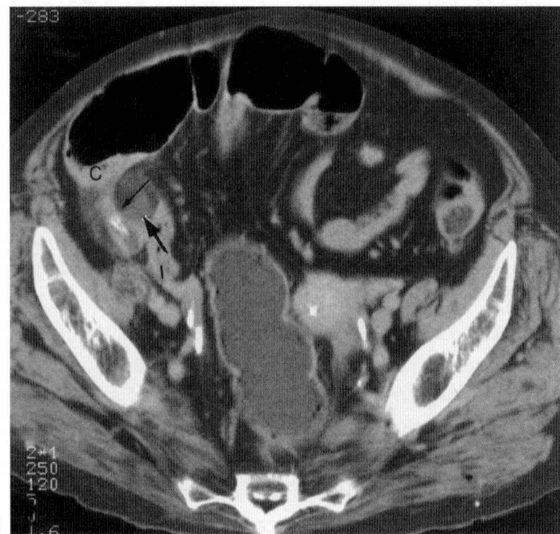

Fig. 6.18A–C. Appendiceal abscess. A Endoluminal, B intramural and C periappendicular fluid collections. Endoluminal calcified appendicolith (C *thin arrow*). Stranding in the periappendicular fat and thickening of surrounding peritoneum owing to extension of the inflammatory process

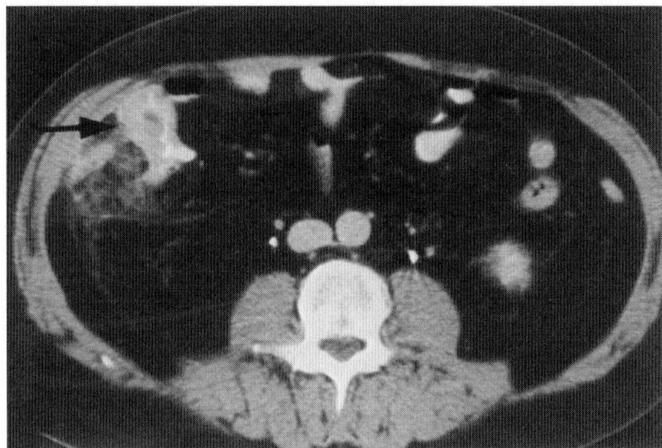

Fig. 6.19. Appendiceal and periappendiceal abscess. Enhancing thick-walled appendix with endoluminal fluid and calcified appendicolith. Fluid, strands and haziness in the periappendiceal fat limited by the thickened peritoneum and the lateroconal fascia

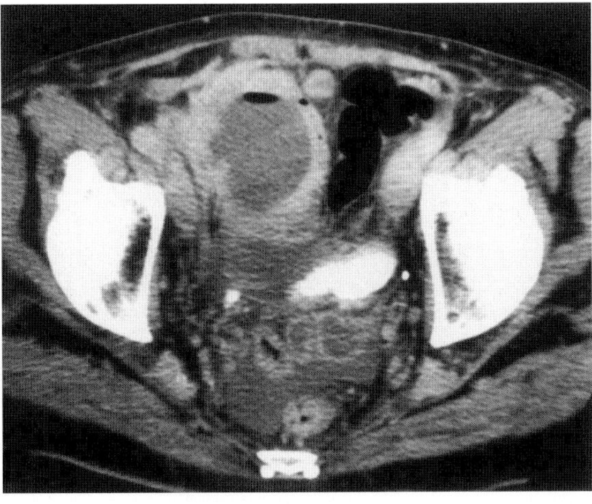
A

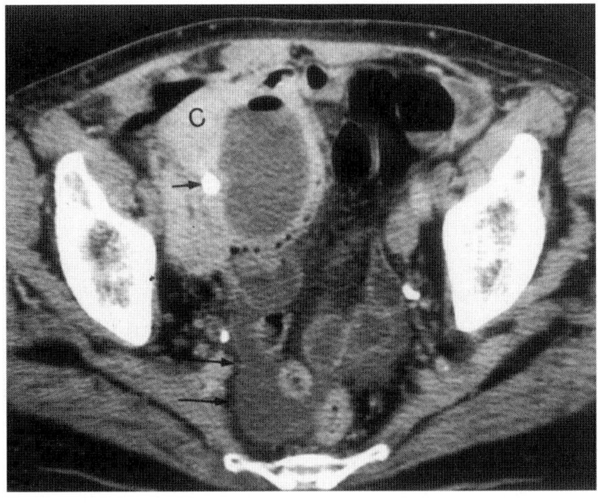

B

Fig. 6.20A, B. Appendiceal abscess. Wide air-fluid collection limited by a thick enhancing capsule. Calcified appendicolith (*small arrow*). Small amount of fluid in the adjacent peritoneal cavity and in the pelvic recesses (*long arrows*)

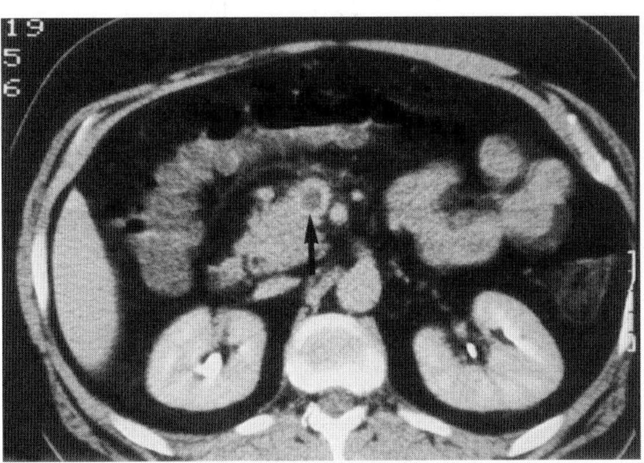

A

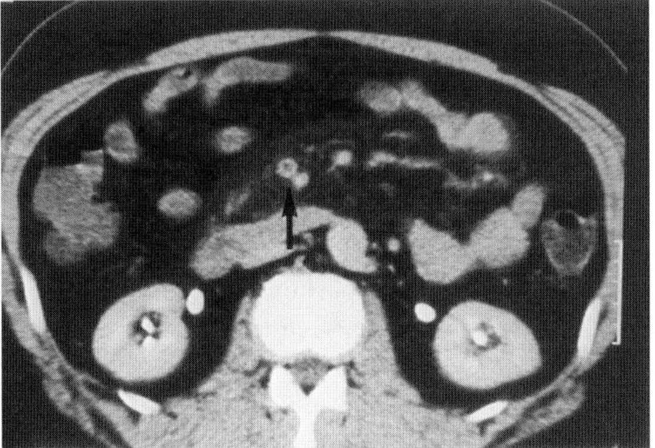
B

Fig. 6.21A, B. Appendicitis complicated by thrombosis of A the superior mesenteric and B the ileocolic vein (*arrows*). Rounded appearance of thickened enhancing wall and central low-attenuation lumen of the thrombosed veins

A possible complication of acute appendicitis is ileocolic, mesenteric and portal venous thrombosis (Fig. 6.21). At present, CT appears to be an accurate method that can be used to confirm or to exclude suspected appendicitis, and perhaps to establish an alternative diagnosis and to assign a grade to the acute appendiceal inflammation, which is essential before appropriate treatment can be selected (Figs. 6.15–6.18). This may be:

1. Simple antibiotic therapy in early appendicitis or when it is complicated by a small abscess (<3 cm) or a phlegmon
2. CT-guided percutaneous drainage in circumscribed periappendiceal abscesses
3. Surgical operation; only in the case of free, diffuse or multilocated collections or of intestinal perforation

In suspected or clinically diagnosed appendicitis this rational therapeutic approach reduces the number of unnecessary operations and lowers both morbidity and mortality rates (Jeffrey et al. 1987, 1988; Jeffrey 1989, 1994; Federle 1997).

6.3 Acute Diverticulitis

"CT has been a superb modality for the diagnosis of diverticulitis. ... It is a noninvasive technique that permits the radiologist to tell the clinician the exact extent of this extramucosal disease. ... CT-guided percutaneous abscess drainage can turn a two- or three-stage surgical sequence into a one-stage sigmoidectomy." This is how NEFF et al. (1987) commented on their study of diverticulitis.

As in the case of appendiceal inflammation, CT has a relevant contribution to make: the sensitivity of CT in the detection of diverticulitis is even higher than that of the double-contrast enema (93% for CT vs 80% for the traditional method). However, CT appears to be particularly useful in the characterization (edema, congestion, phlegmon, abscess, intestinal perforation, fibrosis) and evaluation of the extent (subperitoneal cellular, mesentery, retroperitoneum, peritoneum, urinary bladder, ureters and vagina) of the inflammatory process.

In most cases, CT findings resemble those described under General considerations (section 6.1) and under Appendicitis (section 6.2); therefore, we will only report any correlation between each CT sign and the corresponding lesion in Table 6.2 and illustrate the appearances of the different evolutionary phases (Fig. 6.22–6.28).

When the wall of the large intestine is very thick, so that there is a restricted lumen, an irregular external profile, and pericolic or perisigmoidal cells shaded or crossed by linear bands and lymphoadenomegalies, the most important limitation of CT is the difficulty of distinguishing between inflammatory processes and colic tumors crossing or perforating the wall (this happens in 10% of cases). In such conditions a definitive diagnosis is not possible. NEFF et al. (1987), NEFF and VAN SONNENBERG (1989) and HULNICK et al. (1988)

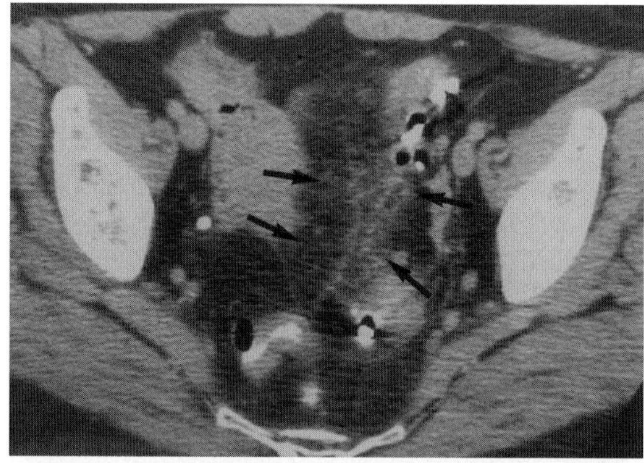

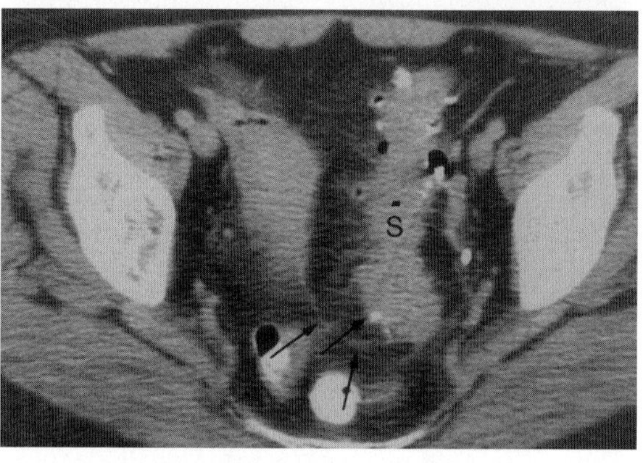

Fig. 6.23A, B. Diverticulitis with peridiverticulitis, stage 1. Hazing of fat of the sigmoid mesocolon (A *thick arrows*), linear strands, extending from the wall of the sigmoid to the peritoneum which limits the mesentery (B *thin arrows*)

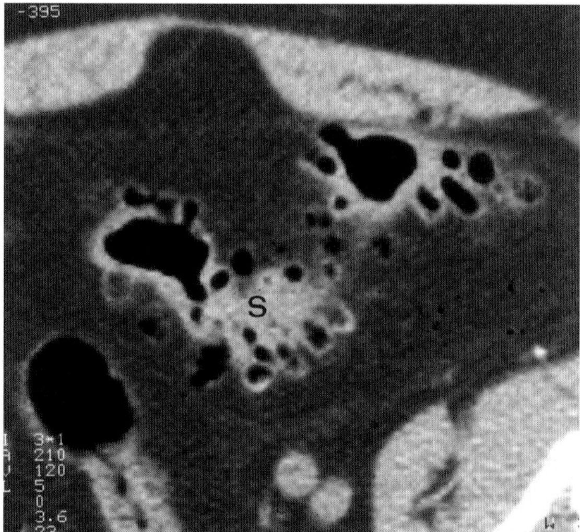

Fig. 6.22. Diverticulosis. Cluster of sigmoidal air-filled diverticula with sharp wall. There are no strands, dimming or fluid in the peridiverticular fat

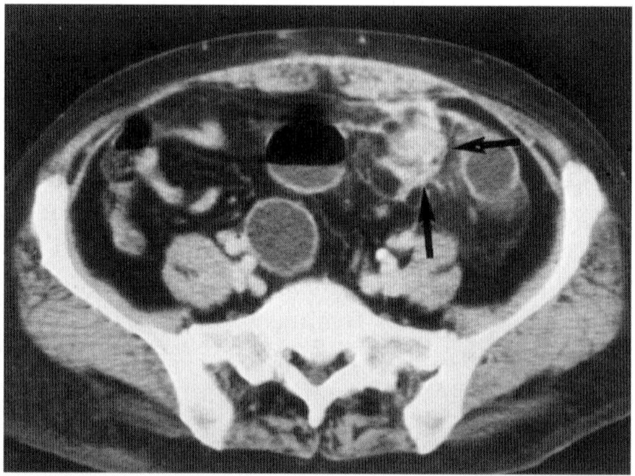

Fig. 6.24. Diverticulitis with peridiverticulitis and small phlegmon, stage 2. Small hyperdense nodule (*arrows*), shading, strands and vascular congestion in the parasigmoidal fat

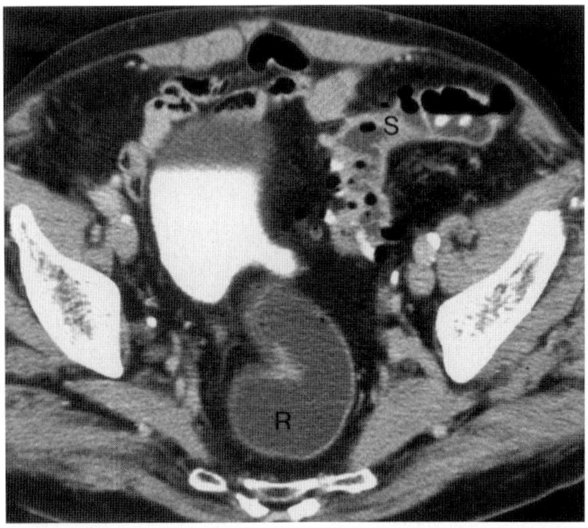

Fig. 6.25A–C. Peridiverticular abscess, stage 3. Small fluid collection encapsulated in the sigmoid mesocolon (*arrows*)

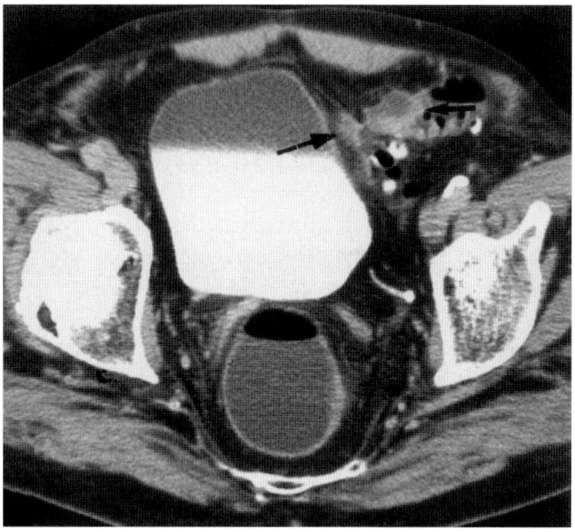

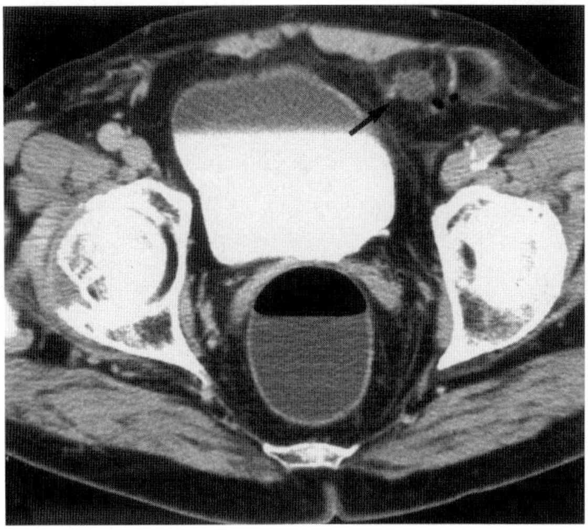

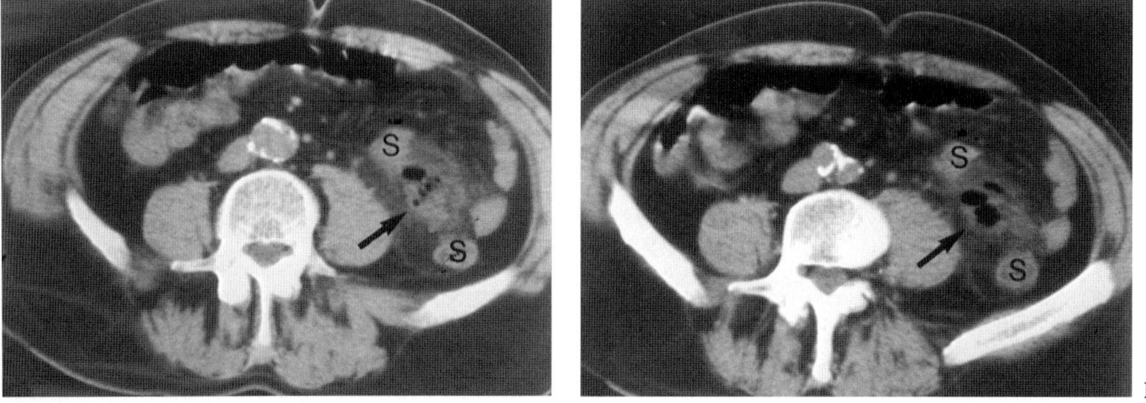

Fig. 6.26A, B. Diverticular perforation, stage 7. Air-fluid collection in the sigmoid mesocolon following extravasation of intestinal material (*arrows*)

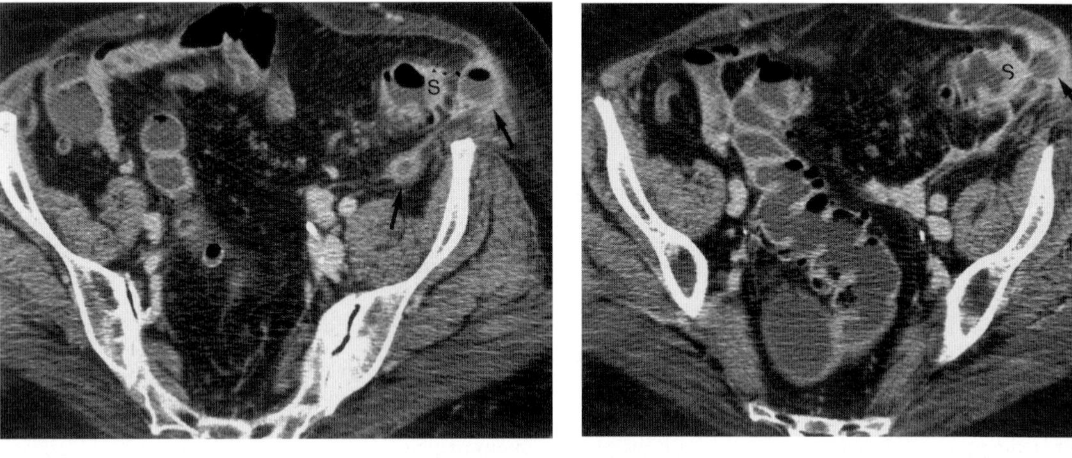

Fig. 6.27A, B. Diverticular perforation into the peritoneal cavity: stage 7. Small air-fluid collection well limited by an enhancing peritoneal capsule (*arrows*) in the retrosigmoidal peritoneal recess

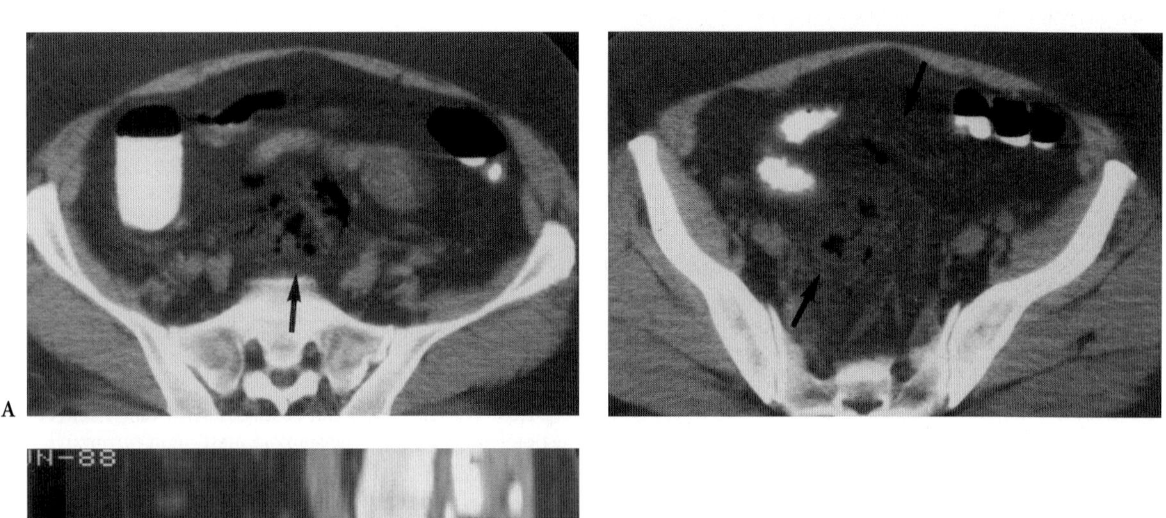

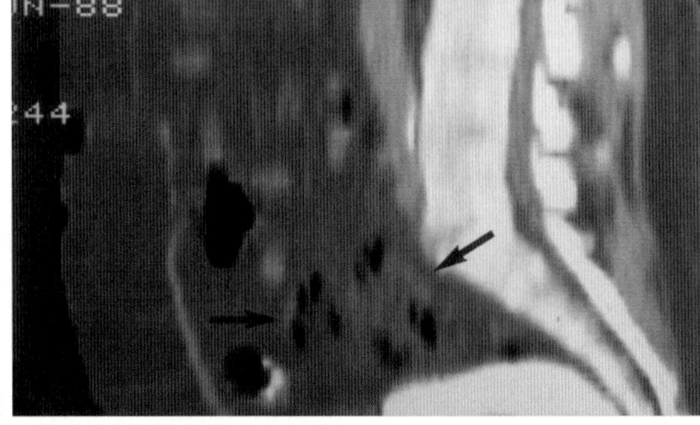

Fig. 6.28A–C. Diverticular perforation extending to the retroperitoneum, stage 8. Diffuse inflammatory soft density changes, with gas bubbles inside, in the sigmoid mesocolon and in the pelvic retroperitoneum (*arrows*)

suggest completing the investigation with an opaque enema in this situation. We prefer to repeat the CT after careful intestinal preparation including a water enema preceded by pharmacological induction of intestinal hypotonia. This method greatly improves the representation of the intestinal wall; in fact, in the case of tumors the wall is clearly seen to be thickening, rigid, unextensible and asymmetrical, whereas diverticulitis is characterized by a progressive thickening of the intestinal wall, which expands during passage of the water enema. Further inflammatory patterns consist in the presence of a fluid collection in the peritoneal parasigmoidal recesses and in the parallel linear strands extending out of the wall and passing through the sigmoid mesocolon because of vascular engorgement (Padidar et al. 1994) (Fig. 6.23).

Table 6.2. Staging of diverticulitisa

Stage	Pathology	CT findings
0	Inflammation limited to the wall	Thickening and enhancing wall
1	Inflammation of the pericolic fat up to the peritoneal serosa	Hazing and stranding of the peridiverticular fat Peritoneal thincking
2	Peridiverticular phlegmon	Paracolic soft-density enhancing mass
3	Peri- or paracolic abscess	Fluid or air-fluid encapsulated collection within the mesocolon
4	Abscess extending to the retroperitoneum	Hazing of the mesocolic and retroperitoneal fat Fluid or air-fluid collection, demarcated by a thin or a thick membrane inside
5	Saccate intraperitoneal abscess	Fluid collection clearly limited by the thickening peritoneum
6	Distant free peritoneal abscess, usually in the pouch of Douglas	Clearly limited peritoneal collection far from diverticulum
7	Intestinal perforation	Fluid, gas bubbles, contrast agent, fecal material in the subperitoneal or peritoneal spaces
8	Intestinal perforation in the retroperitoneum, extending to the mediastinum and to the neck	Bubbles of gas in the retroperitoneum, mediastinum and retrofascial space of the neck
9	Fistulas with urinary or vaginal involvement	Colovesical adhesions. Parallel linear strands or tubular fluid-filled tract. Air in the bladder. Ureteral obstruction
10	Peridiverticular fibrosis	Linear dense strands in the mesenteries

Modified from NEFF et al. (1989)

At present, CT evaluations of the characteristics and extension of the inflammatory process are of fundamental importance for treatment planning, one purpose of which is to reduce the number of surgical operations as far as possible. In fact, a surgical treatment should be performed only in the case of intestinal perforation, large abscesses or fistulae (stages 4–9).

In the early phases of the inflammatory process, when a phlegmon just affects the intestinal wall or also extends to the surrounding fat (stage 0–2), an antibiotic treatment is enough, whereas for circumscribed abscesses with a diameter smaller than 3 cm (stage 3) CT-guided percutaneous drainage must be suggested, because this leads to healing in almost all cases.

6.4 Acute Cholecystitis

Acute cholecystic inflammations are usually associated with lithiasis, which is the main factor in the etiology.

The inflammation produces edematous / congestive thickening of the wall, with the possibility of a suppurative evolution that can go so far as to involve the serosa. An exudative and/or biliary fluid collection caused by a microperforation of the gallbladder wall or to circumscribed peritonitis may grow within the space between the wall and the serosa, where it is confined by the surrounding peritoneum. Further diffusion of the inflammation may involve the gastrohepatic, gastrocolic, and hepatoduodenal ligaments, producing a congestive-edematous response or a collection. Sometimes, these collections may perforate into the peritoneal cavity, producing mixed purulent and biliary peritonitis, which may remain located in the subhepatic space or diffuse into the whole of the peritoneal cavity, particularly into Morrison's recess and the pouch of Douglas.

CT findings in acute cholecystitis (Table 6.3) include:

- Thickening and contrast hyperattenuation of the gallbladder wall, with or without intramural hypodense linear bands (Fig. 6.29) or bulky abscessed areas (Figs. 6.30, 6.32)
- Distension of the gallbladder by high-attenuation fluid at the beginning of the inflammation (Fig. 6.30, 6.32)

Table 6.3. CT findings in acute cholecystitis

Pathology	CT findings
Edema, congestion, hemorrhage from the gallbladder wall	Thickening, contrast-enhancing wall
Dense bile, pus, sludge, gallstones, hemorrhagic fluid which distends the gallbladder	**Intramural low-density layers Gallbladder distended by dense fluid (+20/+35 HU), sludge and gallstones**
Intramural abscess	Intramural fluid or air-fluid collection with enhancing capsule
Pericholecystic involvement	Pericholecystic fluid Peritoneal thickening
Involvement of ligaments	Shading, strands and fluid in the ligamental fat
Peritonitis	Low-density collections in the adjacent recesses or in the whole of the peritoneal cavity

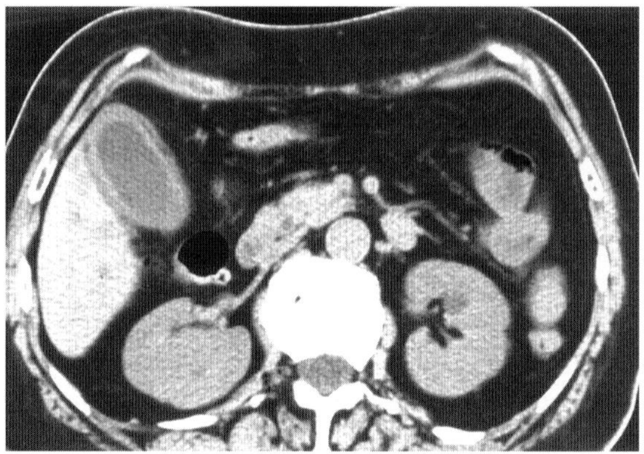

Fig. 6.29. Acute cholecystitis. Thickening and postcontrast enhancing gallbladder walls with thin low-density intramural layer

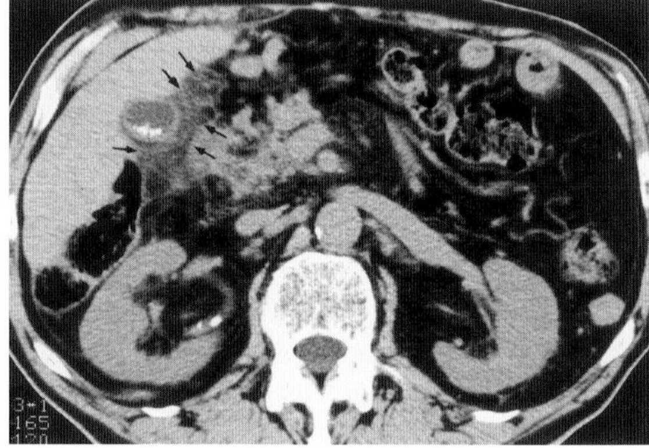

Fig. 6.31. Acute lithiasic cholecystitis with pericholecystitis. Gallbladder with thickening wall, containing calcified calculi. Thin pericholecystic fluid limited by thickened peritoneum. Hazing and stranding of the gastrocolic ligament (*small arrows*)

A 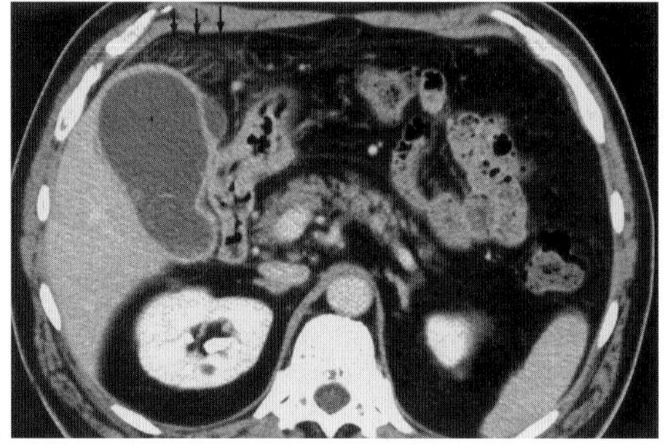

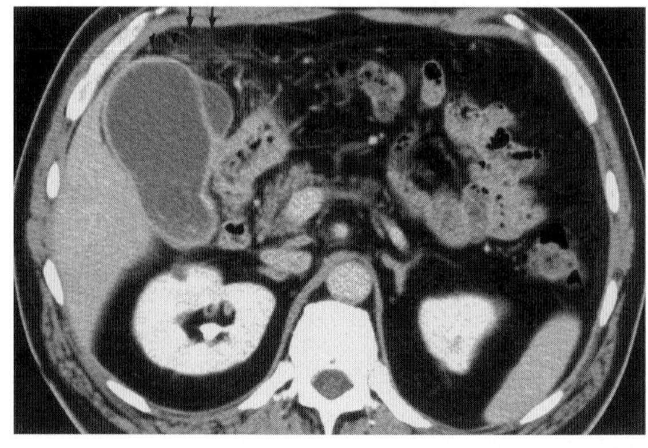 B

Fig. 6.30A, B. Acute cholecystitis with pericholecystitis. Dilated gallbladder with thickening and contrast-enhancing wall. Small intramural collection. Stranding and hazing in the gastrocolic ligament (*arrows*)

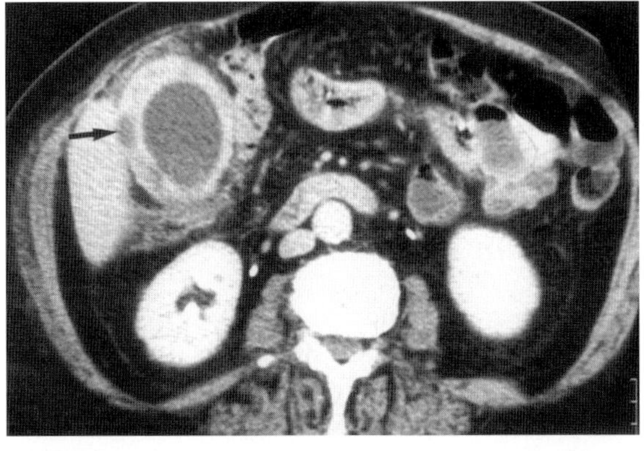
A

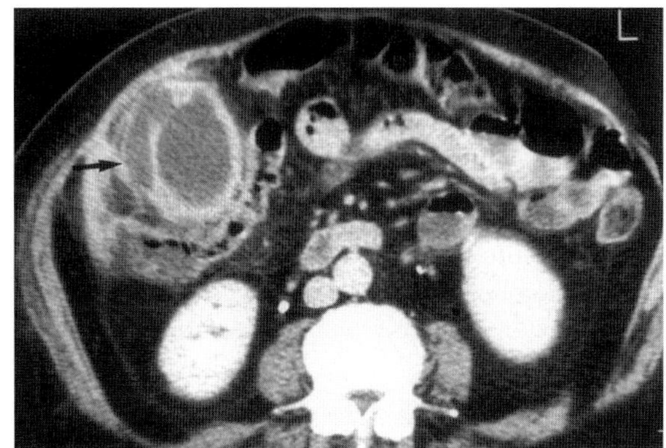
B

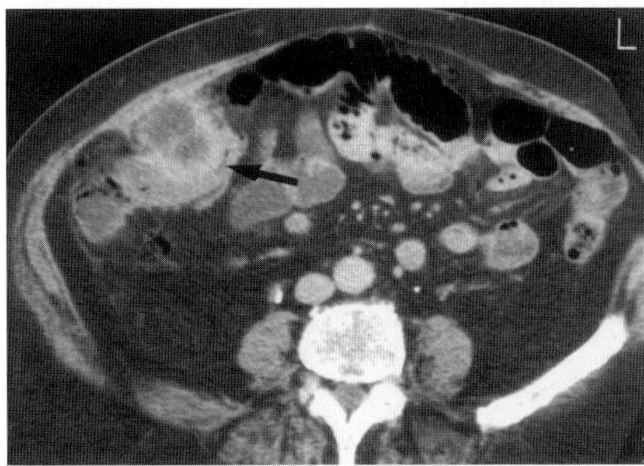
C

Fig. 6.32A–C. Acute cholecystitis with pericholecystitis. Intramural abscess (*arrow*), saccate pericholecystic fluid caused by rupture of the cholecystic wall

- Pericholecystic low-density collections with thickening of the surrounding peritoneum
- Strands of hazing and collections extending to the subperitoneal fat of the hepatoduodenal, gastrohepatic and gastrocolic ligaments (Figs. 6.30–6.32)
- Intraperitoneal collections limited by thickened and enhancing peritoneum, confined in the right subhepatic recesses or extending into the whole peritoneal cavity when the peritoneum is perforated

Acute cholecystitis is usually diagnosed when typical clinical and laboratory findings are present, but it may also be misdiagnosed and confused with an abscess or other abdominal inflammations. With CT it is easy to detects acute cholecystitis; other abdominal diseases can be excluded and the stage and the severity of the inflammatory process, the supervening complications, such as pericholecystic extension, cholecystic perforation and peritonitis can be shown.

6.5 Acute Pancreatitis

During acute pancreatitis, the destructive action of the pancreatic enzymes may lead to the development of necrotic hemorrhagic inflammatory collections, which can spread from the pancreatic compartment over the anterior pararenal, subperitoneal mesocolic and mesenteric spaces and the peritoneal cavity. The fluid follows preexisting pathways, defined by the arrangement of the posterior peritoneum, mesocolon and mesentery and by the contiguity and continuity of these structures with the retroperitoneum. In fact, the anterior face of the pancreas makes close contact with the posterior peritoneum, which constitutes the posterior wall of the bursa omentalis in the upper part, whereas in the lower part it limits the mesenteric-colic cavities; furthermore, the transverse mesocolon extends transversely between the two cavities and, at a lower level, the expansion of the mesenteric adipose tissue continues forward without interposition of laminae and fasciae in the anterior pararenal space. Therefore, the diffusion of collections from the pancreatic compartment involves the lesser sac or the submesocolic cavities because of disruption of the peritoneum, whereas in the mesocolic or mesenteric subperitoneal spaces spread is favored by the simple detachment of the adipose tissue located between the peritoneal layers along the vessels extending from the retroperitoneum to the mesenteries.

At first, the collections occupy the peripancreatic adipose cells (Fig. 6.36) and are generally well limited both anteriorly by the posterior peritoneum and posteriorly by the anterior renal fascia. Then, dissecting the fat in the anterior pararenal space, they may diffuse downward as far as the pelvis, behind the sigmoid and the rectum and at the sides into the lateroconal gutters.

CT plays a significant part in detecting the pathological characters (edematous or necrotic-hemorrhagic) and the peculiarities of the collections in the retroperitoneal, subperitoneal and peritoneal spaces and in establishing the management of acute pancreatitis (follow-up and possible guided percutaneous drainage). In addition, CT can indicate the prognosis with regard to morbidity or mortality.

On CT scans the inflamed gland appears enlarged with focal or segmental low-attenuation nonenhancing areas, or encapsulated fluid collections (pseudocysts), indistinct peripancreatic fat or peripancreatic fluid (Figs. 6.33–6.36).

Involvement of the transverse mesocolon and small bowel mesentery is shown on CT as hazing and streaking of the subperitoneal fat around the middle colic or jejunoileal vessels and collections within it (Figs. 6.37, 6.38, 6.41,6.42).

If gas bubbles develop inside the collections this may be due to an abscess or to an intestinal perforation.

The pancreatic fluid may spread into the lesser sac because of the enzymatic disruption of the posterior layer of the parietal peritoneum, where it may occupy one or both recesses (Figs. 4.26–4.29) or swell the whole cavity, which then appears as a wide oval or semicircular water-density cyst-like process between the anterior renal fascia and the stomach (Fig. 6.39). A wide pancreatic subcapsular or anterior peripancreatic collection may cause similar find-

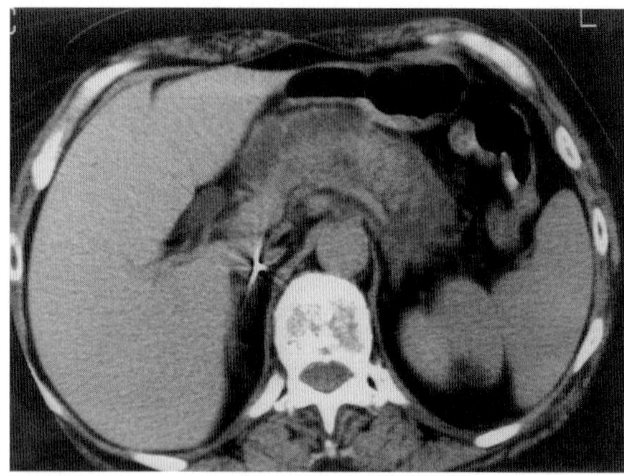

Fig. 6.33. Acute pancreatitis. Diffuse enlargement and nonhomogeneousness of the pancreas with subcapsular fluid collection. The easily seen thin fat-density layer between pancreas and stomach excludes extrapancreatic extension

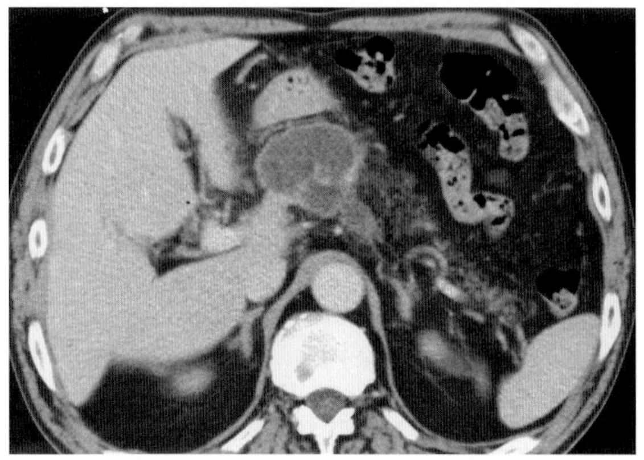

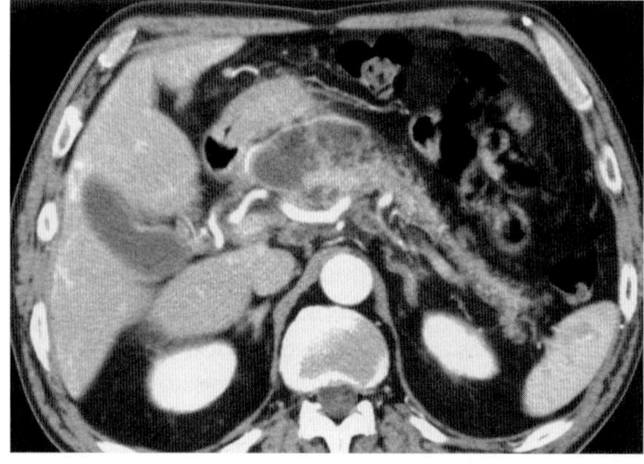

Fig. 6.34A, B. Acute necrotic pancreatitis of the pancreatic head. A Pseudocyst of the pancreatic head. B Normal prepancreatic fat

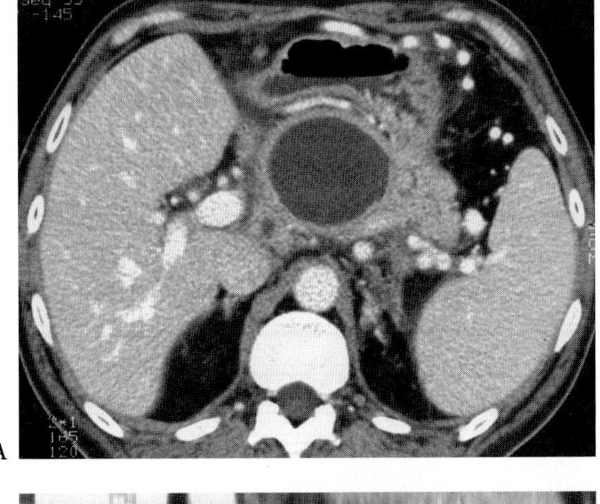

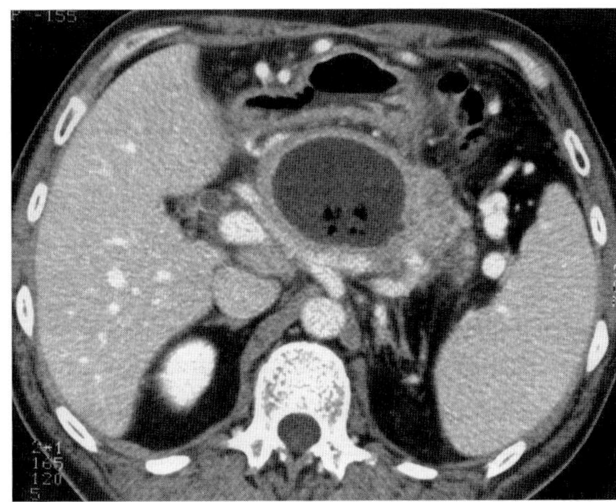

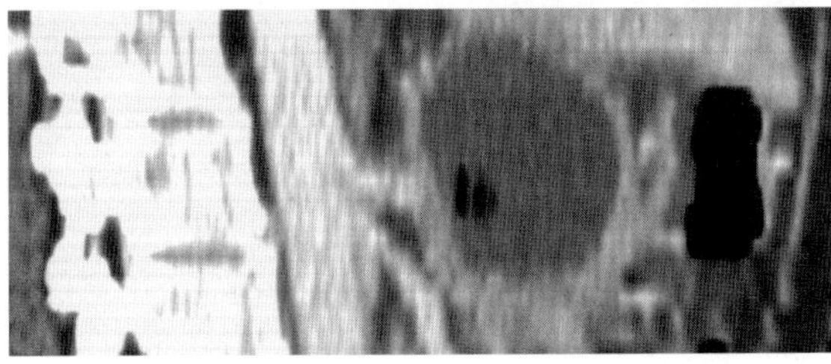

Fig. 6.35A–C. Abscessed necrotic pancreatitis. Fluid collection with gas bubbles inside surrounded by a thick enhancing capsule in the pancreatic isthmus. The presence of a normal gastropancreatic space excludes peritoneal involvement

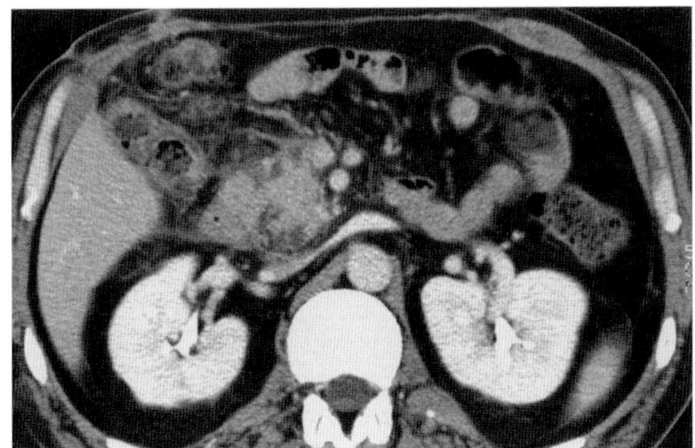

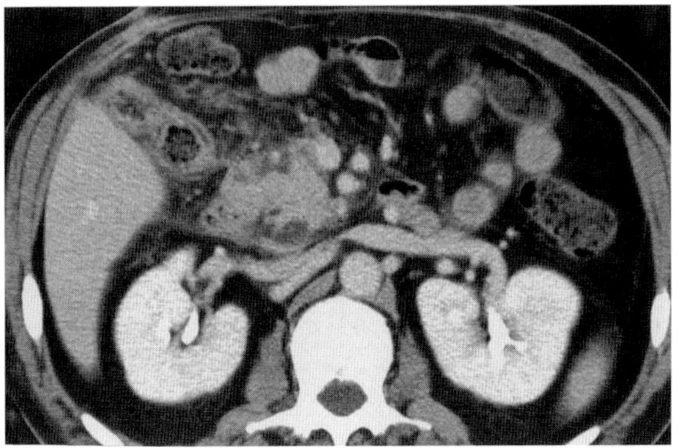

Fig. 6.36A, B. Acute necrotic pancreatitis of the pancreatic head. A Segmental swelling and nonhomogeneous enhancement with low-density areas of the pancreatic head. B Hazing and small pocket of fluid in the pericephalic and right mesocolic fat around the right middle colic vessels between the ascending and the transverse colon

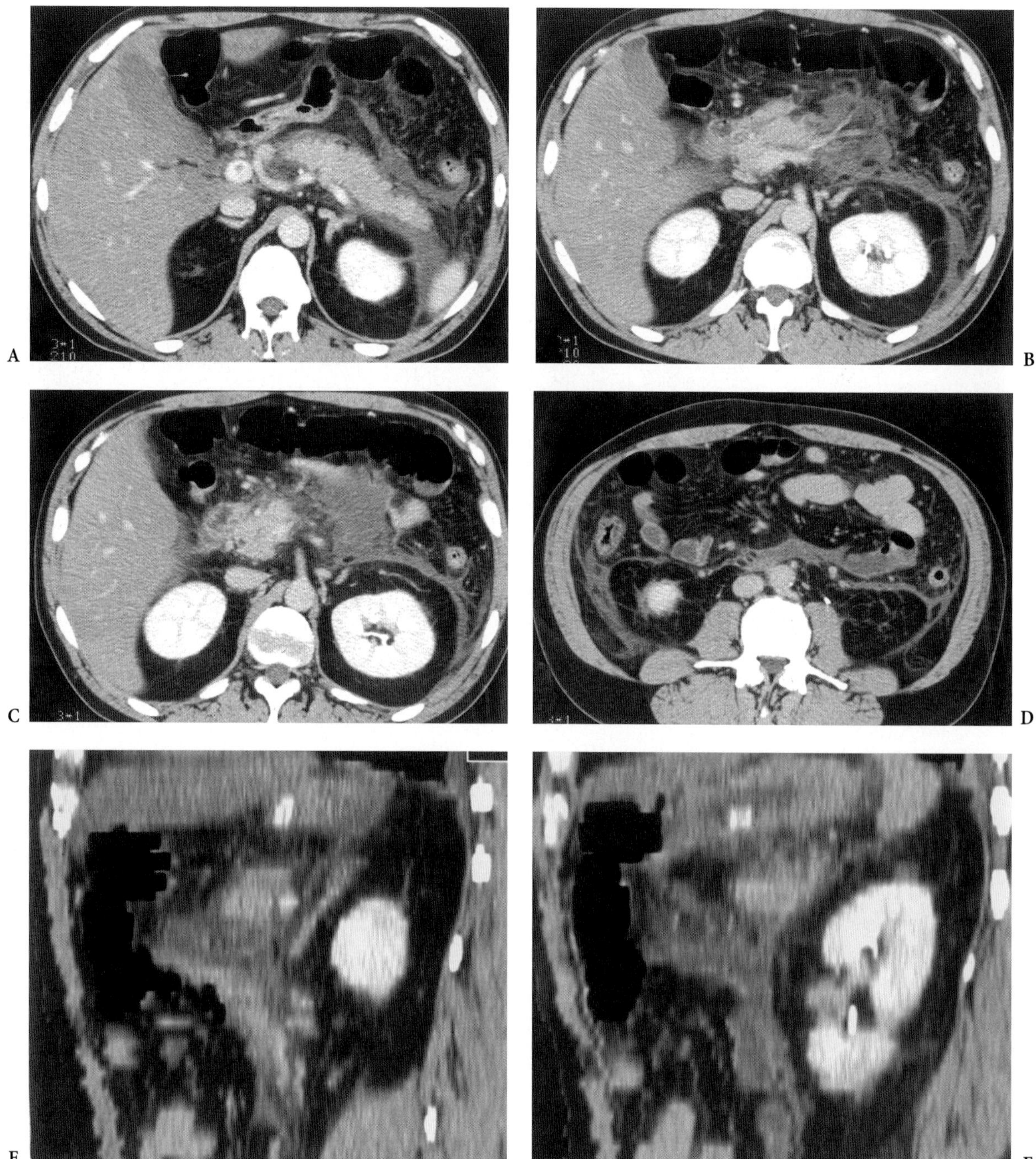

Fig. 6.37A–F. Acute necrotic pancreatitis with retroperitoneal and transverse mesocolic collections. Enlarged and nonhomogeneously enhanced pancreas. A Peripancreatic collection extending downward in the anterior pararenal space and in the lateroconal gutters. B The anterior renal fascia limits the anterior pararenal space behind and separates it from the perirenal compartment. C The collection expands forward within the leaves of the transverse mesocolon around the left middle colic vessels, up to the transverse colon. D–F The sagittal reconstructions give an overall view of the extension of the pancreatic collection

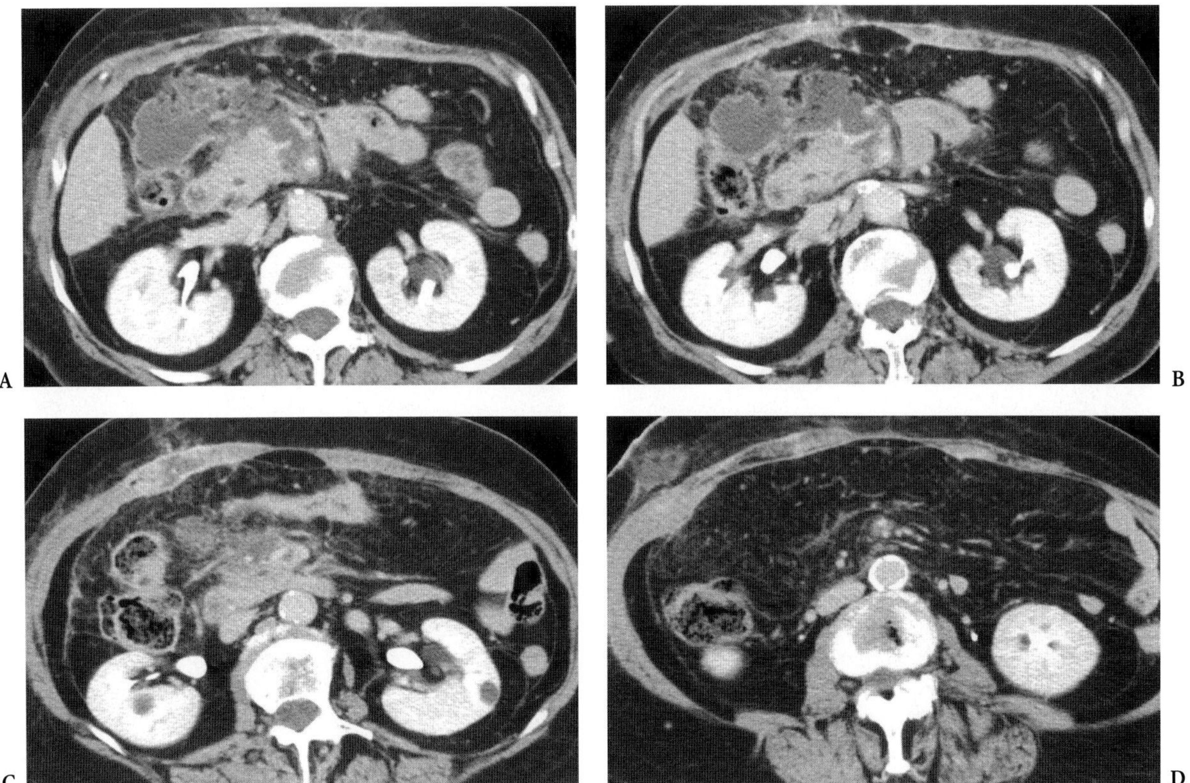

Fig. 6.38A–D. Acute necrotic pancreatitis with fluid collections in the transverse mesocolon, small bowel mesentery and acending mesocolon. Thickening of the peritoneum and of the lateroconal fascia

ings positioned similarly; however, a thin fat-density line between the fluid and the stomach allows the differential diagnosis (Figs. 6.39, 6.40).

Spread through the peritoneal cavity usually occurs into the bursa omentalis because of the discontinuation of its posterior wall. In the bursa omentalis, the fluid takes up a transverse position between the stomach and the pancreas; a single wide semicircular cavity between the anterior renal fascia and the stomach is not rare (Fig. 6.39).

The pancreatic fluid may penetrate the large peritoneal cavity directly, owing to lysis of the posterior peritoneum, or through Winslow's foramen from the lesser sac, and it collects preferentially in the perihepatic or pelvic spaces (Fig. 6.41).

6.6 Typhus

Typhus diffuses to the peritoneum, mesocolic subperitoneal spaces and ligaments through the lymphatic network of the intestinal wall as far as the juxtaintestinal and mesenteric lymph nodes, which become hyperplastic. A nonhomogeneous dense thickening of the transverse mesocolon and of the gastrocolic ligament (Ascenti et al. 1992) is visible on CT.

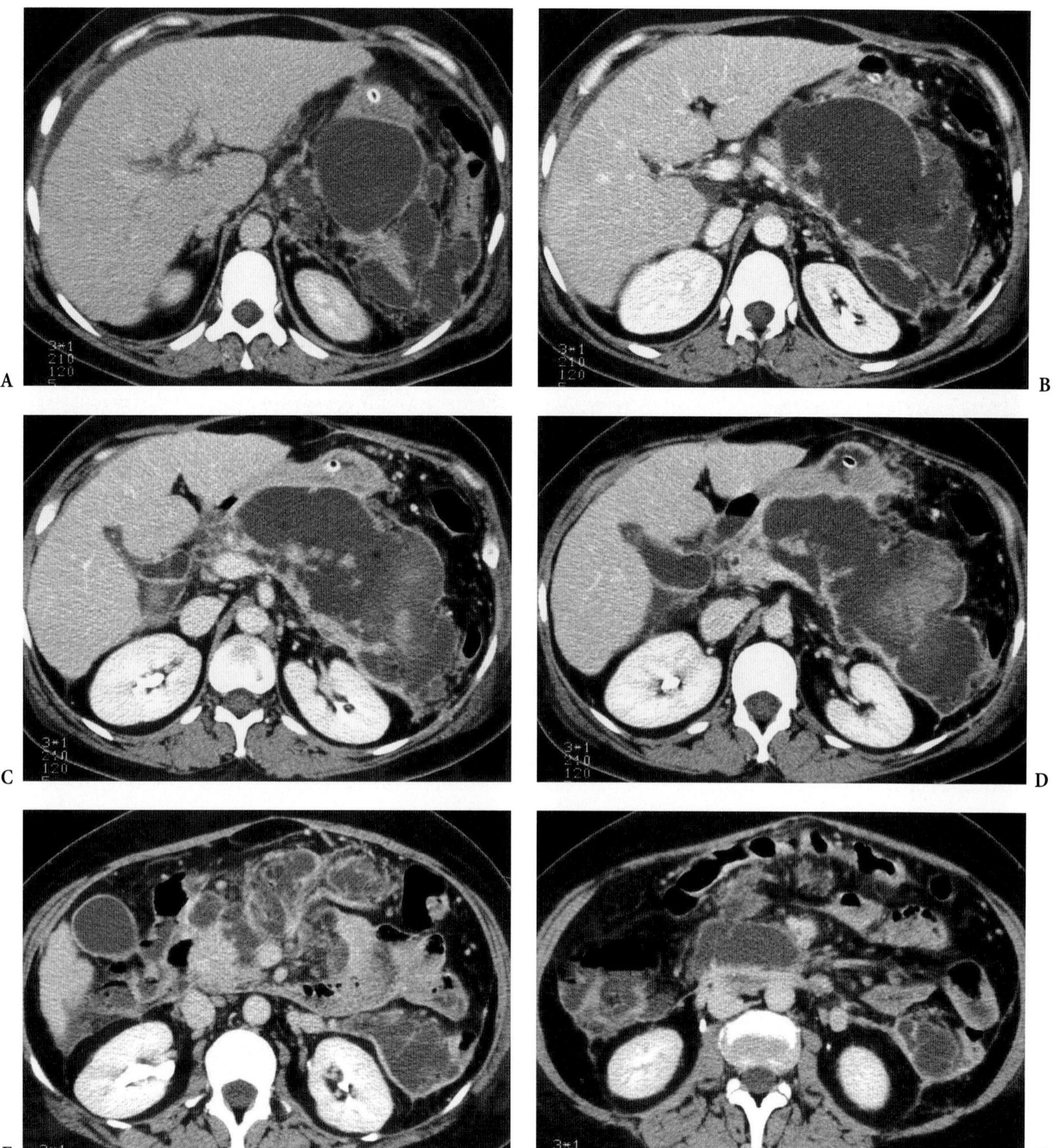

Fig. 6.39A–F. Acute necrotic pancreatitis extending into the transverse mesocolon and the peritoneum. Multiseptate pseudocyst with dense spots of fresh blood inside and thickening enhancing wall, occupying the pancreatic compartment and the lesser sac, in close contact with the stomach wall without interposed fat cleavage plane. From the lesser sac the collection spreads into the perihepatic spaces through Winslow's foramen. The retroperitoneal collection spreads downward, sliding along the anterior renal fascia and the left lateroconal fascia, and diffusing forward between the leaves of the transverse mesocolon

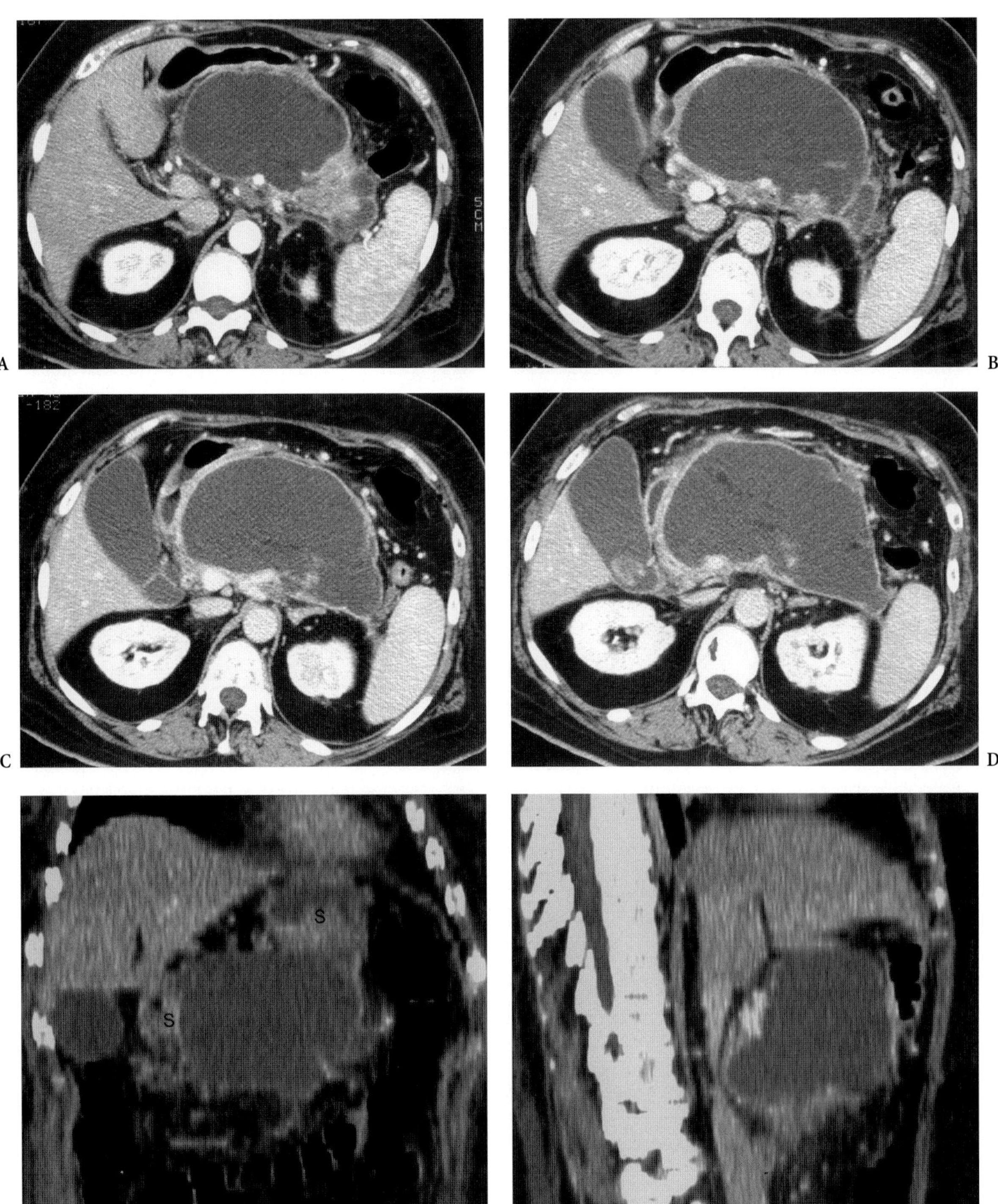

Fig. 6.40A–F. Acute necrotic pancreatitis. Huge pseudocyst with thickening fibrous wall, extending forward, without involvement of the lesser sac, as shown by the fat cleavage layer between the pseudocyst and the stomach. Coronal and sagittal reconstructions

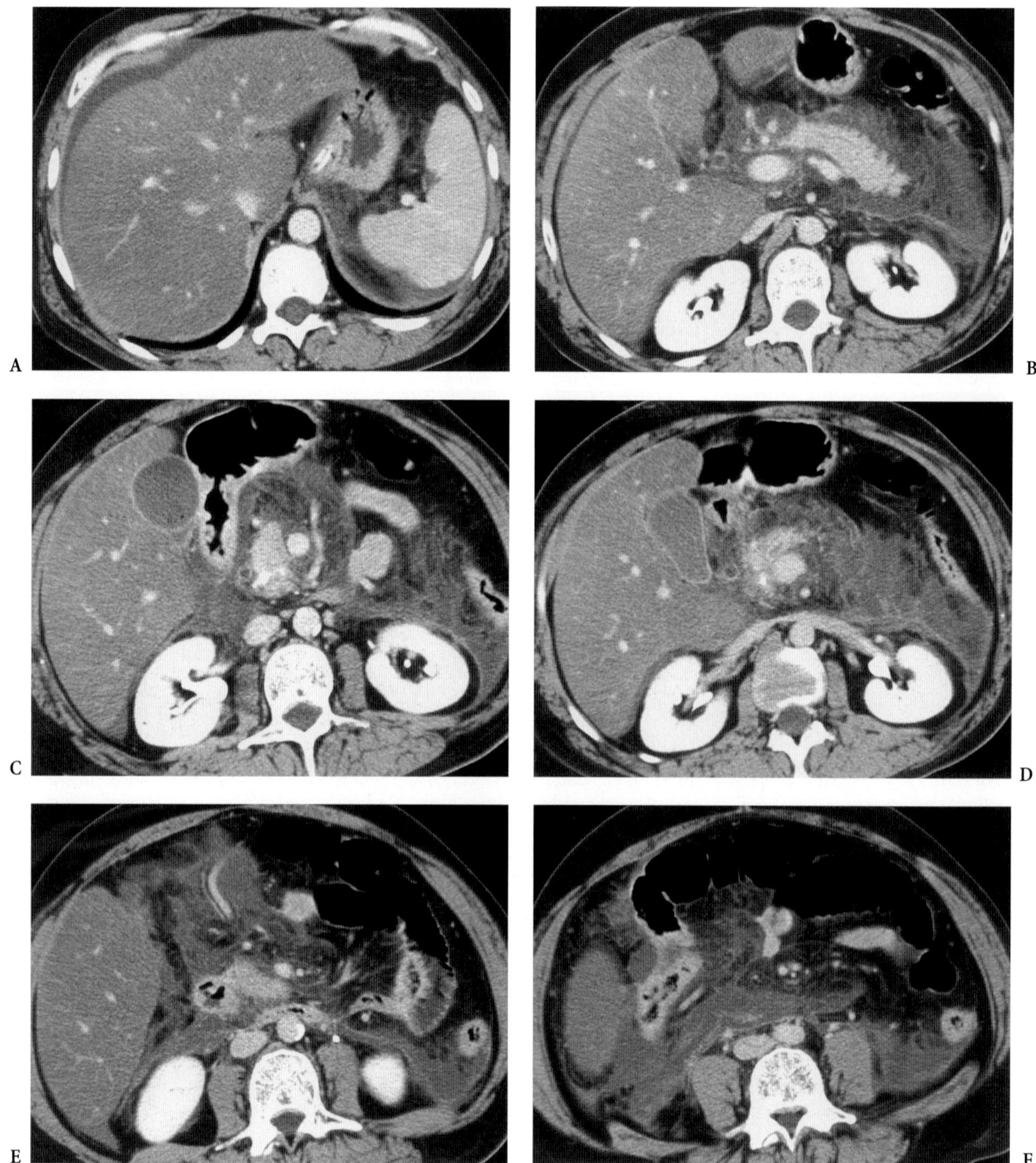
A
B
C
D
E
F

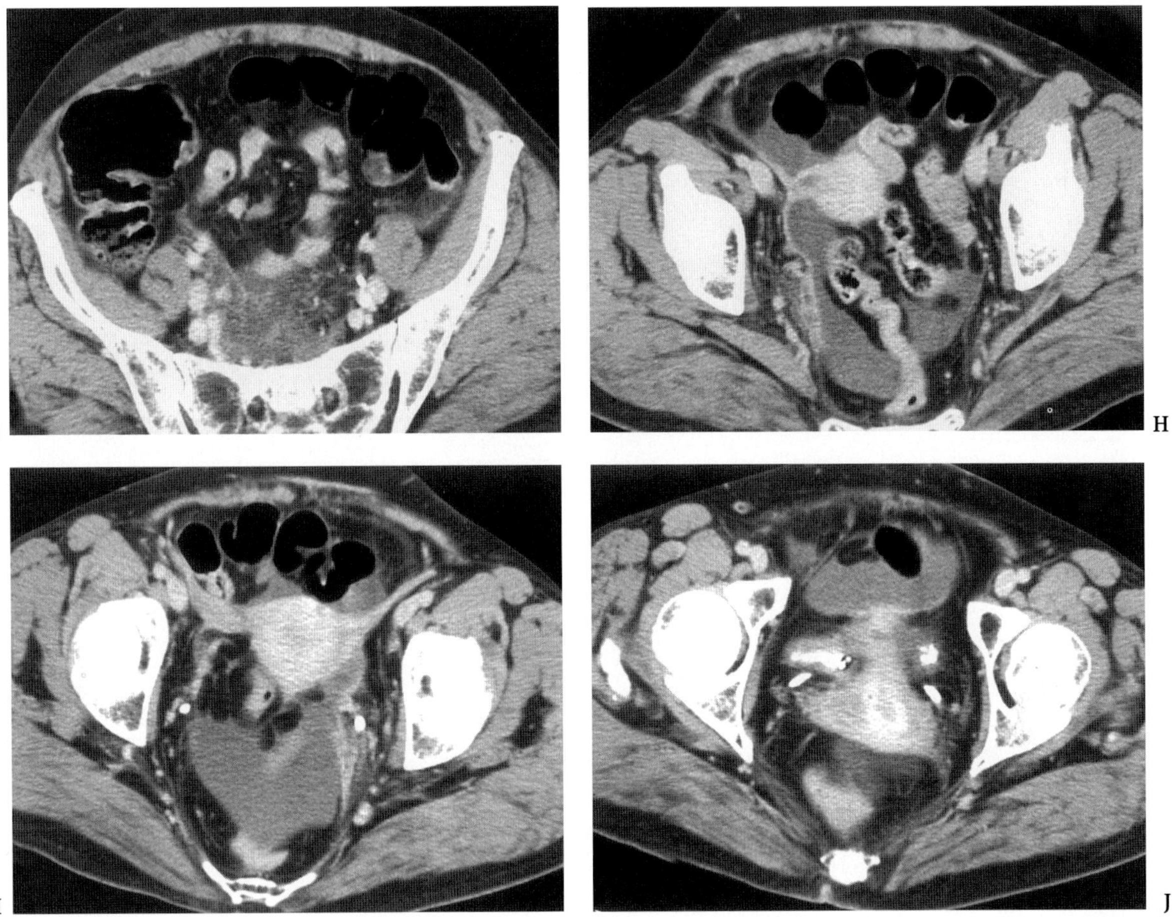

Fig. 6.41A–H. Acute necrotic pancreatitis with large retro- and intraperitoneal collection. In the retroperitoneum, the fluid dissects the adipose tissue and collects around the pancreas; it then diffuses downward in front of the anterior renal fascia in the anterior pararenal space and along the lateroconal gutters up to the pelvic inlet (*H*) and penetrates forward into the transverse mesocolon (*E*) and the small bowel mesentery (*F*). The separation limit between the retroperitoneum and the mesentery is constituted by the superior mesenteric vessels. A small amount of fluid penetrates the peritoneum and collects in the lowest points of the cavity: perihepatic spaces (*A*), parasigmoidal (*C*) and supravesical (*I*) recesses and pouch of Douglas (*J*)

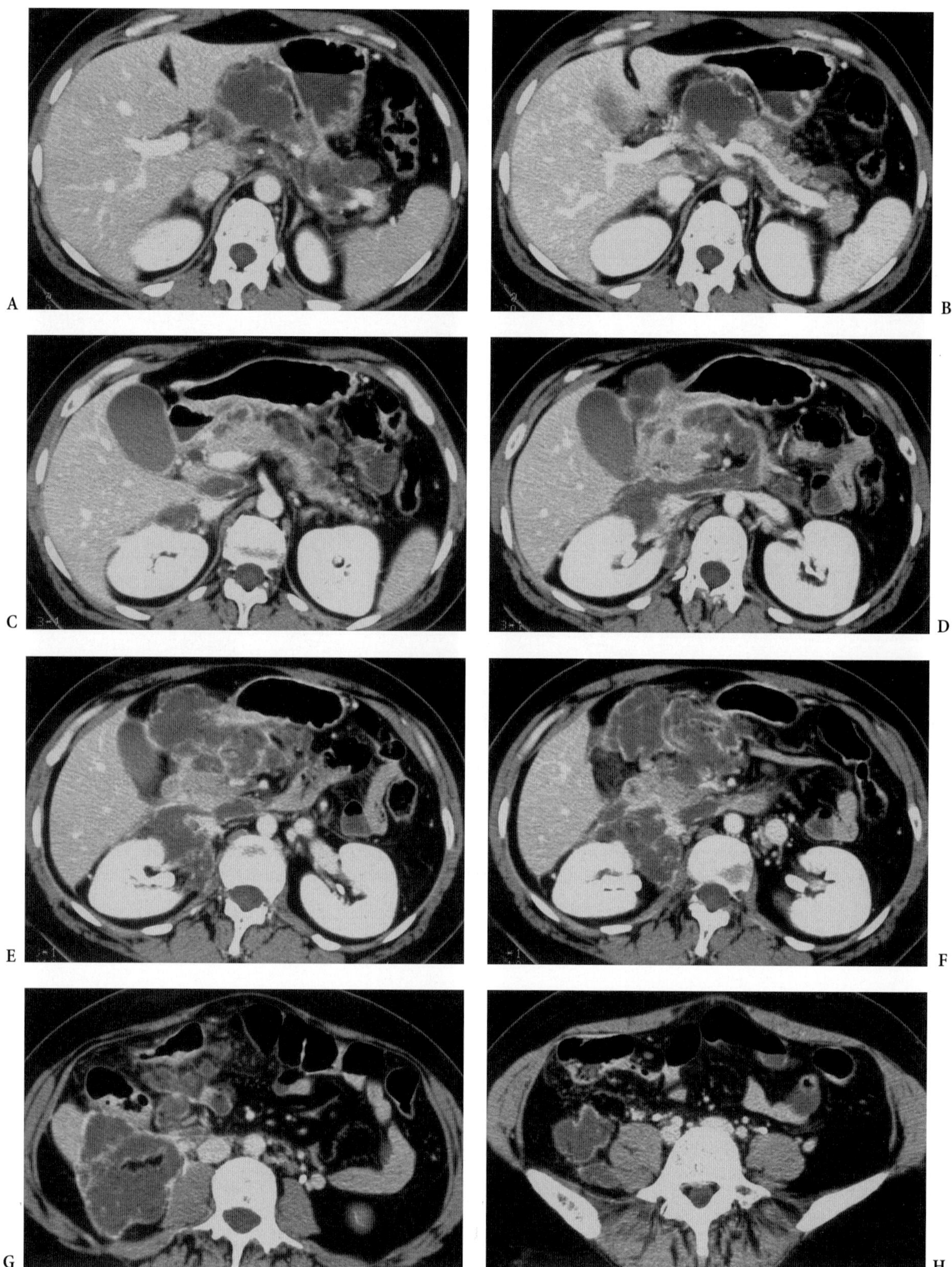

Fig. 6.42A–H. Acute necrotic pancreatitis with mesenteric, mesocolic and perirenal involvement. Wide retroperitoneal collection has extended into the whole of the anterior pararenal space up to the right iliac fossa and forward between the transverse mesocolic and mesenteric leaves in front of the superior mesenteric vessels. It has also penetrated the right perirenal space (D–H), crossing the anterior renal fascia

Bibliography

General Considerations

Alexander ES, Proto AV, Clark RA (1983) CT differentiation of subphrenic abscess and pleural effusion. AJR Am J Roentgenol 140: 47–51

Aronberg DJ, Stanley, Levitt RG, Sagel SS (1978) Evaluation of abdominal abscess by computed tomography. J Comput Assist Tomogr 2:384–387

Balthazar EJ, Chako AC (1992) Computed tomography in acute gastrointestinal disorders. Am J Gastroenterol 85:1445–1452

Biello DR, Levitt RG, Mason GL (1979) The roles of gallium 67 scintigraphy ultrasonography, and computed tomography in the detection of abdominal abscesses. Semin Nucl Med 9:58

Bydder GM, Kreel L (1980) Attenuation values of fluid collections within the abdomen. J Comput Assist Tomogr 4:145–150

Callen PW (1979) Computed tomographic evaluation of abdominal and pelvic abscesses. Radiology 131:171–175

Caron-Poitreau C, Dauvier A, Vialle M, Friess JJ, Rieux D (1981) Apport de la tomodensitométrie dans le diagnostic des suppurations abdominales. J Radiol 62:283–290

Caron-Poitreau C, Rieux D, Dauvier A, Vialle M (1983) Apport de la tomodensitométrie dans la recherche d'un épanchement liquidien abdominal intrapéritonéal. Radiologie 3:11–16

Churchill R, Meyers MA (1986) Intraperitoneal fluid collections. In: Meyers MA (ed) Computed tomography of the gastrointestinal tract including the peritoneal cavity and mesentery. Springer, New York Berlin Heidelberg

Churchill RJ (1989) CT of intraabdominal fluid collections. Radiol Clin North Am 27:653–666

Clark RA, Towbin R (1983) Abscess drainage with CT and ultrasound guidance. Radiol Clin North Am 21:445–459

Cohen JM, Winreb JC, Maravilla KR (1985) Fluid collections in the intraperitoneal and extraperitoneal spaces: comparison of MR and CT. Radiology 155:705–708

Connel TR, Stephens DH, Carlson HC, Brown ML (1980) Upper abdominal abscess: a continuing and deadly problem. AJR Am J Roentgenol 134:759

Feldberg MAM (1983) Computed tomography of the retroperitoneum. Nijhoff, Boston

Filly RA (1979) Detection of abdominal abscesses: a combined approach employing ultrasonography, computed tomography, and gallium-67 scanning. Can Assoc Radiol 30:202–210

Gagliardi PD, Hoffer PB, Rosenfield AT (1988) Correlative imaging in abdominal infection: an algorithmic approach using nuclear medicine, ultrasound, and computed tomography. Semin Nucl Med 18:320

Gazelle GS, Haaga JR, Stellato TA, Gauderer MWL, Plecha DT (1991) Pelvic abscesses: CT-guided transrectal drainage. Gastrointest Radiol 181:49

Gerzof SG, Robbins AH, Birkett DH (1978) Computed tomography in the diagnosis and management of abdominal abscesses. Gastrointest Radiol 3:287–294

Gerzof SG, Robbins AH, Birkett DH (1979) Percutaneous catheter drainage of abdominal abscess guided by ultrasound and computed tomography. AJR Am J Roentgenol 133:1–8

Gerzof SG, Robbins AH, Johnson WC, Burkitt DH, Nabstih DC (1981) Percutaneous catheter drainage of abdominal abscesses. A five year experience. N Engl J Med 305:653–657

Ghahremani GG, Gore RM (1989) CT diagnosis of postoperative abdominal complications. Radiol Clin North Am 27:787

Haaga JR, Alfidi RJ (1978) Peritoneal abscesses and other disorders. In: Haaga IR, Reich NE (eds) Computed tomography of the whole body. Mosby, St Louis

Haaga JR, Alfidi RJ (1983) Peritoneal abscesses and other disorders. In: Haaga JR, Alfidi RJ (eds) Computed tomography of the whole body, 2nd edn. Mosby, St Louis

Haaga JR, Winstein AJ (1980) CT guided percutaneous aspiration and drainage of abscess. AJR Am J Roentgenol 135:1187–1194

Haaga JR, Alfidi RJ, Havrilla TR (1977) CT detection and aspiration of abdominal abscesses. AJR Am J Roentgenol 123: 465–474

Halber MD, Daffner RH, Morgan CL, Trought WS, Thompson WM, Rice RP, Korobkin M (1979) Intraabdominal abscess; current concepts in radiologic evaluation. AJR Am J Roentgenol 133:9

Halvorsen RA, Jonsen MA, Rice RP, Thompson WM (1982) Anterior left subphrenic abscess: characteristic plain film and CT appearance. AJR Am J Roentgenol 139:283–289

Harter LP, Moss AA, Goldberg HI (1983) Computed tomographic guided fine needle aspirations for neoplastic and inflammatory disease. AJR Am J Roentgenol 140:363

Jeffrey RB Jr (1988) Percutaneous drainage of enteric abscesses. Semin Interv Radiol 5:211–222

Jeffrey RB, Federle MP, Laing FC (1983) Computed tomography of mesenteric involvement in fulminant pancreatitis. Radiology 147:185–188

Jeffrey RB, Federle MP, Laing FC (1984) Computed tomography of silent abdominal abscesses. J Comput Assist Tomogr 8:67–70

Khochel JQ, Koehler PR, Lee TG, Welch DM (1980) Diagnosis of abdominal abscesses with computed tomography, ultrasound, and in leukocyte scan. Radiology 137:425–432

Koehler PR, Moss AA (1980) Diagnosis of intra-abdominal and pelvic abscesses by computed tomography. JAMA 244:49–52

Korobkin M, Callen PW, Filly RA, Hoffer PB, Shimshak RR, Kressel HY (1978) Comparison of computed tomography, ultrasonography, and gallium-67 scanning in the evaluation of suspected abdominal abscess. Radiology 129:89

Lambiase RE, Deyoe L, Cronan JJ, Dorfman GS (1992) Percutaneous drainage of 335 consecutive abscesses: results of primary drainage with 1 year follow-up. Radiology 184:167

Levitt RG (1983) Abdominal wall and peritoneal cavity. In: Lee JKT, Sagel SS, Stanley RI (eds) Computed body tomography. Raven Press, New York

Levitt RG, Biello DR, Sagel SS, Stanley RJ, Aronberg DJ, Robinson ML, Siegel BA (1979) CT and 67-Ga-citrate radionuclide imaging for evaluating suspected abdominal abscess. AJR Am J Roentgenol 132:529–534

Lundstedt C, Hederstrom E, Holmin T, Lunderquist A, Navne T, Owman T (1983) Radiological diagnosis in proven intraabdominal abscess formation: a comparison between plain films of the abdomen, ultrasonography and computerized tomography. Gastrointest Radiol 8:261–266

McNeil BJ, Sanders R, Alderson PO, Hessel SJ, Fenberg H, Siegelman SS, Adams DF, Abrams HS (1981) A prospective study of computed tomography, ultrasound and gallium imaging in patients with fever. Radiology 139:647
Meyers MA (1970) The spread and localization of acute intraperitoneal effusions. Radiology 95:547–554
Meyers MA (1988) Intraperitoneal spread of infections. In: Meyers MA (ed) Dynamic radiology of the abdomen: normal and pathologic anatomy. Springer, New York Berlin Heidelberg
Meyers MA (1992) Diffusione intraperitoneale delle infezioni. In: Meyers MA (ed) Radiologia dinamica dell'addome. Verduci, Rome
Meyers MA, Oliphant M, Berne AS, et al (1987) The peritoneal ligaments and mesenteries: pathways of intraabdominal spread of disease. Radiology 163:593–604
Mitchell GAG (1940) The spread of acute intraperitoneal effusions. Br J Surg 28: 291–313
Mueller PR, Simeone JF (1983) Intra-abdominal abscesses: diagnosis by sonography and computed tomography. Radiol Clin North Am 21:425–443
Mueller PR, Simeone JF, Butch RJ, et al (1986) Percutaneous drainage of subphrenic abscess: a review of 62 patients. AJR Am J Roentgenol 147:1237–1240
Mueller PR, van Sonnenberg E (1989) Abscesses and fluid collections: detection and drainage. In: Taveras JM, Ferrucci JT (eds) Radiology diagnosis – imaging – intervention. Lippincott, Philadelphia
Mueller PR, van Sonnenberg E, Ferrucci JT Jr (1984) Percutaneous drainage of 250 abdominal abscesses and fluid collections. II. Current procedural concepts. Radiology 151:343–347
Muro LR (1982) Detection of abdominal abscesses with gallium-67 citrate correlative studies with computed tomography. Semin Nucl Med 12:173–183
Murphy D, Hughes PM, Zammit-Maempel I (1992) Computed tomographic assessment of intraperitoneal fluid distribution prior to intraperitoneal chemotherapy for ovarian cancer. Br J Radiol 65:295
Schneekloth G, Terrier F, Fuchs WA (1982) Computed tomography of intraperitoneal abscesses. Gastrointest Radiol 7:35–41
Seltzer SE (1984) Abnormal intraabdominal gas collections visualized on computed tomography: a clinical and experimental study. Gastrointest Radiol 9:127–131
Siegelman SS, Copeland BE, Saba GP, Cameron JL, Sanders RC, Zerhouni EA (1980) CT of fluid collections associated with pancreatitis. AJR Am J Roentgenol 134:1121–1132
Siewert V, Raptopoulos V (1994) CT of acute abdomen: findings an impact on diagnosis and treatment. AJR Am J Roentgenol 163:1317–1324
Silverman PM, Baker ME, Cooper C, et al (1986) CT appearance of diffuse mesenteric edema. J Comput Assist Tomogr 10:67–70
Sones PJ (1984) Percutaneous drainage of abdominal abscesses. AJR Am J Roentgenol 142:35–39
Stanley RJ (1980) Fluid characterization with computed tomography. In: Moss AA, Goldberg HI (eds) Computed tomography, ultrasound and X-ray: an integrated approach. Academic Press, New York
van Sonnenberg E, Ferrucci JT Jr, Mueller P (1982) Percutaneous drainage of abscesses and fluid collections: technique, results, and applications. Radiology 142:1–10
van Sonnenberg E, Mueller PR, Ferrucci JT Jr (1984) Percutaneous drainage of 250 abdominal abscesses and fluid collections. I. Results, failures, and complications. Radiology 151:337–341
van Sonnenberg E, D'Agostino HB, Sanchez RB, Casola G (1992) Percutaneous abscess drainage (editorial comments). Radiology 184:27
Whalen JP (1976) Anatomy and radiologic diagnosis of perihepatic abscesses. Radiol Clin North Am 14:406–428
Wolverson MK, Jagannadharao B, Sundaram M, Joyce PF, Riaz MA, Shields JB (1979) CT as a primary diagnosis method in evaluating intraabdominal abscess. AJR Am J Roentgenol 133:1089

Appendicitis

Balthazar EJ, Gordon RB (1989) CT of appendicitis. Semin Ultrasound CT MR 10:326–340
Balthazar EJ, Megibow AJ, Hulnick D, Gordon RB, Naidich DP, Birnbaum ER (1986) CT of appendicitis. AJR Am J Roentgenol 147:705–710
Balthazar EJ, Megibow AJ, Gordon RB, et al (1989) Computed tomography of the abnormal appendix. J Comput Assist Tomogr 12:595–601
Balthazar EJ, Megibow AJ, Siegel SE, Birnbaum BA (1991) Appendicitis: prospective evaluation with high-resolution CT. Radiology 180:21–24
Balthazar EJ, Birnbaum BA, Yee J, Megibow AJ, Roshkov J, Gray C (1994) Acute appendicitis: CT and US correlation in 100 patients. Radiology 190:31–35
Barakos JA, Jeffrey RB, Federle MP, Wing VW, Laing FC, High-Tower DR (1986) CT in the management of periappendiceal abscess. AJR Am J Roentgenol 146:1161–1164
Birnbaum BA, Balthazar EJ (1994) CT of appendicitis and diverticulitis. Radiol Clin North Am 32:885–898
Brown JJ (1991) Acute appendicitis. The radiologist's role. Radiology 180:13–14
Catalano O (1995) Interesse diagnostico della tomografia computerizzata nell'appendicite acuta dell'adulto. Radiol Med 89:798–803
Clarke PD (1987) Computed tomography of gangrenous appendicitis. J Comput Assist Tomogr 11:1081–1082
Curtin Kr, Fitzgerald SN, Nemeek AA Jr, et al (1995) CT diagnosis of acute appendicitis: imaging findings. AJR Am J Roentgenol 164:905–909
Federle MP (1997) Focused appendix CT technique: a commentary. Radiology 202:20–21
Feldberg MAM, Hendriks MJ, Van Waes PFGM (1985) Computed tomography in complicated acute appendicitis. Gastrointest Radiol 10:289–295
Fish B, Smulewicz JJ, Barek L (1981) Role of computed tomography in diagnosis of appendiceal disorders. NY State J Med 81:900–904
Gale ME, Birnbaum S, Gerzof SG, Sloan G, Johnson WC, Robbins AH (1985) CT appearance of appendicitis and its local complications. J Comput Assist Tomogr 9:34–37
Ghiatas AA, Chopra S, Chintapalli KN, et al (1996) Computed tomography of the normal appendix and acute appendicitis. Eur Radiol 7:1045–1047
Jeffrey RB (1989) Management of the periappendiceal inflammatory mass. Semin Ultrasound CT MR 10:341–347
Jeffrey RB (1994) Acute appendicitis. In: Gore RM, Levine MS, Laufer I (eds) Textbook of gastrointestinal radiology. Saun-

ders, Philadelphia, pp 2538–2540

Jeffrey RB Jr, Tolentino CS, Federle MP, Laing FC (1987) Percutaneous drainage of periappendiceal abscess: review of twenty patients. AJR Am J Roentgenol 149:59–62

Jeffrey RB Jr, Federle MP, Tolentino CS (1988) Periappendiceal inflammatory masses: CT-directed management and clinical outcome in 70 patients. Radiology 167:13–16

Jones B, Fishman EK, Siegelman SS (1983) Computed tomography and appendiceal abscess: special applicability in the elderly. J Comput Assist Tomogr 7:434–438

Malone AJ Jr, Wolf CR, Malmed AS, Melliere BF (1993) Diagnosis of acute appendicitis: value of unenhanced CT. AJR Am J Roentgenol 160:763–766

Nisolle JF, Bodart E, De Caniere L, et al (1996) Appendicite aigue d'expression clinique gauche: apport diagnostique de la tomodensitometrie. Arch Pediatr 3:47–50

Nunez D Jr, Huber JS, Yrizarry JM, Mendez G, Russel E (1986) Nonsurgical drainage of appendiceal abscesses. AJR Am J Roentgenol 146:587–589

Rao PM. Rhea JT, Novelline RA, et al (1997) Helical CT technique for the diagnosis of appendicitis: prospective evaluation of a focused appendix CT examination. Radiology 202:139–144

Scaglione M, Pinto F, Romano L, Forner AL, et al (1996) L'appendicite acuta complicata: descrizione di un caso diagnosticato con tomografia computerizzata. Radiol Med 92:655–657

Scatarige JC, Yousem DM, Fishman EK, Jones B, Siegelman SS (1987) CT abnormalities in right lower quadrant inflammatory disease: review of findings in 26 patients. Gastrointest Radiol 12:156–162

Shapiro MP, Gale ME, Gerzof SG (1989) CT of appendicitis – Diagnosis and treatment. Radiol Clin North Am 27:753–762

Taourel P, Baron MP, Pradel J, Fabre JM, Seneterre E, Bruel JM (1992) Acute abdomen of unknown origin: impact of CT on diagnosis and management. Gastrointest Radiol 17:287–291

van Sonnenberg E, Wittich GR, Casola G, et al (1987) Periappendiceal abscesses: percutaneous drainage. Radiology 163:23–26

Diverticulitis

Ambrosetti P, Robert J, Witzig JA et al (1992) Prognostic factors from computed tomography in acute left colonic diverticulitis. Br J Surg 79:117–119

Angelelli G, Brindicci D, Macarini L (1991) La TC nello studio dele lesioni della parete dell'apparato digerente. Radiol Med 81:83–89

Balthazar EJ (1994) Diverticular disease. In: Gore RM, Levine MS, Laufer I (eds) Textbook of gastrointestinal radiology. Saunders, Philadelphia, pp 1072–1097

Balthazar EJ, Megibow AJ, Gordon RB, Hulnick D (1987) Cecal diverticulitis: evaluation with CT. Radiology 162:79–81

Balthazar EJ, Megibow AJ, Schinella RA, Gordon R (1990) Limitations in the CT diagnosis of acute diverticulitis: comparison of CT, contrast enema, and pathologic findings in 16 patients. AJR Am J Roentgenol 154:281–285

Bass IS, Goldberg HI, Shea WJ, Jeffrey RB Jr (1988) Evaluation of diverticulitis and its complications. In: Fishman ER, Jones B (eds) Computed tomography of the gastrointestinal tract. Churchill Livingstone, New York

Benya EC, Ghahremani GG, Brosnan JJ (1991) Diverticulitis of the jejunum: clinical and radiological features. Gastrointest Radiol 16:24–28

Bimbaum BA, Balthazar EJ (1994) CT of appendicitis and diverticulitis. Radiol Clin North Am 32:885–898

Catalano O (1996) La tomografia computerizzata nello studio della diverticolite acuta del sigma. Radiol Med 92:588–593

Cho KC, Morehouse HT, Alterman DD, Thornhill BA (1990) Sigmoid diverticulitis: diagnostic role of CT – comparison with barium enema studies. Radiology 176:111–115

Di Nardo R, Capanna G, Iannicelli E et al (1994) Diagnostica per immagini nella valutazione delle complicanze pelviche da malattie intestinali. Radiol Med 88:49–55

Doringer E, Ferner R (1990) Computertomographie der Kolondivertikulitis. Rofo Fortschr Geb Roentgenstr Neuen Bildgeb Verfahr 152:76–79

Ernst S, Wypior HJ, Stark V et al (1996) Computertomographie der akuten Sigmadivertikulitis. Rofo Fortschr Geb Roentgenstr Neuen Bildgeb Verfahr 164:102–107

Feldberg MAM, Hendriks MJ, van Waes PFGM (1985) Role of CT in diagnosis and management of complications of diverticular disease. Gastrointest Radiol 10:370–377

Goldman SM, Fishman EK, Gatewood OMB, Jones B, Brendler C, Siegelman SS (1984) CT demonstration of colovesical fistulae secondary to diverticulitis. J Comput Assist Tomogr 8:462–468

Greenstein S, Jones B, Fishman EK, Cameron JL, Siegelman SS (1986) Small bowel diverticulitis: CT findings. AJR Am J Roentgenol 147:271–274

Griffen WO, Dempsey DT, Caroline DF (1992) Diverticulitis. In: Taylor MB (ed) Gastrointestinal emergencies. Williams & Wilkins, Baltimore, pp 415–425

Hachigian MP, Honickman S, Eisenstat TE, et al (1992) Computed tomography in the initial management of acute left-sided diverticulitis. Dis Colon Rectum 35:1123–1129

Hulnick DH, Megibow AJ, Balthazar EJ, Naidich DP, Bosniac MA (1984) CT in the evaluation of diverticulitis. Radiology 152:491–495

Ide O, van Beers B, Pauls C, et al (1994) Diagnostic des diverticulites aigues du colon: comparaison de l'echographie et de la tomodensitometrie. J Belge Radiol 77:262–267

Jarret TW, Vaughan ED (1995) Accuracy of computerized tomography in the diagnosis of colovesical fistula secondary to diverticular disease. J Urol 153:44–46

Johnson CD, Baker ME, Rice RP, Silverman P, Thompson WM (1987) Diagnosis of acute colonic diverticulitis: comparison of barium enema and CT. AJR Am J Roentgenol 148:541–546

Kanehann LB, Caroline DF, Friedman AC, et al (1988) CT findings in venous intravasation complicating diverticulitis. J Comput Assist Tomogr 12:1047–1049

Labs JD, Sarr MG, Fishman EK, et al (1988) Complications of acute diverticulitis of the colon: improved early diagnosis with computerized tomography. Am Surg 155:331–336

Lieberman JM, Haaga JR (1983) Computed tomography of diverticulitis. J Comput Assist Tomogr 7:431–433

Megibow AJ (1986) Diverticulitis. In: Meyers MA (ed) Computed tomography of the gastrointestinal tract. Springer, New York Berlin Heidelberg, pp 235–252

Minilel G, Chittaro L, Abbona M (1996) Enfisema sottocutaneo, pneumomediastino e pneumoretroperitoneo da perforazione di diverticolo del sigma. Descrizione di un caso

esaminato con tomografia computerizzata spirale. Radiol Med 92:653–655
Mueller PR, Saini S, Wittenburg J, et al (1987) Sigmoid diverticular abscesses: percutaneous drainage as an adjunct to surgical resection in 24 cases. Radiology 164:321–325
Neff CC, van Sonnenberg E (1989) CT of diverticulitis: diagnosis and treatment. Radiol Clin North Am 27:743–752
Neff CC, van Sonnenberg E, Casola G, et al (1987) Diverticular abscess: percutaneous drainage. Radiology 163:15–18
Padidar AM, Jeffrey Jr RB, Mindelzun RE, Dolph JF (1994) Differentiating sigmoid diverticulitis from carcinoma on CT scans: mesenteric inflammation suggests diverticulitis. AJR Am J Roentgenol 163:81–83
Pillari G, Greenspan B, Vernace FM, et al (1984) Computed tomography of diverticulitis. Gastrointest Radiol 9:263–289
Saini S, Mueller PR, Wittenberg J, et al (1986) Percutaneous drainage of diverticular abscess: an adjunct to surgical therapy. Arch Surg 121:475–477
Scatarige JC, Fishman EK, Crist DW, Cameron JL, Siegelman SS (1987) Diverticulitis of the right colon: CT observations. AJR Am J Roentgenol 148:737–739
Stefánsson T, Nyman R, Nilsson S, Ekbom A, Påhlman L (1997) Diverticulitis of the sigmoid colon. A comparison of CT, colonic enema and laparoscopy. Acta Radiol 38:313–319

Acute Cholecystitis

Blankenberg F, Wirth R, Jeffrey RB Jr, Mindelzun R, Francis I (1991) Computed tomography as an adjunct to ultrasound in the diagnosis of acute cholecystitis. Gastrointest Radiol 16:149–153
Fidler J, Paulson EK, Layfield L (1995) CT evaluation of acute cholecystitis. AJR Am J Roentgenol 166:1085–1088
Jenkins M, Golding RH, Cooperberg PL (1983) Sonography and computed tomography of hemorrhagic cholecystitis. AJR Am J Roentgenol 140:1197–1198
Kane RA, Costello P, Duszlak E (1983) Computed tomography in acute cholecystitis: new observations. AJR Am J Roentgenol 141:697–701
Lamki N, Reval B, St. Ville E (1986) Computed tomography of complicated cholecystitis. J Comput Assist Tomogr 319–324
McDonnell CH III, Jeffrey RB Jr, Vierra MA (1994) Inflamed pericholecystic fat: color Doppler flow imaging and clinical features. Radiology 193:547–550
McMillin K (1985) Computed tomography of emphysematous cholecystitis. J Comput Assist Tomogr 9:330–332
Mirvis Se, Vainright JR, Nelson AW, Johnston GS, Shorr R, Rodriguez A, Whiteley NO (1986) The diagnosis of acute acalculous cholecystitis: a comparison of sonography, scintigraphy, and CT. AJR Am J Roentgenol 147:1171–1175
Mirvis SE, Whitley NO, Miller JW (1987) CT diagnosis of acalculous cholecystitis. J Comput Assist Tomogr 11:83–87
Terrier F, Becker CD, Stoller C, Triller JK (1984) Computed tomography in complicated cholecystitis. J Comput Assist Tomogr 8:58–62

Acute Pancreatitis

Balthazar EJ (1987) Prognostic value in CT in acute pancreatitis: is the early CT examination indicated? Radiology 163:876–877
Balthazar EJ (1989) CT diagnosis and staging of acute pancreatitis. Radiol Clin North Am 27:19–37
Balthazar EJ, Ranson JHC, Naidich DP, et al (1985) Acute pancreatitis: prognostic value of CT. Radiology 156:767–772
Balthazar EJ, Robinson DL, Megibow AJ, Ranson JH (1990) Acute pancreatitis: value of CT in establishing prognosis. Radiology 174:331–336
Balthazar EJ, Freeny PC, van Sonnenberg E (1994) Imaging and intervention in acute pancreatitis. Radiology 193:297–306
Benziane KI, Azais O, Carretier M, Vandermarcq G, Gasquet CH (1991) La tomodensitometrie dans la surveillance évolutive des pancréatites aigues. J Radiol 72:591–598
Bottani G, Lucev M, Abelli M, Martino N, Valesi MG, Di Giulio G (1990) "Staging" della pancreatite acuta: utilizzo della TC. Min Chir 45:383–386
D'Anza FM, Cecconi L, Vincenzoni M (1984) La TC nella patologia del peritoneo. Proceedings of the XXXI National Congress of SIRM, vol 3. Monduzzi, Florence, pp 109–112
D'Anza FM, Fusco A, Vincenzoni M, De Cinque M, Valentini AL, Falappa P (1982) La TC nella valutazione delle raccolte liquide intra e peripancreatiche. Impegno Ospedaliero 3:15–19
Freeny PC (1989) Classification of pancreatitis. Radiol Clin North Am 27:1–3
Friedrich JM, Leibing U, Pfeifer T, Schnarkowski P, Buchler M, Malfertheiner P, Beger HG (1994) Zur Früherkennung infizierter Flüssigkeitsansammlungen bei akuter Pankreatitis in der Computer Tomographie. Fortschr Rontgenstr 161:208–213
Heikent JP, Balfe DM, Picus D, Scahrp DW (1984) Radical pancreatectomy. Postoperative evaluation by CT. Radiology 153:211–215
Hill MC, Barking J, Isikoff MB, Silverstein W, Kalser M (1982) Acute pancreatitis: clinical vs CT findings. AJR Am J Roentgenol 139:263–269
Hill MC, Birns MT, Fiedman AC, et al (1987) Pancreatitis. In: Friedman AC (ed) Radiology of the liver, biliary tract, pancreas and spleen. Williams & Wilkins, Baltimore
Jeffrey RB, Federle MP, Laing FC (1983) Computed tomography of mesenteric involvement in fulminant pancreatitis. Radiology 147:185–188
Jeffrey RB Jr, Laing FC, Wing VW (1986) Extrapancreatic spread of acute pancreatitis: new observations with realtime US. Radiology 159:707–711
Meyers MA, Evans JA (1973) Effects of pancreatitis on the small bowl and colon: spread along mesenteric planes. AJR Am J Roentgenol 119:151–165
Procacci C, Graziani R, Bicego E, Mainardi P, Guarise A, Valdom S, Squaranti R (1996) Pancreas. In: Pozzi-Mucelli R (ed) Trattato italiano di tomografia computerizzata. Gnocchi, Naples, pp 980–989
Raptopoulos V, Kleinman PK, Marks S, Snyder M, Silverman

PM (1986) Renal fascial pathway: posterior extension of pancreatic effusions within the anterior pararenal space. Radiology 158:367–374

Rotondo A, Smaltino F (1993) La TC nelle urgenze del pancreas operato. In: Romagnoli R, Del Vecchio E (eds) Diagnostica per immagini nelle "urgenze". Idelson, Naples

Siegelman SS, Copeland BE, Saba GP, Cameron JL, Sanders RC, Zerhouni EA (1980) CT of fluid collections associated with pancreatitis. AJR Am J Roentgenol 134:1121–1132

Simonetti G, Squillaci E, Maspes F, Giuntoli P, Giuliani S, Ronconi R (1993) TC e diagnostica per immagini nell'urgenza non traumatica dell'addome. Le pancreatiti acute. In: Romagnoli R, Del Vecchio E (eds) Diagnosi per immagini nelle "urgenze"". Idelson, Naples

Typhus

Ascenti G, Blandino A, Luciani A, Pandolfo I (1992) Peritonite tifoide focale: studio radiologico e tomodensitometrico. It Curr Radiol 11:121–123

7 Chronic Inflammatory Diseases

CONTENTS

7.1 Crohn's Disease

Granulomatous ileocolitis, or Crohn's disease, is a chronic inflammatory intestinal disease with predominant involvement of the distal small bowel and the cecum-ascending colon; the etiology of the disease is unknown, even though various pathogenetic factors: infective, immunological, genetic, vascular, dietetic, psychological, and environmental, have been hypothesized.

The clinical signs that lead to requests for instrumental examinations are: diarrhea, abdominal pain and the presence of blood in the feces; these signs vary in different subjects in intensity, duration, recovery, and relapse. Abdominal pain is usually located in the lower quadrants of the abdomen; when it is on the right side it often simulates appendicitis, whereas on the left it can resemble the pain of irritable colon syndrome, diverticulitis or ulcerative colitis. However, most symptoms reflect complications, such as abscesses or fistulae, rather than the disease itself.

The abnormalities produced by the disease consist in edema, mural fat infiltration of the intestinal wall, hyperplasia of the lymphatic follicles and development of aphthoid ulcers (1–2 mm deep), which may penetrate the swollen mucosa and join together underneath, forming long intramural longitudinal fistulae running parallel to the visceral lumen.

After a phase of mucosal hyperplasia, after recovery from the pathologic process the wall becomes thin again, and not uncommonly atrophic mucosa, fibrosis of the submucosal and muscular layers, and tubular narrowing of the lumen may be left.

Often the disease involves the mesentery and the mesocolon, producing lesions ranging from simple perivisceral fibrofatty proliferative hyperplasia, to edema, congestion and development of phlegmons, abscesses or fistulae. Internal fistulae originating from the intestinal wall may be stopped by peritoneal, fascial and muscular barriers or penetrate the bladder or vagina. External fistulae communicate with the skin surface of the anterior abdominal wall or the perineum.

The radiologic evaluation of Crohn's disease relies on examination of the small bowel after peroral barium or barium enema, air contrast barium enema or colonoscopy. CT is needed to evaluate the extraparietal extensions.

The CT findings in Crohn's disease reflect the mural intestinal and perivisceral anomalies:

a) Intestinal mural changes (Figs. 7.1–7.5, 7.7). The active phase of the disease is characterized by a homogeneously enhancing wall thickened to between 3 and 10 mm, with an irregular internal profile and lumen narrowing caused by the edematous swollen mucosa and submucosa, mural fat infiltration and aphthoid ulcers Fig. 7.6). The ileal thickening is uniform and affects the entire circumference, whereas in the cecum it is asymmetrical and involves mainly the median wall. A double halo or "target" pattern of mural alternating high- and low-density rings or a "double track" in the i.v. contrast enhancement CT may appear; this is due to a submucosal or subserosal confluence of the ulcers, edema or fat (Figs. 7.1 –7.4).

b) Perivisceral changes:

Widening and increased attenuation of perivisceral and mesenteric fat, with dislocation and separation of the ileal loops, owing to the fibrofatty proliferation, edema and hypervascularity (Figs. 7.1–7.4).

Linear or tortuous stranding owing to vascular dilatation or fibrous tissue in the subperitoneal fat (Fig. 7.5).

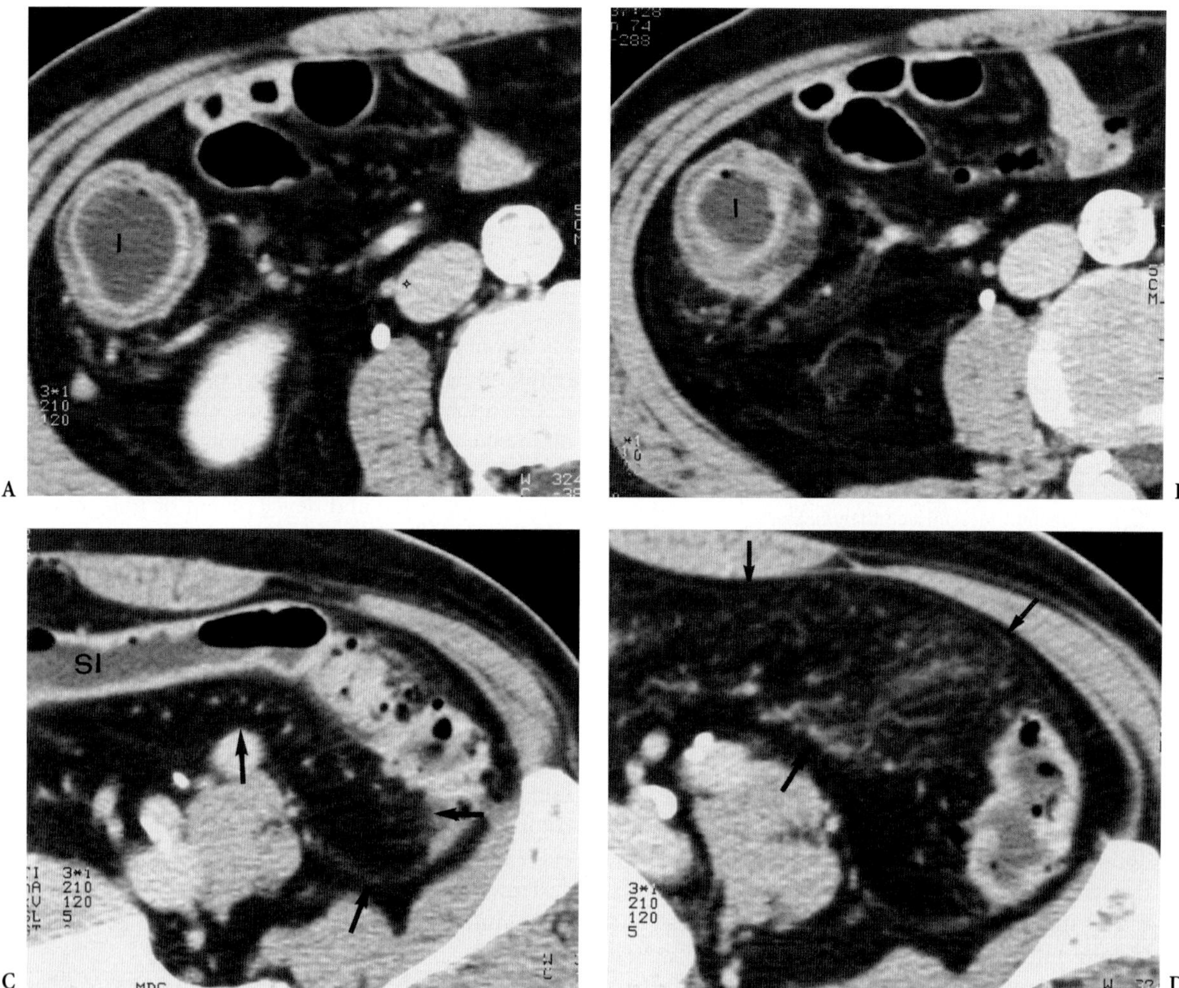

Fig. 7.1A–D. Crohn's ileocolitis. **A, B** Thickening, enhancing ileal wall with double halo or "target sign"(*I*) typical of the active phase of the disease. The low-attenuation ring corresponds to the confluence of the deep ulcers between mucosa and submucosa. Hyperplasia of the mesenteric adipose tissue around the affected loop. **C, D** Thickening and enhancing of the sigmoidal wall (*SI*).Widening and blurring of the sigmoid mesocolon (*arrows*), fat hyperplasia and edema. Perisigmoidal linear stranding owing to vascular dilatation. Thickening of the limiting peritoneum

Thickening of the peritoneum and the lateroconal and anterior renal fasciae owing to edema or fibrosis (Figs. 7.2–7.4).

Mesenteric and retroperitoneal inflammatory or reactive adenopathy, usually 3–8 mm of the shorter axis diameter (Figs. 7.3, 7.5, 7.7), particularly in the ileocolic lymph nodes filtering the lymph flowing out of the cecum and the distal ileal loop.

Phlegmons appearing as soft-tissue enhancing masses with poorly defined limits, and surrounded by hazing fat, adjacent to the intestinal wall or forming a single structure with it.

Abscesses (Figs. 7.5, 7.7) are round or oval water-density or air-fluid collections each limited by a more or less thick and uniform capsule and increasing in density after contrast medium injection.

Fistulae (Figs. 7.4, 7.8) are linear or tortuous tracts extending from the bowel wall to the urinary bladder, vagina, adjacent bowel loops or the cutaneous surface. The fistulous pathway and extent may be better demonstrated after oral administration of a water-soluble contrast medium.

CT may also show associated diseases, such as gallbladder and liver anomalies (Gore et al. 1996).

CT has an important role in both medical and surgical management of the disease, showing up unsuspected abnormalities by identifying and local-

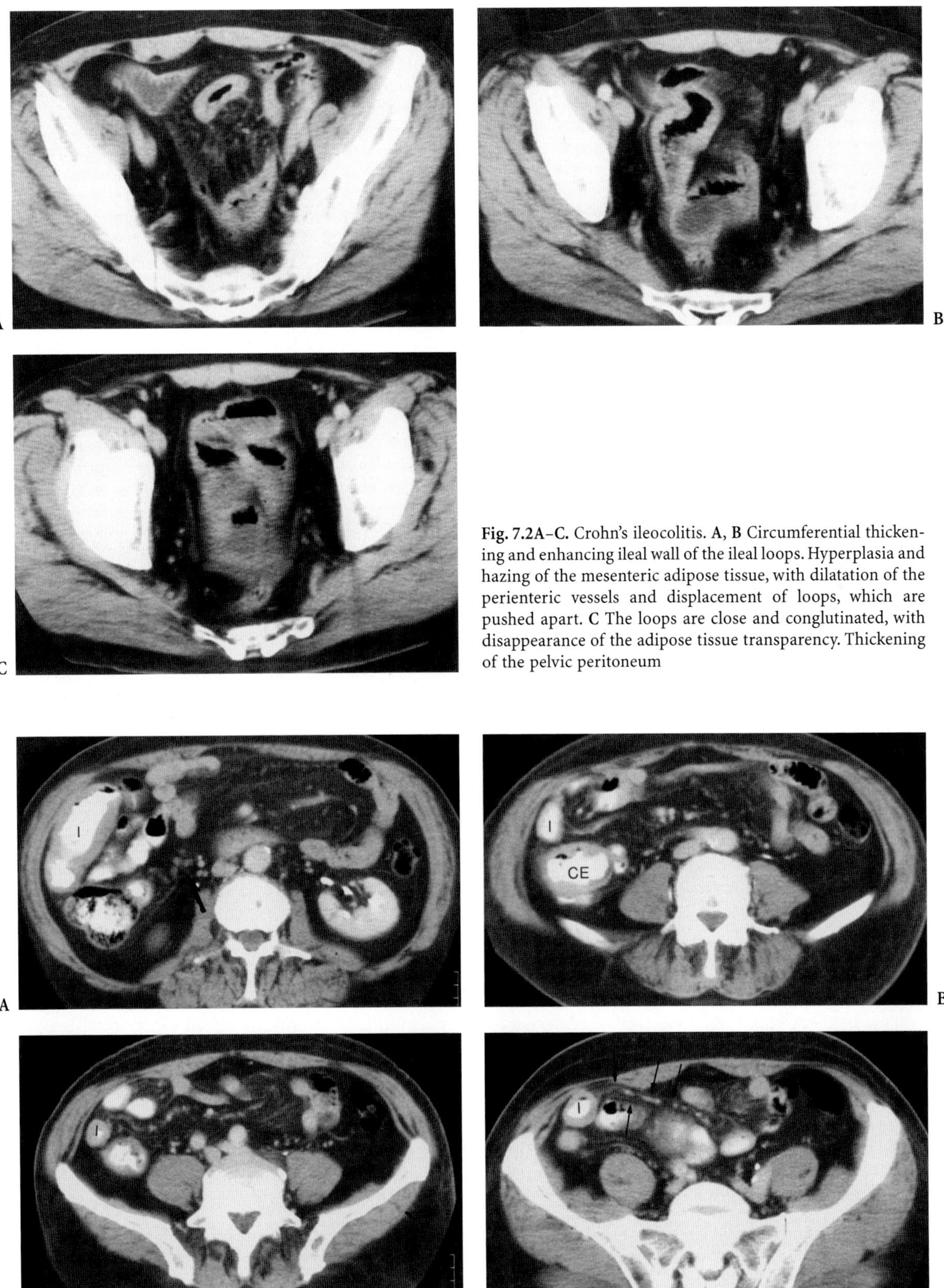

Fig. 7.2A–C. Crohn's ileocolitis. **A, B** Circumferential thickening and enhancing ileal wall of the ileal loops. Hyperplasia and hazing of the mesenteric adipose tissue, with dilatation of the perienteric vessels and displacement of loops, which are pushed apart. **C** The loops are close and conglutinated, with disappearance of the adipose tissue transparency. Thickening of the pelvic peritoneum

Fig. 7.3A–D. Crohn's ileocolitis. Mesenteric edema and fibrosis. **A** Slightly enlarged ileocolic lymph nodes (*thick arrow*). The walls of the ileal and cecal loops show circumferential thickening, contrast enhancing density and irregular internal profile owing to the presence of ulcers in the edematous mucosa. Hyperplastic and shaded edematous fat around the affected loops. **B** The last loop (*I*) enters the cecum from outside and below (**C, D**). **D** "Double track" pattern owing to thickening of mesenteric peritoneum at the sides of the twisted and sinuous vessels (*thin arrows*)

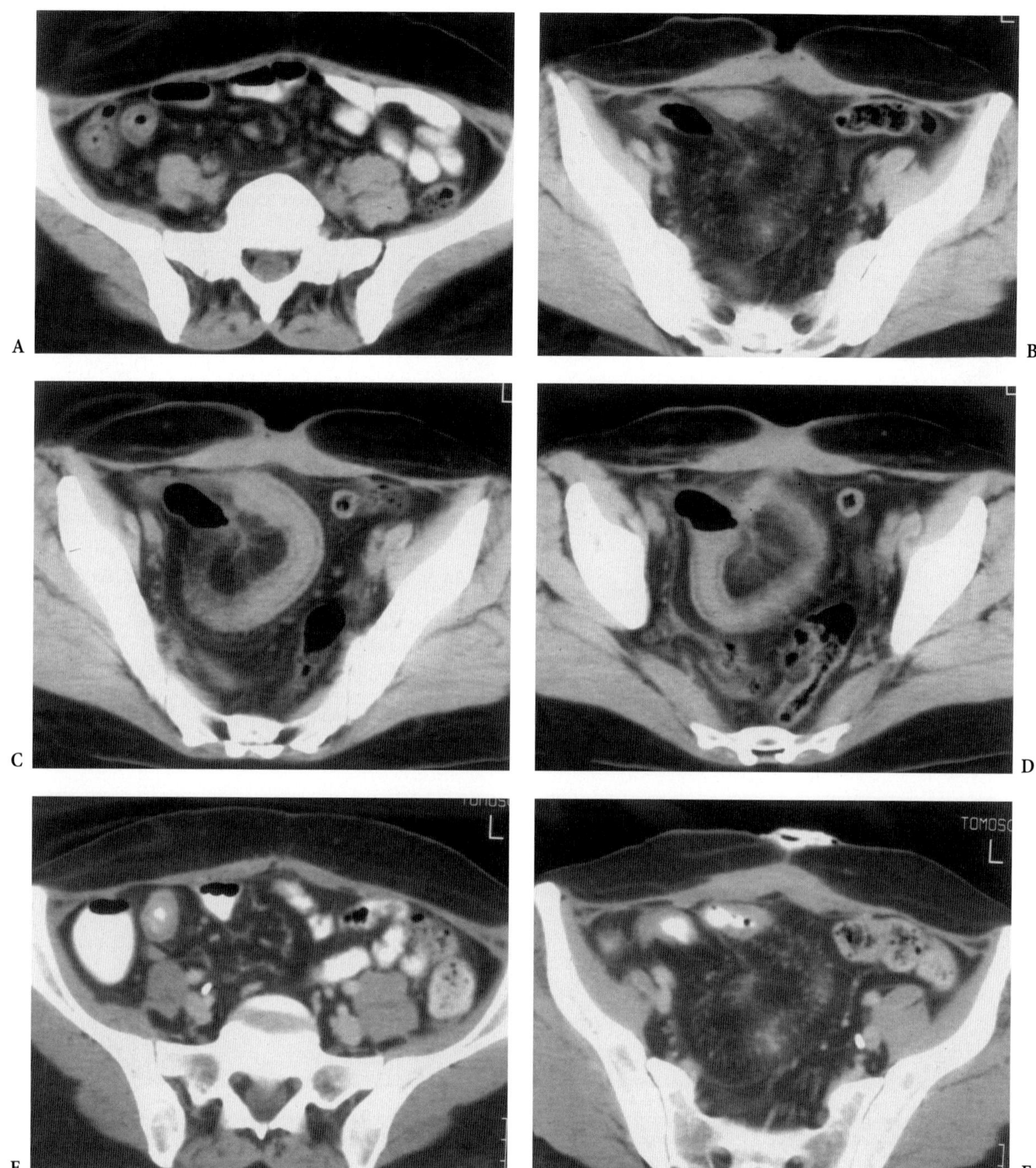

Fig. 7.4A–J. Crohn's ileocolitis. Uniform thickening and contrast enhancing of a long tract of the ileal wall, with a double halo caused by submucous fistulae. The mesenteric adipose tissue is enlarged and pushes the loops away from each other (**B**, **F–H**). Enterocutaneous fistula: the contrast medium coming out of an ileal loop indicates the fistulous tract (**I**, **J** *arrow*). Peritoneal involvement: thickening of the mesenteric peritoneum and fluid collection in the pouch of Douglas (**J** *thin arrow*)

Fig. 7.5A–D. Crohn's ileocolitis. Small abscess; mesenteric and peritoneal fibrosis. Thickening and contrast enhancing of the wall of the last ileal loop and cecum. The surrounding fat is enlarged and hazing and is crossed by vascular and fibrous strandings extending to the peritoneum and to the lateroconal and anterior renal fasciae that are thickened and retracted (**B**). Behind the last ileal loop, a dense nodule with a central area of low attenuation (typical of an abscess) (*arrow*) is visible (**B**, **C**). Slightly enlarged ileocolic lymph nodes (**A**, *thin arrows*). The fibrosis involves the right ureter, without narrowing it, and the anterior renal fascia

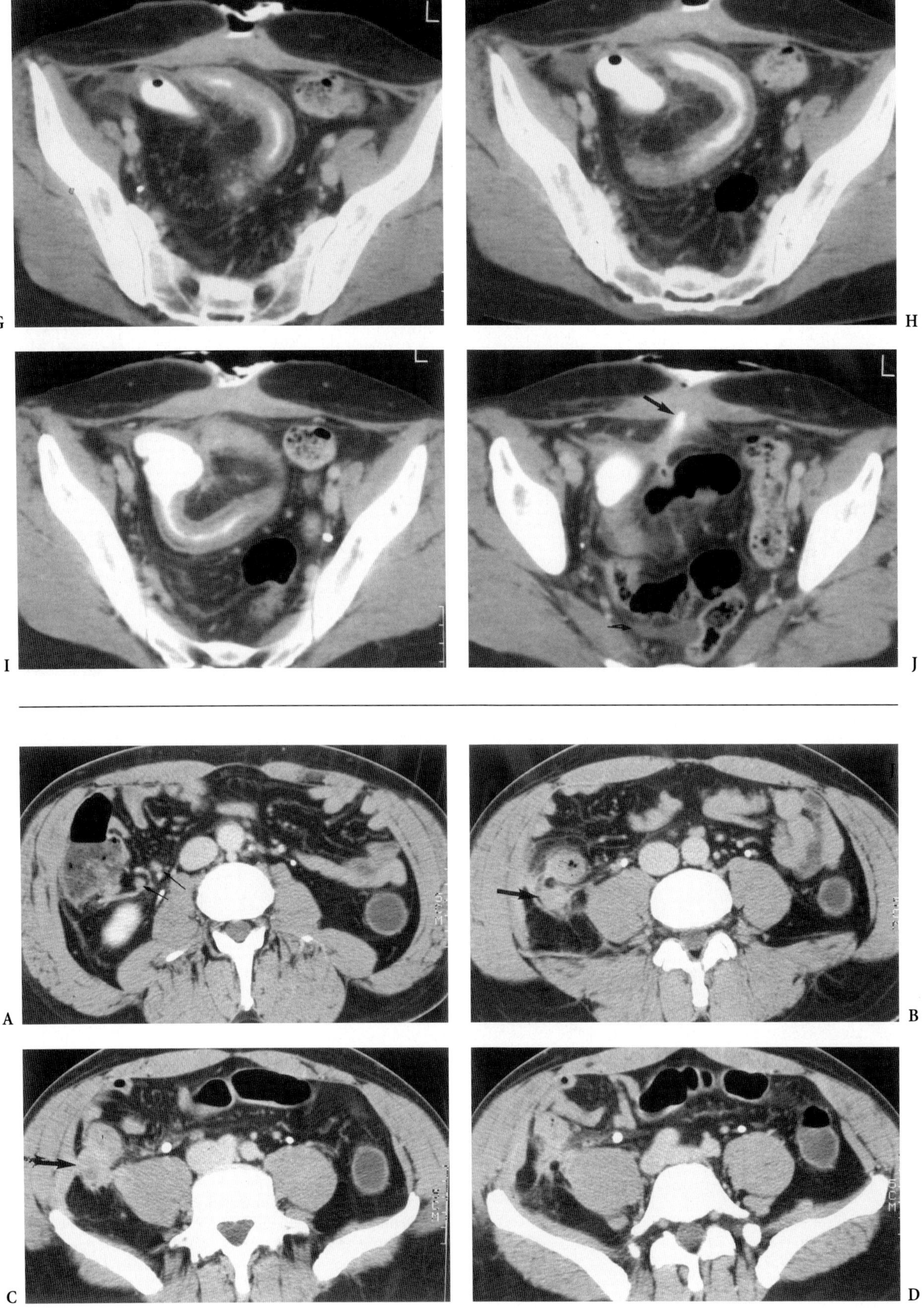

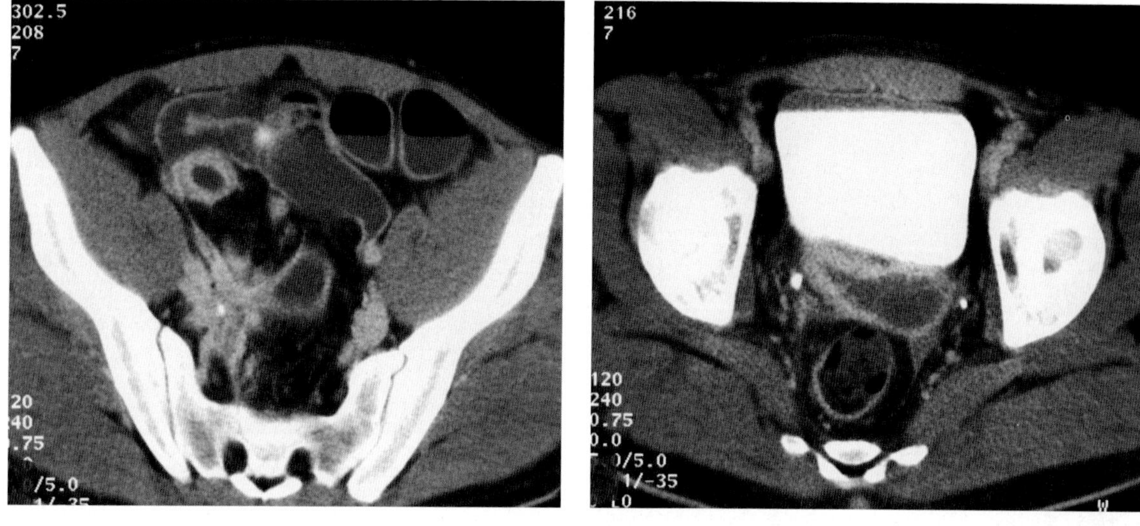

Fig. 7.6A, B. Crohn's ileocolitis. Thickening and enhancing wall of the last ileal loops. Fibrous thickening of the adjacent fat to the point where it involves the retroperitoneum, narrowing, without obstructing, the right ureter (**A**). There is a small amount of fluid in the pelvic space

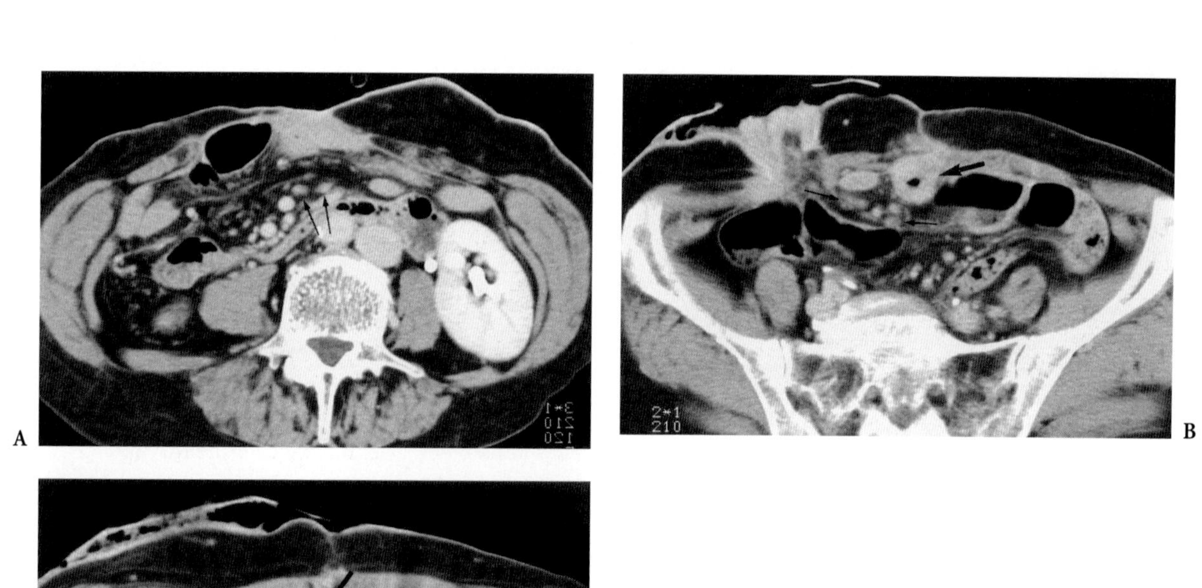

Fig. 7.7A–C. Crohn's ileocolitis. Recurrent disease in a patient who has had a total colectomy with cutaneous right ileostomy. Thickening and contrast enhancement of an ileal loop because of a relapse (**B, C** *thick arrow*). Shading of the mesentery around the loop because of an inflammatory infiltration. Enlargement of the superior mesenteric lymph nodes (**A, B** *thin arrows*)

A
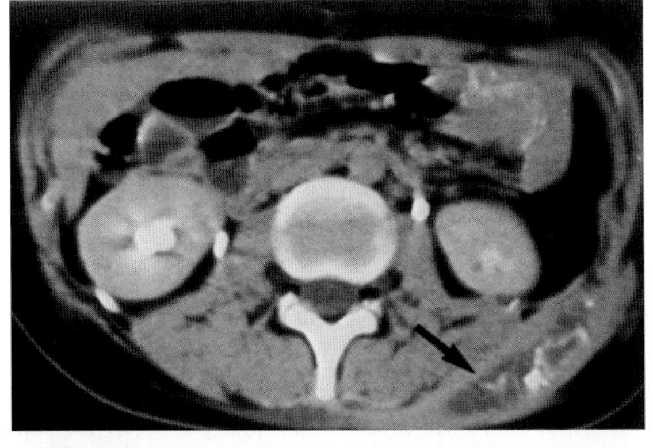

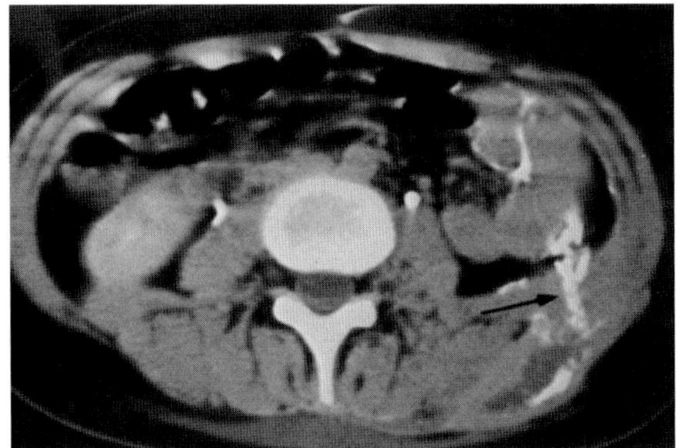
B

C
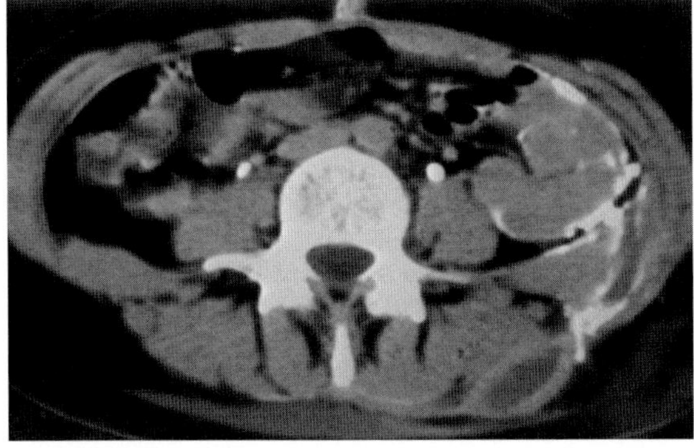

Fig. 7.8A–C. Crohn's ileocolitis. Enterocutaneous fistula in a patient who underwent total colectomy. The opaque contrast medium coming out of the intestine spreads between the peritoneum and the walls of the ileal loops; thereafter, it moves backward and outward through a linear fistulous tract (**B** *thin arrow*), after constituting a wide cavity in the superficial planes of the muscular wall (**A, B** *thick arrow*)

izing the sites of phlegmons, abscesses, intestinal obstructions, and the pathways and extent of fistulae.

CT is also useful for guiding percutaneous aspiration or drainage of abscesses, which may obviate the need for surgery (Wills 1997).

7.2 Tuberculosis

In spite of widespread screening, the availability of effective antituberculous therapy, and the disappearance of the bovine infection, in recent years a renewed rise in the incidence of tuberculosis attributable to *Mycobacterium tuberculosis* and *Mycobacterium avium intracellulare* has been observed, not only in the thoracic region, where the disease is primarily and most frequently located, but also in the abdominal region. This phenomenon is probably related to increasing risk factors, such as acquired immune deficiency syndrome (AIDS), corticosteroid or immunosuppressive therapies, alcoholism, intravenous drug abuse, associated with diabetes mellitus, cancer, to the emergence of drug resistant mycobacteria, and to the direct transmission from infected travelers or immigrants (Hulnick et al. 1985).

The diagnosis of abdominal tuberculosis is often delayed because its clinical presentation is variable and nonspecific, including fever, abdominal distension, obscure abdominal pain, nausea, vomiting, weight loss, diarrhea, and night sweats, with clinical tests often inconclusive or misleading.

The peritoneal, mesenteric and lymph node abnormalities may result from spread of a pleuropulmonary infection through transdiaphragmatic lymphatic connections between pleura and peritoneum and abdominal lymph nodes, from hematic miliary peritoneal seeding, or from lymphatic diffusion of gastroenteric or tubal infections.

Abdominal tuberculosis includes adenopathies, exudative peritonitis and omental involvement.

Lymphadenitis is the most common manifestation of abdominal tuberculosis, with a striking tendency for mesenteric and peripancreatic lymph nodes to be involved (Hulnick et al. 1985). In the center of the lymph nodes the infection develops in the form of granuloma of the epithelioid and Langhans giant cells, followed by caseous necrosis and a peripheral inflammatory reaction rich in vessels. Caseous lymph nodes may adhere to each other in clusters or melt into a conglomerate mass. A fistulous tract in the subperitoneal space may be due to the rupture of these caseous tuberculous lesions.

Healing follows the generation of fibrous sclerosis or calcareous precipitation leading to cicatrization or organization. An analogous evolution is found in the nodules of the internal surface of the peritoneum or in the omentum.

On CT performed during the granulomatous stage of the inflammation, before caseification, the lymph nodes are enlarged, homogeneous and contrast enhancing (Fig. 7.11). After caseous necrosis the enlarged lymph nodes show a low-density center and a peripheral rim enhancing with contrast; typically, caseous lymph nodes join together in clusters or conglomerate with a multiloculate mass appearance (Figs 7.9, 7.10). Healing fibrosclerotic lymph nodes are enlarged, deformed, and very dense, but not contrast enhancing. It is not uncommon for them to be calcified (Fig. 7.11–7.15).

Tuberculous peritonitis is due to the insemination of the internal surface of the peritoneum by granulomatous nodules with a plastic reaction and hypersecretion of serum rich in proteins and blood cells. On CT, it is characterized by free or loculated ascites, thickened and enhanced peritoneum and/or mesentery with dense nodularity on the internal surface. Ascitic fluid may be near water density in the early exudative stage of the immune response (Hulnick et al. 1985) or high density (20–50 HU) when it contains blood cells and elevated proteins (Dahlene et al. 1984; Epstein and Mann 1982; Hulnick et al. 1985).

Omental tuberculosis. In the omentum the tuberculosis may involve lymph nodes or the omental soft tissue. On CT the lymph node involvement appears as round nodules or masses, which are homogeneous and enhancing or of low attenuation with peripheral enhancing rim, or, when healing, calcified (Fig. 7.15). In the area of inflammation in the omen-

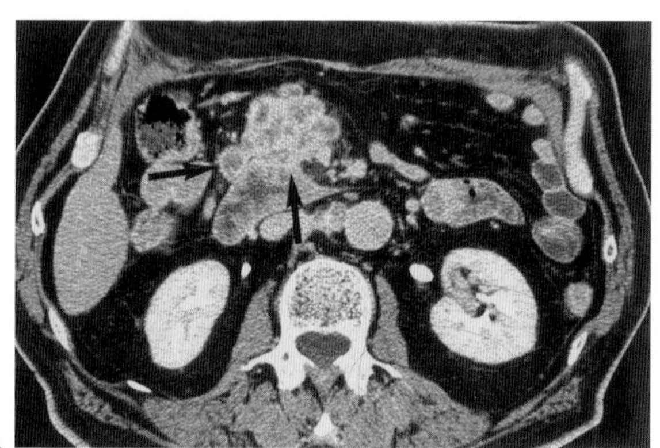
A

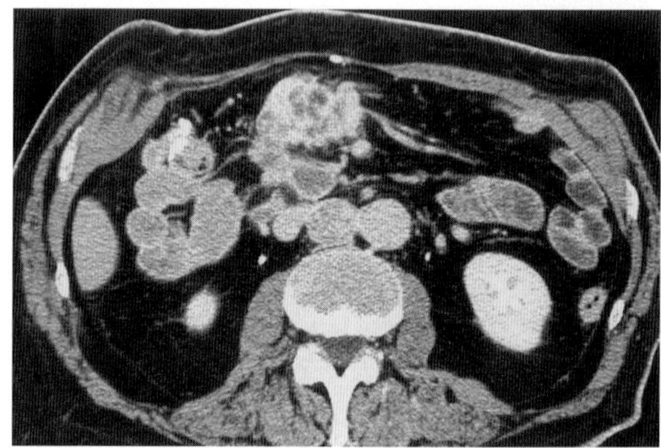
B

Fig. 7.9A, B. Caseous tuberculous adenitis. Cluster of enlarged, low-attenuating mesenteric lymph nodes with enhancing wall

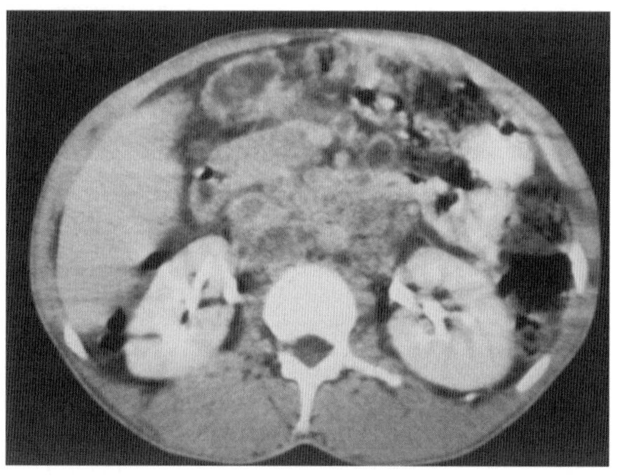
A

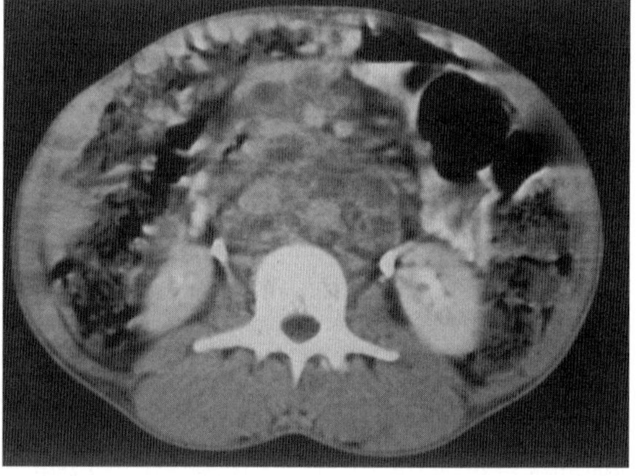
B

Fig. 7.10A, B. Tuberculous adenitis in an AIDS patient. Multiloculated low-density mesenteric and retroperitoneal mass caused by caseous lymph node conglomerate

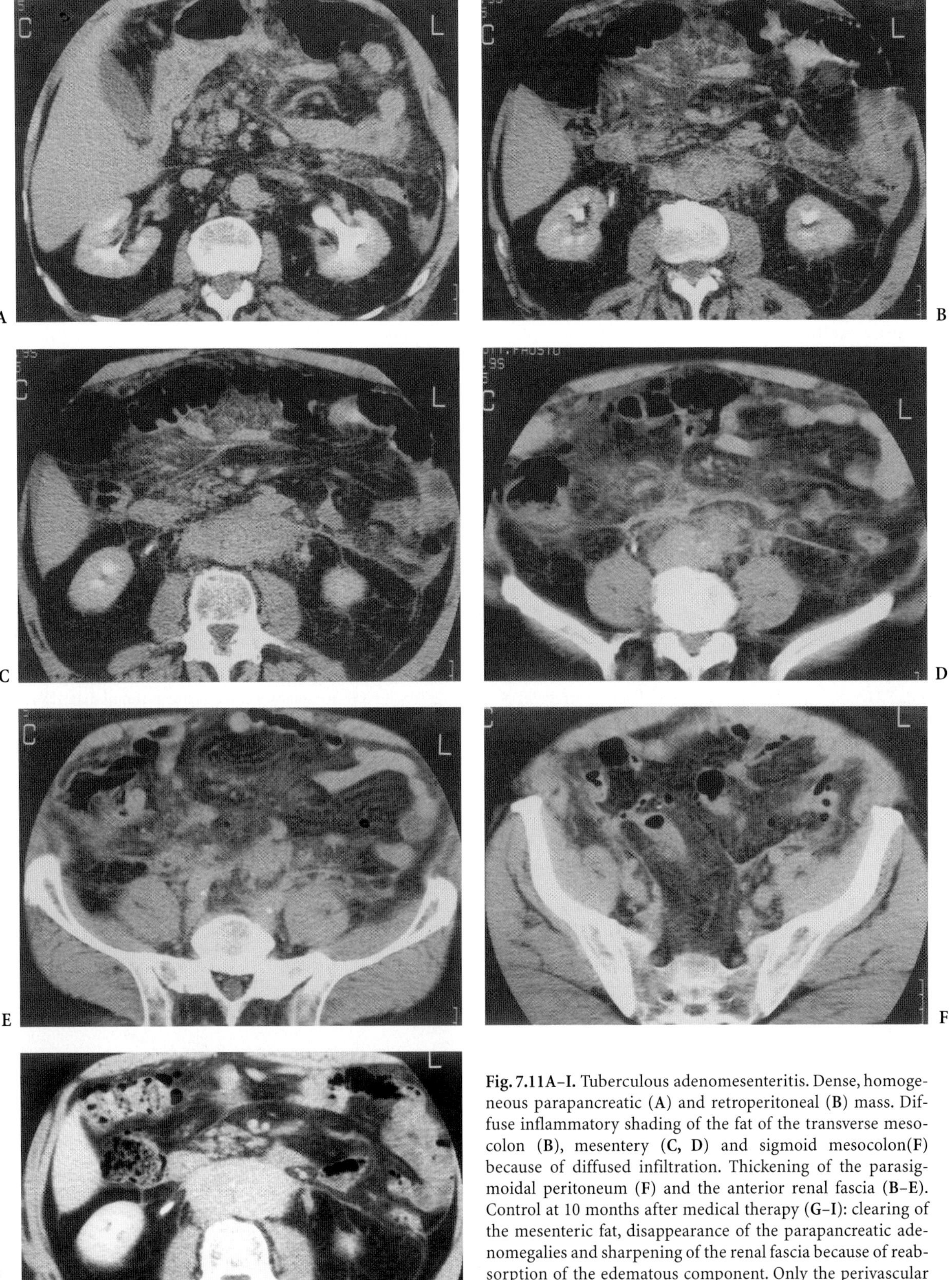

Fig. 7.11A–I. Tuberculous adenomesenteritis. Dense, homogeneous parapancreatic (**A**) and retroperitoneal (**B**) mass. Diffuse inflammatory shading of the fat of the transverse mesocolon (**B**), mesentery (**C, D**) and sigmoid mesocolon(**F**) because of diffused infiltration. Thickening of the parasigmoidal peritoneum (**F**) and the anterior renal fascia (**B–E**). Control at 10 months after medical therapy (**G–I**): clearing of the mesenteric fat, disappearance of the parapancreatic adenomegalies and sharpening of the renal fascia because of reabsorption of the edematous component. Only the perivascular lymph nodal mass is still visible, but it is less dense and its profile is sharper

(**7.11H,I.** see next page)

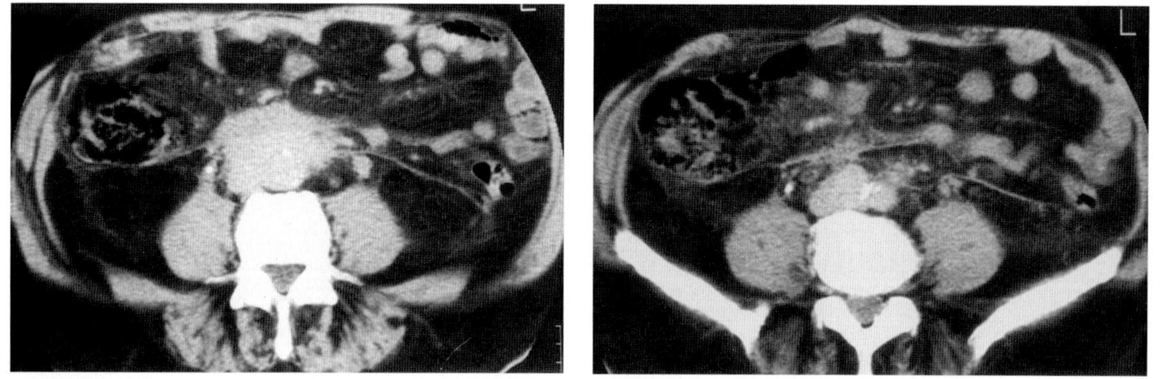

Fig. 7.11A–I. Continued
Clearing of the mesenteric fat, disappearance of the parapancreatic adenomegalies and sharpening of the renal fascia because of reabsorption of the edematous component. Only the perivascular lymph nodal mass is still visible, but it is less dense and its profile is sharper

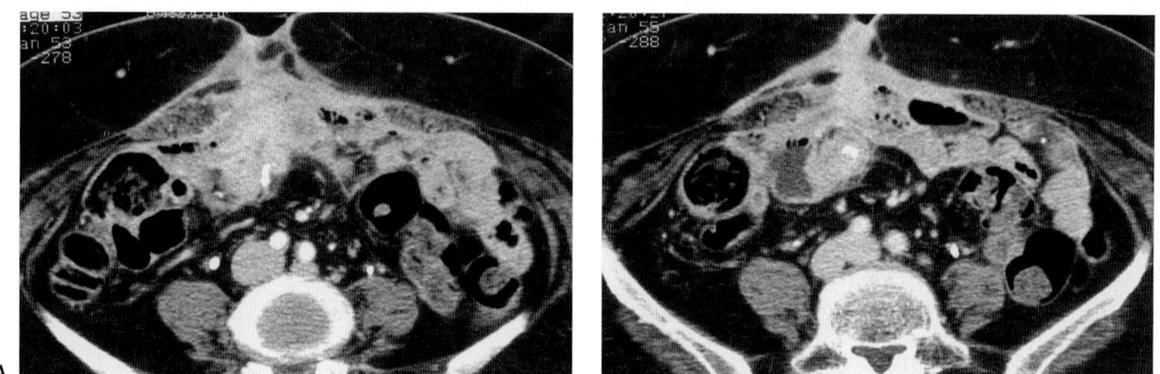

Fig. 7.12A, B. Omental tuberculosis. Enhancing irregular omental mass with low-attenuation caseous areas and nodular calcifications inside spreading backward in the mesentery

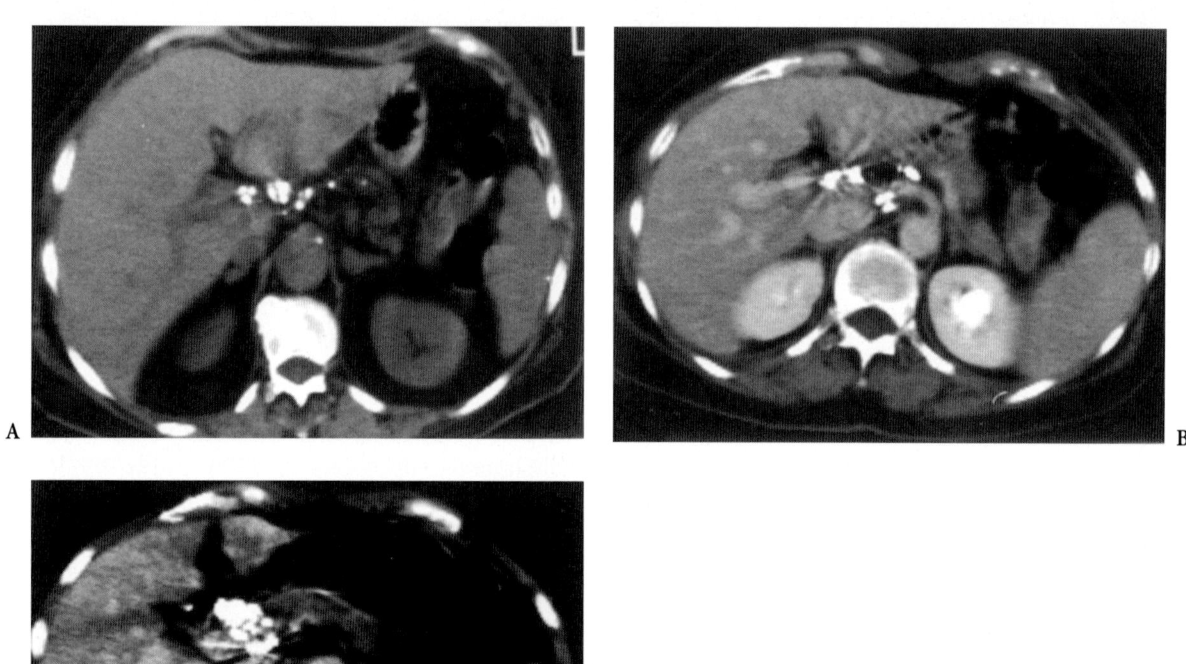

Fig. 7.13A–C. Outcome of tuberculous lymphoadenitis. Deep and superficial hepatic (**A**, **B**) and pancreatoduodenal (**C**) lymph nodes, enlarged and calcified

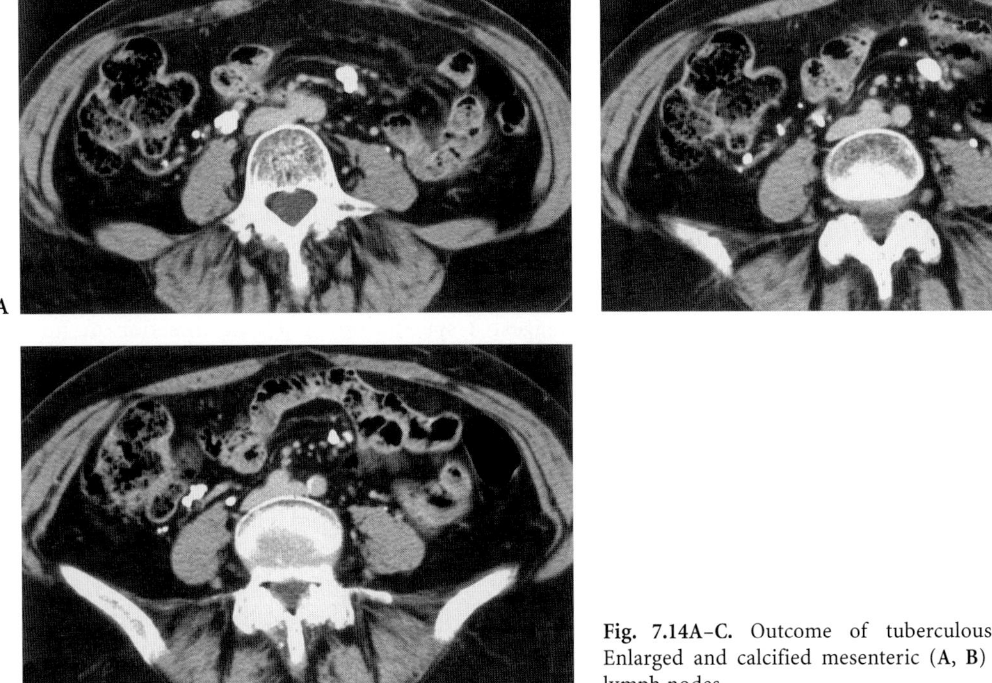

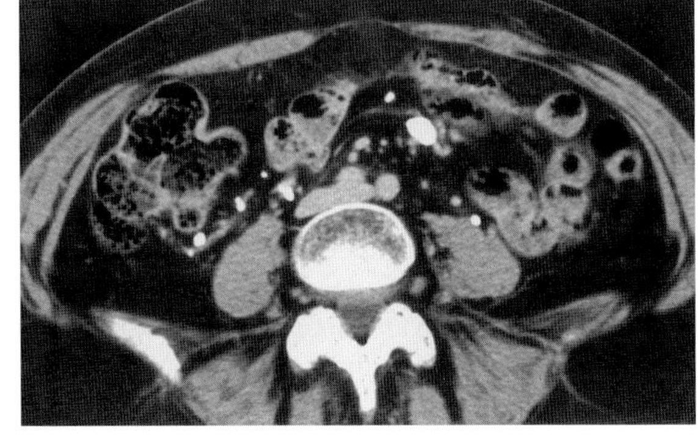

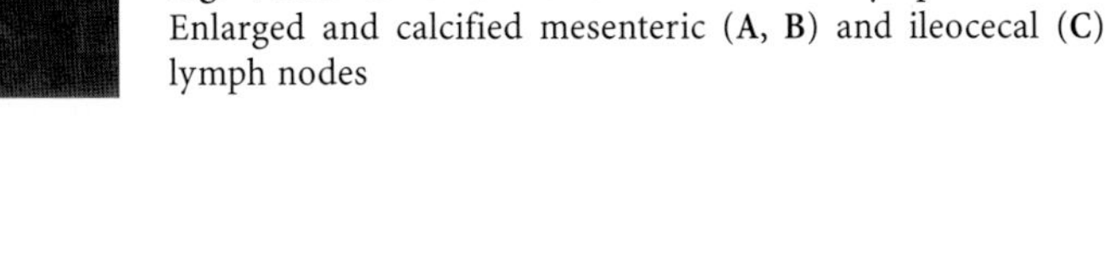

Fig. 7.14A–C. Outcome of tuberculous lymphoadenitis. Enlarged and calcified mesenteric (**A**, **B**) and ileocecal (**C**) lymph nodes

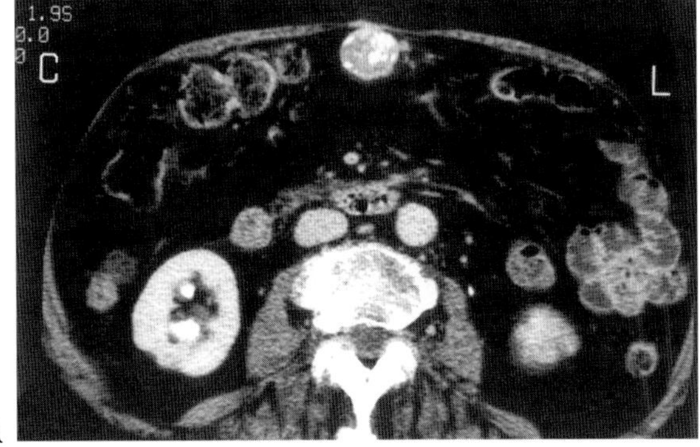

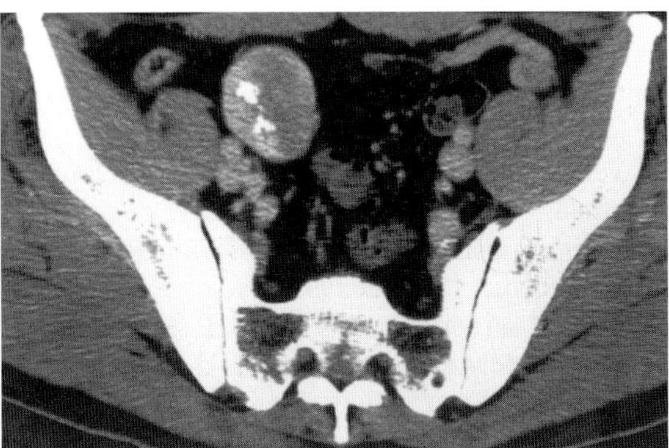

Fig. 7.15A, B. Tuberculous granulomata. Thick, dense, sharply walled ovoid masses with low-density caseous areas and nodular calcifications inside **A** in the omentum and **B** in the right iliac fossa

tum density becomes increasingly higher and non-homogeneous, and strands and thickening appear, making up a transverse omental "cake" (Fig. 7.12).

Granulomatous lesion (tuberculomas) in ligaments, mesenteries or omentum may also leave residual ovoid masses with a well-defined profile and heterogeneous structure made up of low-density areas and amorphous calcifications (Fig. 7.15).

None of the CT findings taken singly is diagnostic of the disease. However, taken together, enlarged lymph nodes with low-density centers and enhancing rims, sited predominantly in the mesenteric or peripancreatic areas, high-density loculated ascites with thin septation, and peritoneal, mesenteric and omental thickening are suggestive of tuberculous disease (Hulnick 1985); however, histological or cytological tests and positive cultures are needed for a conclusive diagnosis (Demirkazik et al. 1996).

7.3 Acquired Immunodeficiency Syndrome and Related Opportunistic Pathologies

The immunodepressive status induced by human immune deficiency virus (HIV) infection favors the development of either infective or tumoral opportunistic pathologies. Usually, it occurs 10 years after the HIV reconversion and before clinical signs of the acquired Immune deficiency syndrome (AIDS) become manifest.

Table 7.1. Pathogenic organisms in AIDS-related infections

Mycobacterium tuberculosis (MTB)
Mycobacterium avium intracellulare (MAI)
Histoplasma capsulatum
Pneumocystis carinii (PC)
Coccidioides immitis
Cryptosporidium
Candida albicans
Cytomegalovirus (CMV)

In the abdomen the opportunistic infective processes are mainly (80%) supported by *Mycobacterium tuberculosis* (MTB) and *Mycobacterium avium* (MBA), and less frequently by *Histoplasma* and *Pneumocystis carinii*; occasionally, infections may be caused by other infective agents (Table 7.1).

Tumors – non-Hodgkin lymphomas and Kaposi's sarcomas – account for approximately one-third of the opportunistic abdominal pathology, with a 3-to-1 ratio (RADIN 1991a, b, 1995).

In HIV seropositive patients CT shows hepatomegaly, slightly enlarged lymph nodes (shorter axis diameter <0.5 cm) and, in homosexuals, rectal wall thickening with perirectal hazing (WALL et al. 1994).

In HIV patients whose disease has progressed to clinical AIDS, CT findings may show abdominal opportunistic pathology, including adenopathy, gastroenteric, hepatic and splenic abnormalities, ascites, and omental and peritoneal involvement.

Adenopathy takes the form of a large lymph node with the diameter of the minor axis >1.5 cm; it may have a homogeneous attenuation as high as or higher than that of the iliopsoas muscle with central or diffuse low attenuation on contrast enhanced CT scans (Fig. 7.10).

None of these CT findings can be correlated with a specific pathology. However, some patterns may suggest a specific opportunistic infection or neoplasm: CT findings suggesting various opportunistic pathologies are schematized in Table 7.2.

Lymph nodes with short axis diameter greater than 30 mm are associated with NH lymphoma in 90% of cases (RADIN 1991a, b, 1995). The high attenuation of slightly enlarged lymph nodes on dynamic sequential boluses is associated with disseminated Kaposi's sarcoma in nearly 80% of cases (HERTS et al. 1992). Lymph nodes isolated or grouped in clusters with central or diffuse low attenuation on contrast-enhanced CT appear in disseminated MTB infection (RADIN 1991a, 1995). Clusters of enlarged lymph nodes may be due to MTB infection or to NH lymphoma.

A conclusive diagnosis of specific infections or neoplasms is needed to decide on an appropriate therapy; however, a percutaneous fine-needle lymph node biopsy or an aspiration under CT guidance followed by histological examination and/or mycobacterium, fungal and viral organism cultures must be performed (WALL et al. 1994; RADIN 1991a, 1995).

Gastrointestinal abnormalities. Focal or diffuse circumferential wall thickening or a mass affects the stomach, small bowel, proximal colon and rectum in infective or tumoral opportunistic diseases (RADIN 1995). Perirectal thickening and/or increased attenuation, often associated with isolate or multiple mural nodules, are present in Kaposi's sarcoma.

Table 7.2. CT findings in lymph nodes in AIDS-related syndromes

Pathology	Solid	Central or diffuse low density	Contrast enhanced	Confluence	Diameter
Tuberculosis	+	+	+	+	
Other opportunistic infections	+				
Non-Hodgkin's lymphoma	+	+[a]		+	>3 cm
Kaposi's sarcoma	+		+++		<1 cm

[a] Only after treatment

Hepatic and splenic abnormalities. These consist of moderate or marked hepatomegaly and splenomegaly, with or without focal low attenuation, almost always small multiple lesions that are due to opportunistic infective abscesses or tumors (lymphomas or Kaposi's sarcoma).

Ascites. Small, moderate or large amounts of fluid may be present in 30% of AIDS-related infections or tumors, particularly in the case of MTB infection (RADIN 1995).

Omental involvement. Thickening, linear stranding, omental cake or masses are the common abnormalities revealed by CT and due to lymphomatous infiltration.

7.4 Mesenteric Panniculitis

Panniculitis (otherwise known as mesenteric lipodystrophy, retractile or sclerosing mesenteritis) is an unusual chronic inflammatory process of the mesenteric adipose tissue, whose etiology is unknown. It has been considered as an idiopathic form or a manifestation of an isolated or systemic disorder of the connective tissue, associated with retroperitoneal fibrosis or retractile mediastinitis, or with surgery, abdominal trauma, infection, gastroduodenal ulcer, foreign body, pancreatitis. Therefore, it can be hypothesized that the disease is not caused by a single factor. An autoimmune response with ischemia has also been hypothesized.

The lesion consists in fatty infiltration, chronic lymphoreticular inflammation and fibrosis of the small bowel mesentery, especially at the root, which may also involve the vasculo-nervous fascia, the sigmoid mesocolon and the intestinal wall.

According to the predominant pathologic process, the disease is called lipodystrophy when the major feature is the fatty infiltration, panniculitis when chronic inflammation is the dominant component, and retractile mesenteritis when fibrosis is the main histological finding. The three different pathologic features seem more likely to be successive stages of the same inflammatory process (MATA 1987).

Abdominal pain, anorexia, nausea, vomiting, fever, weight loss and constipation are the most frequent manifestations, which usually go on for a long time before the diagnosis is made. Macroscopically the mesenteric panniculitis appears as an infiltrating or pseudotumoral mass for which there are two different corresponding CT findings.

In the infiltrating pattern, lipodystrophy and liponecrosis are predominant; a slight increase in the density of the adipose tissue of the mesenteric root may be observed around the vasculo-nervous bundle, which is limited by a thin ring (fat ring sign) constituted by the thickening of the mesenteric perivascular fascia (MINDELZUN et al. 1996; SABATÈ et al. 1999) (Fig. 7.16).After liposclerotic evolution, the infiltrated area increases in density and extension and is limited by dense radiating linear strandings, probably fibrous bands that may combine to form a mass or a plaque with lumpy contours; hence, linear radial striations project forward or to the sides along the vasculo-nervous fasciae. The ileal loops are pulled backwards. This form may also extend to the retroperitoneum, incorporating ureters and great vessels, where they may simulate a retroperitoneal fibrosis, and to the omentum, forming a thick plaque (omental cake) in the anterior abdominal quadrant, which resembles those observed in carcinosis and tuberculosis (WARSHAUER et al 1997).

In pseudotumoral panniculitis CT reveals a nonhomogeneous mass containing areas of fat, water and soft density and calcification corresponding to necrotic or liquefied fat, inflammatory infiltration, hemorrhage and fibrosis. It is limited by a well-defined, thick, uniform and enhancing wall formed by the fibrous capsule (KATZ et al. 1985).

The pseudotumoral mass pushes and divides the intestinal loops without infiltrating or narrowing them, and may incorporate the mesenteric vasculo-nervous bundle without producing alterations. It is separated from the thin bundle by the perivascular fascia.

The major differential diagnoses are carcinoid, lipoma, liposarcoma and gossypiboma.

A nodular carcinoid with dense radiating linear strandings may simulate sclerosing mesenteritis, but the absence of typical clinical manifestations of carcinoid, of liver contrast enhancing metastases, of positive scintigraphy with meta-iodo-benzyl-guanidina, and normal 5-hydroxindoleacetic levels make the differential diagnosis easy.

Lipoma can be differentiated from pseudotumoral mesenteritis with predominant adipose component slightly denser than the adjacent fat because of the different relative positions of the abdominal vessels: a lipoma displaces the vessels, whereas the panniculitis incorporates them.

Myxoid liposarcoma can also mimic pseudotumoral mesenteric lipodystrophy. It is not always possible to distinguish between these two entities with certainty on CT examination. In such cases a CT-

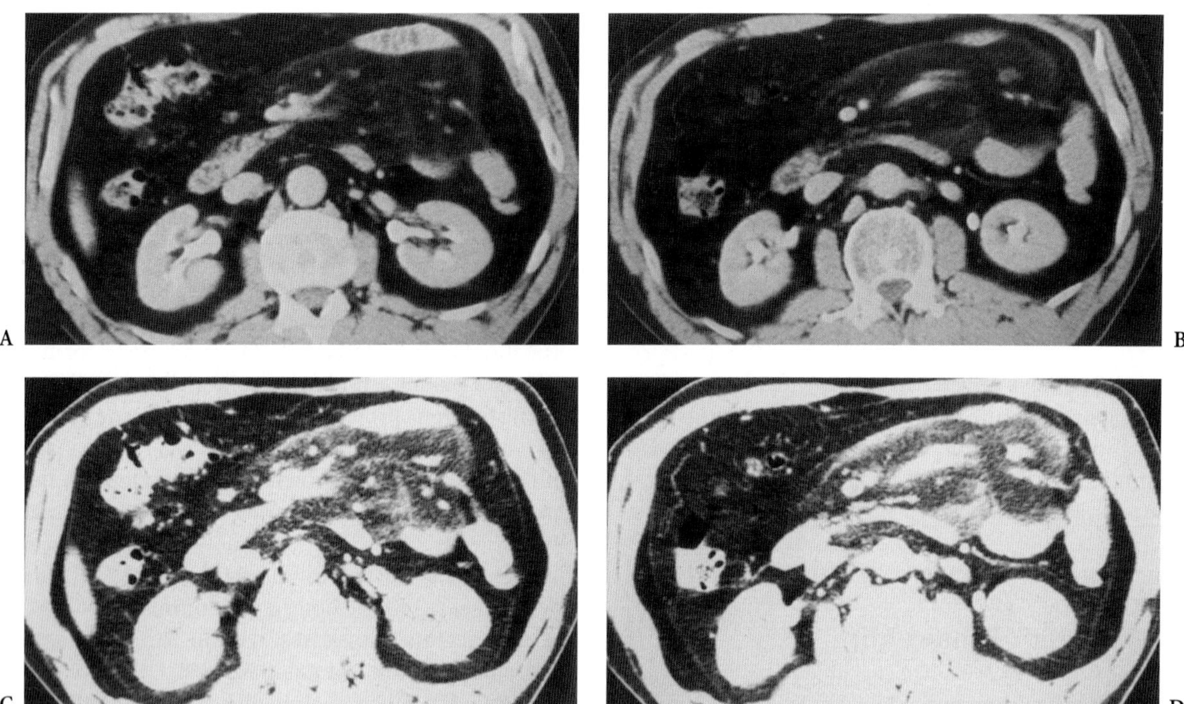

Fig. 7.16A–D. Infiltrating type of retractile mesenteritis. Slight increase in the attenuation of the mesentery surrounding the superior mesenteric vessels (**A**, **B**), more evident when a narrow window is used (**C**, **D**)

guided needle biopsy or a laparotomy is unavoidable (Katz et al. 1985).

When the gossypiboma has the appearance of a nonhomogeneous well-encapsulated mass, it is similar to a pseudotumoral form of mesenteric panniculitis, because both these forms are granulomata. An element favoring the diagnosis of gossypiboma is represented by the persistent perifocal contrast enhancement and by the absence of negative fat density inside.

7.5 Omental-Mesenteric Inflammatory Pseudotumor

The omental-mesenteric inflammatory pseudotumor is a rare benign lesion of unknown etiology and histogenesis, observed in preadolescent children. It has only recently been identified as a pathological and clinical entity, after being variously named in the past: benign myofibroblastoma, fibrous xanthoma, plasma cell granuloma, myofibrohistiocytic inflammatory proliferation, lymphoid hamartoma, myxoid hamartoma, xanthomatous pseudotumor, pseudosarcoma, inflammatory fibrosarcoma.

Macroscopically, it looks like a large, nonencapsulated, vascular mass arising from the mesentery or from the omentum. Sections have a homogeneous or trabecular grayish myxoid appearance, without necrotic areas, hemorrhages or cysts inside (Day et al. 1986).

Histologically, the pseudotumor is constituted by bundles of large, elongate and poorly arranged nonpleiomorphic spindle cells, with ultrastructural and immunohistochemical characteristics of myofibroblasts. The fibroxanthomatous stroma is often densely infiltrated by mature plasma cells, small lymphocytes and other inflammatory cells (Treissman et al. 1994).

Inflammatory pseudotumor is usually an incidental finding in children suffering from atypical disturbances such as fever, growth retardation and loss of weight. It is seen as a large, mobile abdominal mass with a nodular surface. Laboratory tests indicate microcytic hypochromic anemia, thrombocytosis, polyclonal hypergammaglobulinemia, and elevated erythrocyte sedimentation rate.

CT findings of the pseudotumoral mass are aspecific, either when it shows a homogeneous, slightly enhancing soft tissue density (Day et al. 1986), or when it appears nonhomogeneous, with hypodense areas within a solid tissue irregularly enhancing with contrast medium (TREISSMAN et al. 1994).

The exact diagnosis of the nature of this unusual process is not generally taken into account even when the age of the patient (under 16 years), the clinical manifestations, the laboratory data and the radiological findings should suggest it. Only a histopathological study and ultrastructural and immunohistochemical tests can make it possible to recognize it.

Bibliography

Crohn's Disease

Angelelli G, Brindicci D, Macarini L, Favia V (1990) Interesse della tomografia computerizzata nello studio del morbo di Crohn. Radiol Med 79:65–69

Berliner L, Redmond P, Purow E, Megna D, Sottile V (1982) Computed tomography in Crohn's disease. Am J Gastroenterol 77:548–553

Casola G, vanSonnenberg E, Neff CC, Saba RM, Withers C, Emarine CW (1987) Abscesses in Crohn's disease: percutaneous drainage. Radiology 163:19–22

Fishman EK, Wolf EJ, Jones B, Bayless TM, Siegelmann SS (1987) CT evaluation of Crohn's disease: effect on patient management. AJR Am J Roentgenol 148:537–549

Frager DH, Goldman M, Beneventano TC (1983) Computed tomography in Crohn disease. J Comput Assist Tomogr 7:819–824

Frick W, Persingehl M, Klase KC (1986) Inflammatory bowel disease and related conditions. In: Meyer MA (ed) Computed tomography of the gastrointestinal tract including the peritoneal cavity and mesentery. Springer, New York Berlin Heidelberg

Goldberg HI, Gore RM, Margulis AR, Moss AA, Baker EL (1983) Computed tomography in the evaluation of Crohn disease. AJR Am J Roentgenol 140:277–282

Gore RM, Marn CS, Kirby DF, Vogelzang RL, Neiman HL (1984) CT Findings in ulcerative, granulomatous, and indeterminate colitis. AJR Am J Roentgenol 143:279–284

Gore RM, Cohen MI, Vogelzang RL, Neiman HL, Tsang TK (1985) Value of computed tomography in the detection of complications of Crohn's disease. Dig Dis Sci 30:701–709

Gore RM, Balthazar EJ, Ghahremami GG, Miller FH (1996) CT features of the ulcerative colitis and Crohn's disease. AJR Am J Roentgenol 167:3–15

Gossios KJ, Tsianos EV (1997) Crohn disease: CT findings after treatment. Abdom Imaging 22:160

Jacobs JE, Birnbaum BA (1995) CT of inflammatory disease of the colon. Semin Ultrasound CT MRI 16:91–101

Jones B, Fishman EK, Hamilton SR et al (1986) Submucosal accumulation of fat inflammatory bowel disease: CT pathological correlation. J Comput Assist Tomogr 10:759–763

Kerber GW, Geenberg M, Rubin JM (1984) Computed tomographic evaluation of local and extraintestinal complications of Crohn's disease. Gastrointest Radiol 9:143–148

Megibow AJ, Bosniak MA, Ambos MA, Redmond PE (1981) Crohn's disease causing hydronephrosis. J Comput Assist Tomogr 5:909–911

Merine D, Fishman EK, Kuhlman JE, Jones B, Bayless TM, Siegelman S (1989) Bladder involvement in Crohn disease: role of CT in detection and evaluation. J Comput Assist Tomogr 13:90–93

Orel SG, Rubesin SE, Jones B, Fishman EK, Bayless TM, Siegelman SS (1987) Computed tomography vs barium studies in the acutely symptomatic patient with Crohn disease. J Comput Assist Tomogr 11:1009–1016

Pompili GC, Damiani G, Mariani P, Matacena G, Ardizzone S, Bianchi Porro G, Cornalba G (1994) Contributo della tomografia computerizzata alla diagnosi del morbo di Crohn. Radiol Med 88:44–48

Raptopoulos V, Schwartz RK, McNicholas MMJ, et al (1997) Multiplanar helical enterography in patients with Crohn's disease. AJR Am J Roentgenol 169:1545

Riddlesberger MM Jr (1985) CT of complicated inflammatory bowel disease in children. Pediatr Radiol 15:384–387

Simpkins KC, Gore RM (1994) Crohn's disease. In: Gore RM, Levine MS, Laufer I (eds) Textbook of gastroenterology. Saunders, Philadelphia, pp 2660–2681

Usewils R, Dumoulin P, Vossen P, et al (1986) CT signs of Crohn's disease. J Belge Radiol 69:151–155

Wilhelm JP, Bresson A, Claudon M, Regent D, Champigneulle B, Bigard MA, Gaucher P (1988) Study of the small bowel and mesentery in Crohn's disease: comparison of ultrasonics, X-ray computed tomography and small bowel transit in 18 patients. Ann Gastrol Hepatol 24:49–54

Wills JS, Lobis IF, Deustman FI (1997) Crohn disease: state of the art. Radiology 202:597–610

Tuberculosis

Ablin DS, Jain KA, Azourz EM (1994) Abdominal tuberculosis in children. Pediatr Radiol 24:473–477

Bankier AA, Fleischmann D, Wiesmayr MN, Puts D, Kontrus M, Hübsch P, Herold CJ (1995) Update: abdominal tuberculosis – unusual findings on CT. Clin Radiol 50:223–228

Cremin BJ (1995) Tuberculosis: the resurgence of our most lethal infectious disease – a review. Pediatr Radiol 25:620–626

Dahlene DH Jr, Stanley RJ, Koehler RE, Shin MS, Tishler JMA (1984) Abdominal tuberculosis: CT findings. J Comput Assist Tomogr 8:223–225

Demirkazik FB, Akhan O, Özmen MN, Akata D (1996) US and CT findings in the diagnosis of tuberculous peritonitis. Acta Radiol 37:517–520

Denath FM (1990) Abdominal tuberculosis in children: CT findings. Gastrointest Radiol 15:303–306

Denton T, Hossain J (1993) A radiological study of abdominal tuberculosis in a Saudi population, with special reference to ultrasound and computed tomography. Clin Radiol 47:409–414

Deutch S, Sandler M, Alpern M (1987) Abdominal lymphadenopathy in benign diseases. CT detection. Radiology 163:355–338

Epstein BM, Mann JH (1982) CT of abdominal tuberculosis. AJR 139: 861–866

Gufler H, Meyer E (1992) Intraabdominal calcifications. Lymph node calcifications following mesenterial tuberculosis. Radiologe 32:185–186

Ha HK, Jung JI, Lee MS, Choi BG, Lee MG, Kim YH, Kim PN, Auh YH (1996) CT differentiation of tuberculous peritoni-

tis and peritoneal carcinomatosis. AJR Am J Roentgenol 167:743–748
Hanson RD, Hunter TB (1985) Tuberculous peritonitis: CT appearance. AJR Am J Roentgenol 144:931–932
Hulnick DH, Megibow AJ, Naidich DP, Hilton S, Cho KC, Balthazar EJ (1985) Abdominal tuberculosis: CT evaluation. Radiology 157:199–204
Hunter TB (1985) Tuberculous peritonitis: CT appearance. AJR Am J Roentgenol 144: 931–932
Jeffrey RB, Nyberg DA, Bottles K, et al (1986) Abdominal CT in acquired immunodeficiency syndrome. AJR Am J Roentgenol 146:7–13
Mehta JB, Eapen T, Gubler R, et al (1985) Abdominal tuberculosis mimicking neoplasia on computed tomography. South Med J 78:1385–1386
Nyberg DA, Federle MP, Jeffrey RB, Bottles K, Wofsy CB (1985) Abdominal CT findings of disseminated *Mycobacterium avium intracellulare* in AIDS. AJR Am J Roentgenol 145: 297–299
Perich J, Ayuso MC, Vilana R, Ayuso JR Cardenal, Mallofré C (1990) Disseminated lymphatic tuberculosis in acquired immuno-deficiency syndrome: computed tomographic findings. Can Assoc Radiol J 51:353–357
Pombo F, Rodriquez E, Mato J, Pere-Fontan J, Rivera E, Valvuena L (1992) Patterns of contrast enhancement of tuberculous lymph nodes demonstrated by computed tomography. Clin Radiol 46:13–17
Radin DR (1991) Intraabdominal *Mycobacterium tuberculosis* vs *Mycobacterium avium intracellulare* infections in patients with AIDS: distinction based on CT findings. AJR Am J Roentgenol 156:487–491
Soriano V, Tor J, Domenech E, Gabarre E, Muga R, Inaraja L, Casas D, Olazabal J, Clotet B (1991) Abdominal tuberculosis in patients with acquired immunodeficiency syndrome. Med Clin (Barc) 97:121–124
Suri S, Gupta S, Suri R (1999) Computed tomography in abdominal tuberculosis. Br J Radiol 72:92
Yang Z-G, Min P-Q, Sone S, et al (1999) Tuberculosis versus lymphoma in the abdominal lymph node: evaluation with contrast-enhanced CT. AJR Am J Roentgenol 172:619
Zirinsky K, Auh YH, Kneeland JB, Rubenstein WA, Kazam E (1985) Computed tomography, sonography, and MR imaging of abdominal tuberculosis. J Comput Assist Tomogr 9:961–963

AIDS and AIDS-related Syndromes

Alterman DD, Cho KC (1988) Histoplasmosis involving the omentum in an AIDS patient: CT demonstration (case report). J Comput Assist Tomogr 12:664–665
Balthazar EJ, Megibow AJ, Barry M, Opulencia JF (1993) Histoplasmosis of the colon in patients with AIDS: imaging findings in four cases. AJR Am J Roentgenol 161:585–587
Balthazar EJ, Noordhoorn M, Megibow AJ, Gordon RB (1996) CT of small-bowel lymphoma in immunocompetent patients and patients with AIDS: comparison of findings. AJR Am J Roentgenol 168:675–680
Bennum RR, Costello P (1983) CT findings in angioimmunoblastic lymphadenopathy. J Comput Assist Tomogr 7:454–456
Brooke R, Nyberg D, Bottles K, et al (1986) Abdominal CT in AIDS. AJR Am J Roentgenol 146:7–13
Cohen D, Fields S (1988) CT findings in visceral leishmaniasis mimicking lymphoma. Comput Med Imaging Graph 12:325
Ha HK, Jung Ji, Lee MS, Choi BG, Lee MG, Kim YH, Kim PN, Auh YH (1996) CT differentiation of tuberculous peritonitis and peritoneal carcinomatosis. AJR Am J Roentgenol 167:743–748
Herts BR, Megibow AJ, Birnbaum BA, Kanzer GK, Noz ME (1992) High-attenuation lymphadenopathy in AIDS patients: significance of findings at CT. Radiology 185:777–781
Jeffrey RB, Nyberg DA, Bottles K, et al (1986) Abdominal CT in acquired immunodeficiency syndrome. AJR Am J Roentgenol 146:7–13
Knollmann FD, Maurer J, Grunenwald T, et al (1997) Abdominal CT features and survival in acquired immunodeficiency. Acta Radiol 38:970
Meyers SA, Kuhlman JE, Fishman EK (1990) Enterovesical fistula in a patient with cryptosporidiosis and AIDS. CT demonstration. Clin Imaging 14:143–145
Moon KL, Federle MP, Abrams DL, Volberding P, Lewis BJ (1984) Kaposi sarcoma and lymphadenopathy syndrome: limitations of abdominal CT in acquired immunodeficiency syndrome. Radiology 150:479–483
Radin DR (1991a) Intraabdominal *Mycobacterium tuberculosis* vs *Mycobacterium avium-intracellulare* infections in patients with AIDS: distinction based on CT findings. AJR Am J Roentgenol 156:487–491
Radin DR (1991b) Disseminated histoplasmosis: abdominal CT findings in 16 patients. AJR Am J Roentgenol 157:955–958
Radin R (1995) HIV infection: analysis in 259 consecutive patients with abnormal abdominal CT findings. Radiology 197:712–722
Radin DR, Esplin JA, Levine AM, Ralls PW (1993) AIDS related non Hodgkin's lymphoma: abdominal CT findings in 112 patients. AJR Am J Roentgenol 160:1133–1139
Wall SD (1994) Gastrointestinal manifestation of acquired immunodeficiency syndrome. In: Gore RM, Levine MS, Laufer I (eds) Text book of gastrointestinal radiology. Saunders, Philadelphia
Wan YL, Ng SH, Les TY, Tsai CC (1989)Actinomycosis of the greater omentum. Gastrointest Radiol 14:38–40

Panniculitis-mesenteritis

Badiola Varella CM, Sussman SK, Glickstein MF (1991) Mesenteric panniculitis: findings on CT, MRI, and angiography (case report). Clin Imaging 265–267
De Giovanni L, Amato A, Civello IM (1988) Mesenteric fibromatosis. Minerva Chir 31:1757–1759
Forte MD, Brant WE (1988) Spontaneous isolated mesenteric fibromatosis. Report of a case. Dis Colon Rectum 31:315–317
Frouge C, Hoang C, Soulez G, Chagnon S, Blery M (1990) X-ray computed tomographic aspects of mesenteric panniculitis. J Radiol 71:19–21
Fujiyoshi F, Ichinari N, Kajiya Y, et al (1997) Retractile mesenteritis: small bowel radiography, CT and MR imaging. AJR Am J Roentgenol 169:791
Grenier N, Dorsier F, Le Bastard E, Perez T, Goussot JF, Grelet P (1986) La panniculite pseudo-tumorale intra-abdominale. J Radiol 67:411–414
Gudinchet F, Schnyder P (1987) Mesenteric panniculitis. Acta Radiol 28:727–729

Hailemariam S, Jaeger P, Goebel N, Grant JW (1988) Mesenteric fibromatosis with ureteric stenosis. Postgrad Med J 64:79–81

Harbrecht PJ (1966) Variants of retroperitoneal fibrosis. Ann Surg 165:388–401

Hayashi S, Oyama K, Hirakawa K, Oda M, Kogure T (1982) Mesenteric panniculitis, case report and its radiological diagnosis including CT. Rinsho-Hoshasen 27:143–146

Holland P (1990) Sclerosing encapsulating peritonitis in chronic ambulatory peritoneal dialysis. Clin Radiol 41:19

Katz ME, Heiken JP, Glazer HS, Lee JKT (1985) Intraabdominal panniculitis: clinical, radiographic, and CT features. AJR Am J Roentgenol 145:293–296

Kopecky KK, Lappas JC, Baker MK, Madura JA (1988) Mesenteric panniculitis: CT appearance. Gastrointest Radiol 13:273–274

Mata JM, Inarasa L, Martin J, Olazabal A, Castilla MT (1987) CT features of mesenteric panniculitis. J Comput Assist Tomogr 11:1021–1023

Monahan DW, Poston WK Jr, Brown GJ (1989) Mesenteric panniculitis. South Med J 82:782–784

Murayama T, Imoto S, Ito M, Matsushita K, Matozaki S, Nakagawa T, Kanbara Y, Kono N, Sashikata T (1992) Mesenteric fibromatosis presenting as fever of unknown origin. Am J Gastroenterol 87:1503–1505

Ng SH, Wong HF, Ko SF, Tsai CC (1992) Retractile mesenteritis with colon and retroperitoneum involvement: CT findings. Gastrointest Radiol 17:333–335

Paris A Jr, Willing SJ (1991) CT appearance of mesenteric saponification. Clin Imaging 15:213–215

Perez Fontan JF, Soler R, Sanchez J, Iglesias P, Sanjurgo P, Ruiz J (1986) Retractile mesenteritis involving the colon: barium enema, sonographic and CT findings. AJR Am J Roentgenol 147: 937–940

Roscher R, Gaedicke G, Mohr W (1988) Mesenteric fibromatosis in childhood. Monatsschr Kinderheilkd 136:393–396

Seigel RS, Kuhns LR, Borlaza GS, McCormick TL, Simmons JL (1980) Computed tomography and angiography in ileal carcinoid tumor and retractile mesenteritis. Radiology 134:437–440

Silverman PM, Baker ME, Cooper C, Kelvin FM (1987) Computed tomography of mesenteric disease. Radiographics 7:309–320

Sussman SK, Glickstein MF (1991) Mesenteric panniculitis – findings on CT, MRI, and angiography. Clin Imaging 15:265–267

Tanaka N, Nakanishi T, Suga K, Nagatomi Y (1990) A case of mesenteric panniculitis of the transverse colon. Rinsho-Hoshasen 35:415–418

Trautwein C, Herman E, Rambow A, Lohr H, Klose P, Gabbert H, Poralla T (1990) Retractile mesenteritis. Diagnostic and therapeutic aspect. Dtsch Med Wochenschr 115:174–178

Whitley NO, Bohlman ME, Baker LP (1982) CT patterns of mesenteric disease. J Comput Assist Tomogr 6:490–495

Will CH, Nitsch J, Buschfort R (1993) The radiological findings in mesenteric lipodystrophy. Rofo Fortschr Geb Rontgenstr Neuen Bildgeb Verfahr 158:78–79

Omental-mesenteric Inflammatory Pseudotumor

Day DL, Sane S, Dehner LP (1986) Inflammatory pseudotumor of the mesentery and small intestine. Pediatr Radiol 16:210–215

Goodman K, Baim R, Clair MR, Perkes EA (1983) Angiomatous lymphoid hamartoma of the pelvis. Radiology 146:728

Jeffrey RB, Fishman EK (1996) Spiral TC of the body. A teaching file. Lippincott-Raven, Philadelphia

Meis JM, Enzinger FM (1991) Inflammatory fibrosarcoma of the mesentery and retroperitoneum: a tumor closely simulating inflammatory pseudotumor. Am J Surg Pathol 15:1146–1156

Tang TT, Segura AD, Oechler MD, Harb JM, Adair SE, Gregg DC, et al (1990) Inflammatory myofibrohistiocytic proliferation simulating sarcoma in children. Cancer 65:1626–1634

Treissman SP, Gillis DA, Lee CLY, Giacomantonio M, Resch L (1994) Omental-mesenteric inflammatory pseudotumor. Cancer 73:1433–1437

Wu JP, Yunis EJ, Jaeschke WF, Gilbert EF (1973) Inflammatory pseudotumors of the abdomen: plasma cell granulomas. J Clin Pathol 26:943–948

8 Peritoneal and Mesenteric Trauma

Abdominopelvic traumas can produce contusions, dilacerations, peritoneal and ligamental avulsions, fractures of parenchymatous organs, perforation of the bowel, rupture of the biliary and urinary tracts, and tear or rupture of vessels with penetration of fluid (blood, urine, bile) or gas into the peritoneal cavity and the subperitoneal spaces.

Helical CT is a quick way of providing accurate information to supplement clinical and hemodynamic investigations, with the aim of deciding on the best treatments, avoiding dangerous and unnecessary laparotomies (in about 95% of all patients who undergo laparotomy after blunt traumas because of suspected bowel or mesenteric injuries these are found not to be present) (Rizzo et al.1989) in the case of simple or limited injuries to organs and/or viscera in patients with hemodynamic alterations but without abdominal lesions. In addition, it may be an alternative to angiography alone followed by selective embolization even in patients with an abundant hemoperitoneum. Conversely, in patients who are hemodynamically stable, but have severe multiple-organ injuries or active bleeding and thus need surgery, CT gives the surgeon an accurate indication of the localization and extent of the injuries or of the active bleeding (Shuman 1997).

CT findings in the case of peritoneal and mesenteric injuries include linear soft-dense strandings within the mesentery, diffuse higher attenuation of the mesenteric fat, soft or highly dense focal or cake-like masses, and air, fluid and clot in the peritoneal cavity or between the leaves of the mesentery. These lesions are often present simultaneously and associated with hollow or solid organs injuries.

- Linear soft-density strandings and higher attenuation mesenteric fat in the first days after abdominal trauma correspond to a contusive edematous or hemorrhagic areolar tissue infiltration (Figs. 8.1, 8.2).
- Streaky density greater then 3 mm within the mesentery adjacent to a small bowel loop detected in the early period following a blunt abdominal trauma is a significant sign of intestinal rupture and is related to perivascular bleeding and to cellular infiltration caused by direct mesenteric injury or chemical irritation from spilled intestinal material (Hagiwara et al. 1993, 1995). Focal thickening of the small bowel wall is due to an intramural hematoma, and is a significant sign of intestinal rupture when associated with mesenteric manifestations (Hagiwara et al. 1993, 1995).
- According to the position of the high-density stripes in the mesentery can be seen as an indicator of the location of small bowel rupture: this is found within the first 90 cm of the small bowel if the stripes are located in the upper part of the abdomen, in the ileal loops up to 230–280 cm from Treitz's ligament if they are concentrated in the middle part of the abdomen, and in the last 50 cm of the ileum if they are situated in the lower part of the abdomen (Hagiwara et al. 1993, 1995).
- A focal area of high attenuation (60–90 HU) (Fig. 8.3) detected in the mesentery by CT 24–36 h after an abdominal trauma corresponds to a hematoma with high hemoglobin content (Chintapalli et al. 1998; Orwig and Federle 1989). When it is adjacent to the thickening of the bowel wall or the solid organ injured it indicates the presence and the origin of hemorrhage (sentinel clot) and requires immediate surgical exploration.

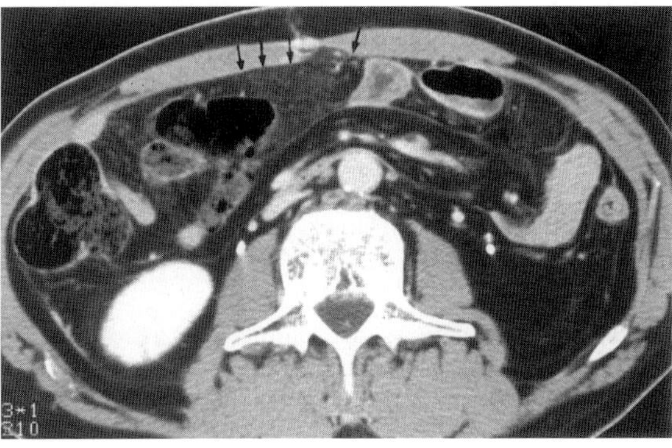

Fig. 8.1. Omental and mesenteric contusion. Edematous increase in density of fat in the anterior abdominal planes (*arrows*)

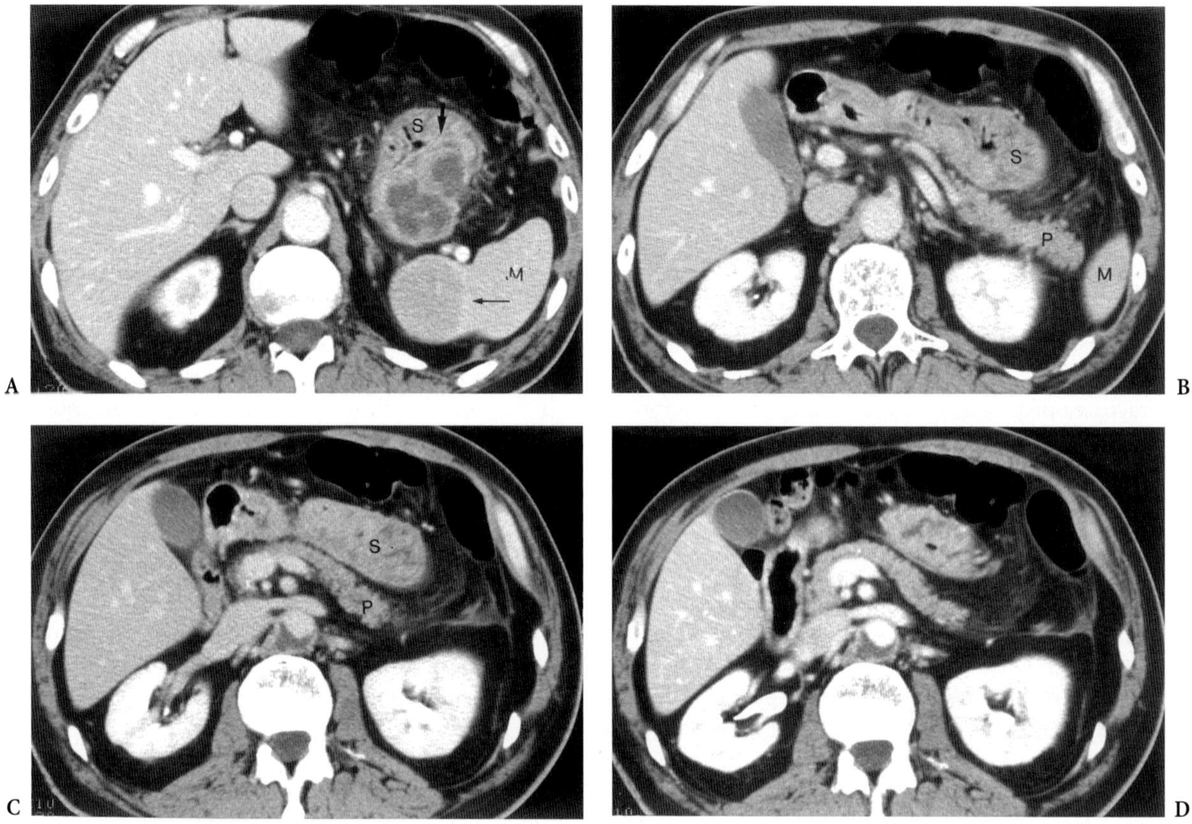

Fig. 8.2A–D. Ligamental and peritoneal contusion and gastric and splenic hematomas. Edematous increase in attenuation and soft density streaks in the gastrohepatic (**A**), gastrosplenic (**A, B**) and gastrocolic (**A–C**) ligaments. Thickening of the posterior peritoneum and of the left lateroconal and anterior renal fasciae (**C–D**), with very thin hemorrhagic fluid between peritoneum and fasciae. Gastric intramural (**A** *thick arrow*) and splenic (**A** *thin arrow*) hematomas

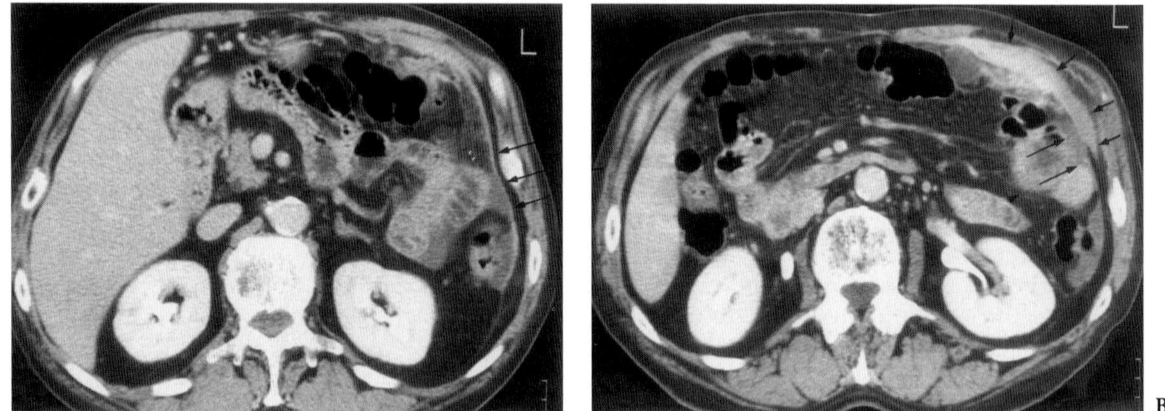

Fig. 8.3A, B. Traumatic jejunal rupture. Jejunal loop dilated with thickened and enhancing wall. Small amount of fluid in the surrounding peritoneal leaves (*long arrows*). Absence of free air. Left extrafascial hematoma (*small arrows*) between the abdominal muscular wall and the transversalis fascia

- Air in the peritoneal cavity (pneumoperitoneum) (Fig. 8.8) is a classic sign of intestinal perforation; however, cannot always be observed shortly after the trauma and must be searched for with suitable windows (for example those used in the evaluation of the pulmonary parenchyma), and possibly with a repeat of the CT a few hours if the suspicion of an intestinal rupture persists. In the case of pneumoperitoneum, when the patient is in a recumbent position the air is preferentially located in the right subphrenic space, between the diaphragm and the anterior face of the liver, but it can also spread in front of the stomach on the left side or into the inflection of the abdominal wall between or outside the rectus abdominis muscle.
- Free air observed in the mesenteric interstices (Fig. 8.9) in the case of subperitoneal perforation is contained at the point of rupture of the intestinal wall, where it forms small bubbles.

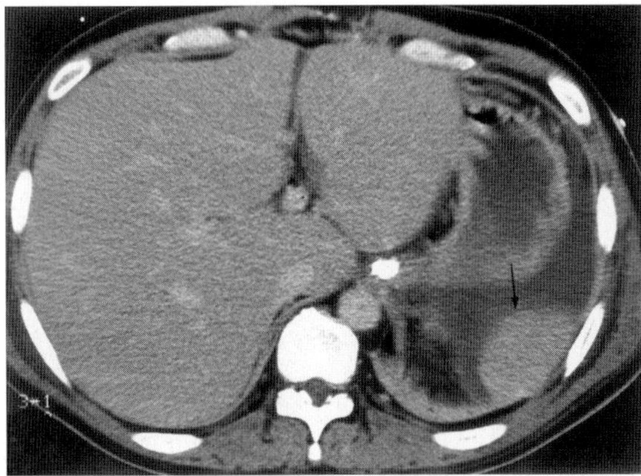

Fig. 8.4. Recent hemorrhage. Unenhanced CT in a patient affected by shock after splenectomy because of traumatic rupture of the spleen. Wide and mostly hyperdense (*arrow*) hemorrhagic collection in the splenic recesses

- Low-attenuation intraperitoneal fluid (less than 20 HU) is often found, even in small amounts, on CT performed in patients who have sustained abdominal traumas. Possible causes for this are peritoneal lavage, leakage of bile, extravasation of urine, rupture of the small bowel, and extravasation of blood or lymph. Recognizing the nature of the single peritoneal fluid is rather difficult.
- Intraperitoneal hematic collections (hemoperitoneum) are usually due to splenic or hepatic rupture. CT findings have been described in chapter 5 (sect. 5.3).

Small-volume blood collections within the peritoneal cavity are deposited in the recess surrounding the organ from which the bleeding originates (Roberts 1996) at an early stage and indicate the site of the hemorrhage. Gravity causes larger volumes of hemorrhagic fluid to spread quickly into the lowest space: collections from the upper abdomen into Morrison's pouch and submesocolic hemorrhages into the pelvic space. Supramesocolic collections may also extend into the pelvic spaces through the right paracolic gutter or, when they are abundant, through the left paracolic gutter overflowing the phrenicocolic ligament. Because of this possible localization of the blood exclusively in the pelvis, CT scanning should always be extended to the pelvis (Roberts 1996) (Fig. 8.6).

Subperitoneal mesenteric massive hemorrhage may also result from avulsion of the root of the mesentery and from laceration of the mesenteric vessels. Contrast medium extravasation in the mesentery or in the peritoneal cavity indicates active bleeding caused by vascular injury sustained during the CT scan. It starts 30 s after i.v. contrast injection and is better defined in the venous phase as a very high attenuation area (>85 HU), surrounded by clotted

A

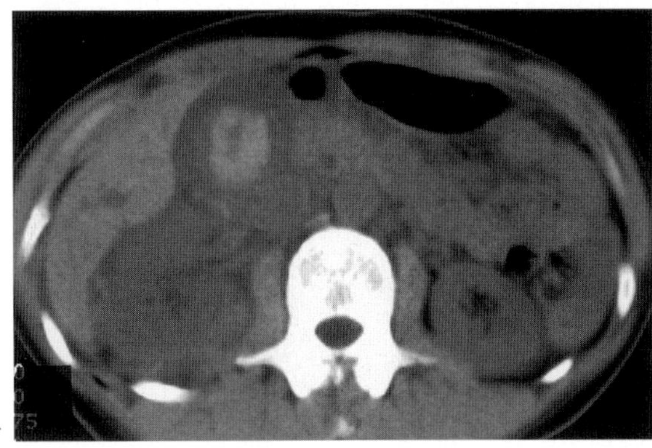

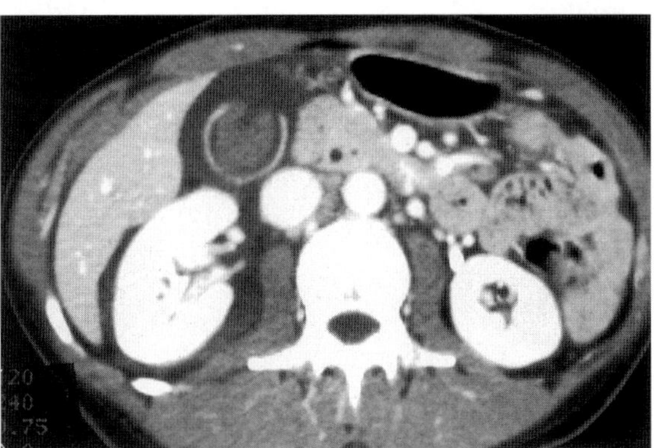

B

Fig. 8.5. Gallbladder rupture. Interruption of the thickened and enhancing cholecystic wall with intraluminal hemorrhagic high-attenuation fluid surrounded by low-density fluid

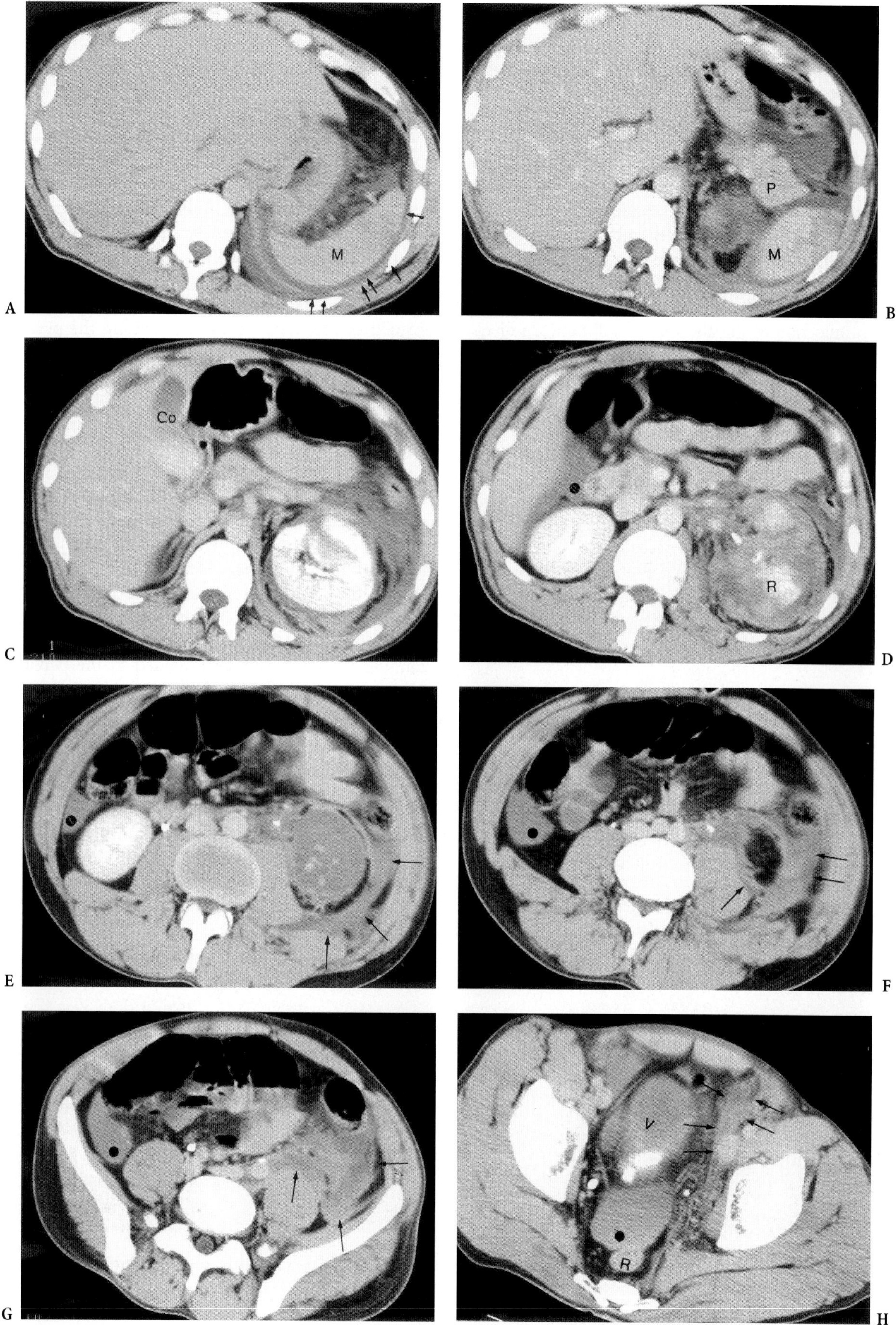
A
M
B
P
M
C
Co
D
R
E
F
G
H
V
R

blood with lower density. In later scans it may be possible to differentiate pelvic vascular extravasation from a urine leak because of the higher density of the extravasated contrast and because of the surrounding lower attenuation hematoma (Mirvis 1989; Shanmuganathan et al. 1993, 1995). CT findings indicate the presence and the source of the vascular bleeding requiring immediate angiographic embolization.

Trauma to the gallbladder may result in contusion, laceration and disruption with luminal hemorrhage and pericholecystic collection (Erb et al. 1994) Contusion is characterized by ill defined contours. A gallbladder laceration with biliary leakage is seen as an interruption of the contour of a thickened and enhanced cholecystic wall, with pericholecystic low-attenuation fluid (Fig. 8.5). This section of the gallbladder wall is suggested by a double contour. The disruption appears as collapsed cholecystic lumen. An intraluminal high-density area in the gallbladder is due to a recent hemorrhage, which may have been caused by an injury of either the gallbladder or the liver (hemobilia). It may show layering, with low-attenuation bile over denser clotted blood. Pericholecystic fluid alone, whether the cholecystic wall is well or ill defined, is likely to reflect a microperforation of the gallbladder.

When biliary leakage is suspected, associated CT i.v. cholangiography with delayed images, or alternatively a cholangio-cholecystoscintigraphy, helps to confirm that the gallbladder or the biliary tract is ruptured or to exclude this possibility.

A diffuse increase in attenuation of the hepatoduodenal ligament, the presence of intraperitoneal fluid in the subhepatic spaces and concomitant hepatoduodenal injury must raise the suspicion of dilaceration of the main biliary tract.

The goal of CT evaluation of cholecystic traumas is quick acquisition of the information needed to direct clinical management. Lacerations and avulsions require immediate surgical treatment; contusions demand only medical wait-and-see" management, perhaps with repeat CT or US examination to exclude an increasing volume of the pericholecystic collection (Erb et al. 1994).

Rupture of the urinary bladder produces an outflow of urine into the peritoneum if the visceral dome is injured, or into the subperitoneal spaces if the lateral walls or the floor are ruptured. Rapid detailed recognition of the rupture and its site is needed to make it possible to perform the correct treatment: conservative if the lesion is subperitoneal, or surgery if the lesion is intraperitoneal. Any delay in repairing lesions of the dome can be fatal (Levine et al 1995).

CT detects (even in precontrast scans) the presence of low-density (attenuation values: 0–20 HU) collections in the vesical compartment, which is suggestive of a rupture. An outflow of radiopaque urine from the urinary bladder after contrast medium administration provides the opportunity to determine the site of the visceral rupture easily; this is at the level of the dome if the contrast medium penetrates the paravesical peritoneal recesses, and in the perineal part of the wall if radiopaque urine spreads into the subperitoneal spaces. In the case of rupture of the dome, the urine flows upward from the peritoneal paravesical recesses into the inframesocolic cavities surrounding the ileal loops or, following the right paracolic gutter, spreads up to the supramesocolic peritoneal spaces (subphrenic and right subhepatic recesses).

On the other hand, the subperitoneal urinary collections may spread upward into the prevesical space along the anterior abdominal wall, backward into the retroperitoneum or downward between the perineal muscles and the root of the thigh or into the scrotum.

CT findings of "hypoperfusion complex" related to the hypovolemic shock in patients with both serious hemodynamic instability attributable to reduced cardiac output and peripheral vasoconstriction and poor diagnosis have been described by Taylor et al. (1987) and confirmed by Jeffrey and Federle (1988), Shin et al. (1990) and Sivit et al. (1992) (Fig. 8.8). These findings consist in an intense and persistent enhancement of the spleen, kidneys, adrenal glands, pancreas and bowel wall, in a marked and diffuse luminal fluid dilatation of the ileal loops, in small aortae and slit-like inferior cava, and in fluid collections inside the peritoneum. " These findings " emphasizes Taylor, "may help direct attention to the patient's serious hemodynamic abnormality as much as to individual organ defect."

Fig. 8.6A–H. Severe left thoracoabdominal trauma: intra- and retroperitoneal hemorrhage. **A** Left pleural collection. **B** Fracture of the spleen with **A–C** peritoneal hemorrhage in the perisplenic recess (*small arrows*). The hemorrhagic fluid (*small circles*) descends initially into the right subhepatic recess (**D**) then, following the right paracolic gutter, as far as the right paravesical recesses (**H**).High-density streaks and areas in the gastrosplenic ligament, caused by dilaceration and hemorrhage (**A, B**). Intracholecystic hemorrhage (*C*) with layering of low attenuating bile over denser clotted blood. Fracture of the left kidney, with hemorrhage in the perirenal compartment and limited by the renal fascia and by the septa of the adipose tissue. Retroperitoneal hematic collection that from the left posterior pararenal space (*long thin arrows*) spreads downward as far as the pelvic laterorectal extraperitoneal space (**B–H**)

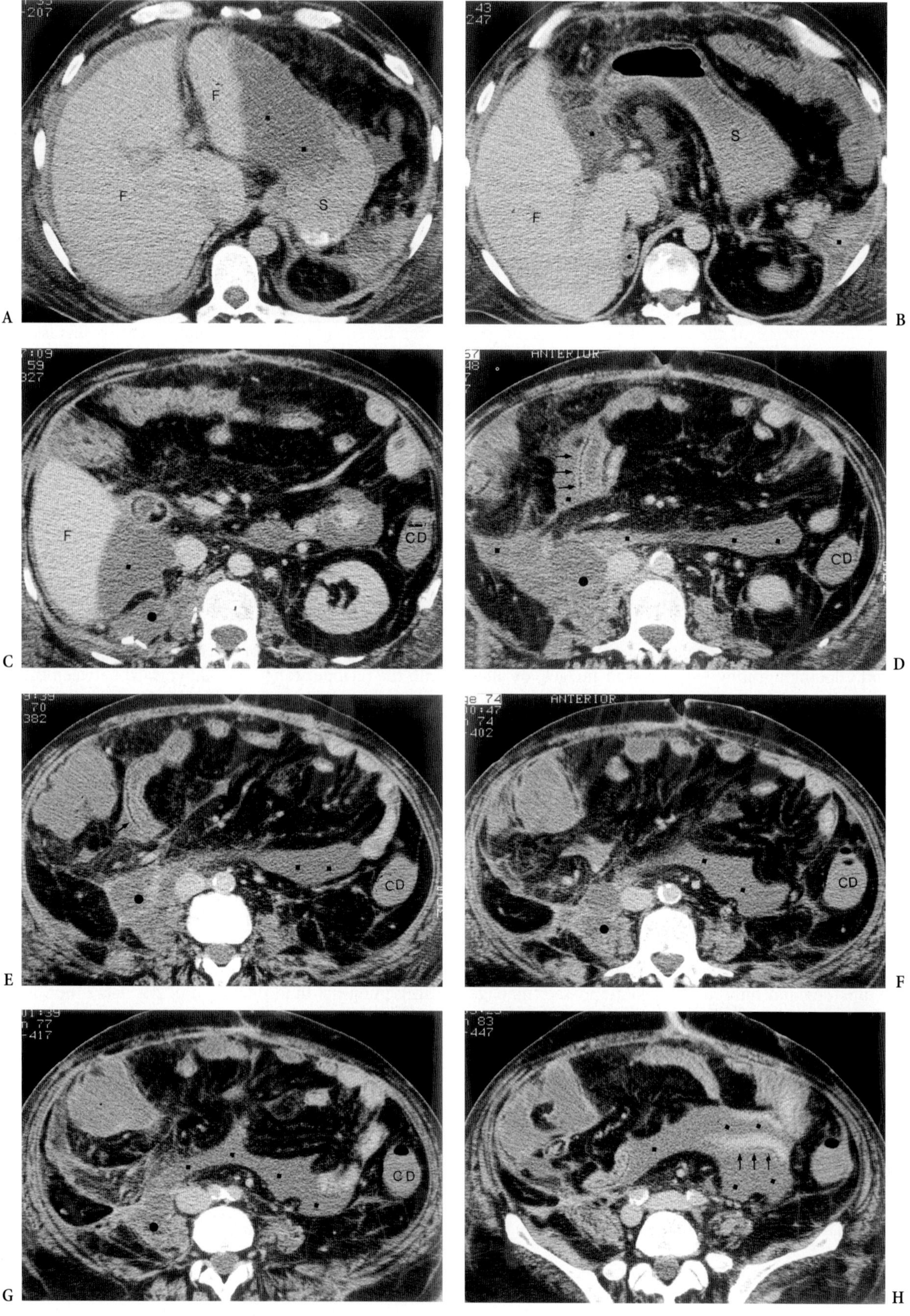
A
F
F
S
B
F
S
C
F
CD
D
ANTERIOR
CD
E
CD
F
ANTERIOR
CD
G
CD
H

Fig. 8.7A–D. Outcome at 15 days after cholecystectomy, splenectomy and right nephrectomy necessitated by serious thoracoabdominal trauma. The ligaments and the omentum appear widely shaded and moiré because of contusion and dilaceration. Perihepatic peritoneal effusion is wider in the right subhepatic and gastrohepatic recesses (**A**), in the splenic (**A, B**) and the submesocolic spaces (*small squares*) (**D–H**).A high-density area due to fluid in the splenic space suggests a recent small bleeding. Wide collection occupying the right renal compartment (*circles*)

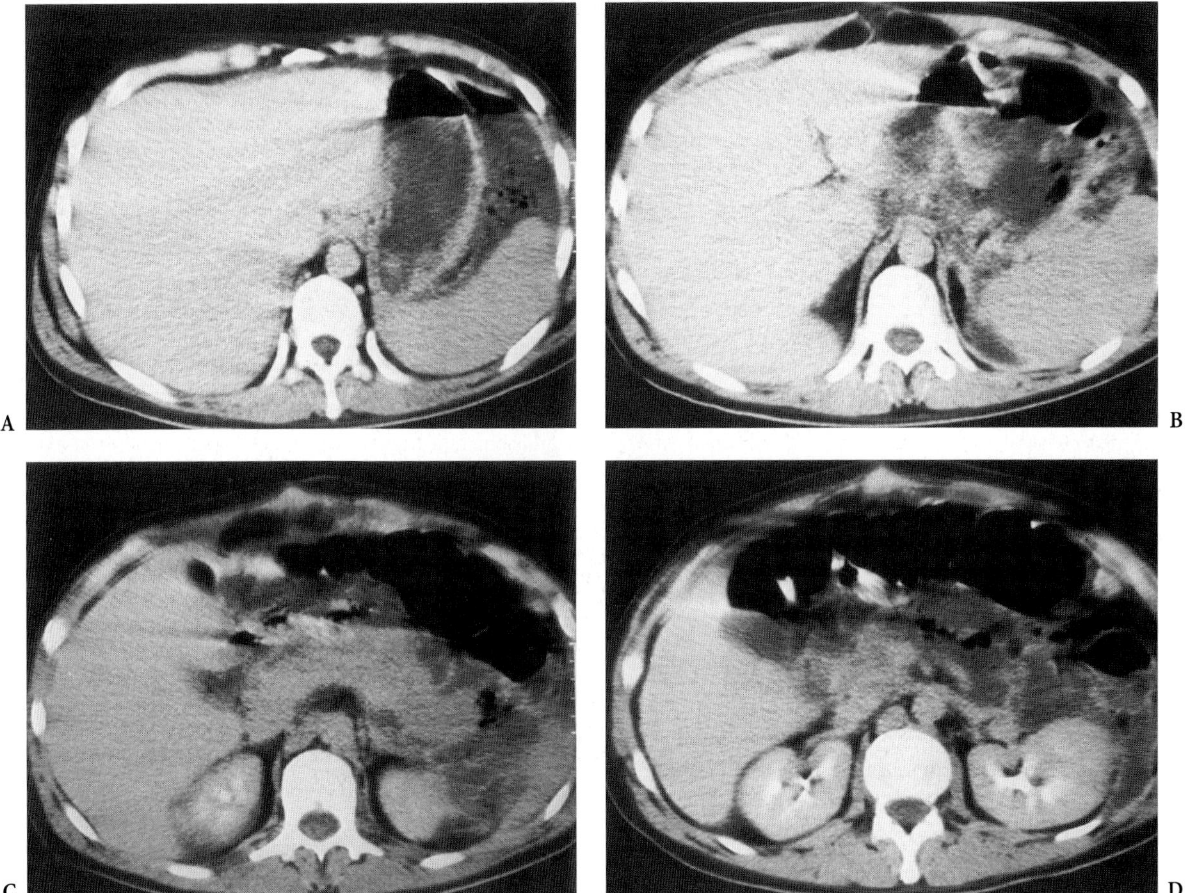

Fig. 8.8A–D. Blunt trauma of the left hypochondrium: intestinal perforation. Rupture in the splenic flexure of the colon with air-fluid level in the gastrocolic ligament (**A**). Collection in the mesentery and in the left lateroconal space (**D**)

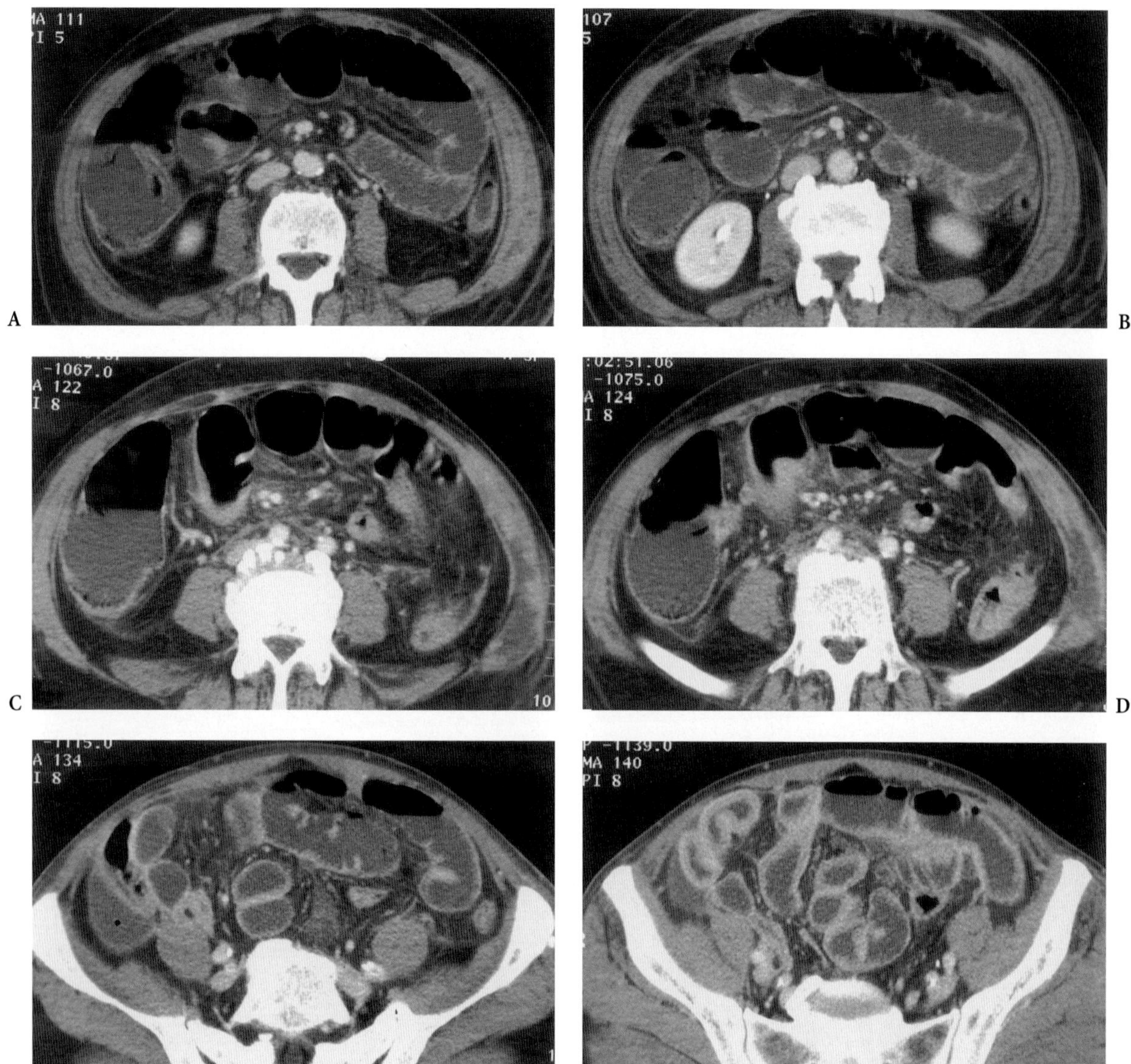

Fig. 8.9A–K. Abdominopelvic trauma with intestinal perforation, contusion of the transverse mesocolon and the mesentery, and abdominal parietal hematoma. Dilated ileal loops in the right hypochondrium with air-fluid level. Gas bubble in the adjacent mesentery due to median ileal perforation (**A, B**).Contusive increase of attenuation of the transverse mesocolon (**C**) and the mesentery (**D, E**).Free effusion (*small squares*) (**F, H–K**) with air bubbles (*small arrows*) (**H, J**) in the pelvic peritoneal spaces due to perforation of last ileal loops. High and persistent wall enhancement of distended ileal loops due to hypoperfusion produced by peripheral vasoconstriction and paralytic ileus (**F–H**).Hematic collection between the fasciae of the left oblique muscles (**C, D**)

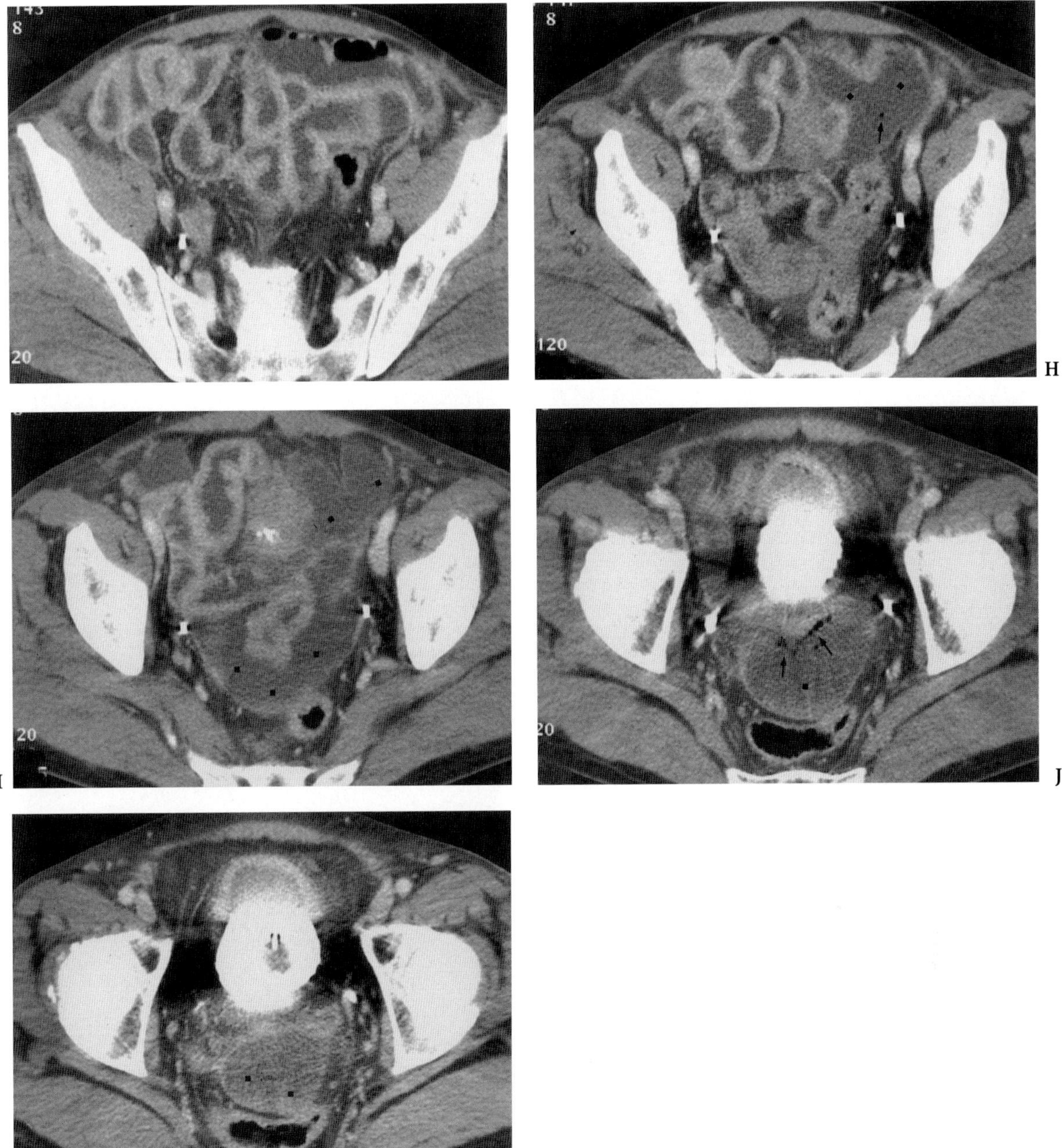
G
H
I
J
K

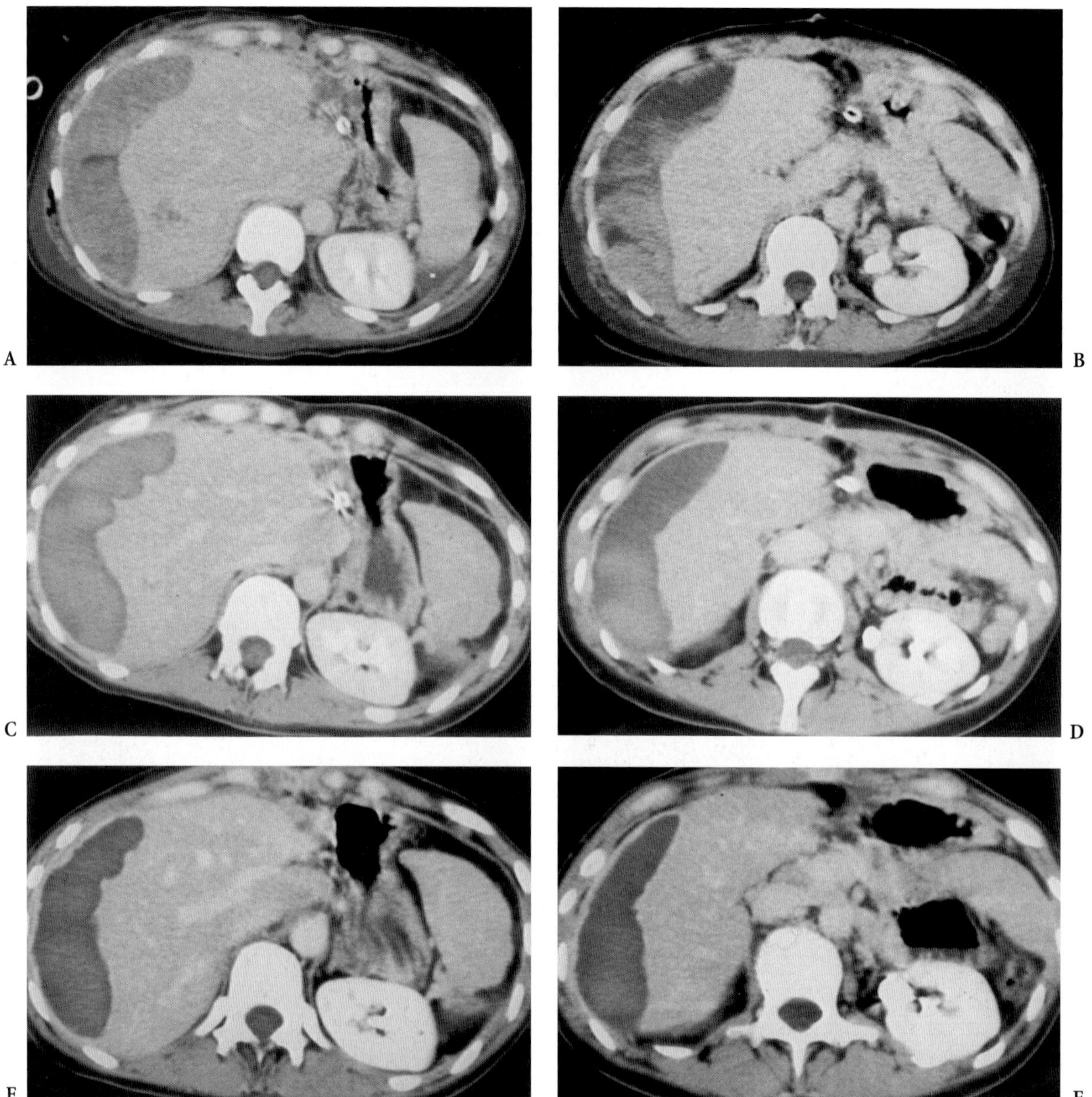

Fig. 8.10A–F. Evolution of a traumatic blood subcapsular hepatic collection. **A, B** Just after trauma: nonhomogeneous density with parahydric and hyperdense areas. **C,D** After 13 days: central homogeneously high density with thin peripheral low-density halo, where hemolysis is already in progress. A richly vascularized contrast enhancing pseudocapsule surrounds the collection. **E, F** One month later: widening of the peripheral low-density halo, but with persistence of the central hyperdensity owing to slow reabsorption of the clot

→

Fig. 8.12A–F. Traumatic anterior abdominal hematoma. Contusion with dilaceration of the rectus abdominis muscle and extrafascial collection, predominantly hyperdense. The fluid is limited inside by the transversalis fascia and by the aponeurosis of the rectus muscle and extends from the epigastrium to the pelvis. Under Douglas' subumbilical arcuate line, the collection spreads into the right subperitoneal prevesical space (**C–E**), extending in the pelvis between the sacro-recto-genito-pubic fascia and the extraperitoneal laterorectal fat outside and the umbilicovesical ligament inside (**F**)

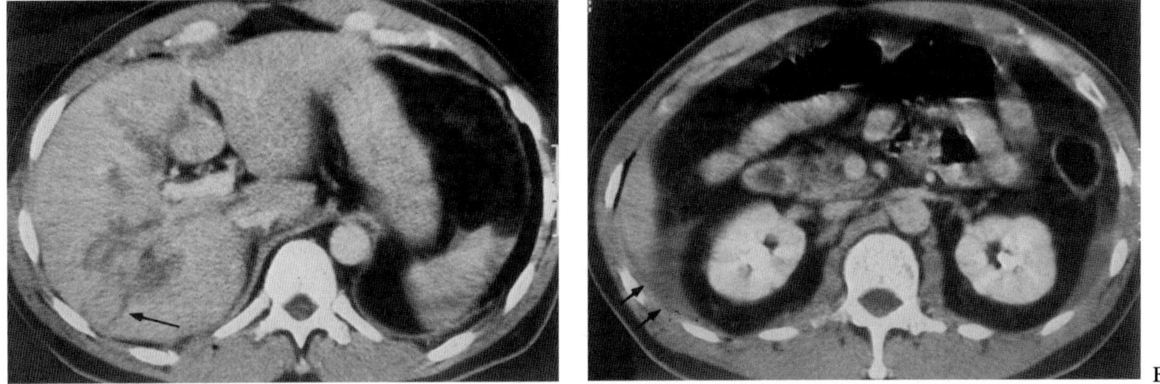

Fig. 8.11. A Fracture of the right lobe of the liver (*arrow*) has caused fluid collection in Morrison's recess (**B** *small arrows*)

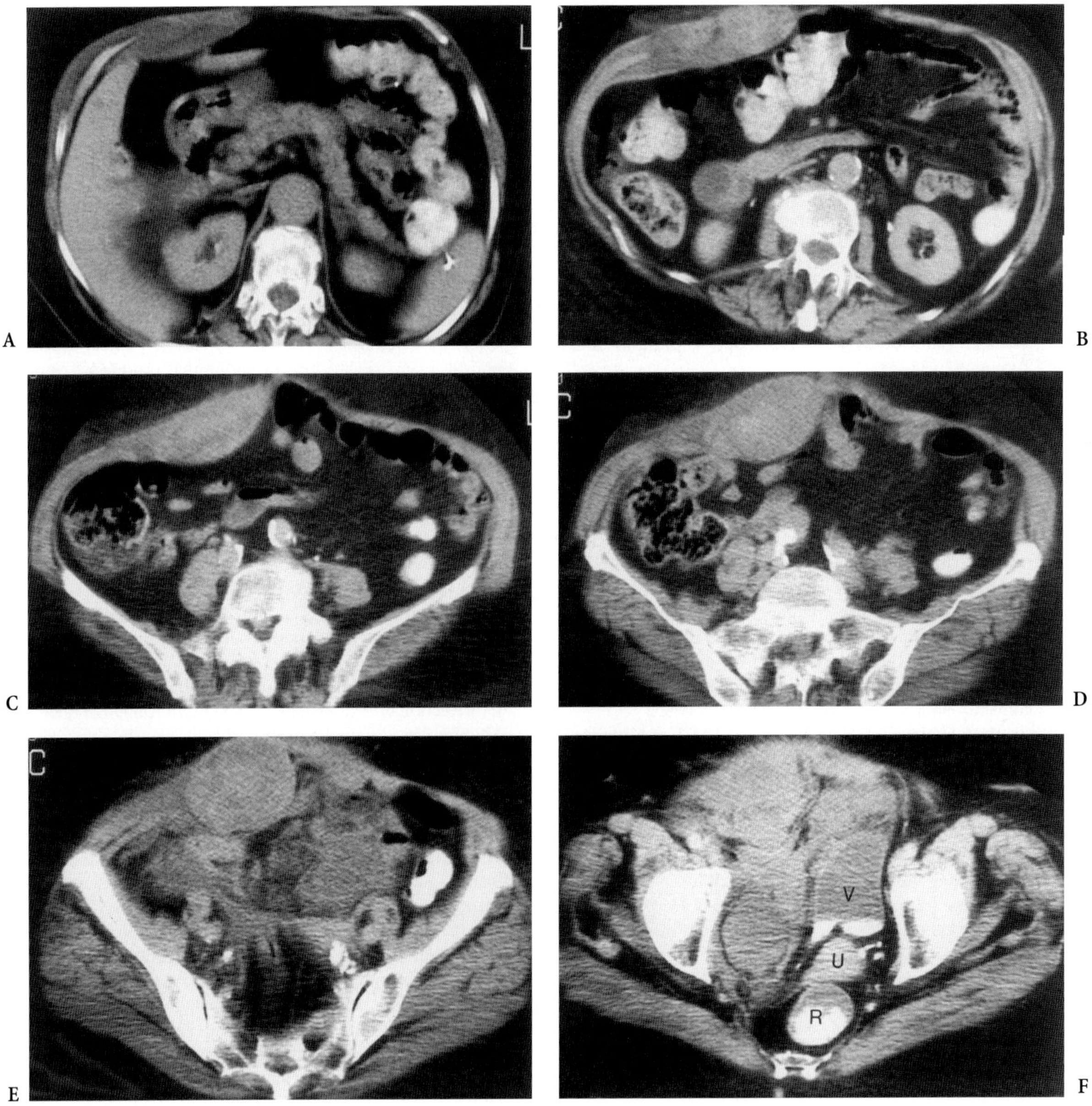

A B

C D

E F

V
U
R

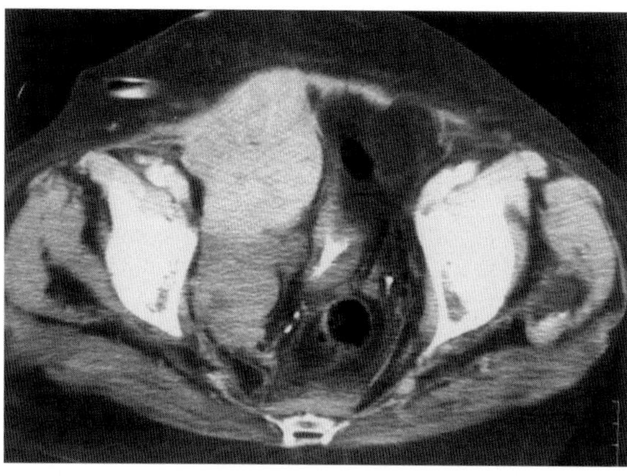

Fig. 8.13. Traumatic pelvic hematoma. Unenhanced CT: wide high-density subperitoneal collection in right prevesical space

Bibliography

Albanese CT, Meza MP, Gardner MJ, et al (1996) Is computed tomography a useful adjunct to the clinical examination for the diagnosis of pediatric gastrointestinal perforation from blunt abdominal trauma in children? J Trauma Injury Infect Crit Care 40:417–421

Alexander ES, Clark RA (1982) Computed tomography in the diagnosis of abdominal hemorrhage. JAMA 248:1104–1107

Ball DS, Friedman AC, Radecki PD, Caroline DF (1988) Avulsed gallbladder: CT appearance. J Comput Assist Tomogr 12:538–539

Berger PE, Kuhn JP (1981) CT of blunt abdominal trauma in childhood. AJR Am J Roentgenol 136:105–110

Berland LL, Doust BD, Foley WD (1980) Acute hemorrhage into the gallbladder diagnosed by computed tomography and ultrasonography. J Comput Assist Tomogr 4:260–262

Borchers HD, Heller M (1986) Iatrogenic injuries. In: Heller M, Jend HH, Genant HK (eds) Computed tomography of trauma. Thieme, Stuttgart New York

Breen DJ, Janzen DL, Zwirewich CV, et al (1997) Blunt bowel and mesenteric injury: diagnostic performance of CT signs. J Comput Assist Tomogr 21:706–712

Brody AS, Seidel FG, Kuhn JP (1989) CT evaluation of blunt abdominal trauma in children comparison of ultrafast and conventional CT. AJR Am J Roentgenol 159:803

Brody JM, Leighton DM, Murphy BL (2000) CT of blunt trauma bowel and mesenteric injury: typical findings and pitfalls in diagnosis. Radiographics 20:1253–1536

Brunsting LA, Morton JH (1987) Gastric rupture from blunt abdominal trauma. J Trauma 27:887–890

Bulas DI, Taylor GA, Eichelberger MR (1989) The value of CT in detecting bowel perforation in children after blunt abdominal trauma. AJR Am J Roentgenol 153:561–564

Catalano O (1995) Il pneumoperitoneo da trauma toracico. Radiol Med 89:72–75

Cerva DS Jr, Mirvis SE, Shanmunganathan K, Kelley IM, Pais SO (1996) Detection of bleeding in patients with major pelvic fractures; value of contrast-enhanced CT. AJR Am J Roentgenol 166:131–135

Chandler JG, Berk RN, Golden GT (1977) Misleading pneumoperitoneum. Surg Gynecol Obstet 144:163–174

Chintapalli K, Dodds WJ, Olson DL (1988) Computed tomography characteristics of intermesenteric hematomas. CT Comput Tomogr 12:122–128

Cook DE, Walsh JW, Vick CW, Brewer WH (1986) Upper abdominal trauma: pitfalls in CT diagnosis. Radiology 159:65–69

Cox TD, Kuhn JP (1996) CT scan of bowel trauma in the pediatric patient. Radiol Clin North Am 34:807–818

Daneman A, Matzinger MA, Martin DJ (1983) Posttraumatic hemorrhage into the gallbladder. J Comput Assist Tomogr 7:59–61

Danne FD (1988) A perspective on the early management of abdominal trauma. Aust N Z J Surg 58:851–858

Donohue JH, Federle MP, Griffiths BG, Trunkey DD (1987) Computed tomography in the diagnosis of blunt intestinal and mesenteric injuries. J Trauma 27:11–17

Druy EM, Rubin BE (1979) Computed tomography in the evaluation of abdominal trauma. J Comput Assist Tomogr 3:40–44

Erb RE, Mirvis SE, Shanmuganathan (1994) Gallbladder injury secondary to blunt trauma: CT findings. J Comput Assist Tomogr 18:778–784

Fabian TC, Mangiante EC, White TJ, Patterson CR, Boldreghini S, Britt LG (1986) A prospective study of 91 patients undergoing both computed tomography and peritoneal lavage following blunt abdominal trauma. J Trauma 26:602–608

Federle MP (1984) CT of upper abdominal trauma. Semin Roentgenol 19:269–280

Federle MP (1994) Abdominal trauma. In: Gore RM, Levine MS, Laufer I (eds) Textbook of gastrointestinal radiology. Saunders, Philadelphia pp 2600–2606

Federle MP, Jeffrey RB (1983) Hemoperitoneum studied by computed tomography. Radiology 148:187–192

Federle MP, Goldberg HI, Kaiser JA, Moss AA, Jeffrey RB Jr, Mall JC (1981) Evaluation of abdominal trauma by computed tomography. Radiology 138:637–644

Federle MP, Crass RA, Jeffrey RB, Trunkey DD (1982) Computed tomography in blunt abdominal trauma. Arch Surg 117:645–650

Federle MP, Yagan N, Peitzman AB, Krugh J (1997) Abdominal trauma: use of contrast material for CT is safe. Radiology 205:91–93

Foley WD, Cates JD, Kellman GM, et al (1987) Treatment of blunt hepatic injuries: role of CT. Radiology 164:635–638

Gay SB, Sistrom CL (1992) Computed tomography evaluation of blunt abdominal trauma. Radiol Clin North Am 30:367–387

Glazer GM, Buy JN, Moss AA, Goldberg HI, Federle MP (1981) CT detection of duodenal perforation. AJR Am J Roentgenol 137:333–336

Goldstein AS, Sclafani SJA, Kupferstein NH, et al (1985) The diagnostic superiority of computerized tomography. J Trauma 25:938–944

Gottesman L, Marks RA, Khoury PT, Moallem AG, Wichern WA Jr (1984) Diagnosis of isolated perforation of the gallbladder following blunt trauma using sonography and CT scan. J Trauma 23:280–281

Hagiwara A, Yukioka T, Katayama M (1993) Streaky soft tissue infiltration appearance ("streaky appearance") of the mesentery by enhanced CT scan in two patients with traumatic intestinal perforation. Jpn Assoc Acute Med 4:144

Hagiwara A, Yukioka T, Satou M, et al (1995) Early diagnosis of small intestine rupture from blunt abdominal trauma using computed tomography: significance of the streaky density within the mesentery. J Trauma 38:630–633

Hamilton P, Rizoli P, McLellan B, Murphy J (1995) Significance of intra-abdominal extraluminal air detected by CT scan in blunt abdominal trauma. J Tauma 39:331–333
Hara H, Babyn PS, Bourgeois D (1992) Significance of bowel wall enhancement on CT following blunt abdominal trauma in childhood. J Comput Assist Tomogr 16:94–98
Haugen SG, Walsh JW, Thompson WM (1995) Imaging of abdominal trauma. Imaging 7:22–32
Hidaka H, Irie H, Hirata H, Shigematsu A, Matsukuma K, Tatsuma T, Era S (1990) Mesenteric hematoma; a pediatric case. Rinsho-Hoshasen 35:525–528
Hofer GA, Cohen AJ (1989) CT signs of duodenal perforation secondary to blunt abdominal trauma. J Comput Assist Tomogr 13:430–432
Jamieson DH, Babyn PS, Pearl R (1996) Imaging gastrointestinal perforation in pediatric blunt abdominal trauma. Pediatr Radiol 26:188–194
Jeffrey RB (1989) CT and sonograph of the acute abdomen. Raven Press, New York
Jeffrey RB Jr, Federle MP (1988) The collapsed inferior vena cava: CT evidence of hypovolemia. AJR Am J Roentgenol 50: 431–432
Jeffrey RB Jr, Federle MP, Wall S (1983) Value of computed tomography in detecting occult gastrointestinal perforation. J Comput Assist Tomogr 7:825–827
Jeffrey RB Jr, Federle MP, Laing FC, Wing VW (1986) Computed tomography of blunt trauma to the gallbladder. J Comput Assist Tomogr 10:756–758
Jeffrey RB Jr, Cardoza JD, Olcott EW (1991) Detention of active intraabdominal arterial hemorrhage: value of dynamic contrast-enhanced CT. AJR Am J Roentgenol 156:725–729
Kane NM, Dorfman GS, Cronan JJ (1987) Efficacy of CT following peritoneal lavage in abdominal trauma. J Comput Assist Tomogr 11:998–1002
Kane NM, Cronan JJ, Dorfman GS, et al (1989) Pediatric abdominal trauma: evaluation by computed tomography. Radiology 170:591
Kane NM, Francis JR, Ellis JH (1989) The value of CT in the detection of bladder and posterior urethral injuries. AJR Am J Roentgenol 153:1243–1246
Kane NM, Francis IR, Burney RE, Wheatley MJ, Ellis JH, Korobkin M (1991) Traumatic pneumoperitoneum: implications of computed tomography diagnosis. Invest Radiol 26:574
Karnaze GC, Sheedy PF II, Stephen DH, McLeod RA (1981) Computed tomography in duodenal rupture due to blunt abdominal trauma. J Comput Assist Tomogr 5:267–269
Karp MP, Cooney Dr, Berger PE, Kuhn JP, Jewett TC (1981) Role of computed tomography in evaluation of blunt abdominal trauma in children. J Pediatr Surg 16:316–323
Kaufman RA, Towbin R, Babcock DS, et al (1984) Upper abdominal trauma in children: imaging evaluation. AJR Am J Roentgenol 142:449–460
Kearney PA Jr, Vahey T, Burney RE, Glazer G (1989) Computed tomography and diagnostic peritoneal lavage in blunt abdominal trauma: their combined role. Arch Surg 124:344–347
Kelly J, Raptopoulos V, Davidoff A, Waite R, Norton R (1989) The value of non-contrast-enhanced CT in blunt abdominal trauma. AJR Am J Roentgenol 152:41–46
Kirks DR, Caron KH, Bisset GS III (1992) CT of blunt abdominal trauma in children: an anatomic "snapshot in time." Radiology 182:633–632
Krudy AG, Doppman JL, Bissonette MB, Girton M (1983) Hemobilia: computed tomographic diagnosis. Radiology 148:785–789
Kunin JR, Korobkin M, Ellis JH, et al (1993) Duodenal injuries caused by blunt abdominal trauma: value of CT in differentiating perforation from hematoma. AJR Am J Roentgenol 160:1221–1223
Lang EK (1990) Intra-abdominal and retroperitoneal organ injuries diagnosed on dynamic computed tomograms obtained for assessment of renal trauma. J Trauma 30:1161–1168
Levine CD, Patel UJ, Wachsberg RH, et al (1995) CT in patients with blunt abdominal trauma: clinical significance of intraperitoneal fluid detected on a scan with otherwise normal findings. AJR Am J Roentgenol 164:1381–1385
Levine CD, Patel UJ, Silverman PM, Wachsberg RH (1996) Low attenuation of acute traumatic hemoperitoneum on CT scans. AJR Am J Roentgenol 166:1089–1093
Lewin JR, Patterson EA (1980) CT recognition of spontaneous intraperitoneal hemorrhage complicating anticoagulant therapy. AJR Am J Roentgenol 134:1271–1272
Lis LE, Cohen AJ (1990) CT cystography in the evaluation of bladder trauma. J Comput Assist Tomogr 14:386–389
Livingston DH, Lavery RF, Passannante MR, et al (1998) Admission or observation is not necessary after a negative abdominal computer scan in patients with suspected blunt abdominal trauma: result of a prospective, multi-institutional trial. J Trauma 44:273–282
Lopez FM, Bloncourt J, Eynius F, et al (1988) Traumatismes abdominaux. In: Lamarque J, Pujol J, Rouanet J (eds)Tomodensitométrie abdominale et pelvienne. Axone, Montpellier
Lowe FC, Fishman EK, Oesterling JE, et al (1989) Computed tomography in diagnosis of bladder rupture. Urology 33:341–343
Maas R, Gurtler KF (1986) Trauma-induced space-occupying lesions. In: Heller M, Jend HH, Genant JK (eds) Computed tomography of trauma. Thieme, Stuttgart New York
Madura MJ, Craig RM, Shields TW (1982) Unusual causes of spontaneous pneumoperitoneum. Surg Gynecol Obstet 154:417–420
Marx JA, Moore EE, Jorden RC, Eule J Jr (1985) Limitations of computed tomography in the evaluation of acute abdominal trauma: a prospective comparison with diagnostic peritoneal lavage. J Trauma 25:933–937
McCort J (1976) Intraperitoneal and retroperitoneal hemorrhage. Radiol Clin North Am 14:391–405
McCort JJ (1987) Caring for the major trauma victim: the role of radiology. Radiology 163:1–9
Mee S, McAninch J, Federle, et al (1987) Computerized tomography in bladder rupture: diagnostic limitations. J Urol 137:207–209
Mindell HJ (1989) On the value of non-contrast-enhanced CT in blunt abdominal trauma. AJR Am J Roentgenol 152:47–48
Mirvis SE (1989) Diagnostic imaging of the urinary system following blunt trauma. Clin Imaging 13:269–280
Mirvis SE, Shanmuganathan K (1992) Computed tomography in blunt trauma. Semin Roentgenol 28:150–183
Mirvis SE, Gens DR, Shanmuganathan K (1992) Rupture of the bowel after blunt abdominal trauma: diagnosis with CT. AJR Am J Roentgenol 159:1217–1221
Miyakawa K, Kaji T, Wakabayashi M, Hoshikawa Y, Tani I, Ashida H, Ishikawa T (1992) CT of intestinal injuries following blunt trauma. Nippon Igaku Hoshasen Gakkai Zasshi 52:1653–60

Motateanu M, Mirescu D, Schwieger AF, Laverriere C (1992) Computed tomography of retroperitoneal duodenal rupture in blunt abdominal trauma. Eur J Radiol 15:163–165

New PFJ, Aronow S (1976) Attenuation measurements of whole blood fractions in computed tomography. Radiology 121:635–640

Nghiem HV, Jeffrey RB Jr, Mindelzun RE (1993) CT of blunt trauma to the bowel and mesentery. AJR Am J Roentgenol 160:53–58

Nghiem HV, Jeffrey RB, Mindelzun RE (1995) CT of blunt trauma to the bowel and mesentery. Semin US CT MRI 16:82–90

Orwig D, Federle MP (1989) Localized clotted blood as evidence of visceral trauma on CT: the sentinel clot sign. AJR Am J Roentgenol 153:747–749

Peitzman AB, Makaroun MS, Slasky BS, Ritter P (1986) Prospective study of computed tomography in initial management of blunt abdominal trauma. J Trauma 26:585–592

Pombo F, Arrojo L, Perez Fonta J (1991) Haemoperitoneum secondary to spontaneous rupture of hepatocellular carcinoma: CT diagnosis. Clin Radiol 43:321

Procacci C, Bicego E, Domperi P, Zimbardo L, Minniti S, Laganà D (1991) La TAC nell'imaging integrato dei traumi dei visceri pelvici. In: Romagnoli R, Del Vecchio E (eds) Diagnostica per immagini nelle urgenze. Idelson, Naples

Radin DR (1991) Intramural and intraperitoneal hemorrhage due to duodenal ulcer. AJR Am J Roentgenol 157:45

Raghavendra BN, Grieco AJ, Balthazar EJ, Megibow AJ, Subramanyam BR (1982) Diagnostic utility of sonograph and computed tomography in spontaneous mesenteric hematoma. Am J Gastroenterol 77:570–573

Rizzo MJ, Federle MP, Griffiths BG (1989) Bowel and mesenteric injury following blunt abdominal trauma: evaluation with CT. Radiology 173:143–148

Roberts JL (1996) CT of abdominal and pelvic trauma. Semin Ultrasound CT MRI 17:142–169

Rozler MH, Saxe J, MC Carroll KA (1995) Detection of free intraperitoneal air on computed tomography after blunt abdominal trauma. Emerg Radiol 2:84–89

Rubin GD, Jeffrey RB Jr, Walter JF (1991) Pancreatic microcystic adenoma presenting with acute hemoperitoneum: CT diagnosis. AJR Am J Roentgenol 156:749

Sandler CM, Hall JT, Rodriguez MB, et al (1986) Bladder injury in blunt pelvic trauma. Radiology 158:633–638

Shanmuganathan K, Mirvis S, Sover E (1993) Value of contrast enhanced CT in detecting active hemorrhage in patients with blunt abdominal or pelvic trauma. AJR Am J Roentgenol 161:65–69

Shanmuganathan K, Mirvis S, Reaney SM (1995) Pictorial review: CT appearances of contrast medium extravasation associated with injury sustained from blunt abdominal trauma. Clin Radiology 50:182–187

Shanmuganathan K, Mirvis S, Sherbourne CD, Chiu WC, Rodriguez A (1999) Hemoperitoneum as the sole indicator of abdominal visceral injuries: a potential limitation of screening abdominal US for trauma. Radiology 212:423–430

Sher R, Frydman GM, Russell TJ, O'Donnell C (1996) Computed tomography detection of active mesenteric hemorrhage following blunt abdominal trauma. Trauma Injury Infect Crit Care 40:469–471

Sherck JP, Oakes DD (1990) Intestinal injuries missed by computed tomography. J Trauma 30:1–7

Shin MS, Berland LL, Ho KJ (1990) Small aorta: CT detection and clinical significance. J Comput Assist Tomogr 14:102–103

Shuman WP (1997) CT of blunt abdominal trauma in adults. Radiology 205:297–306

Sivit CJ, Peclet M, Taylor GA (1989) Life threatening intraperitoneal bleeding: demonstration with CT. Radiology 171:430

Sivit CJ, Taylor GA, Bulas DI, et al (1991a) Blunt trauma in children: significance of peritoneal fluid. Radiology 178:185

Sivit CJ, Taylor GA, Bulas DI, Bowman LM, Eichelberger MR (1991b) Blunt trauma in children: significance of peritoneal fluid. Radiology 178:185–188

Sivit CJ, Taylor GA, Bulas DI, Kushner DC, Potter BM, Eichelberger MR (1992) Post traumatic shock in children: CT findings associated with hemodynamic instability. Radiology 182:723–726

Sivit CJ, Eichelberger MR, Taylor GA (1994) CT in children with rupture of the bowel caused by blunt trauma: Diagnostic efficacy and comparison with hypoperfusion complex. AJR Am J Roentgenol 193:1195

Sivit CJ, Frazier AA, Eichelberger MR (1995a) Prevalence and distribution of hemorrhage associated with splenic injury in children. Radiology 197:298

Sivit CJ, Cutting JP, Eichelberger MR (1995b) CT diagnosis and localisation of rupture of the bladder in children with blunt abdominal trauma: significance of contrast extravasation in pelvis. AJR Am J Roentgenol 1243–1246

Skala J, Witte C, Bruna J, Case T, Finley P (1992) Chyle leakage after blunt trauma. Lymphology 25:62–68

Sorkey AJ, Farnell MB, Williams HJ Jr, et al (1990) Complementary roles of diagnostic peritoneal lavage and computed tomography in the evaluation of blunt abdominal trauma. Radiology 175:289

Strouse PJ, Close BJ, Marshall KW, et al (1999) CT of bowel and mesenteric trauma in children. Radiographics 19:1237–1250

Taylor GA, Fallat ME, Eichelberger MR (1987) Hypovolemic shock in children: abdominal CT manifestations. Radiology 165:643–646

Taylor GA, Fallat ME, Potter BM, Eichelberger ME (1988)The role of computed tomography in blunt abdominal trauma in children. J Trauma 28:1660–1664

Taylor GA, Guion CJ, Potter BM, Eichelberger MR (1989) CT of blunt abdominal trauma in children. AJR Am J Roentgenol 153:555–559

Taylor GA, Kaufman RA, Sivit CJ (1994) Active hemorrhage in children after thoracoabdominal trauma: Clinical and CT features. AJR Am J Roentgenol 162:401

Trerotola SO, Kuhlman JE, Fishman EK (1990) Bleeding complications of femoral catheterization: CT evaluation. Radiology 174:37

Watanabe AT, Jeffrey RB (1987) CT diagnosis of traumatic rupture of the cisterna chyli. J Comput Assist Tomogr 11:175–176

Wing VW, Federle MP, Morris JA Jr, Jeffrey RB, Bluth R (1985) The clinical impact of CT for blunt abdominal trauma. AJR Am J Roentgenol 145:1191–1194

Wolfman NT, Bechtold RE, Scharling ES, Meredith JW (1992) Blunt upper abdominal trauma: evaluation by CT. AJR Am J Roentgenol 158:493–501

Wolverson MK, Crepps LF, Sundaram M, Heiberg E, Vas WG, Shields JB (1983) Hyperdensity of recent hemorrhage at body computed tomography: incidence and morphologic variation. Radiology 148:779–784

9 Other Nonneoplastic Pathologies

CONTENTS

9.1 Diffused Mesenteric Amyloidosis

Amyloidosis is a multisystemic disease of unknown etiology, characterized by extracellular deposits of amyloid protein and by fibrosis around and inside the walls of the vessels located in one or more organs or tissues.

It may be a primary disease (LA amyloidosis), in which case the amyloid protein is a light chain monoclonal immunoglobulin and it is related to multiple myeloma, or a secondary disease (AA amyloidosis), which is a reactive phenomenon during infections or chronic inflammatory processes.

Only two cases of amyloidosis with a mesenteric localization (Allen et al. 1985; Raffi et al. 1985) have been observed on CT examination. CT revealed a diffuse soft-tissue infiltration of the mesentery with encasement of mesenteric vessels. An exploratory laparotomy showed a diffuse and uniform thickening of the mesentery, the omentum and the peritoneal surface.

The authors compared this CT image with that of peritoneal carcinosis. We believe that the clinical manifestations considered together with the observed mesenteric (not peritoneal) location, the absence of ascites, the uniform orientation, the spread over the entire mesentery and the vascular involvement should have led to the suspicion of amyloidosis.

9.2 Omental Infarction

Omental infarction is a rare, but well-defined, acute abdominal pathology, which preferentially affects the right side of the omentum; it is due to reduced vascularization induced by an arterial or venous obstruction. It may be idiopathic or can be caused by torsion of the greater omentum or by traumatic or surgical adhesions; it can also occur during chronic pancreatitis.

The infarcted omental segment varies in extension and may show different levels of pathological alteration, such as congestion, hemorrhage, liponecrosis, peritoneal serohematic effusion, or inflammatory infiltration. The lesions tend to remain circumscribed or to heal spontaneously without residua or with retracting fibrous scars; autoamputation also sometimes occurs (Puylaert 1992), and occasionally an omental abscess develops (Balthazar and Lefkowitz 1993).

Patients suffer acute or subacute pain, usually located in the right inferior abdominal region; moderate leukocytosis and sometimes fever are present. On clinical examination, omental infarction is usually confused with acute appendicitis or, less frequently, with cholecystitis. Echographic and CT examinations exclude these latter pathologies and indicate the correct diagnosis (Balthazar and Lefkowitz 1993; Ceuterick et al 1987; Puylaert 1992).

The echographic examination shows the omental infarction as a well-limited, noncompressible ovoid or cake-like flat solid mass, which is moderately hyperechogenic, located behind the anterior abdominal wall. The mass is painful when it is directly pressed with the transducer.

CT shows the omental infarct as a solid circumscribed mass, which is slightly denser than adipose tissue and is crossed by streaks of hyperattenuation. The definition of its contours varies, and it makes close contact with the abdominal wall, pushing the intestinal loops backward. When an abscess develops inside the mass, a fluid area becomes visible (Fig. 9.1).

After exclusion of inflammatory diseases of visceral origin (appendicitis, cholecystitis, diverticulitis, pancreatitis), no other problems of differential diagnosis against abdominal pathologies characterized by acute onset must be expected.

If the omental infarction has been caused by torsion of the omentum, the mass shows a complex shape: a fibrous structure concentrically around the point of torsion with interposed hypodense necrotic areas and fat (GRASSI et al. 1996).

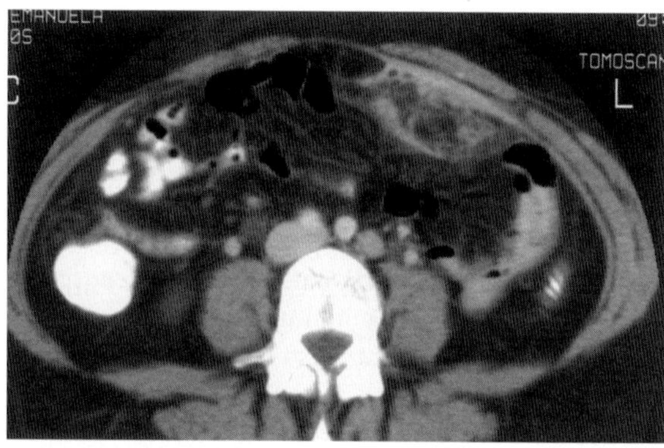

Fig. 9.1. Omental infarction with purulent and necrotic areas. Well-limited nonhomogeneous left paramedian mesogastric mass containing omental fat, dense spots and a purulent collection surrounded by a thin capsule

9.3 Focal Necrosis of the Omentum

During the evolution of acute pancreatitis, besides the well-known retro- and intraperitoneal alterations, focal necrosis of the omental adipose tissue may occur. This phenomenon is seen clinically as an indolent epigastric swelling with echographic aspects of a well-limited mass with a mixed solid and cystic structure. CT does not only confirm this structure, but also localizes it to the omental site next to the anterior abdominal wall (HAYNES et al. 1985).

The diagnosis is usually suggested by the concomitant presence of a nonhomogeneous omental mass with acute and recurrent pancreatitis.

9.4 Foreign Bodies

9.4.1 Gossypibomas

Intraabdominal foreign bodies are almost always retained surgical towels or sponges made of cotton or synthetic fibers and surrounded by a reaction, by which they tend to be isolated or encysted.

The retained sponges or towels, being made of inert materials, do not undergo any degradation, specific decomposition, or biochemical process and they produce two types of body response: an aseptic fibrinous reaction with complete fibrous encapsulation and formation of a foreign body granuloma (CHOI et al. 1988; SHEWARD et al. 1986) and a nonspecific exudative reaction, which often leads to abscess formation resulting from secondary bacterial invasion (CHOI et al. 1988). This latter response represents an attempt to expel the foreign body, but it may cause postsurgical complications, such as external or intestinal fistulae with perforation and/or obstruction.

Foreign body granulomas are usually asymptomatic, unless secondary inflammatory complications occur, and may be found occasionally (even years after surgery) when a CT of the abdomen is performed for other reasons.

In contrast, the exudative reactions produce precocious and often severe clinical symptoms; septic complications are not rare.

The CT image of a gossypiboma reflects the pathological aspect. The foreign body granuloma may resemble that of the original tissue that has formed it (laparotomic towel or surgical sponge); in contrast, it may show a completely aspecific shape. In the former case, a sharply outlined low-density (20–30) spherical or ovoid mass may be observed with denser, structured (even calcified) images inside, which are sometimes recognizable only with narrow windows. These structures have been described as spoked-wheel, whirl-like, spongiform (PARIENTY et al. 1981), whorled (STEWARD et al. 1986), having multiple linear infolded density (BUY et al. 1989), wavy and striped (CHOI et al. 1988), and spotted (CHOI et al. 1988). The wall of the mass may be extremely thin and undetectable, or it may be seen as a thin border, enhancing only slightly or not at all, surrounding the gossypiboma (Fig. 9.2). Older gossypibomas have a thick and high-attenuation capsule, whose contrast enhancement is marked and persistent After many years the capsule may calcify.

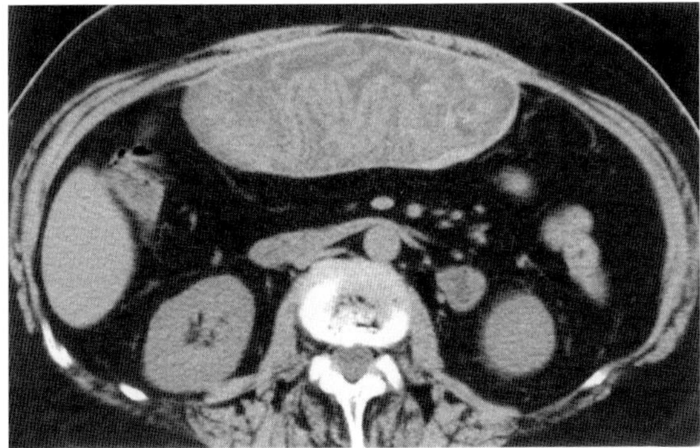

Fig. 9.2. Gossypiboma. Typical serpiginous strands of the gauze, well limited by thin dense rim

Furthermore, the presence of a foreign body granuloma is also suggested by a spongiform pattern, characterized by small air bubbles trapped between sponges or towels in a fluid environment, and by a well-encapsulated mass with a denser fibrous tissue. Some authors regard this appearance as a sign of abscessed gossypiboma. Kopka et al. (1996) believe that the bubbles are a characteristic sign of gossypiboma owing to the persistence of air, which may go on for as much as 6 months after surgery (Kopka et al. 1996).

Granulomatous gossypibomas may also show aspecific non diagnostic findings: mass with large nonhomogeneous low-density core without typical spongiform structures inside surrounded by a thick dense, strong and prolonged contrast enhancing wall. According to Kokuba et al. (1987), this pattern is suggestive of gossypiboma in asymptomatic patients with a history of surgery. Only the clinical manifestations permit the differentiation with an abdominal abscess. Kopka et al. (1996) reported similar findings, but without a strongly enhancing rim, very probably due to fibrous and poorly vascularized tissue.

When a gossypiboma is characterized by an aspecific exudative reaction, it appears as a large mass made up of a nonhomogeneous increase in the density of the adipose tissue that has been incorporated. The mass is crossed by strips, some of which appear to be characteristic of the gauze fibers; as in a foreign body granuloma, these strips are wavy, whirl-like, spiral, linear or spoke-wheel. The wall is made up of a thin dense linear image around the swelling mass. The abscessed collection that has developed inside the granuloma has a homogeneous water density (Fig. 9.3). The omental adipose cellular around the mass is often slightly shaded.

There are no problems with differential diagnosis in typical cases, whereas the atypical forms must be specifically distinguished from postsurgical encysted hematomas. These structures resemble gossypibomas with a pseudocystic aspect; differences are evident in the case of calcareous deposits, which are peripheral in the hematoma and central in the gossypiboma.

The granulomatous masses with a thick and regular wall and a water-density content may be confused with lymph node colliquative metastases. When present, the unique differential element is represented by the persistent increased density of the wall.

A dense nonhomogeneous mass may resemble the nodular form of panniculitis, from which the gossypiboma can be distinguished especially because it shows a characteristic persistence of the postcontrast peripheral density; on the other hand, the presence of negative attenuation areas is typical of the adipose component of panniculitis.

The forms containing small gas bubbles may be confused with fecal material. Differential elements are the usual location of the scatomas and the thickness of the wall: the intestinal wall is thin and uniform with a sharp profile, whereas that of the gossypiboma is thickened and hyperenhancing after contrast medium (Choi et al. 1988).

In the case of infections, the clinical pattern and the CT aspect of a gossypiboma resemble those of an

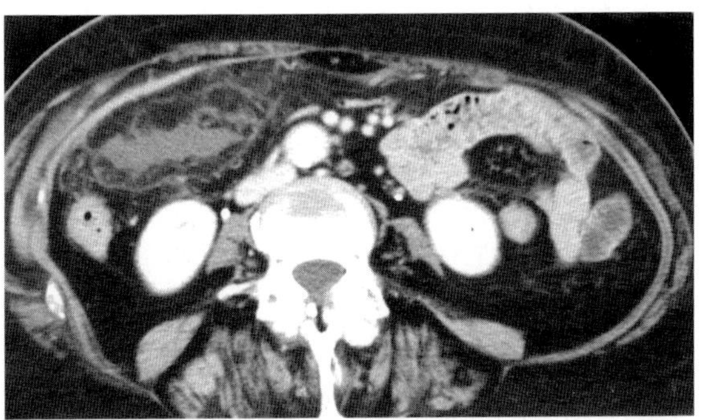

A

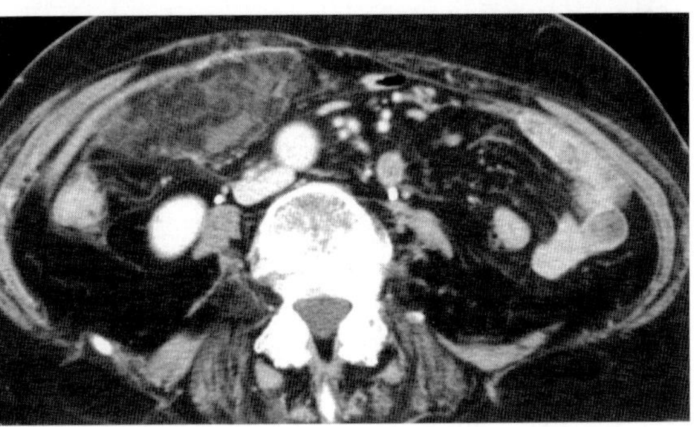

B

Fig. 9.3A, B. Abscessed exudative gossypiboma. Omental ovoid mass well limited by a dense and thin capsule showing a serpiginous structure and a wide near water-density area

abscess, except for the presence of the foreign body inside the collection.

Finally, a gossypiboma perforating the intestinal wall cannot be distinguished from the omental or subperitoneal collections secondary to dehiscence of anastomoses or postsurgical dilacerations of the intestinal wall, because both pathological conditions have the same CT aspect.

9.4.2 Gallstones and Intraperitoneal Clips (Cliptomas)

Gallstones or surgical clips used to clamp the cystic artery or the cystic duct may slip during laparoscopic cholecystectomy in the peritoneum and fall preferentially into the pelvis, Morrison's recess and/or the right iliac fossa, inducing an aseptic reaction with development of foreign body granulomas, fibrosis, or adhesions. These may be asymptomatic and be detected incidentally during CT studies done postoperatively or they may cause recurrent abdominal or back pain, simulating ureteral calculi or appendicitis.

Both gallstones or clip granulomas (clip granulomas) are easily recognizable on CT. Gallstones are suggested by intraperitoneal low density or more often opaque, or by stratified nodules surrounded by dense tissue. The cliptomas have a characteristic metallic high attenuation that permit their identification.

9.5 Castleman's Disease

Castleman's disease is a lymphoproliferative disorder reported under many different terms, including giant lymph node hyperplasia, lymphoid hamartoma, and angiomatous lymphoid hyperplasia. It is mostly located in the mediastinum and rarely in other sites.

Macroscopically, the lymph nodes affected by the disease make up a single spherical or ovoid mass with a smooth surface.

Histologically, it is characterized by hyperplasia of lymphoid follicles with vascular proliferation (hyaline vascular type) or with mature plasma cells and relativity few capillaries (plasma cell type). The hyaline vascular kind is the most common solitary type (80–90%) and has a benign course. The plasma cell type may be solitary or may have multicentric involvement; it is associated with fever, weight loss, multifocal lymphadenopathy, and splenomegaly. Its clinical course is either variable, with periods of remission and exacerbation, or aggressive, and often fatal.

At the abdominal level, it appears as a mass, which is usually isolated and asymptomatic; it is occasionally found during echographic or CT examinations.

Only five cases of a mesenteric localization of this disease examined with CT have been reported in the literature (Ferreiros et al. 1989; Iida et al. 1983; Libson et al. 1988). They have been described as homogeneous, solid and well-defined lymph nodal masses, which may have an early marked enhancement (Ferreiros et al. 1989; Iida et al. 1983) or low or absent increase in attenuation after i.v. contrast injection (Libson et al. 1988). The former correspond to the hyaline vascular and the latter, to the poorly vascularized plasmacellular type, respectively.

9.6 Whipple's Disease

Whipple's disease is a rare multisystemic bacterial process that mostly affects the small bowel, joint capsules, lymph nodes, and central nervous system. Clinically it is characterized by malabsorption, intermittent diarrhea, steatorrhea, abdominal pain, weight loss often preceded by arthralgia, and fever. It is associated with abdominal and pelvic masses and peripheral lymphadenopathies.

Macroscopically, Whipple's disease is characterized by thickening of the small bowel folds and enlargement of the mesenteric lymph nodes. Thickening of the folds is due to dilatation of the lymphatics filled with macrophages containing Whipple's bacilli. The enlargement of the mesenteric lymph nodes is caused by massive fatty acid infiltration of the marginal sinus, which obstructs the lymphatic flux and contributes to a further lymphangiomatous distension of the intestinal lymphatic collectors. The enlarged lymph nodes may blend in a voluminous mass (Rijke al. 1983; de Wazières et al. 1993).

Radiological examination of the gastrointestinal tract characteristically shows prominent mucosal folds of the small bowel and nodularities, mostly in the distal duodenum and in the jejunum, which are due to lymphangectasiae.

In patients affected by malabsorption syndrome, the disease may be suggested by the echographic finding of multiple enlarged hyperechoic mesenteric lymph nodes and by the CT pattern of numerous enlarged lymph nodes with a low-attenuation center (-4/+10 HU) and denser rim. These lymph nodes may reach 3–4 cm in diameter, remaining isolated or joining together in larger masses. The echographic and CT aspects of the adenopathies reflect the massive lipidic infiltration of the lymph nodes.

Enlarged and hollow mesenteric lymph nodes are not specific for Whipple's disease, because they may be found in AIDS-related tuberculosis, in treated lymphomas, and in metastases.

A peroral biopsy of the distal duodenal mucosa can confirm the hypotheses suggested by imaging examinations, showing numerous macrophages that contain large granules of glycoproteins in the cytoplasm and *Tropheryma whippelii* (the bacillus responsible for the disease) in various disintegration phases and are positive to periodic acid–Schiff reagent (PAS) in the lamina propria. Bacilli and macrophages are present in all tissues; they decrease in frequency and disappear after antibiotic treatment.

9.7 Intestinal Perforation

Perforation of the intestinal wall may be caused by any of several lesions: gastroduodenal peptic ulcers, diverticula, tumors (especially of the sigmoid colon), dehiscence of anastomoses, traumas, Crohn's disease. The perforation allows the passage of air, gastric secretions, food, bile, and pancreatic fluid into the peritoneal cavity or the subperitoneal spaces. The initial irritation of the peritoneum or of the subperitoneal cellular is followed by an inflammatory process after 36–48 h. The perforation into the peritoneal cavity may be blocked by a reactive response, which surround it with a limiting barrier, or may extend further. Therefore, the intraperitoneal fluid collections tend to spread into the lowest spaces (right subhepatic recess, right paracolic gutter, pelvic cavities), whereas the subperitoneal collections expand slowly, detaching the fat as far as necessary for them to penetrate the retroperitoneum.

An acute perforation produces very violent pain and tension of the abdominal wall, and this makes it difficult to establish the site of the pain by means of abdominal palpation. A perforation may also occur slowly and insidiously, with unspecific clinical signs, and be masked by the general pattern of the underlying disease or simulate an inflammatory process (cholecystitis, pancreatitis or acute appendicitis). When it is possible, a careful history provides the opportunity to make a correct diagnosis, or at least suggests it when gastric or duodenal ulcer, Crohn's disease, or colon-sigmoidal diverticula are present. Analogously, a slight recovery, the presence of fever, a focal pain or the development of acute symptoms of peritonitis in a patient who has recently undergone an operation must suggest the possibility of an abscessed collection or dehiscence of an anastomosis.

The *CT findings* in intestinal perforation are summarized in Table 9.1. Free air outside the intestinal loops in the peritoneal cavity or in the sub- or retroperitoneal spaces is a specific sign of intestinal perforation, and allows it to be correctly recognized in 100% of cases (Angelelli and Macarini 1996; Donohue et al. 1987; Rizzo et al. 1989; Stapakis and Thickman 1992). However, it is seen only in under 50% of intestinal perforations. CT can show quite small amounts of extraluminal air, which must be carefully searched for with wide or lung-setting windows in the sites where it usually spreads (Fig. 9.4). In the peritoneal cavity the gas is rarely blocked at the site of the perforation, but it rapidly reaches the anterosuperior part of the compartment it has penetrated. Therefore, the position of the air may suggest the site of the perforation (Table 9.1). The air located in the subphrenic spaces and in front of the liver is usually released by a lesion of the anterior gastric or duodenal wall or by a perforation of the submesocolic organs, mostly of the appendix (Figs. 9.5, 9.6). In the latter case, we also observe the presence of gas and fluids around the cecum and in the right paracolic gutter (Fig. 9.5). Care must be taken, because a

Table 9.1. Preferential positions of gas and collections according to site of intestinal perforation

Gas and collections	Site of lesion
Subphrenic peritoneal space	Gastric and duodenal anterior wall Appendix
Lesser sac	Posterior wall of the stomach
Gastrohepatic ligament	Lesser curvature of the stomach
Gastrosplenic or gastrocolic ligament	Greater curvature of the stomach
Retroperitoneum	Postbulbar duodenum
Transverse mesocolon	Transverse colon
Mesenteric folds	Small bowel
Lateroconal space	Ascending or descending colon Appendix
Paracolic gutter	Ascending or descending colon Appendix
Sigmoid mesocolon	Sigmoid
Parasigmoidal or pelvic peritoneal cavity	Colon-sigmoid Appendix

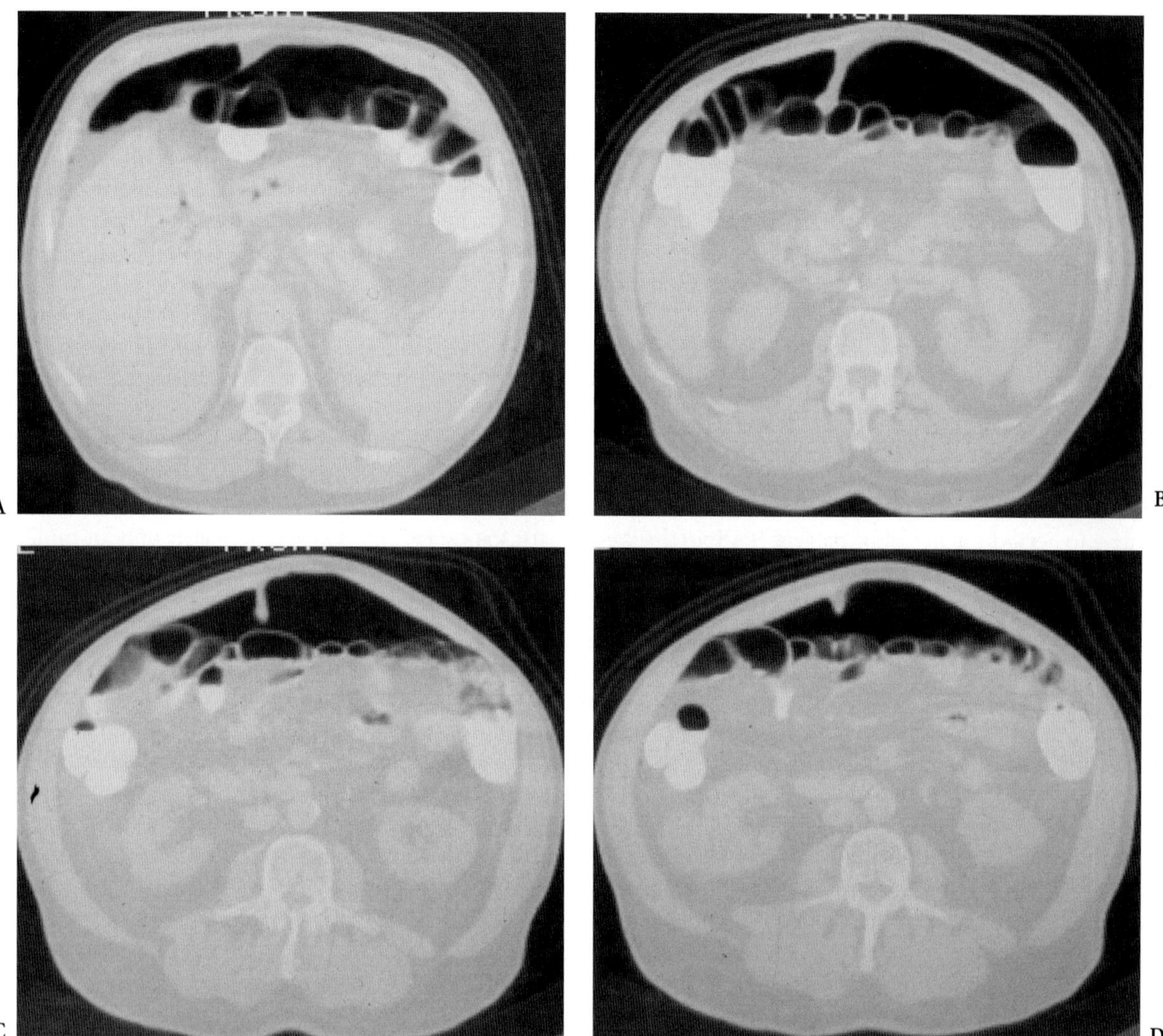

Fig. 9.4A–D. Spontaneous relapsing pneumoperitoneum. Gas occupies and swells the right and left supramesocolic cavities, which are separated at a high level by the falciform ligament and by the ligamentum teres (**A**, **B**); these cavities freely communicate at a low level where these ligaments are not present (**C**, **D**)

subphrenic gas accumulation may be confused with a pneumothorax or with an emphysematous hyperexpansion of the lung that penetrates between the anterior thoracic wall and the diaphragm. However, a correct identification can be obtained just by following the continuation and orientation of the falciform images in the different scans. Air in the lesser sac is typical of perforations of the posterior gastric wall.

It is most common for peritoneal submesocolic perforations to occur at the appendicular and sigmoidal level, with initial penetration of gas into the paracecal and parasigmoidal recess, respectively, and subsequent rapid spread behind the anterior abdominal wall into the median recess between the expansions of the rectus muscles and/or in the pararectal recesses on both sides of these muscles (Fig. 9.10).

When perforations go through into the ligamental or mesenteric subperitoneal spaces small bubbles of gas tend to remain in a circumscribed space next to the lesion of the intestinal wall, suggesting the site of the lesion (Table 9.1). This is placed along the lesser curvature of the stomach if the gas is located in the gastrohepatic ligament; along the greater curvature if it has penetrated the gastrosplenic or the gastrocolic ligament; in the cecum or in the sigmoid if the gas is found in the pericecal (Fig. 9.8) or perisigmoidal (Fig. 9.9) fat, respectively.

When the perforation is in the ascending or the descending colon, the gas preferentially penetrates

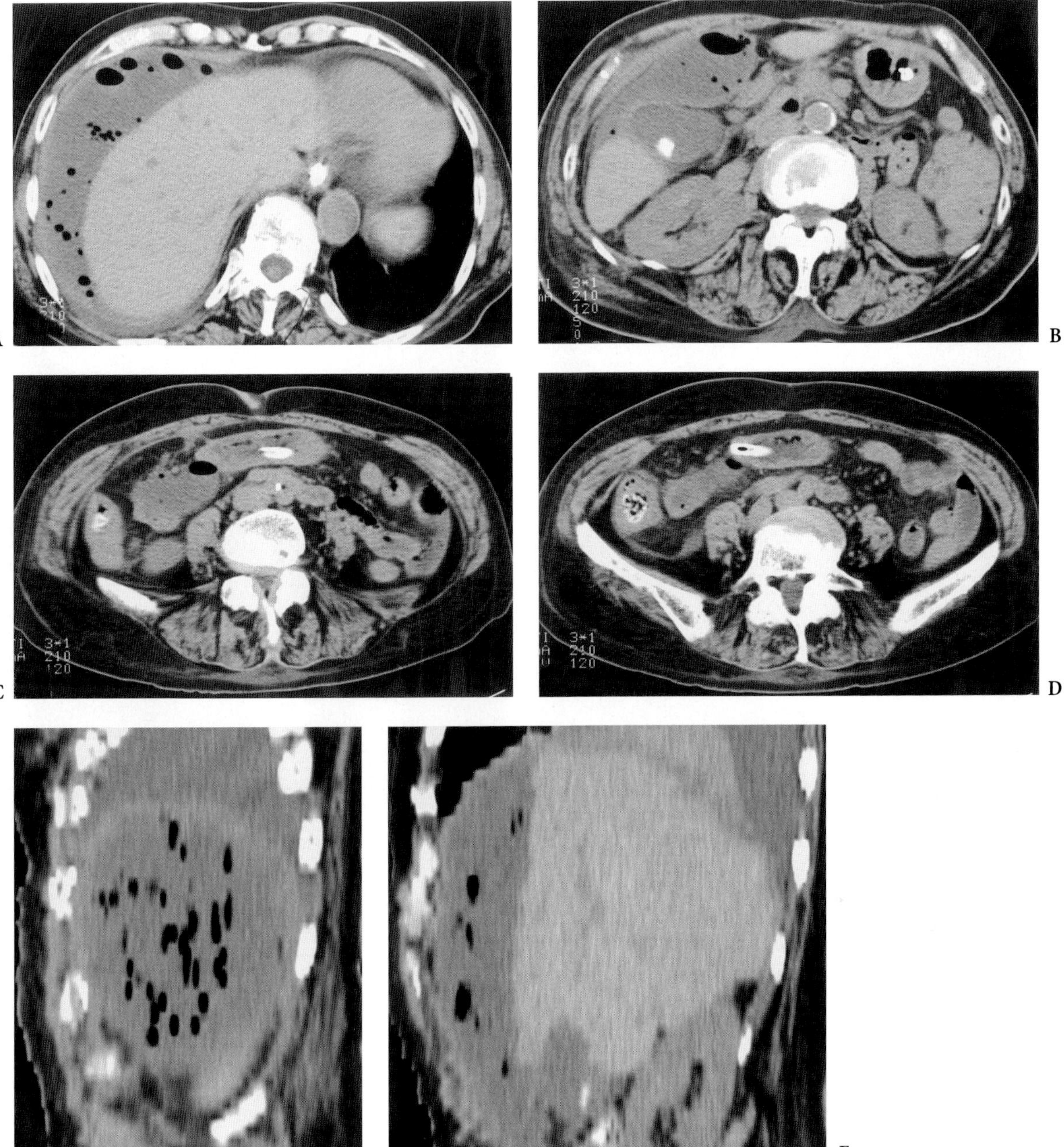

Fig. 9.5. A–D Perforated appendicitis with large abscessed collection in the perihepatic spaces, paracolic gutter and right mesenterocolic cavity. **E, F** The sagittal reconstruction in the right lateral planes shows the continuity of the collection in the supra- and submesocolic spaces

the pericolic retroperitoneal space (lateroconal compartments), and occasionally the mesocolon (when it is well developed), or spreads into the peritoneal cavity (Fig. 9.10).

Small bowel perforations usually do not involve any free air in the mesentery or in the peritoneal cavity, because it is almost completely absent from these viscera.

In the postbulbar duodenal perforations, the gas accumulates in the retroperitoneal spaces around this intestinal tract, next to the pancreatic head (Fig. 9.11). Furthermore, the gas may also spread into the retroperitoneum from the subperitoneal spaces after perforation of the hollow organs located in the subperitoneal spaces, because of detachment of the fat at the sides of the vessels, or direct-

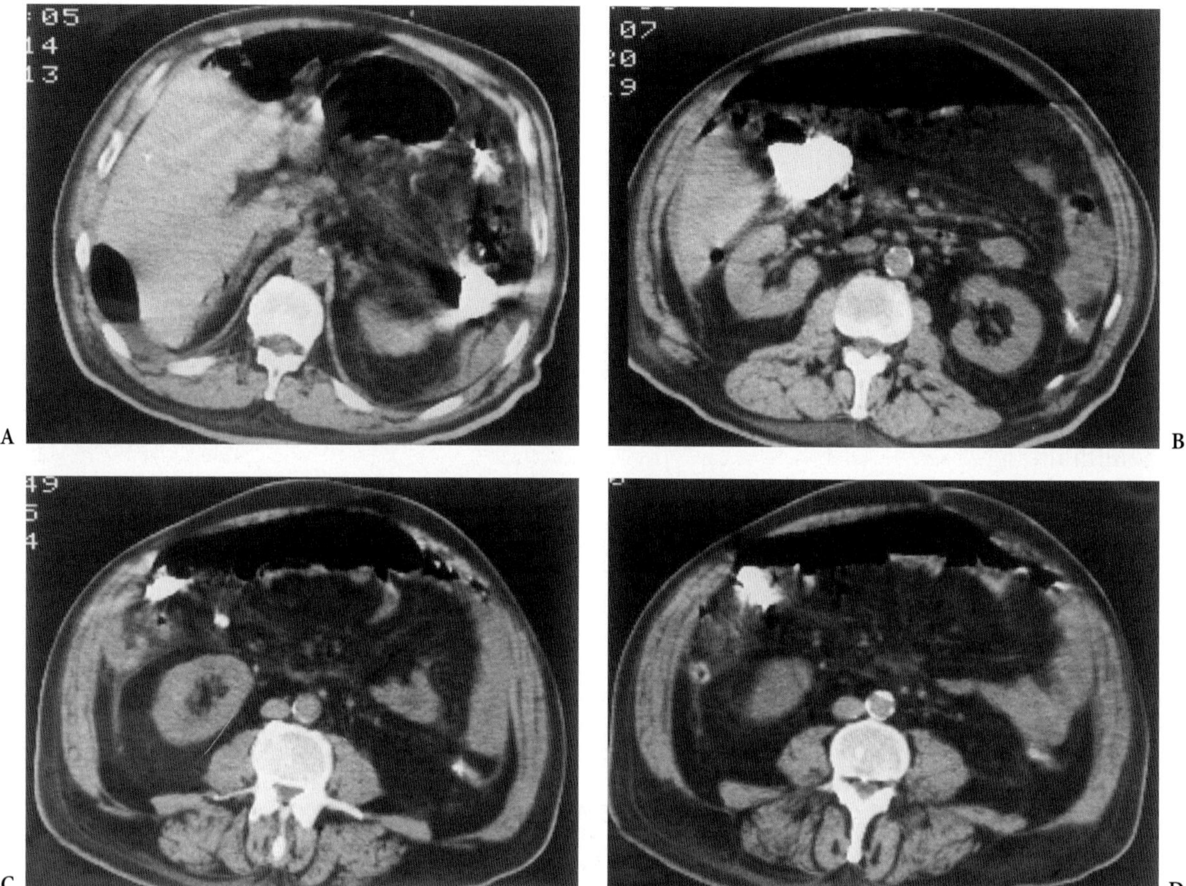

Fig. 9.6A–D. Retrocecal acute appendicitis with perforation into the peritoneal cavity. Transversely sectioned appendix, which appears as a hyperdense ring. (**D**) Increased density of the periappendiceal fat anteriorly. Wide collection with air-fluid level throughout the anterior peritoneal spaces

ly after dehiscence of enteroenteric anastomoses (Fig. 9.12).

Another sign of intestinal perforation is the presence of fluid collections in the peritoneal cavity or in the sub- or retroperitoneal spaces at mesenteric level. Sometimes, this may be the only sign of a perforation, as it usually occurs after a trauma of the small bowel; however, in the large intestine the collections are more often associated with bubbles or air-fluid levels.

Fluid collections in the peritoneal cavity tend to descend quickly to the lowest parts of the compartment in which the perforation has occurred: in the subhepatic Morrison's recess following supramesocolic perforations; in the pelvic spaces, particularly in the pouch of Douglas, in the case of submesocolic lesions. However, the wide communication inside the peritoneal cavity, especially on the right, allows fluid collections of submesocolic (e.g. appendicular) origin to spread into the subhepatic and subphrenic recesses (Figs. 9.5, 9.6) and those of supramesocolic (e.g., gastric or duodenal) origin downward into the pelvic spaces (Figs. 9.12).

Perforations of the posterior gastric wall when the stomach is full may cause gas-free, fluid or dense collections in the lesser sac (Fig. 9.7).

When the outflow of gas and liquids from the bowel after perforation is abundant, the resulting wide swelling of the peritoneal cavity, with air-fluid levels in all planes between the diaphragm and the pelvis (Fig. 9.6), makes it impossible to establish the site and the cause of the perforation; it may be suspected only when a known pathology is present or after recent surgery (dehiscence of anastomosis).

In most cases, the fluid collections located in the subperitoneal spaces are mixed with gas bubbles. However, an isolated juxtaintestinal collection at the mesenteric level is often the only sign of a perforation, because of the virtual absence of air in the jejunoileal tract. A perforation may also occur in extrafascial spaces or structures (Fig. 9.13).

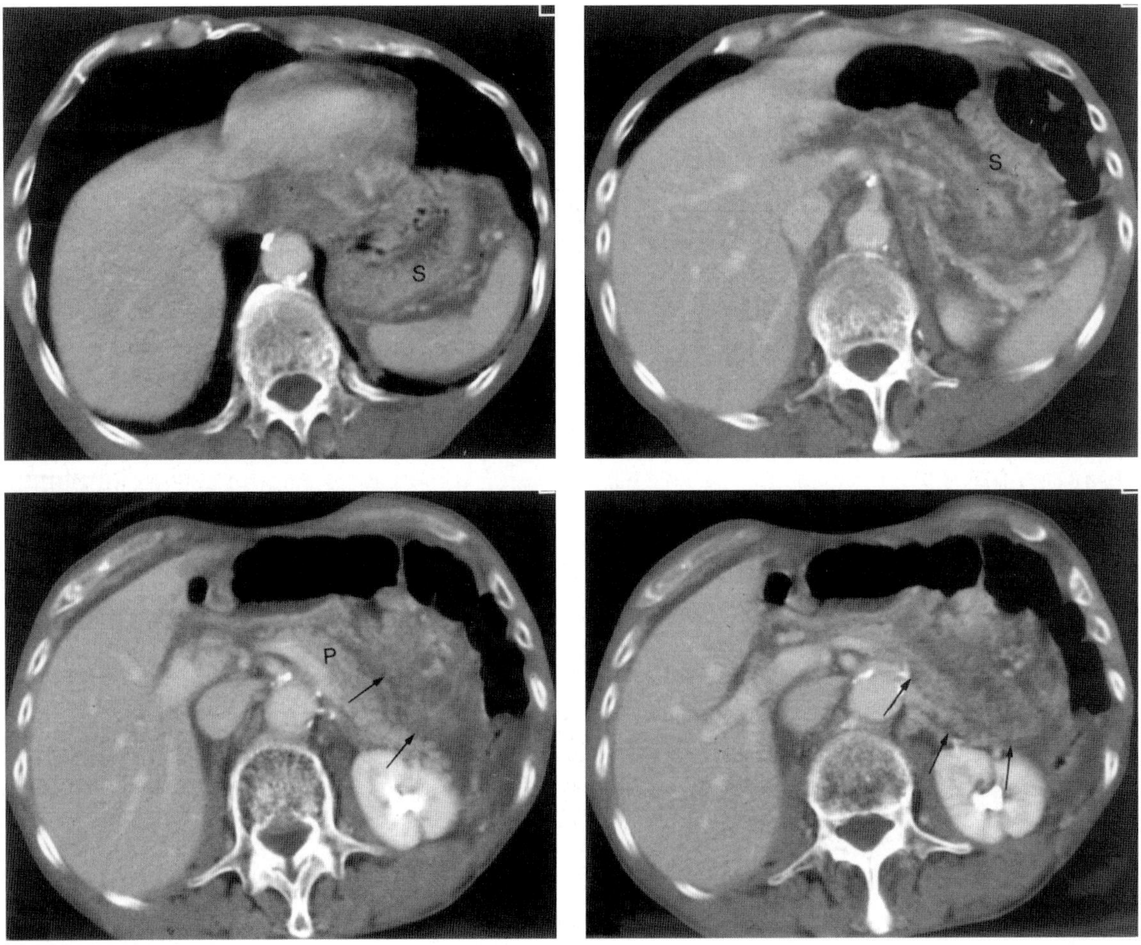

Fig. 9.7A–D. Posterior gastric wall ulcer that has perforated into the lesser sac. Wide collection (*arrows*) in the lesser sac. A small amount of fluid has penetrated the right subhepatic recesses through Winslow's foramen

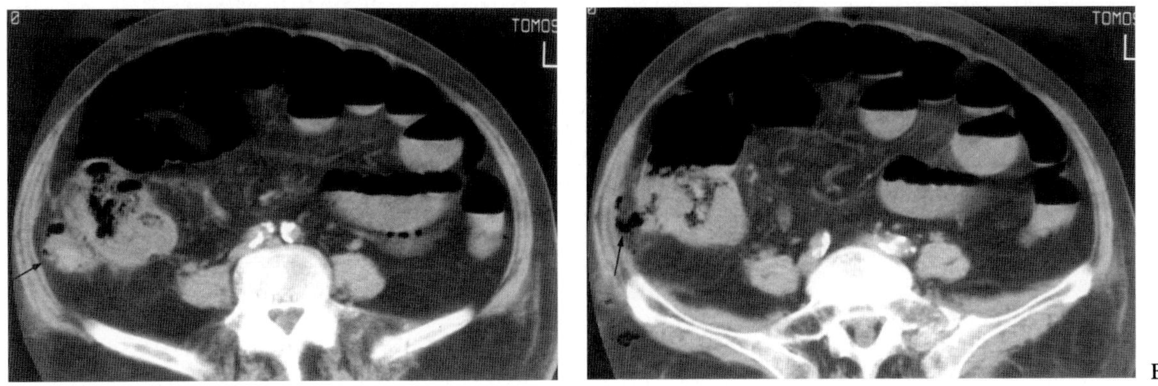

Fig. 9.8A, B. Perforation of the cecum. Small air-fluid collection (*arrow*) in the adipose tissue outside the cecum

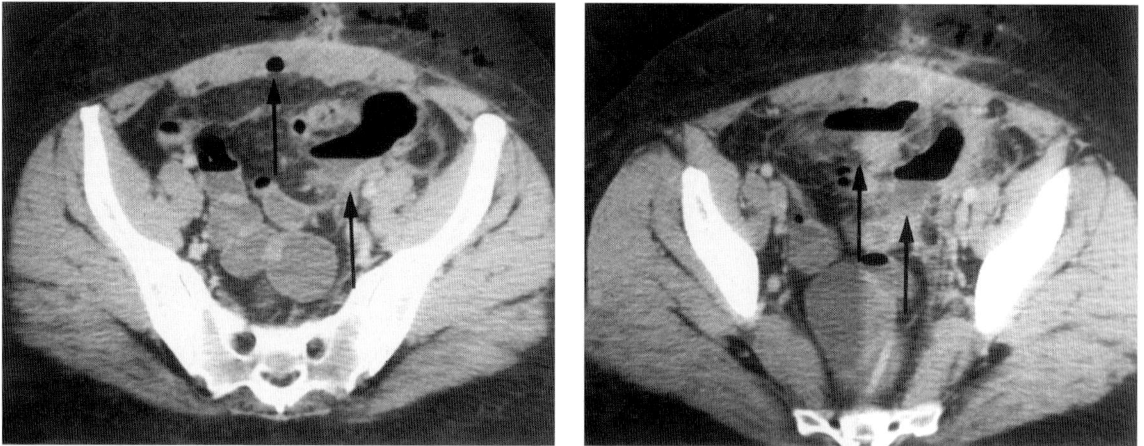

Fig. 9.9A, B. Subperitoneal sigmoidal perforation. Air-fluid collection in the sigmoid mesosigma (*arrows*). Enterocutaneous fistula

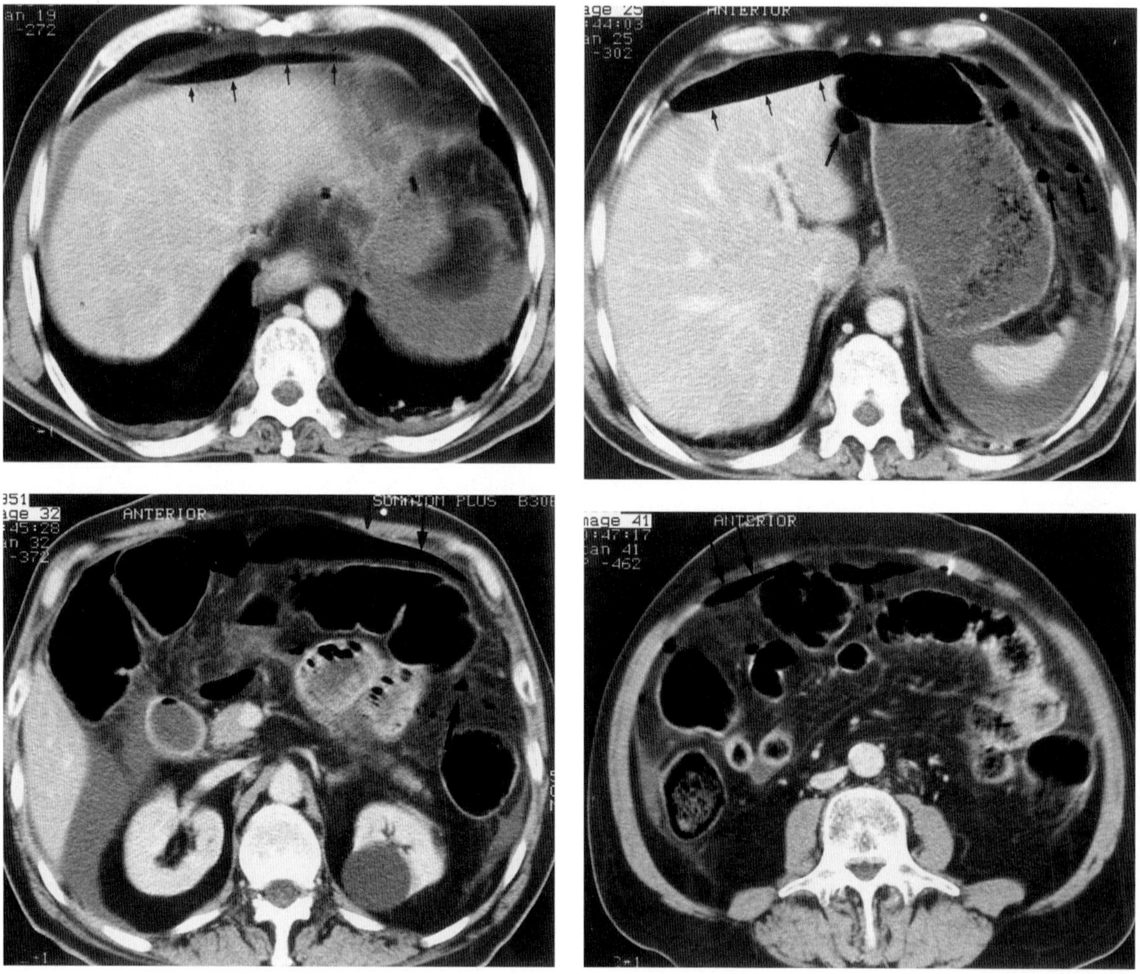

Fig. 9.10A–D. Colonic diverticulum that has perforated into the peritoneal cavity and the subperitoneal spaces. There is air in the right and left subphrenic peritoneal spaces (**A, B** *small arrows*) and behind the rectus abdominis muscle (**C, D** *long arrows*). Fluid can be seen in the subhepatic (**C**) and perisplenic recesses (**A, B**). There is air in the subperitoneal cellular layers of the gastrocolic ligament (**B** *thick arrows*) and of the descending mesocolon (**C** *long thick arrow*)

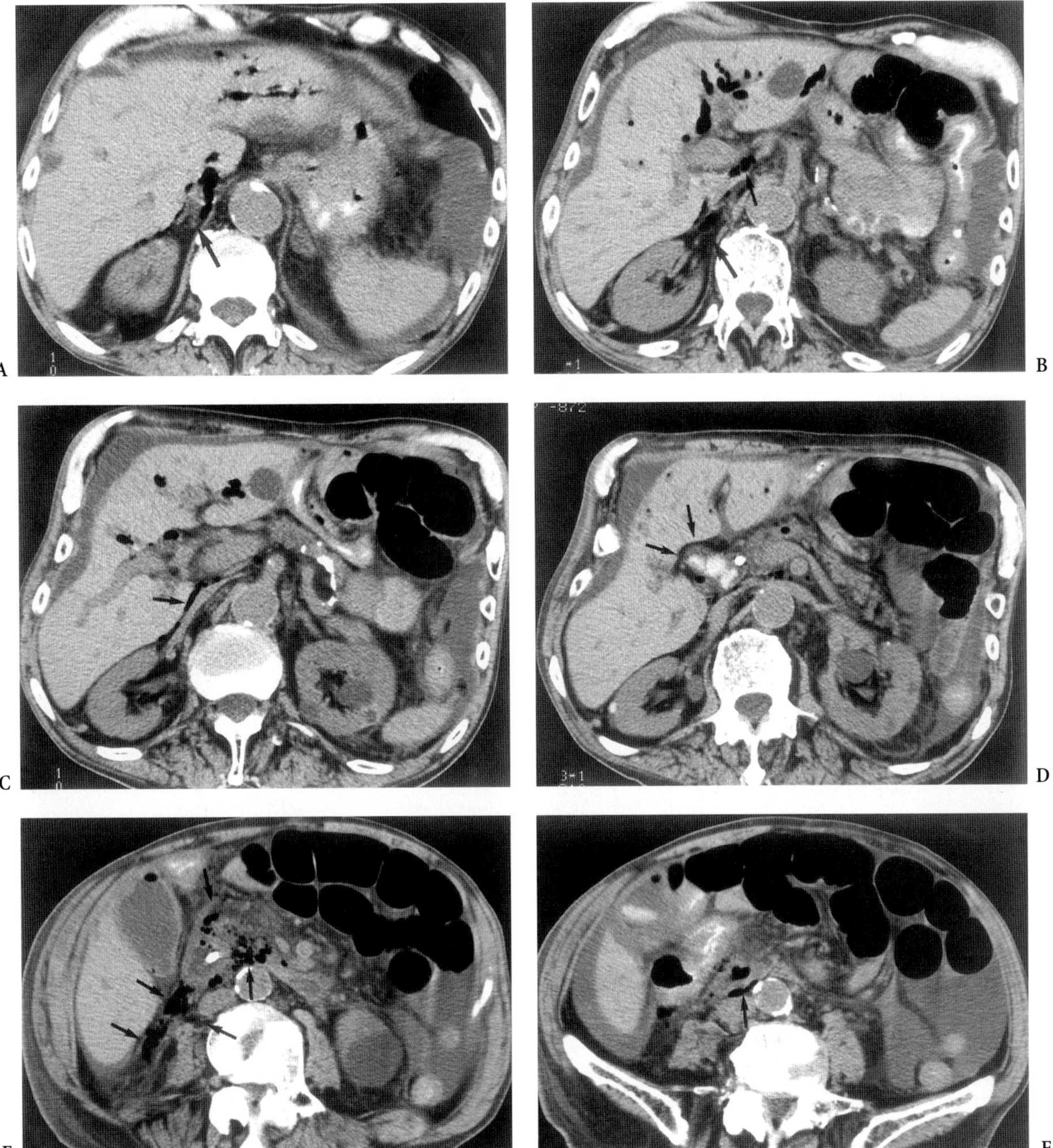

Fig. 9.11A–F. Iatrogenic duodenocholedochal perforation. Air in the hepatoduodenal ligament (*arrows*), in the anterior pararenal space around the head of the pancreas, in the right perirenal compartment around the adrenal gland (**A, B** *large arrow*), and in the biliary tree. Air and fluid in the supramesocolic peritoneal spaces (**C, D** *arrows*)

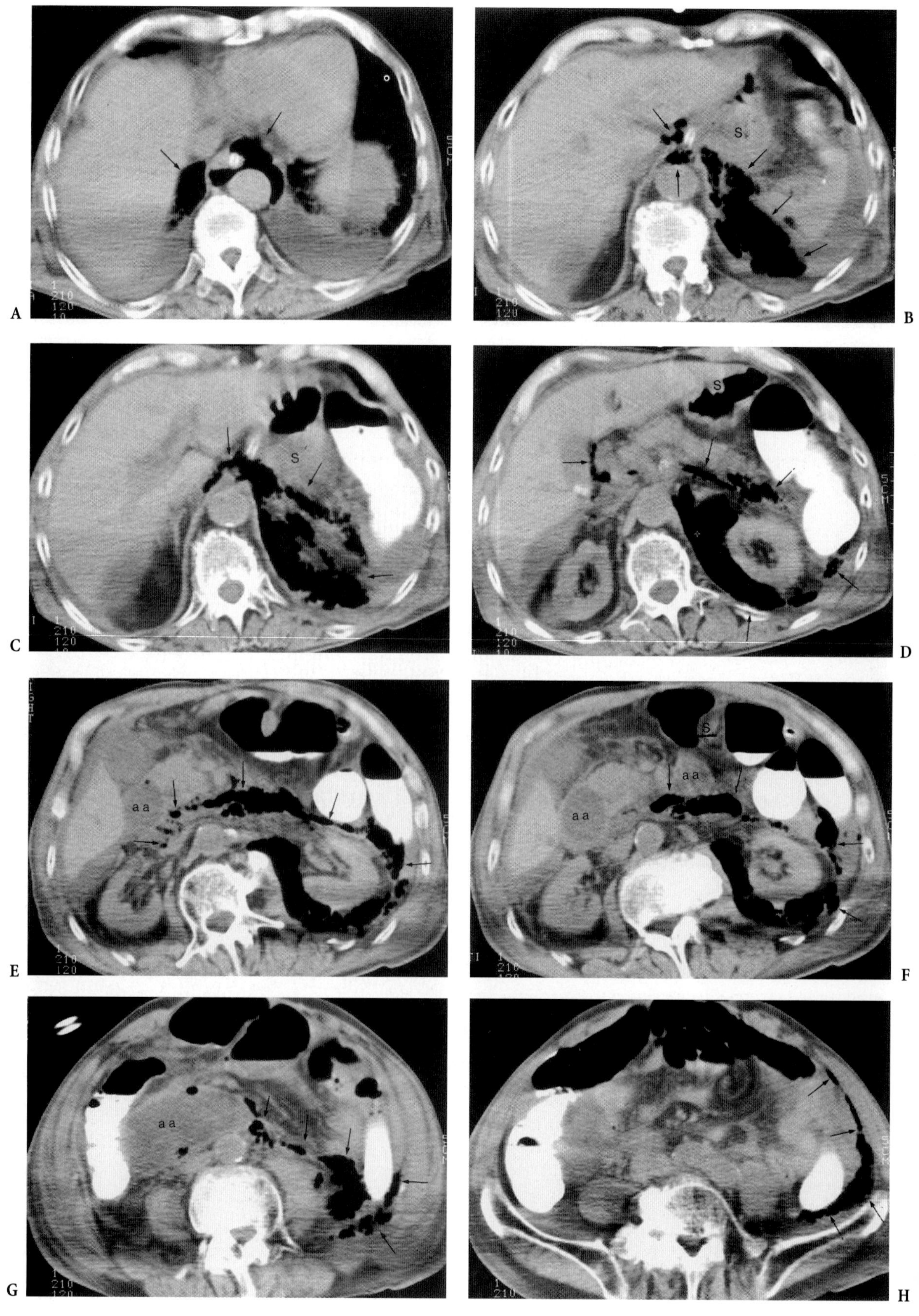
A
B
C
D
E
F
G
H
S
aa

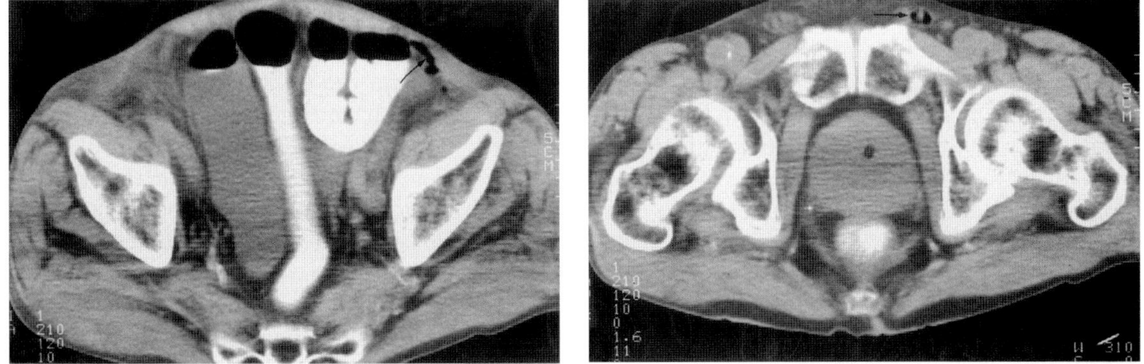

Fig. 9.12A–J. Dehiscence of a gastroduodenal anastomosis. The air coming out from the bowel (*arrows*) spreads into retroperitoneal spaces from the diaphragm (**A, B**) to the pelvis, where it detaches the extraperitoneal fat and reaches the inguinal canal around the funiculum (**I, J**). In addition, the air penetrates the left perirenal space directly through the interruption of the anterior renal fascia, or from below, through the inferior aperture of this compartment, which allows a communication between this compartment and the retroperitoneal pelvic space (**B–G**). Peritoneal fluid collections in the perihepatic, perisplenic and parasigmoidal spaces. Distension of the afferent duodenal loop due to obstruction (**E–G** *aa*)

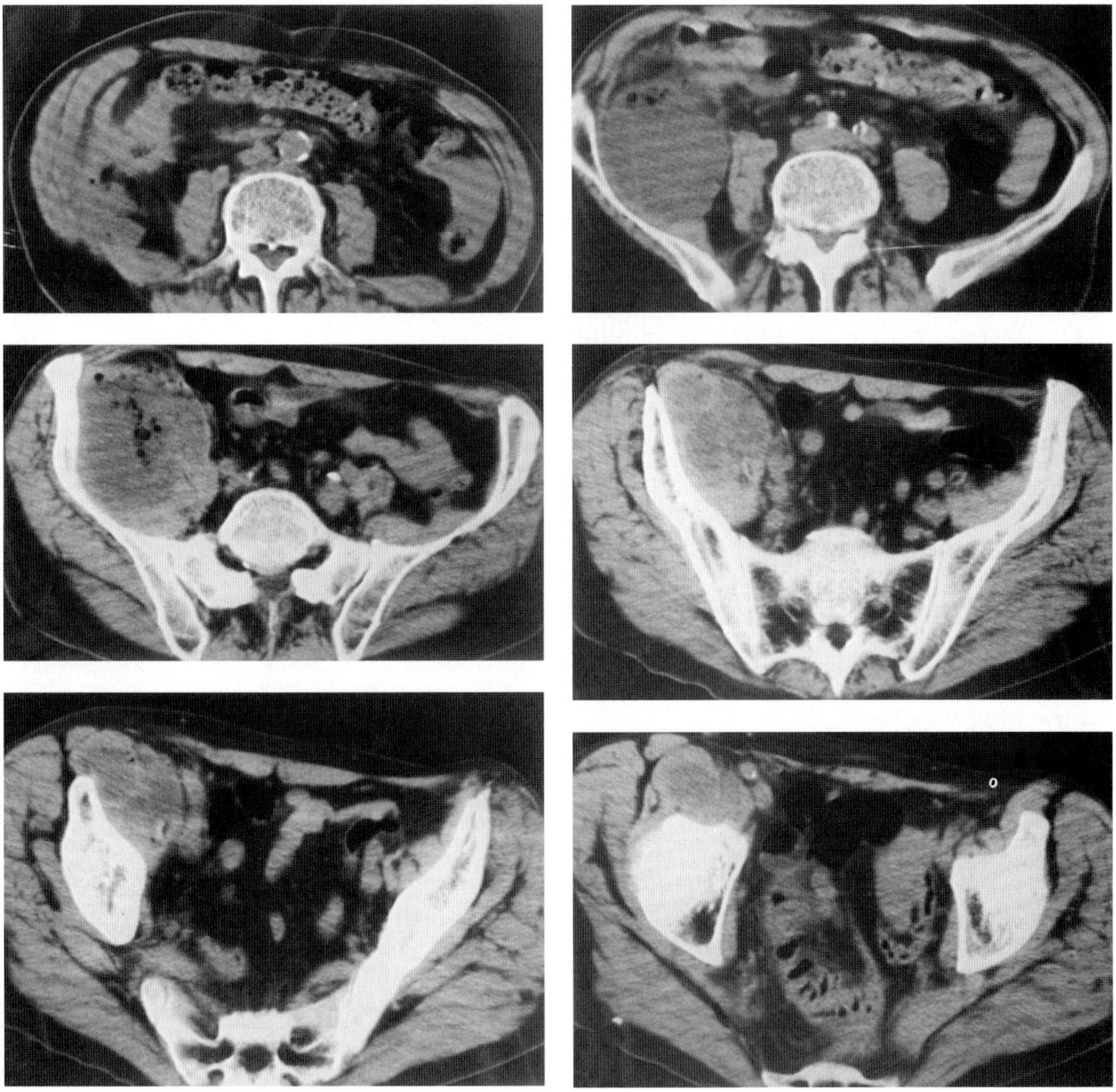

Fig. 9.13A–F. Extrafascial perforation of a tumor in the ascending colon. Wide abscessed collection outside the abdominal transversalis fascia and inside the iliopsoas muscle

Water-soluble contrast material given orally or as an enema may help to confirm the presence and clarify the nature and the site of the perforation. Extravasation of contrast medium from the intestinal wall is a specific sign of perforation, although it is seen in few cases. In fact, the absence of extravasation does not exclude bowel perforation.

9.8 Radiation-induced Injuries

The injuries induced by radiation to the peritoneum, fasciae and subperitoneal adipose cellular tissue are usually sustained as the result of treatment for pelvic tumors or retroperitoneal lymphomas. They have variable onset, damage, duration and recovery and are related to the total radiation dose, to the field shape and width, to the irradiated volume, to the fractionation scheme, and to the individual response. In an early acute stage, such injuries are characterized by inflammatory edema, congestion and cellular infiltration, which are followed by ischemic and vascular lesions and by cellular necrosis. The process may recover and heal in most cases within 6 months after treatment or may lead to fibrotic reactions with thickening of the peritoneum and fasciae and hypertrophy of the adipose cellular tissue.

The evolution of the radiation-induced injuries in the peritoneum and in sub- or retroperitoneal tissue may be followed by means of CT examinations:

1) In the early acute phase, about 6 weeks after radiation therapy, an increase in fat density and a thickening of the peritoneum, ligaments and fasciae, whose profiles become shaded, are seen (Figs. 9.14, 9.15).
2) In the recovery phase, the adipose tissue widens out and brightens, and thin linear strands appear inside. The thickness and density of the peritoneum and of the fasciae decrease, while the profiles become smoother and more regular (Fig. 9.16).

However, when a high radiation dose has been administered, the adipose cellular tissue remains completely and intensely opaque, because of the considerable fibrosis, and it is not distinguishable from the limiting fasciae and the peritoneum (Fig. 9.17).

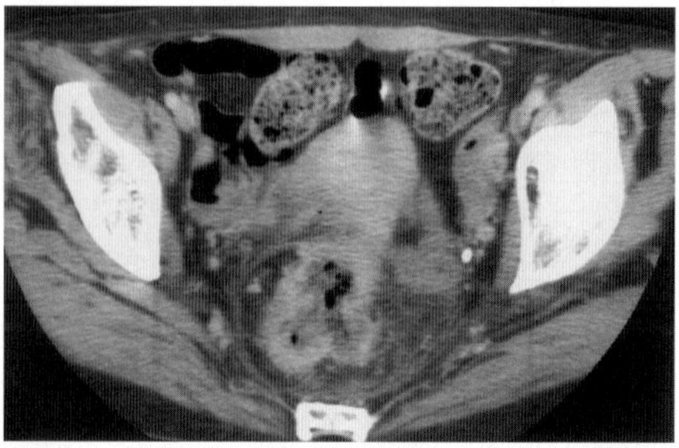

Fig. 9.14. Radiation-induced injuries. Early acute phase after treatment of a rectal carcinoma. Hazy perirectal fat and thickening of ligaments and fasciae

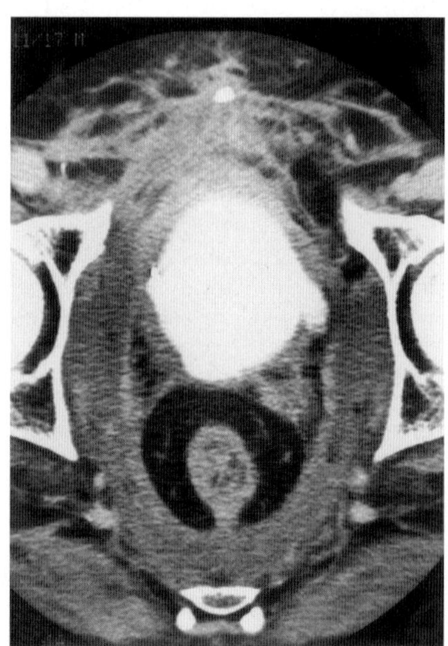

Fig. 9.15. Radiation-induced injuries. Acute phase 2 months after radiotherapy of a relapsing vesical carcinoma. Intense and wide edematous interstitial infiltration of the prevesical and the laterorectal spaces. Thickening of the internal fascia

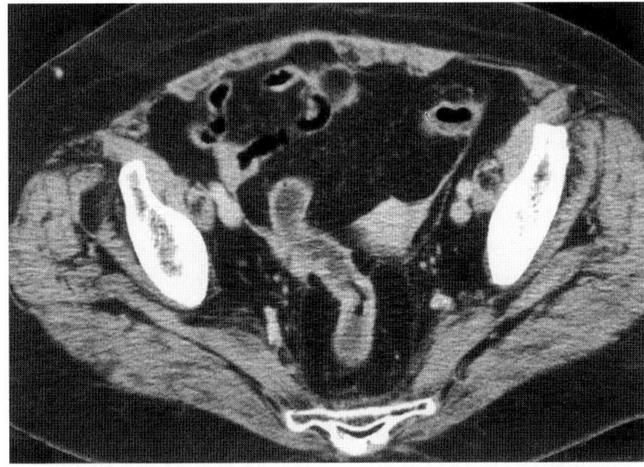
A

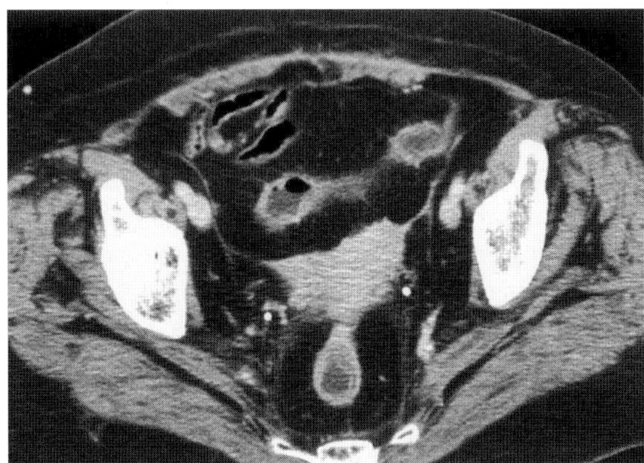
B

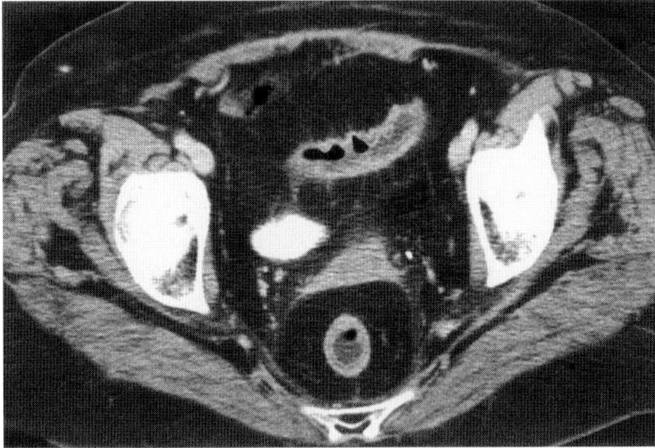
C

Fig. 9.16A–C. Radiation-induced injuries. Fibrosclerotic reparative phase at 6 months after treatment of a relapsing sigmoidal adenocarcinoma. Widening of the pelvic adipose tissue. The sigmoidal and uterine walls are dentated and joined together by thin linear bands. Dense and thin round ligaments show a very sharp profile. The one on the left is retracted and pulls forward the homolateral cornu of the fundus uteri

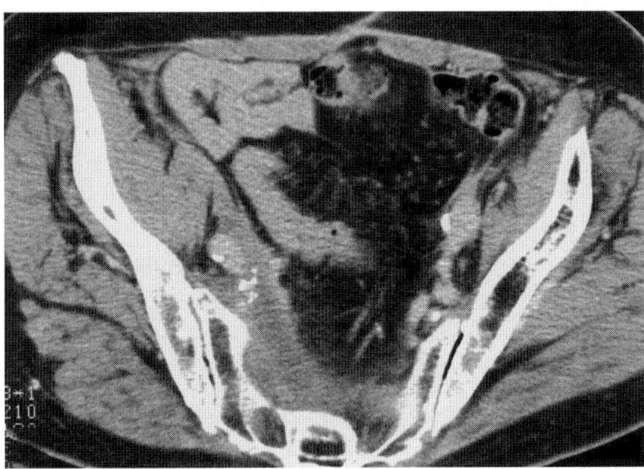
A

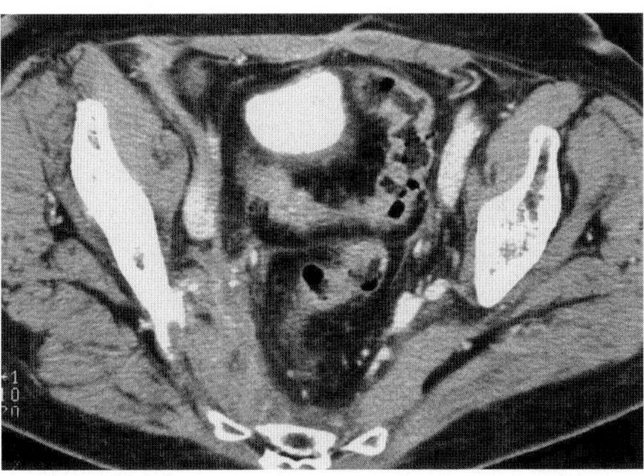
B

Fig. 9.17A, B. Radiation-induced injuries. Recovering fibrotic phase after treatment of a uterine carcinoma. Conspicuous thickening and increased density of the posterior extraperitoneal pelvic space and of the right laterorectal space up to the anterior abdominal wall. Widening of the perisigmoidal and retrovesical adipose tissue

9.9 Peritoneal and Subperitoneal Fibrosis

Peritoneal and subperitoneal fibrosis represents the reparative evolution or the fibrotic involution of peritoneal and subperitoneal lesions of various origin that have primarily or secondarily involved these structures: previous pancreatic, biliary, appendicular, diverticular and lymph nodal inflammatory processes; residua of surgical operations, intestinal perforations, trauma, lymphomas located in the mesentery, peritoneal dialytic treatments, radiation therapy.

The fibrotic alterations consist in a sclerotic network inside the adipose tissue, with reticula that are dense and thick to varying degrees and which confine the omental and the sub- or extraperitoneal fat; they also take the form of thick peritoneal laminae or plaques.

At sites corresponding to these alterations, CT shows an increase in density of the subperitoneal fat, crossed by linear and mostly converging bands, and a thickening of the peritoneum. The intestinal loops are pulled toward these fibrotic scars, but they are not generally obstructed, whereas the vessels are not involved. In most cases, fibroses are circumscribed within a small area, whose site often allows determination of the pathologic cause (Fig. 9.18). For example, the shading and the retraction of the sigmoidal mesocolic fat in the presence of sigmoidal diverticula suggest a previous perforation of a diverticulum and/or a long-lasting peridiverticular inflammatory response; the thickening of the fat surrounding calcified lymph nodes usually represents a residuum of earlier lymphadenitis, which is generally of tuberculous origin and silent. In this case, there may be associated thickening of the peritoneum, with very small nodules or plaques of high or mean density. These alterations are minimal and may be overlooked unless carefully searched for; however, they may indicate the cause and the site of indefinite, but continuous, abdominal pain, which is often confused with neurovegetative disturbances.

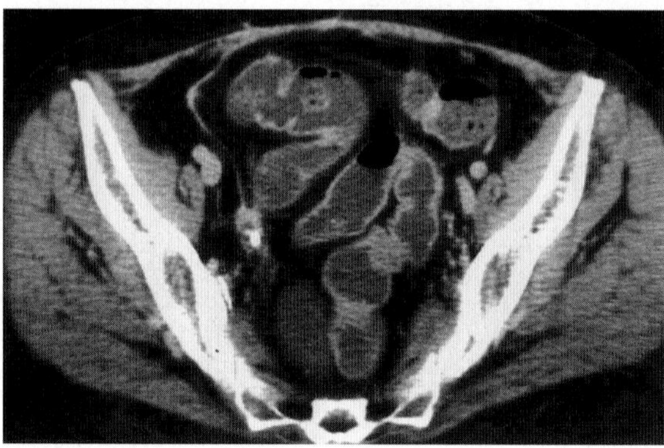

Fig. 9.18. Fibrosis. Fibrous thickening of the right round ligament (residua of adnexectomy)

9.10 Continuous Ambulatory Peritoneal Dialysis

In patients with advanced nephropathies and severe renal failure, substitutive therapy is performed through hemodialysis (in about two-thirds of cases) or by continuous ambulatory peritoneal dialysis (CAPD). This latter treatment is particularly indicated for children who are on a waiting list for renal transplantation, for patients with a difficult vascular route and for diabetic or cardiopathic patients. Peritoneal dialysis is effective when the fluid is uniformly distributed over the entire peritoneal cavity. This correct distribution may already be prevented at the time of the first administration of fluids into the peritoneal cavity, or it can be blocked by subsequently developing complications, adhesions or postperitonitic or postsurgical bridles (Fig. 9.20), which reduce the surface area of the dialyzing peritoneal membrane and induce the production of fluid collections into small spaces and recesses.

Complications can also develop during the treatment, such as abdominal or puboscrotal or vulvar subcutaneous edema, a blockade in the flow of the dialytic fluid secondary to malposition, obstruction or rupture of the catheter, or umbilical, ventral or inguinal herniae.

Therefore, we must face up to the problems concerned with correct introduction and distribution of the fluid and recognize the factors that reduce the efficacy of the treatment or produce complications.

In the search for a solution to these problems, a CT associated with positive-contrast peritoneography has proved demonstrably very accurate and reliable in the selection of the patients who need dialysis and in the discovery of the cause and the site of the complications (reduction of peritoneal spaces, alterations in the catheter, herniae); once these factors have been eliminated, the treatment can be continued without involving CAPD.

A nonuniform distribution of the dialytic fluid in the peritoneal cavity, with collections in sacs or limited spaces, indicates the presence of adhesions (Fig. 9.20), which reduce the surface of the peritoneal dialytic membrane and thus decrease the efficacy of the treatment. Furthermore, the observation of intraperitoneal fluid pockets not penetrated by opaque dialytic liquid may indicate the presence of infected collections or pseudocysts.

In addition, CT positive-contrast peritoneography easily identifies the presence of alterations in the regular flow of the dialysis fluid caused by fibrinous occlusion of the terminal hole of the catheter, by omental wrapping, rupture, kinking or displacement of a nonopaque catheter, or by the site of dialysate leakage.

Finally, in the presence of swelling in the abdominal wall, CT is capable of showing hernial extroflections and distinguishing them from edema that

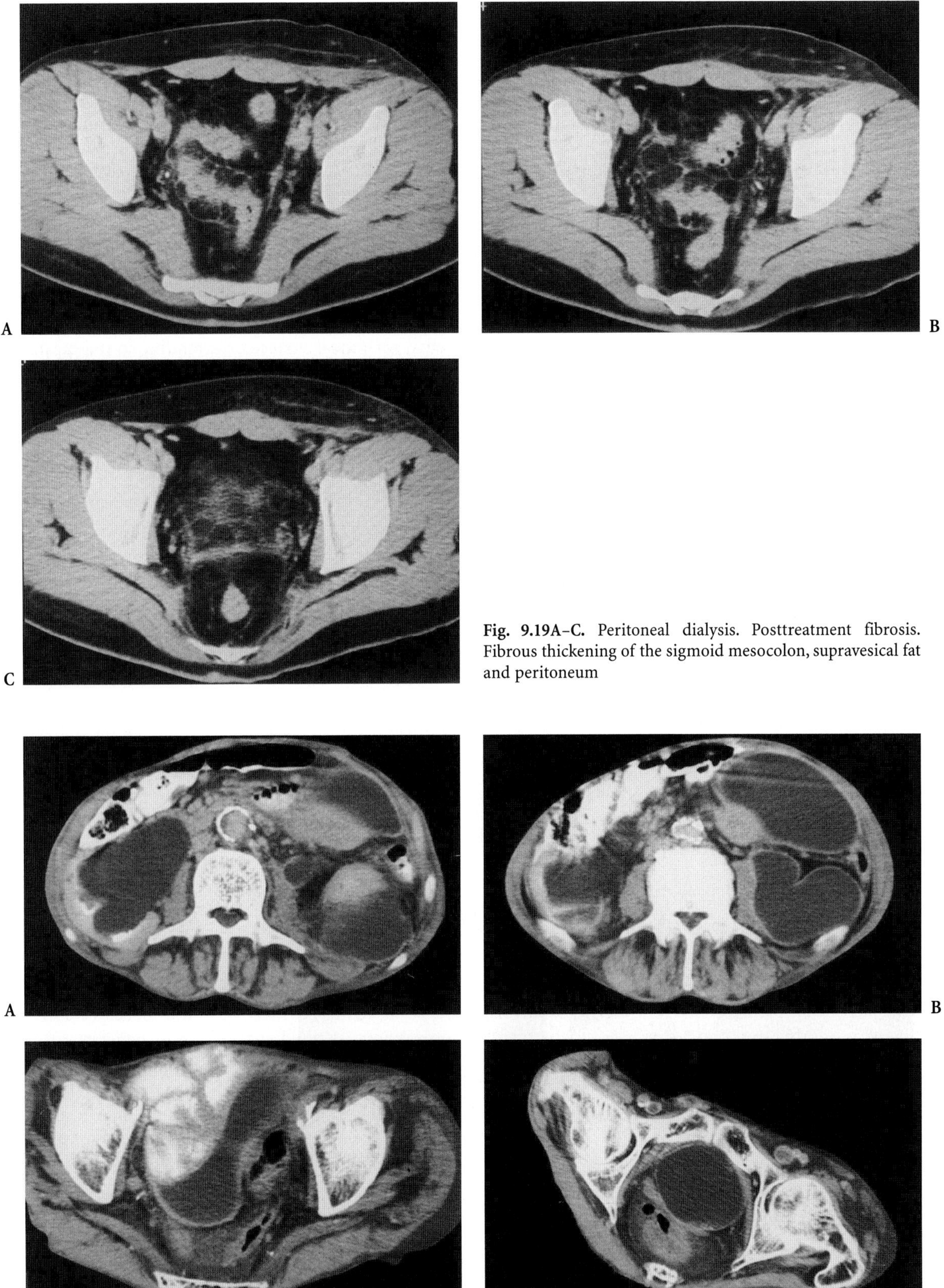

Fig. 9.19A–C. Peritoneal dialysis. Posttreatment fibrosis. Fibrous thickening of the sigmoid mesocolon, supravesical fat and peritoneum

Fig. 9.20A–D. Peritoneal dialysis. Irregular distribution of the dialytic fluid in the peritoneum, owing to adhesions

might have formed as a result of rupture or malpositioning of the catheter.

9.11 Endometriosis

Endometriosis is a heterotopic growth of functioning endometrial tissue in premenopausal women, involving pelvic peritoneum, ovaries, urinary bladder, rectovaginal and uterosacral ligaments, with possible extension to the peritoneal surface, the mesentery, and the omentum and along laparotomy incisions.

Etiologically, endometriosis can be explained as retrograde transtubal menstruation or metaplasia of peritoneal endothelial cells. Hormonal stimulation produces a periodic proliferation of extrauterine endometrioid tissue, cyclic bleeding and hematic lysis, with the development of an inflammatory or fibrous tissue, a solid mass and blood-filled chocolate cysts (endometriomas).

CT is a highly accurate means of detecting occult pathologic processes in women with unexplained pain and of evaluating endometriotic involvement of pelvic tissue and its extension to the peritoneal surface, the omentum and the mesentery.

CT features of endometriosis reflect the various endometriotic alterations, ranging from a simple or thick-walled cyst (Fig. 9.21) to a complex cystic and solid element and to the solid multinodular single or multiple mass (Fishman et al. 1983),involving the pelvic peritoneal surface or extending to the greater omentum and to the mesentery and mimicking peritoneal carcinosis (Nardi and Ruchman 1989).The cystic density varies from that of water to that of recent bleeding (Sawyer and Walsh 1988).The solid elements enhance after i.v. injection of contrast medium. A thickening soft-density tissue may com-

A

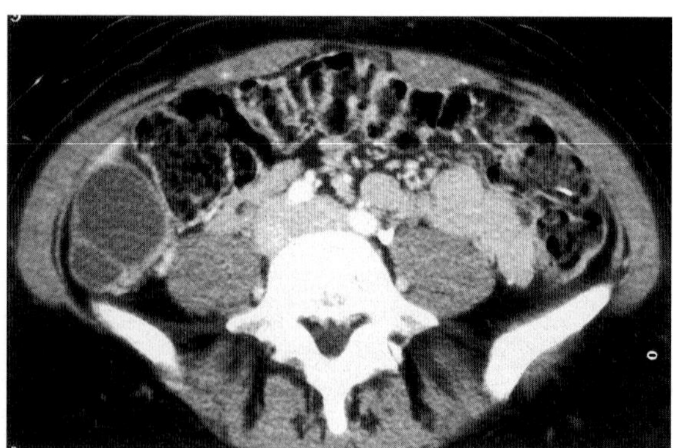

B

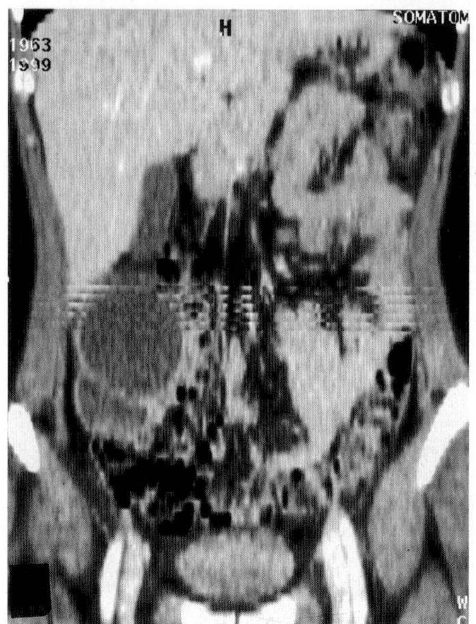

C

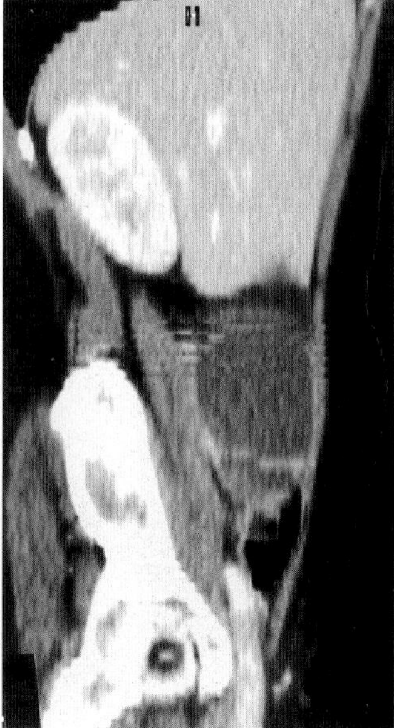

Fig. 9.21. Endometriotic peritoneal cyst. Subhepatic thick-walled septate cyst with slightly higher density than water

press or constrict the rectosigmoid, the urinary bladder, or the distal part of the ureter, or may involve the uterus and the adnexa.

Bibliography

Amyloidosis

Allen HA III, Vick CW, Messmer JM, Parker GA (1985) Diffuse mesenteric amyloidosis: CT, sonographic, and pathologic findings. J Comput Assist Tomogr 9:196–198

Raffi F, Cuillère P, Ruodier JM, Le Bodic L, Rymer R (1985) Amilose péritonéale au cours d'une macroglobulinémie de Waldenstrom. J Radiol 66:735–738

Omental Infarction

Balthazar EJ, Lefkowitz RA (1993) Left-sided omental infarction with associated omental abscess: CT diagnosis. J Comput Assist Tomogr 17:379–381

Ceuterick L, Baert AL, Marchal G, Kerremans R, Geboes K (1987) CT diagnosis of primary torsion of greater omentum. J Comput Assist Tomogr 11:1083–1084

Grassi R, Romano L, Catalano O, Pinto A, Violini M, Rotondo A (1996) Torsione del grande omento. Descrizione di un caso. Radiol Med 91:141–142

Haynes JW, Brewer WH, Walsh JW (1985) Focal fat necrosis presenting as a palpable abdominal mass: CT evaluation. J Comput Assist Tomogr 9:568–569

Kopp W, Becker H, Kullnig P, Fotter R (1987) Spontaninfarkt des Omentum majus: computertomographische Darstellung. Radiologe 27:303–305

Ortore P (1986) Quadro ecografico di infarto emorragico idiopatico dell'omento. Radiol Med 72:328–329

Puylaert JBCM (1992) Right-sided segmental infarction of the omentum: clinical. US and CT findings. Radiology 185:169–172

Foreign Bodies

Apter S, Hertz M, Rubinstein ZJ, et al (1990) Gossypiboma in the early post-operative period: a diagnostic problem. Clin Radiol 42:128–129

Braude P, Van Gansbeke D, Aguilera C, Cassart M, Lalmand B, Struyven J (1992) Gosspibome enkysté du petit épiploon: complementarité de l'échographie et de la tomodensitométrie computérisée. J Belge Radiol 75:125–128

Buy JN, Hubert C, Ghossain MA, Malbec L, Bethoux JP, Ecoiffier J (1989) Computed tomography of retained abdominal sponges and towels. Gastrointest Radiol 14:41–45

Caprio E, Lanza R, Amoroso L, Cerioni M, Carotti L (1993) CT findings of surgically retained sponges and towels (gossypibomas). Eur Radiol 3:383–385

Catalano D, Lapiccirella G (1987) Erosion of the duodenal wall caused by the migration of a retained surgical sponge into the duodenal lumen. Radiologe 301–302

Choi BI, Kim SH, Yu ES, Chung HS, Han MC, Kim CW (1988) Retained surgical sponge: diagnosis with CT and sonography. AJR Am J Roentgenol 150: 1047–1050

Coche G, Pardonnet MH, Chanois AM, Rohmer P, Weill FS, Etienne G, Didier D (1988) Apport de l'échographie et de la scanographie dans le diagnostic des textilomes intraabdominaux. A propos de 12 cas. J Radiol 69:243–251

Cochran ST, Do HM, Ronaghi A, Nissenson AR, Kadell BM (1997) Complication of peritoneal dialysis: evaluation with CT peritoneography. Radiographics 17:869–878

Gallotti N, Granger N, Dorcier F, Laurent F, Guibert JL, Richard O, Brassin J (1987) Le petit épiploon. Aspect normal et pathologie tumorale en échographie et tomodensitométrie. J Radiol 68:13–21

Kokubo T, Itai Y, Ohtomo K, Yoshikawa K, Lio M, Atomi Y (1987) Retained surgical sponges: CT and US appearance. Radiology 165:415–418

Kopka L, Fisher U, Gross AJ, Funke M, Oestermann JW, Grabbe E (1996) CT of retained surgical sponges (texilomas): pitfalls in detection and evaluation. J Comput Assist Tomogr 20:919–923

La Fianza A, Campani R, Dore R, Tateo S (1991) La tomografia computerizzata nei "garzomi" intraperitoneali. Radiol Med 82:706–710

Liessi G, Semisa M, Sandini F, et al (1989) Retained surgical gauzes: acute and chronic CT and US findings. Eur J Radiol 9:182–186

Mantovani G, Volpe E, Soardi GA, Menini F, Thabet O, Bissoli S, Rossetti G (1992) La diagnostica per immagini delle garze ritenute nell'addome. Radiol Med 84:164–168

Parienty RA, Pradel J, Lepreux JF, Nicodeme CH, Dologa M (1981) Computed tomography of sponges retained after laparotomy. J Comput Assist Tomogr 5:187–189

Pascal-Suisse P, Castinel B, Peyron JP, Vergne R, Pringot J (1982) Textile foreign bodies: echotomography and computed tomography of five cases. J Belge Radiol 65:355–361

Reinke J, Biermann FJ, Bosse U, Krings W (1992) Unclear abdominal tumor. Radiologe 32:525–527

Revesz G, Siddiqi T, Buchheit WA, Bonitatibus M (1983) Detection of retained surgical sponges. Radiology 149:411–413

Schild H, v Bülow M (1983) Computertomographie bei der Suche nach iatrogenen Fremdkörpern. CT Sonogr 3:22–24

Schmitt R, Helmberger T, Spindler-Thiele S, Loitzsch RM (1992) Sonographie und Computertomographie bei intraperitoneal belassenen Bauchtüchern. Fortschr Rontgenstr 157:520–522

Sheward SE, Williams AG, Mettler FA, Lacey SR (1986) CT appearance of a surgically retained towel (gossypiboma). J Comput Assist Tomogr 10:343–345

Tonarelli A, Lizzadro A, Garbocci S, Colagrande S (1991) Ascesso da corpo estraneo chirurgico. Riscontri ecografici e tomodensitometrici. Radiol Med 82:710–713

Williams RG, Bragg DG, Nelson JA (1978) Gossypiboma, the problem of the retained surgical sponge. Radiology 129:323–326

Yamato M, Ido K, Izutsu M, Narimatsu Y, Hiramatsu K (1987) CT and ultrasound findings of surgically retained sponges and towels. J Comput Assist Tomogr 11:1003–1006

Castleman's Disease

Ferreirós J, Gómez León N, Mata MI, Casanova R, Pedrosa CS, Cuevas A (1989) Computed tomography in abdominal Castleman disease. J Comput Assist Tomogr 13:433–436

Garber SJ, Shaw DG (1991) Case report: the ultrasound and computed tomography appearance of mesenteric Castleman disease. Clin Radiol 43:429–430

Greenstein S, Fishman EK, Kaufman SL, Kadir S, Siegelman SS (1986) Castleman disease of the retroperitoneum: CT demonstration. J Comput Assist Tomogr 10:547–548
Iida E, Kohno A, Mikami T, Kumekawa H, Akimoto S, Hamano K (1983) Mesenteric Castleman tumor. J Comput Assist Tomogr 7:338–340
Johkoh T, Muller NL, Ichikado K, Nishimoto N, et al (1998) Intrathoracic multicentric Castleman disease: CT findings in 12 patients. Radiology 209: 477–481
Libson E, Fields S, Strauss S, et al (1988) Widespread Castleman disease: CT and US findings. Radiology 166:753–755
Onik G, Goodman PC (1983) CT of Castleman disease. AJR Am J Roentgenol 140:191–192
Riba PO (1979) Castleman's disease. Angiofollicular benign lymph-node hyperplasia. Radiological features in the differential diagnosis of vascular tumours of the pelvis. Br J Radiol 52:412–414

Whipple's Disease

Bi JC, Crosetti EE, Maurino EC, et al (1991) Short-term antibiotic treatment in Whipple's disease. J Clin Gastroenterol 13:303–307
Davis SJ, Patel A (1990) Case report: distinctive echogenic lymphadenopathy in Whipple's disease. Clin Radiol 42:60–62
Dobbins WO III (1982) Current concepts of Whipple's disease (editorial). J Clin Gastroenterol 4:205–208
Dobbins WO III, Kawanishi H (1981) Bacillary characteristics in Whipple's disease: an electron microscopic study. Gastroenterology 80:1468–1475
Jones B, Bauless TM, Fishman EK, Siegelman SS (1984) Lymphadenopathy in celiac disease: computed tomographic observations. AJR Am J Roentgenol 142:1127–1132
Li DKB, Rennie CS (1981) Abdominal computed tomography in Whipple's disease. J Comput Assist Tomogr 5:249–252
Rijke AM, Falke THM, de Vries RRP (1983) Computed tomography in Whipple disease. J Comput Assist Tomogr 7:1101–1102
Wazières B, Fest T, Litzler JF, Simon G, Rohmer P, Dupond JL (1993) Cavitations ganglionnaires mésénteriques dans la malarie de Whipple. J Radiol 12:661–663
Whipple GH (1907) A hitherto undescribed disease characterized anatomically by deposits of fat and fatty acids in the intestinal and mesenteric lymphatic tissues. Bull Johns Hopkins Hosp 18:382

Intestinal Perforation

Alexander ES, Weinberg S, Clark RA, Belkin RD (1982) Fistulas and sinus tracts: radiologic evaluation, management and outcome. Gastrointest Radiol 7:135
Allen KS, Siskind BN, Burrel MI (1986) Perforation of distal esophagus with lesser sac extension: CT demonstration. J Comput Assist Tomogr 10:612–614
Angelelli G, Macarini L (1992) TC del tratto gastroenterico. Minerva Medica, Turin
Angelelli G, Magliocca MA, Zaccheo N (1996) Tomografia computerizzata. Proceedings of the 37th National Congress of SIRM, Milan, 18–22 May 1996
Blake M, Mendelson R, Field S (1993) Pneumo-omentum following perforated greater curvature gastric ulcer. Clin Radiol 47:119–120
Bray JF, MB, Ch B (1984) The "inverted V" sign of pneumoperitoneum. Radiology 151:45–46
Catalano D (1996) Contributo della tomografia computerizzata nello studio della perforazione intestinale. Radiol Med 91:247–252
Catalano D, Traianiello B (1984) Left side abdominal abscess from a retroperitoneal perforation of a duodenal ulcer. Rofo Fortschr Geb Rontgenstr Neuen Bildgeb Verfahr 141:111–113
Chintapalli K, Thorsen MK, Foley WP, Unger GF (1983) Abdominal abscesses with enteric communications: CT findings. AJR Am J Roentgenol 141:27–28
Cho KC, Baker SR (1994) Extraluminal air: diagnosis and significance. Radiol Clin North Am 32:829–844
Donohue J, Federle M, Griffiths B, Trunkey DD (1987) Computer tomography in the diagnosis of blunt intestinal and mesenteric injury. J Trauma 27:11–17
Earls JP, Dechaman AH, Colon E, et al (1993) Prevalence and duration of postoperative pneumoperitoneum: sensitivity of CT vs left lateral decubitus radiography. AJR Am J Roentgenol 161:781–785
Fanucci A, Alessi V, Cucchiara G et al (1988) L'addome acuto. (Proceedings of the XXXIIIrd National Congress on Radiology, Rome, vol 3) Monduzzi, Bologna, pp 1151–1164
Ferrero A, Céspedes M, Cantarero JM, et al (1990) Peritonitis due to rupture of retroperitoneal teratoma: computed tomography diagnosis. Gastrointest Radiol 15:251
Frick MP, Feinberg SB, Stenlund RR, Gedgaudas E (1982) Evaluation of abdominal fistulas with computed body tomography. Comput Radiol 16:17
Fultw PJ, Skucas J, Weiss SL (1992) CT in upper gastrointestinal tract perforations to peptic ulcer disease. Gastrointest Radiol 17:5–8
Ghahremani GG (1993) Radiologic evaluation of suspected gastrointestinal perforations. Radiol Clin North Am 31:1219–1234
Goldman SN, Fishman EK, Gatewood OMB, et al (1985) CT in the diagnosis of enterovesical fistulas. AJR Am J Roentgenol 144:1229–1233
Gonzalez JG, Gonzalez RR, Patino JV, Garcia AT, Alvarez CP, Pedrosa CSA (1988) CT findings in gastrointestinal perforation by ingested fish bones. J Comput Assist Tomogr 12:88–90
Goodwin CA, Lewicki AM (1977) Sigmoid colon perforation into the lesser sac. AJR Am J Roentgenol 128: 491–492
Grassi R, Ragozzino A, Romano L (1996) Il pneumoperitoneo e il retroperitoneo. Proceedings of the 37th National Congress of SIRM, Milan, 18–22 May 1996
Heavey LR, Glazer GM, Francis IR, Fugenschuh D, Jasinki R (1987) Abscesses with enteric communication: a potential pitfall in computed tomography. J Comput Assist Tomogr 11:470–473
Hughes JJ, Blunck CE (1987) CT demonstration of gastropancreatic fistula due to penetrating gastric ulcer. J Comput Assist Tomogr 11:709–711
Jeffrey RB, Federle MP, Wall S (1983) Value of computed tomography in detecting occult gastrointestinal perforation. J Comput Assist Tomogr 7:825–827
Kerlan RB Jr, Jeffrey RB Jr, Pogany AC, Ring EJ (1985) Abdominal abscess with low-output fistula: Successful percutaneous drainage. Radiology 155:73–75

Lee H, Vibhakar SD, Bellon EM (1983) Gastrointestinal perforation: early diagnosis by computed tomography. J Comput Assist Tomogr 7:226–229
Nguywn-BD, Beckman-I (1992) Silent rectal perforation after endoscopic polypectomy: CT features. Gastrointest Radiol 17:271–273
Pappas TN, Debas HT (1992) Complications of peptic ulcer disease: perforation and obstruction. In: Taylor RM (ed) Gastrointestinal emergencies. Williams & Wilkins, Baltimore
Pathak MG, Frank SJ, Ellis JJ (1984) Computed tomography of bowel perforation. Gastrointest Radiol 9:133–135
Ranschaert E, Rigauts H (1993) Confined gastric perforation: ultrasound and computed tomographic diagnosis. Abdom Imaging 18:318–319
Rizzo M, Federle M, Griffiths B (1989) Bowel and mesenteric injury following blunt abdominal trauma: evaluation with CT. Radiology 173:143–148
Sanders LM, Premkumar A, Levy HM, et al (1989) Pneumoperitoneum resembling air in the biliary tree: CT features. J Comput Assist Tomogr 13:817–820
Seigel RS, Kuhns LR, Borlanza GS, et al (1980) Computed tomography and angiography in ileal carcinoid tumor and retractile mesenteritis. Radiology 134:437–440
Shuck JM, Lowe RG (1978) Intestinal disruption due to blunt abdominal trauma. Am J Surg 136:668
Siewert B, Raptopoulos V (1994) CT of the acute abdomen: findings and impact on diagnosis and treatment. AJR Am J Roentgenol 163:1317–1324
Stapakis JC, Thickman D (1992) Diagnosis of pneumoperitoneum: abdominal CT vs upright chest film. J Comput Assist Tomogr 16:713–716

Radiation-induced Injuries

Doubleday LC, Bernardino ME (1980) CT findings in the perirectal area following radiation therapy. J Comput Assist Tomogr 4:634–638
Fishman EK, Zinreich ES, Jones B, Siegelman SS (1984)Computed tomographic diagnosis of radiation ileitis. Gastrointest Radiol 9:149–152
Libshitz HI, Du Brow RA, Loyer EM, Charnsangavej C (1996) Radiation change in normal organs: an overview of body imaging. Eur Radiol 6:786–795

Peritoneal Dialysis

Brown DL, Johnson JB, Kraus AP, Duke RA, Barrett MR (1987) Computed tomography with intraperitoneal contrast medium for localisation of peritoneal dialysis leaks. J Comput Assist Tomogr 11:276–278
Caimi F, Rovere G, Philippson M, Battaglia E (1991) Contributo della peritoneografia in associazione alla tomografia computerizzata, nella valutazione delle complicanze addominali in pazienti sottoposti a dialisi peritoneale continua. Radiol Med 81:656–659
Cochran ST, Do HM, Ronaghi A, Nissenson AR, Kadell BM (1997) Complications of peritoneal dialysis: evaluation with CT peritoneography. Radiographics 17:869
Cooper JC, Nicholls AJ, Simms JM, et al (1983) Genital oedema in patients treated by continuous ambulatory peritoneal dialysis: an unusual presentation of inguinal hernia. BMJ 286:1923–1924
Holland P (1990) Sclerosing encapsulating peritonitis in chronic ambulatory peritoneal dialysis. Clin Radiol 41:19
Hollett MD, Marn CS, Ellis JH, et al (1992) Complications of continuous ambulatory peritoneal dialysis: evaluation with CT peritoneography. AJR Am J Roentgenol 159:983–989
Lee FT Jr, Leahy-Gross KM, Hammond TG, Wakeen MT, Zimmerman SW (1994) Pneumoperitoneum in peritoneal dialysis patients: significance of diagnosis by CT. J Comput Assist Tomogr 18: 439–442
Litherland J, Gibson M, Sambrook P, Lupton E, Beaman M, Ackrill P (1992) Investigation and treatment of poor drains of dialysate fluid associated with anterior abdominal wall leaks in patients on chronic ambulatory peritoneal dialysis. Nephrol Dial Transplant 7:1030–1040
Magill HL, Roy SH, et al (1986) CT peritoneography in evaluation of pediatric dialysis complications. AJR Am J Roentgenol 147:325–328
Maxwell AJ, Boggis CR, Sambrook P (1990) Computed tomographic peritoneography in the investigation of abdominal wall and genital swelling in patients on continuous ambulatory peritoneal dialysis. Clin Radiol 41:100–104
Renzo S, Beatrice D, Giuliano R, Francesco C (1990) Peritoneal x-ray and computerized tomography in evaluating abdominal complications in CAPD. Adv Perit Dial 6:62–63
Roub LW, Drayer BP, Orr DP, et al (1979) Computed tomographic positive contrast peritoneography. Radiology 131:699–704
Scanziani R, Dozio B, Caimi F, De Rossi N, Magri F, Surian M (1992) Peritoneography and peritoneal computerized tomography: a new approach to non-infectious complications of CAPD. Nephrol Dial Transplant 7:1035–1038
Schultz SG, Harmon TM, Nachtnebel KL (1984) Computerized tomographic scanning with intraperitoneal contrast enhancement in a CAPD patient with localized oedema. Perit Dial Bull 4:253–254
Stafford-Johnson DB, Wilson TE, Francis IR, et al (1998) CT appearance of sclerosing peritonitis in patients on chronic ambulatory peritoneal dialysis. J Comput Assist Tomogr 22:295
Twardowski ZJ, Tully RJ, Kirt Nichols W, Sinderrajon S (1984) Computerised tomography (CT) in the diagnosis of subcutaneous leak sites during continuous ambulatory peritoneal dialysis (CAPD). Perit Dial Bull 4:163–166
Twardowski ZJ, Tully RJ, Ersoy FF, Dedhia NM (1990) Computerised tomography with and without intraperitoneal contrast for determination of intra-abdominal fluid distribution and diagnosis of complications in peritoneal dialysis patients. Am Soc Artif Intern Organs 36:95–103
Winek TG, Mosely HS, Grout G, Luallin D (1988) Pneumoperitoneum and its association with ruptured abdominal viscus. Arch Surg 123:709–712

Endometriosis

Clement PB, Young RH, Scully RE (1988) Necrotic pseudoxanthomatous nodules of ovary and peritoneum in endometriosis. Radiology 169:290
Fishman EK, Scatarige JC, Saksouk FA, Rosenshein NB, Siegelman SS (1983) Computed tomography of endometriosis. J Comput Assist Tomogr 7:257–264

Nardi PM, Ruchman RB (1989) CT appearance of diffuse peritoneal endometriosis. J Comput Assist Tomogr 13:1075

Prystowsky JB, Stryker SJ, Ujiki GT, et al (1989) Gastrointestinal endometriosis: incidence and indications for research. Radiology 170:286

Sawyer RW, Walsh JW (1988) CT in gynecologic pelvic disease. Semin Ultrasound CT MR 9:122–142

Stringfellow JM, Hawnaur JM (1998) CT and MRI appearances of sarcomatous change in chronic pelvic endometriosis. Br J Radiol 71:90

Togashi K, Nishimura K, Kimura I, Tsuda Y, Yamanashita K, Shibata T, Nakano Y, Konishi J, Konishi I, Mori T (1991) Endometrial cysts: diagnosis with MR imaging. Radiology 180:73

Weinfield RM, Johnson SC, Lucas CE, et al (1998) CT diagnosis of perihepatic endometriosis complicated by malignant transformation. Abdom Imaging 23: 183

10 Abdominal Herniae

CONTENTS

A hernia is a protrusion, through discontinuities in the parietal wall or in diaphragmatic muscles or along vascular canals, of preperitoneal fat, omentum, peritoneum and abdominal viscera with their ligaments or mesenteries. It is made up of a porta, a sac and its content.

The hernial porta is an aperture in the musculoaponeurotic abdominal or diaphragmatic wall, or a widening anatomical canal giving passage to preperitoneal adipose tissue, peritoneum, and then abdominal viscera.

The hernial sac is formed by the evagination of the peritoneal serosa surrounding the herniated viscera. The content of the sac varies according to the site of the hernial porta. The omentum, the stomach, the small bowel loops, and the colon are the structures most frequently present inside the hernial sac.

Depending on the hernial porta, herniae are classified as: parietal, of the vascular canal, diaphragmatic or internal (Table 10.1).

10.1 Herniae of Abdominal Wall and Vascular Canals

Abdominal wall and inguinocrural herniae cause variable clinical symptoms; they are often asymptomatic, but sometimes produce tenderness or mild abdominal pain at intervals. On the other hand, acute and sometimes severe subobstructive or obstructive manifestations can occur as results of incarceration, strangulation and ischemia.

CT is useful in the solution of numerous problems associated with the presence of a hernia. First, it makes it possible to confirm or refute the clinical hypothesis set up, because in about 10% of cases a physical examination does not clarify the diagnosis, especially in subjects with an excessive amount of fat masking the hernial evagination. Secondly, CT provides the opportunity to clarify the nature and the characteristics of a swelling mass in the abdominal wall; finally, it gives valuable preoperative information to the surgeon and makes the operation easier, especially when previous surgical operations have modified the anatomical structures

Table 10.1. Abdominal herniae

Abdominal wall	Vascular canals	Diaphragmatic	Internal
Spigelian	Inguinal	Morgagni's foramen	Paraduodenal
Umbilical	Crural	Esophageal hiatus	Winslow's foramen
Paraumbilical		Bochdalek's foramen	Paracecal
Lumbar		Traumatic	
Incisional			

morphologically and topographically. This information concerns:

1) The site and width of the hernial porta. This may be narrow or wide; those in the abdominal wall may be located at a site that is different from that of the maximal expansion of the sac.
2) The content of the hernial sac (omental fat, viscera), with particular attention to the vessels that nourish the herniated viscera, which may be unintentionally injured during surgery.
3) The consistency and thickening of the adjacent musculoaponeurotic wall and its relationships with the hernial porta.
4) The complications of the incarceration of hollow viscera, such as obstructive manifestation, inflammation of the wall of the sac and of the surrounding tissues, adhesions, bridles or membranes.

CT provides a detailed representation of the anatomical structures of the anterior abdominal wall, the fasciae and the umbilical folds, and of the extent of the inguinal, femoral and obturator herniae.

CT images are very clear and easy to understand:

- The hernial porta is recognized as an interruption in the continuity of the anterior (Figs. 10.1–10.7) or posterior (Fig. 10.8) abdominal wall or a widening of foramina or anatomical inguinal (Figs. 10.17–10.19) or femoral canals (Fig. 10.21).
- The hernial sac can be recognized by the thin arcuate line of the evaginated peritoneal serosa of which it is made up. This line is easily visible, because it is located between the subcutaneous and the preperitoneal adipose tissue and the omental and subperitoneal fat (Figs. 10.4, 10.6, 10.17). The

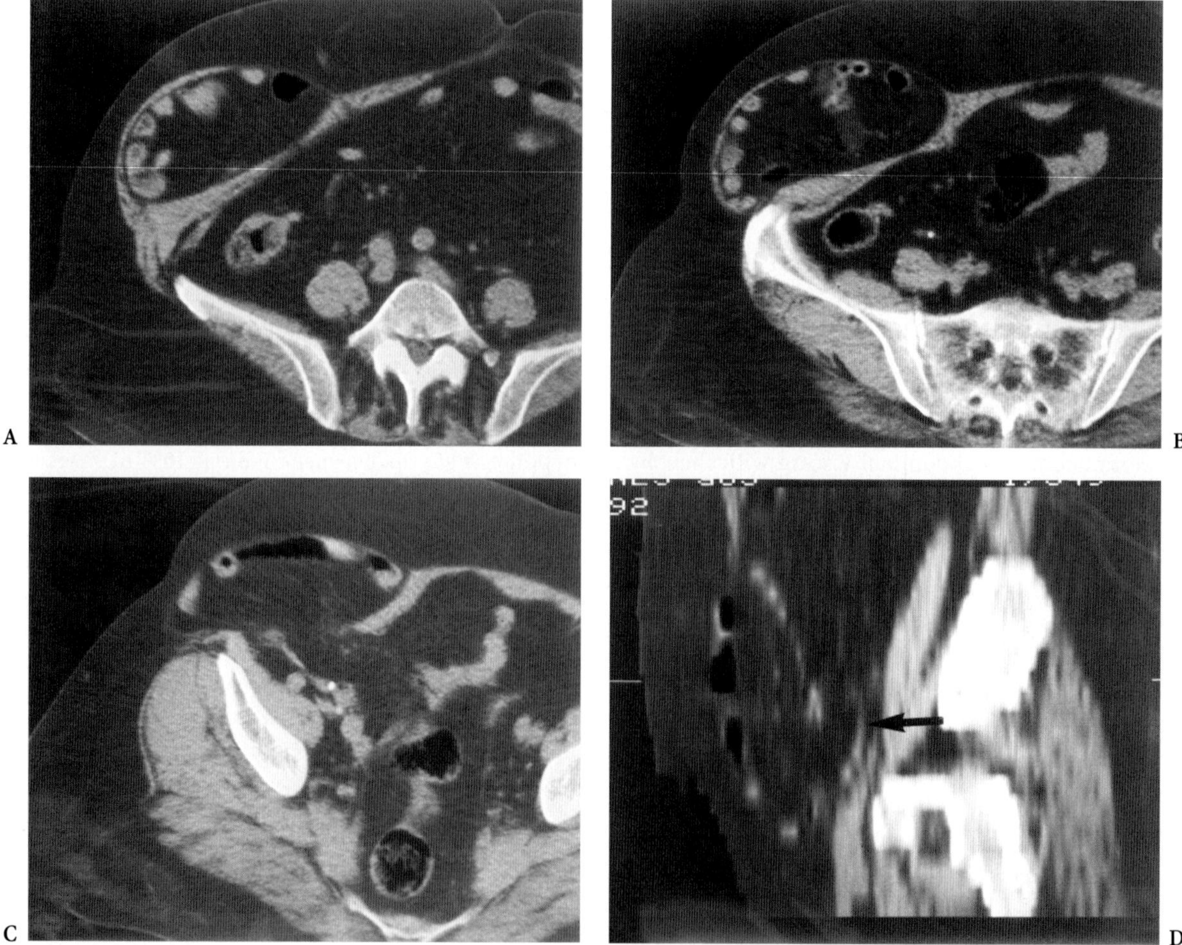

Fig. 10.1A–D. Right spigelian hernia. Wide hernial sac protruding through a parietal defect at the lateral border of the right rectus muscle into subcutaneous fat and containing omentum and ileal loops. The sagittal reconstruction shows the anterolateral hernial porta (*arrow*) and the extension of the sac upward

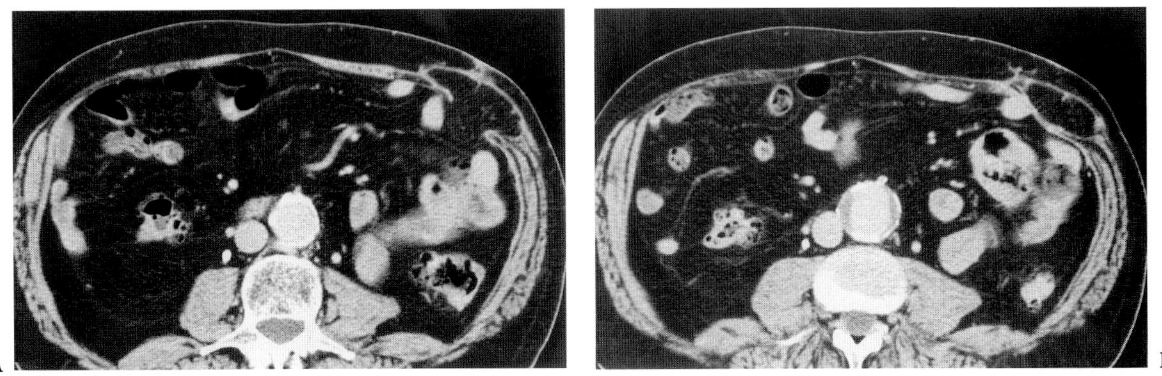

Fig. 10.2A, B. Left spigelian hernia. Hernial porta between the rectus and the iliacus muscles at a high subumbilical level. The sac contains only omentum

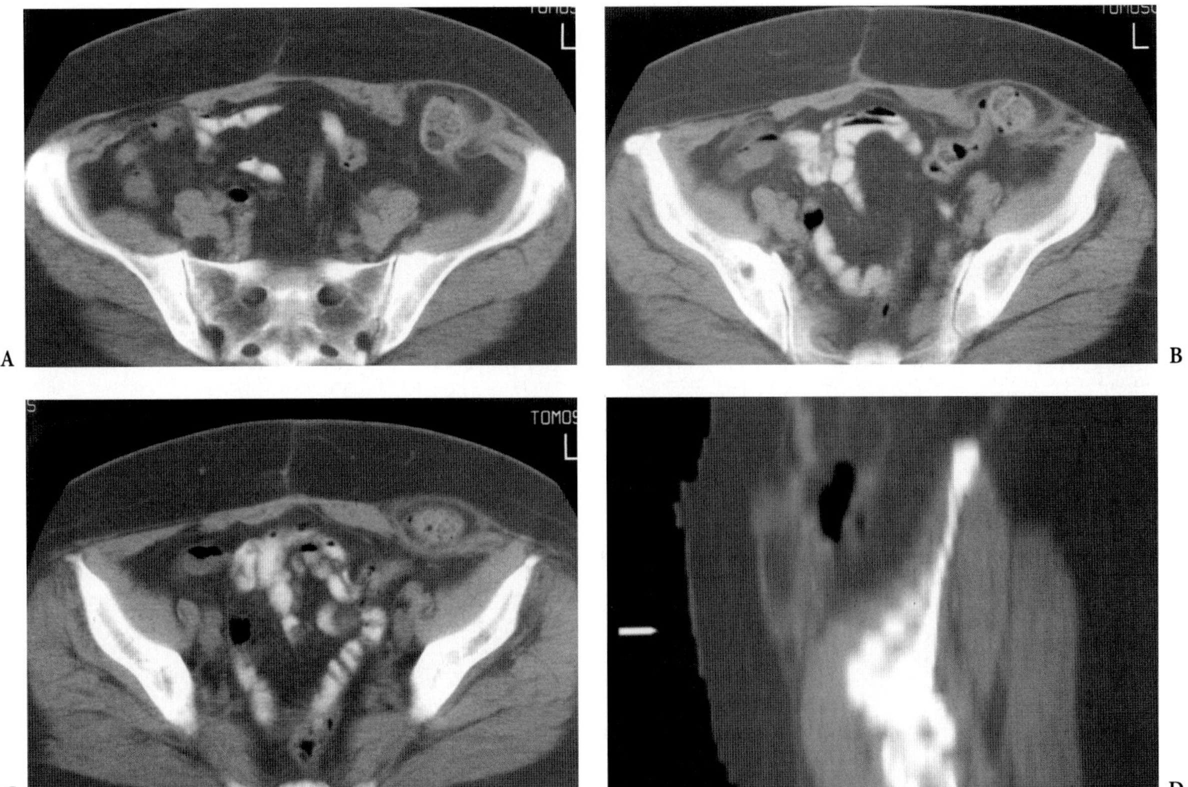

Fig. 10.3A–D. Left spigelian hernia. Hernial porta between the rectus and the obliquus externus muscles. The sac extends between the aponeurotic fascia of the obliquus major muscle anteriorly and the obliquus minor muscle posteriorly; it contains the colon–sigmoid junction

site and width determine how well the images of the vessels located in the omentum and in the inguinal and femoral canals stand out (Figs. 10.4, 10.6, 10.11).

The hollow viscera located inside the sac stand out clearly, because of their thick wall and their gaseous or fluid content. Examination of the contiguous scans (Figs. 10.4, 10.7, 10.16, 10.18), or better, those with reconstructions (Figs. 10.1, 10.3, 10.9, 10.13–10.14) also makes it possible to establish which bowel tract is herniated.

In obstructions of the herniated viscera, the intestinal loops before the occlusion are expanded and show air-fluid levels, whereas the loops after the obstruction are empty or contain very small amounts of air and feces.

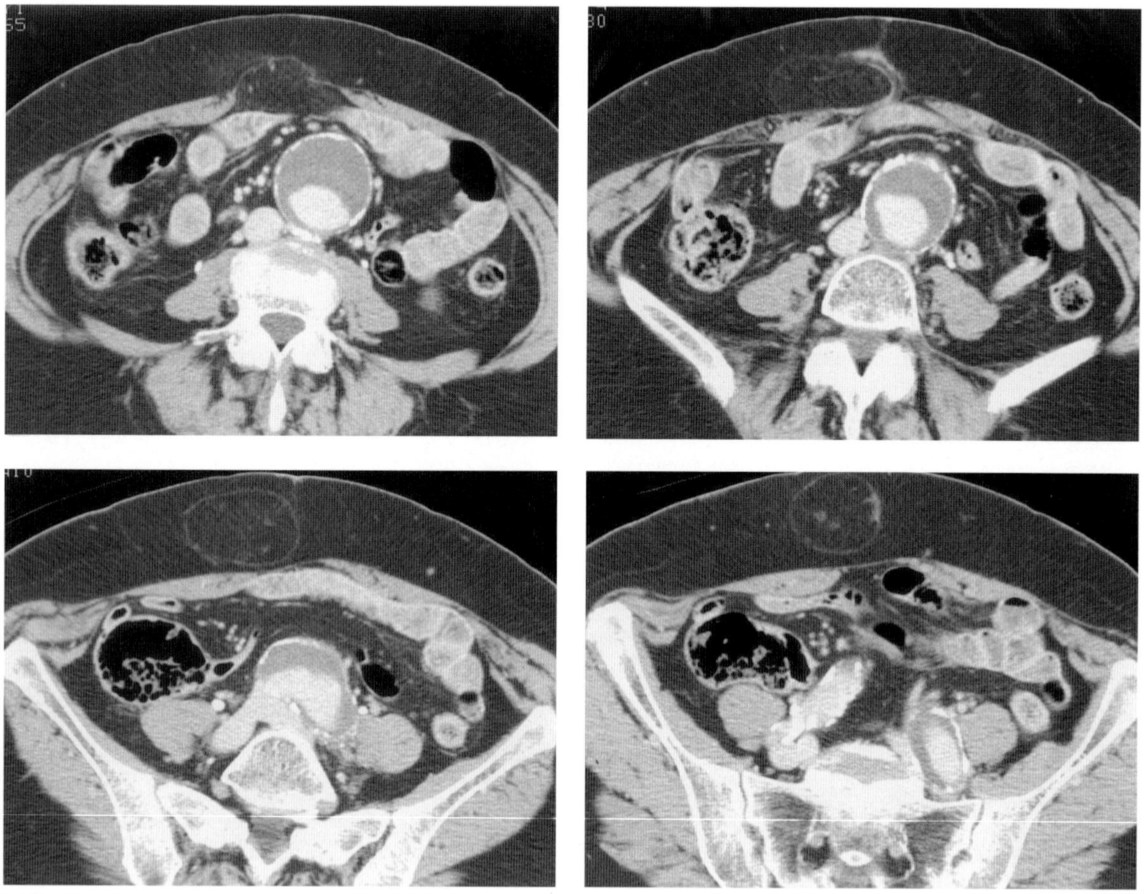

Fig. 10.4A–D. Paraumbilical hernia with omental content. Hernial sac protruding through a wall defect just above the umbilicus extending downward into the subcutaneous fat, impressing and displacing the umbilicus. Circular linear image of the peritoneum that constitutes the wall of the sac. Negative attenuation of the omental content, with the punctiform images of the vessels

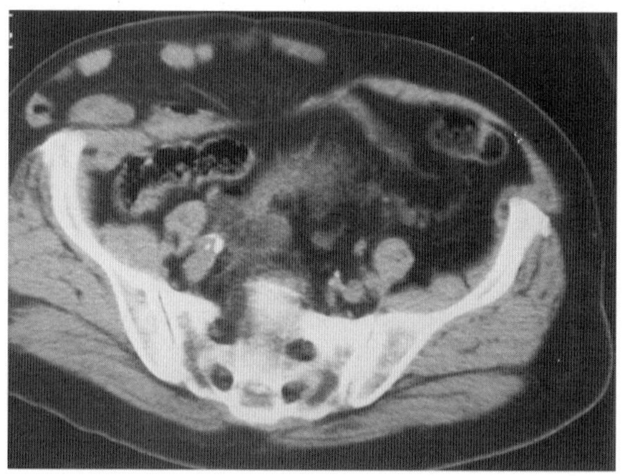

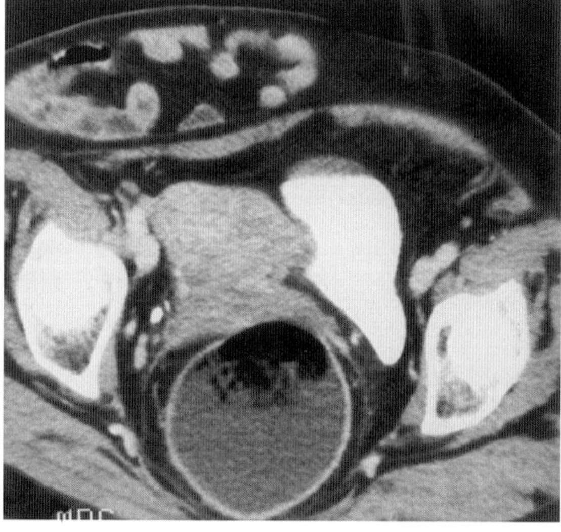

Fig. 10.5A, B. Right paramedian subumbilical hernia. Large hernial porta owing to hypoplasia of the right rectus muscle. Wide hernial sac containing omentum and ileal loops

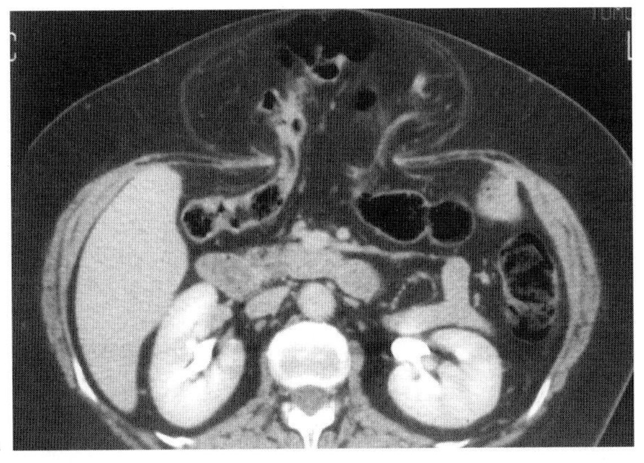

A

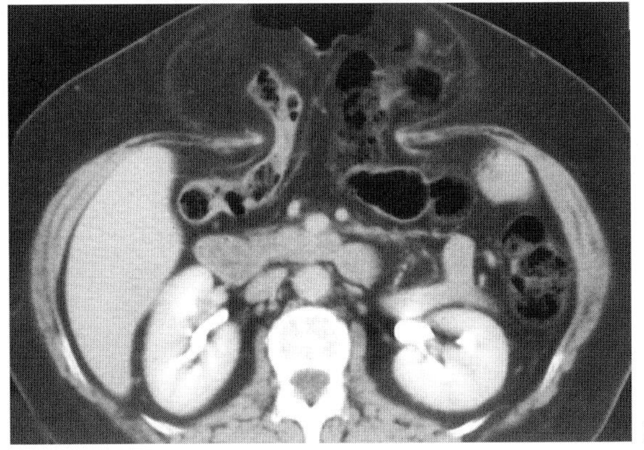

B

Fig. 10.6A, B. Median parasupraumbilical hernia. Hernial sac (*arrow*) containing omentum and transverse colon with the corresponding vessels. Hypoplasia of the rectus abdominis muscle

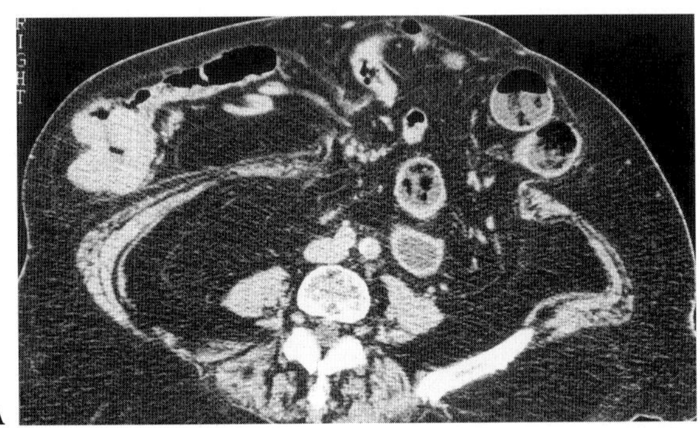

A

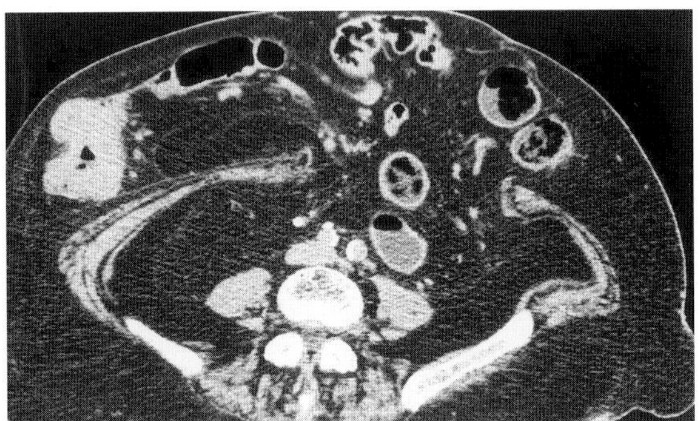

B

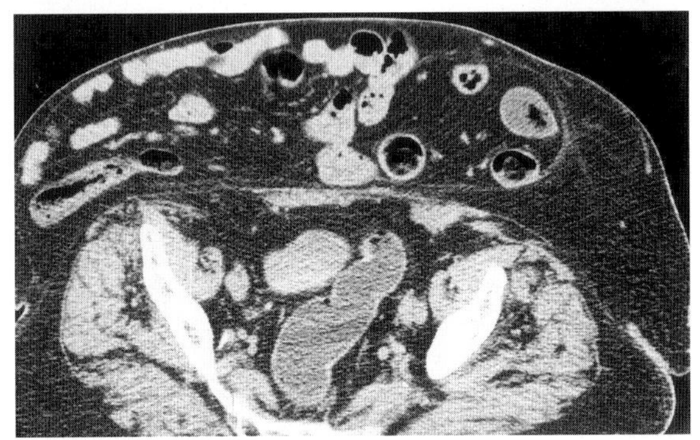

C

Fig. 10.7A–C. Left paramedian subumbilical hernia. Huge hernial sac containing omentum and ileocolic loops. Herniated tumor of the cecum–ascending colon

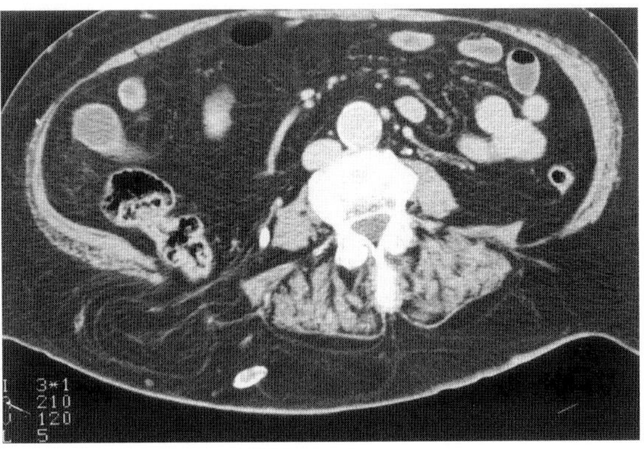

Fig. 10.8. Right lumbar hernia. Large hernial porta between the obliquus internus muscle laterally and the quadratus lumborum muscle medially. Wide hernial sac containing adipose tissue. The cecum stands on the hernial porta without penetrating it

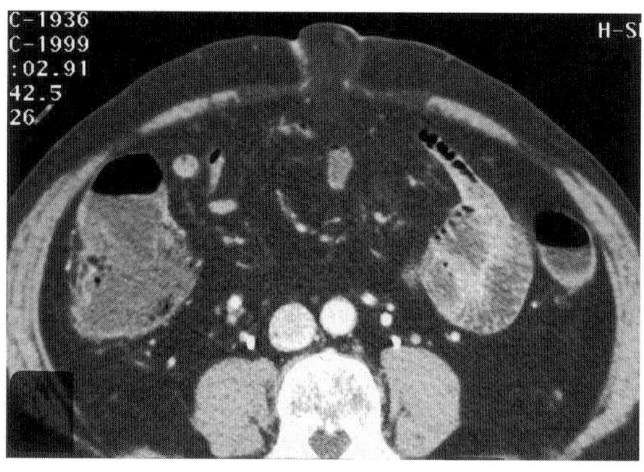

A

B

Fig. 10.9A, B. Umbilical hernia. Small sac containing preperitoneal fat and omentum protruding through the umbilical ring

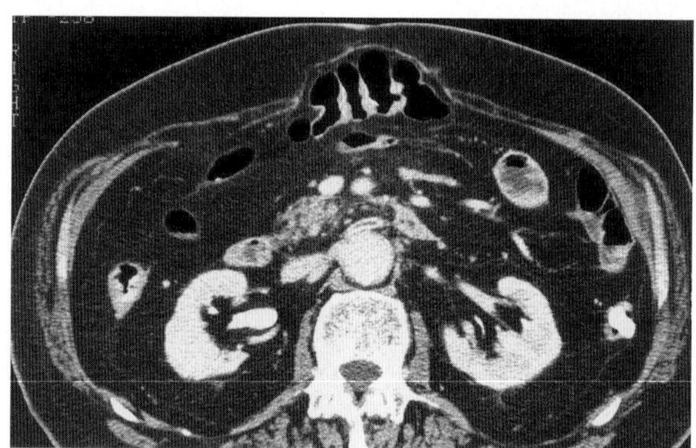

Fig. 10.10. Median incisional hernia. Transverse colon and omentum protruding through a healed midline incision and atrophy of the rectus muscle

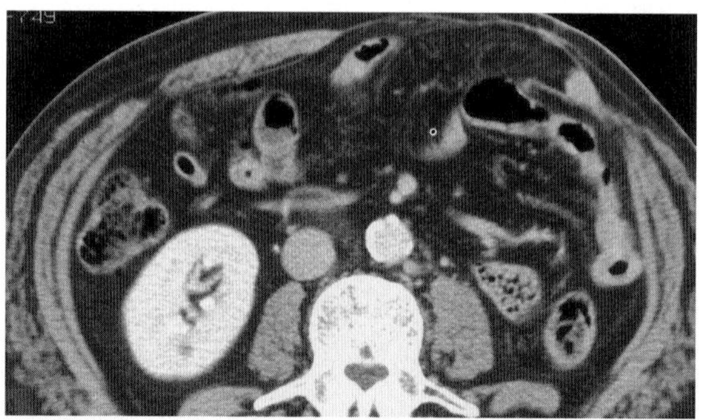

A

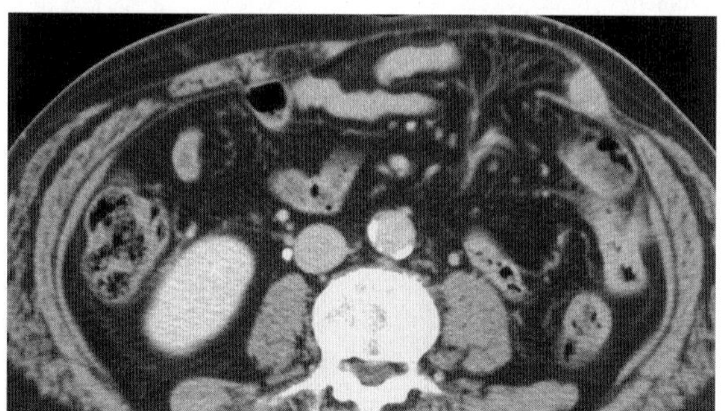

B

Fig. 10.11A, B. Left paraumbilical incisional hernia. Hernial sac containing omentum and small bowel loops with the relative vessels. Hypotrophy of the left rectus muscle

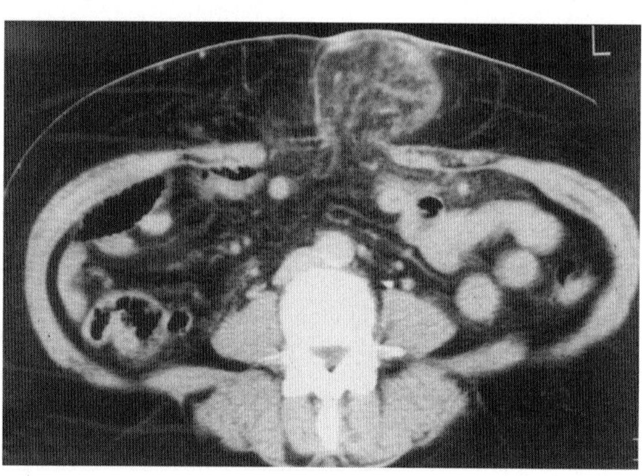

Fig. 10.12. Paraumbilical incisional hernia. Hernial sac containing nothing but thickened and enhancing inflamed omentum protruding into the subcutaneous fat through a midline incisional defect

Fig. 10.15A–D. Left para- and subumbilical incisional hernia. Protrusion of the omentum, the ileum and the ascending colon. Thick subumbilical fibrous mass

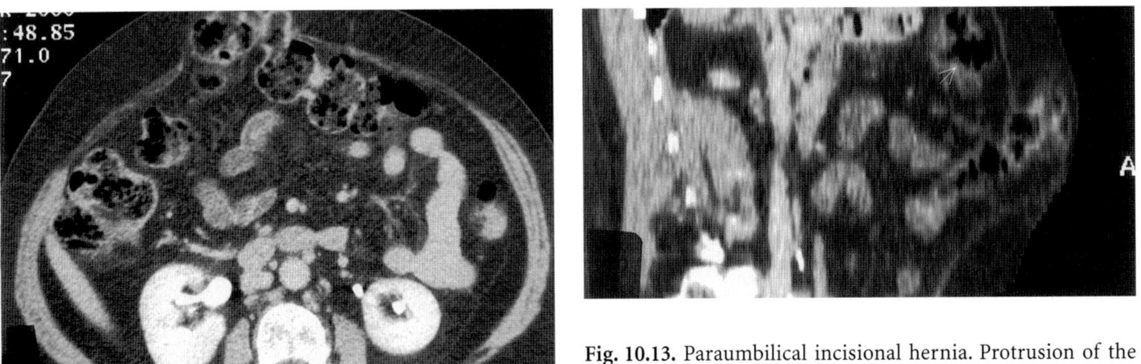

Fig. 10.13. Paraumbilical incisional hernia. Protrusion of the transverse colon through a midline incisional defect

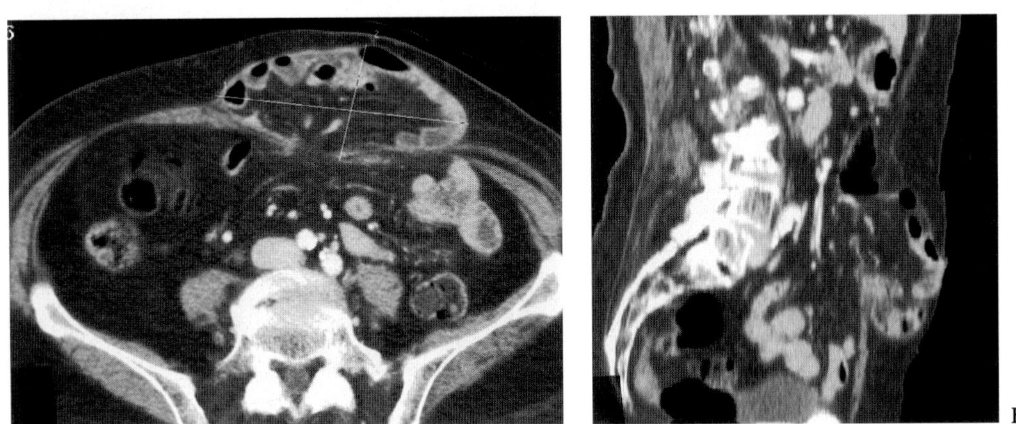

Fig. 10.14. Subumbilical incisional hernia. Hernial sac containing ileal loops protruding through a large defect in the anterior abdominal wall extending downwards into the subcutaneous fat

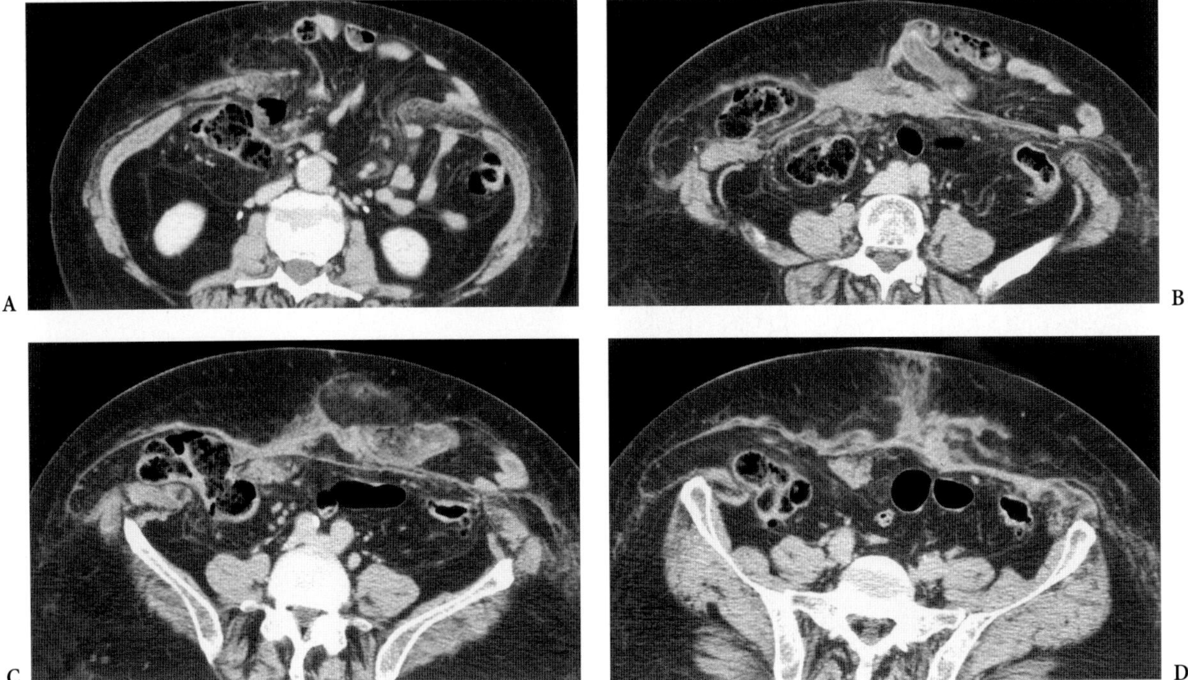

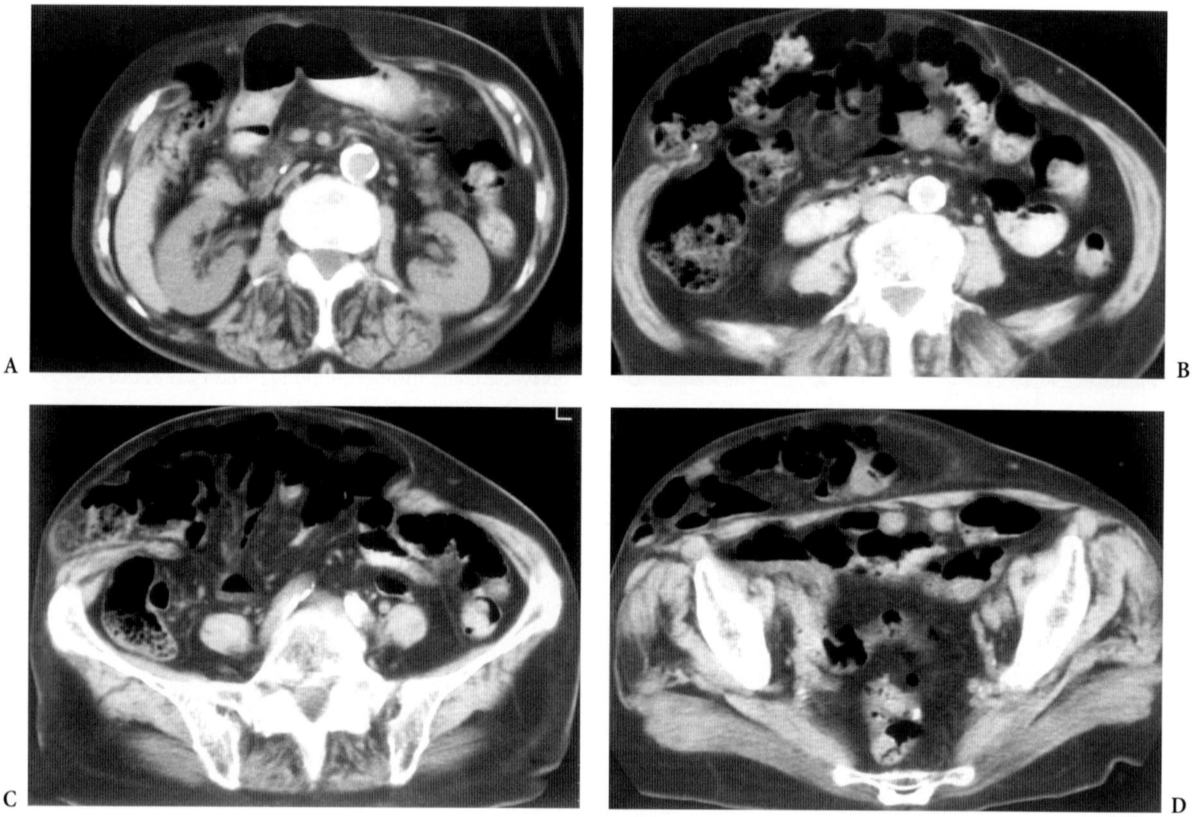

A B C D

Fig. 10.16A–D. Median incisional hernia. Massive herniation of the stomach, the transverse colon and the ileum through a wide defect in the anterior abdominal wall

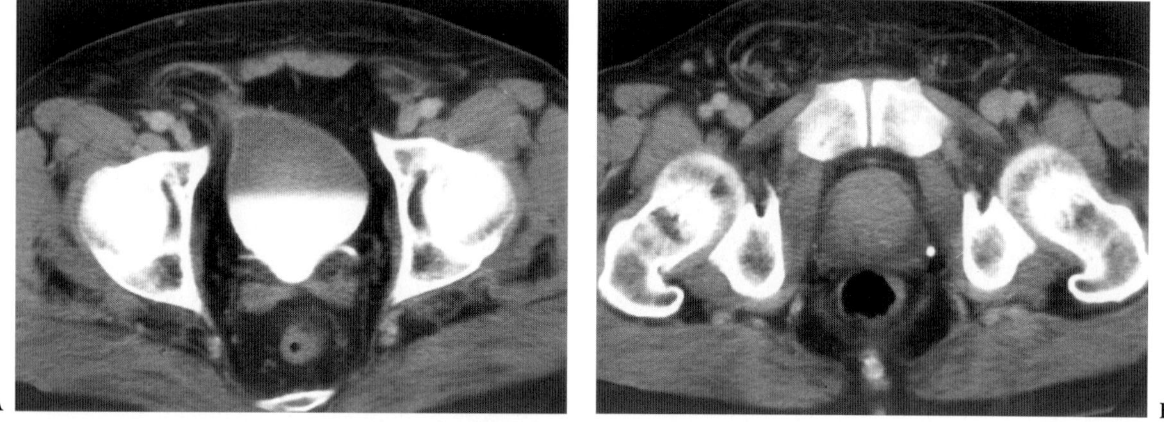

Fig. 10.17A, B. Bilateral external oblique inguinal hernia. **A** Hernial portae. **B** Prepubic tract: the hernial sacs contain preperitoneal and omental fat expanding the inguinal canal and compressing the deferential vessels and ducts

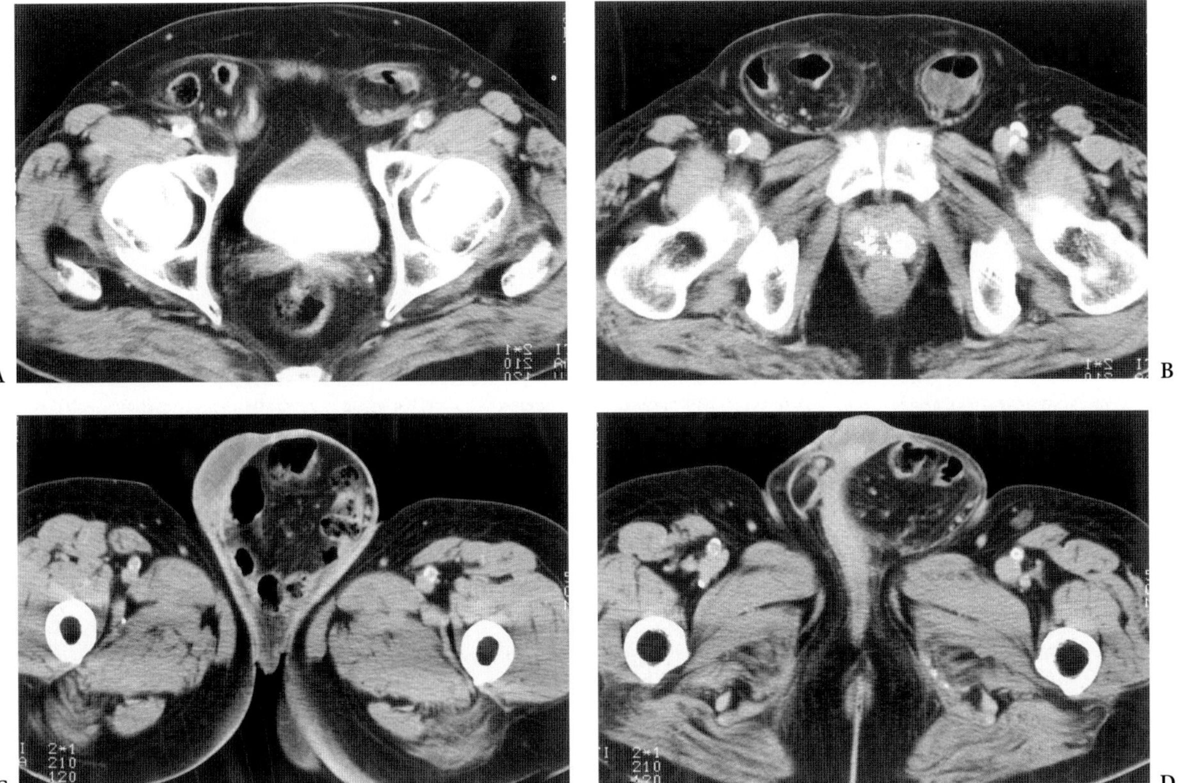

Fig. 10.18A–D. Right external oblique inguinal hernia and left inguinoscrotal hernia. Wide inguinal portae (A) crossed by the hernial sacs containing ileal loops on the right and the sigmoid on the left. The spermatic vessels are pushed in the posterior part of the hernial sacs

In the case of inflammation of the hernia, the walls of the sac and the surrounding tissue become thicker and denser after i.v. contrast medium injection, because of the rich vascularization of the inflammatory tissue (Fig. 10.12).

Adhesions and bridles may form a thick wall around the sac, with linear extensions radiating and intersecting irregularly within the adipose connective tissue; these structures show a moderately high density that does not change after contrast medium injection (Figs. 10.15, 10.20).

10.1.1 Spigelian or Ventral Lateral Herniae

Spigelian herniae develop at the hypogastric level, between the umbilicus and the anterosuperior iliac spine, on the sides of the rectus muscle and under the obliquus externus muscle along the linea semilunaris or spigelian line, which represents the fibrous union of the aponeurosis of the three large muscles of the abdomen with the rectus sheath. The hernial sac may contain omentum and ileal and/or colic loops.

CT shows the defect in the wall between the lateral border of the rectus abdominis muscle and the medial border of the obliquus and transversus muscles (Figs. 10.1–10.3).

10.1.2 Umbilical and Paraumbilical Herniae

Umbilical and paraumbilical herniae develop along the median line at the umbilical level, above or below the umbilicus (Figs. 10.4–10.7).

10.1.3 Lumbar Herniae

Lumbar herniae develop in the posterolateral abdominal wall, i.e. in the spaces of Petit and Grynfelt-Krause, where the wall is weak. The triangular

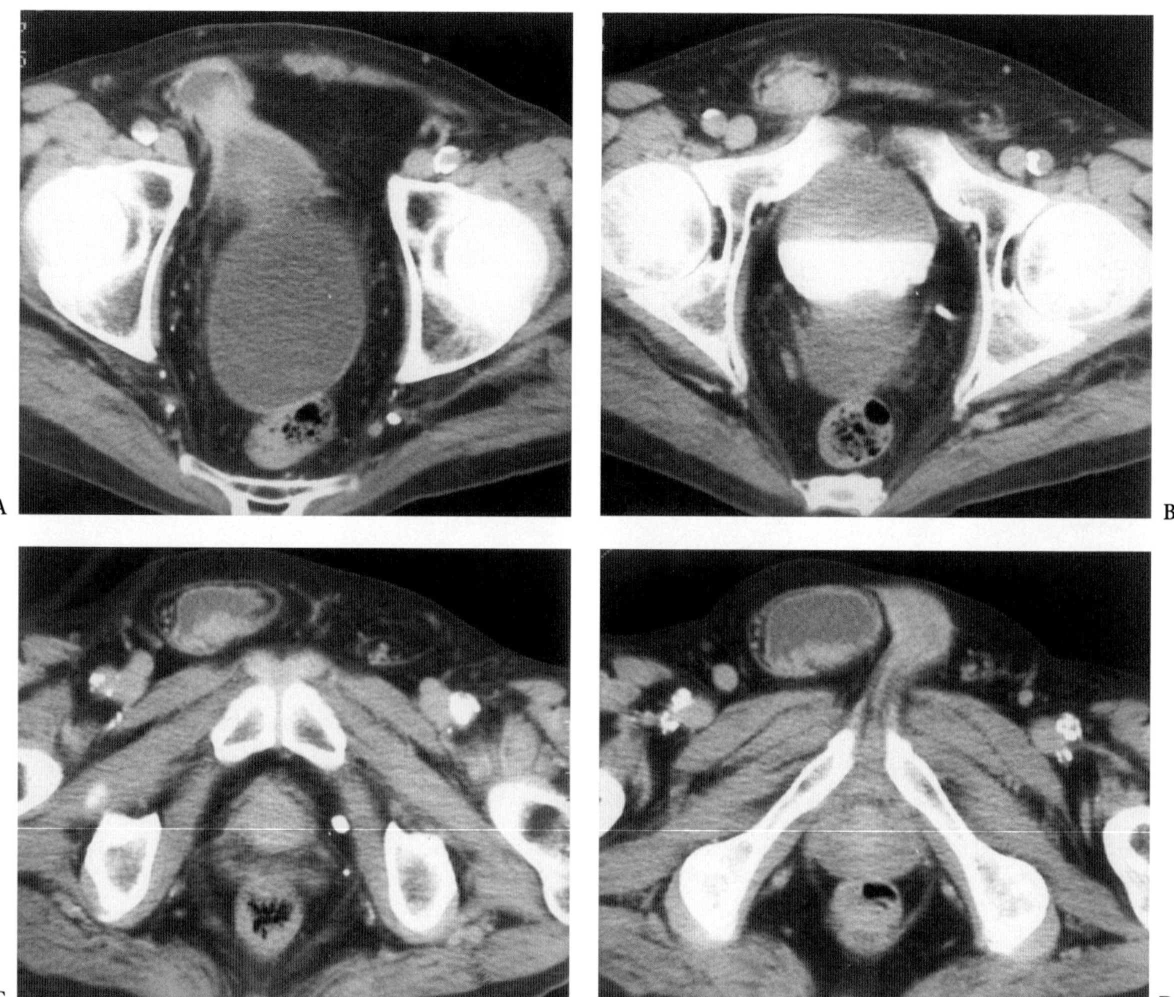

Fig. 10.19A–D. Right external oblique inguinal hernia. Protrusion of ascitic fluid filled peritoneal cavity in the inguinal canal. Deferential vessels located in the external part of the hernial sac

space of Petit is bordered by the iliac crest below, the greater oblique muscle anteriorly and the greater dorsal muscle posteriorly. Grynfelt-Krause's quadrilateral space is bordered at the top by the 12th rib, anteriorly by the posterior border of the internal oblique muscle, and posteriorly by the latissimus dorsi muscle and the quadratus lumborum muscle; it is closed below by the transversus muscle.

These herniae usually develop after surgery, and less frequently after trauma; in rare cases they are congenital. They may contain preperitoneal fat, omentum, ileal loops, the ascending or descending colon, the kidney, the stomach, the spleen or the appendix.

CT shows the interruption in the posterior abdominal wall, the site and the width of the hernial porta, the hernial sac and its content (Fig. 10.8).

10.1.4 Incisional Herniae

Incisional herniae are a protrusion into subcutaneous fat through the abdominal wall consequent on a surgical incision, most frequently located along the median or paramedian abdominopelvic line, where incisions are commonly made. These herniae may be small when they are the result of a simple anterior evagination of the preperitoneal adipose tissue between two muscular bundles and are still contained within the abdominal cavity by a fascia or an aponeurosis; in contrast, they may be voluminous and give rise to a wide sac extending through a large gap in the musculoaponeurotic wall and containing the intestinal loops. A feature peculiar to incisional

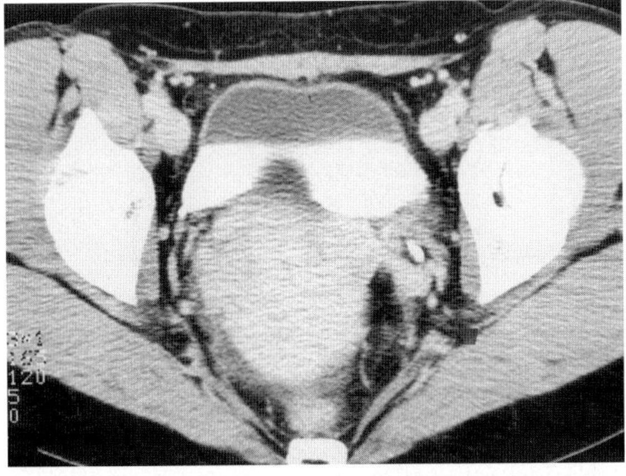

A

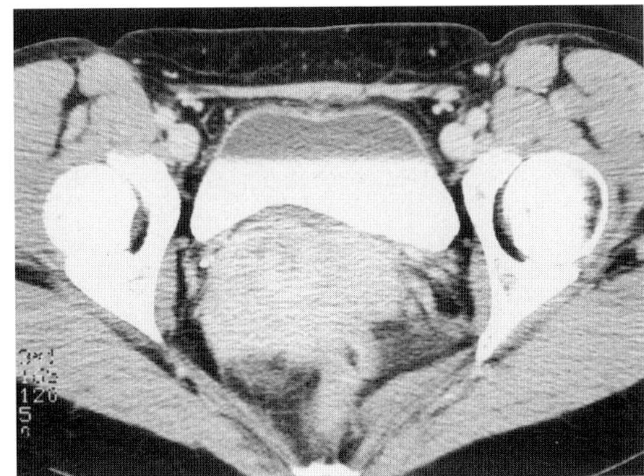

B

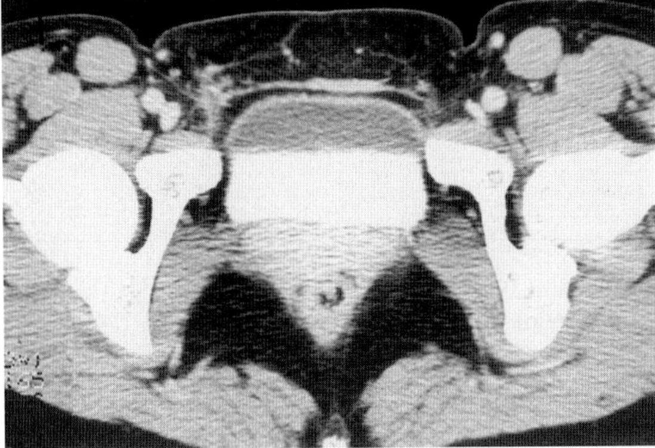

C

Fig. 10.20A–C. Outcome of reduction of right inguinal hernia. Cicatricial fibrous thickening of the surgical incision. A small peritoneal and omental evagination causing pain remains incarcerated in the inguinal canal

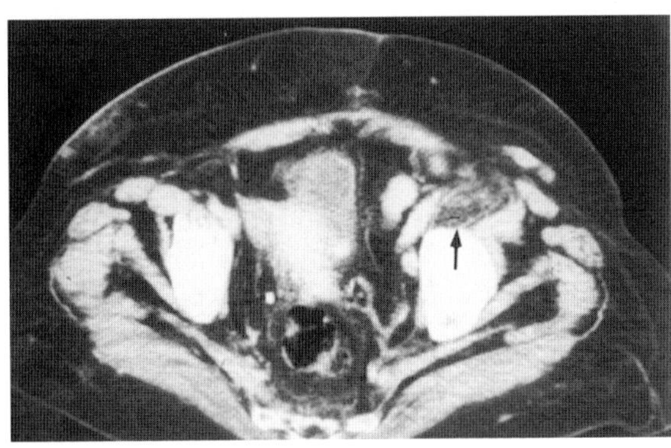

A

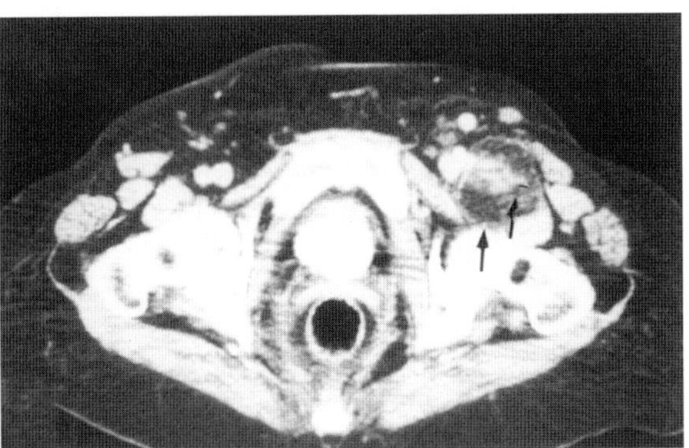

B

Fig. 10.21A, B. Crural hernia. Retroperitoneal liposarcoma herniated between the femoral vessels inside and the iliopsoas muscle outside

herniae is their progressive expansion during the first year after the operation.

In the case of suprapubic incisional herniae the urinary bladder may protrude, even though it is firmly joined to the pelvic floor.

Most incisional herniae can be easily recognized by inspection and palpation, but they can remain undiscovered in various circumstances: in the case of obesity, because of the abundant fat covering the hernial evagination; when a thick, rigid scar is located over a small, deep hernia; or when the herniated segments are positioned among the fascial, aponeurotic and/or muscular layers of the abdominal wall.

CT clearly shows the defect in the abdominal wall, the site and width of the hernia, the hernial sac and its content (Figs. 10.10, 10.11, 10.13–10.16).

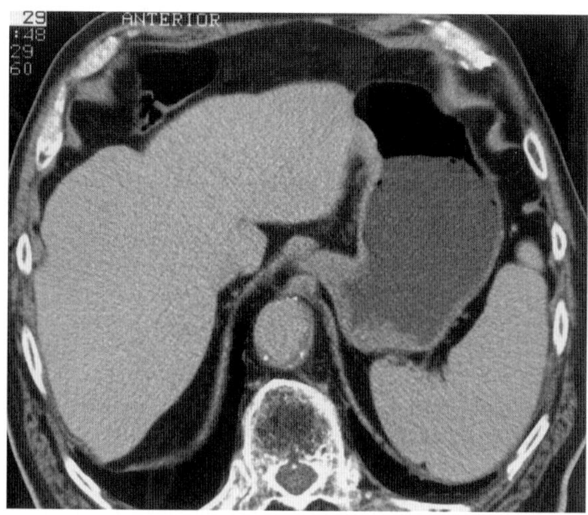

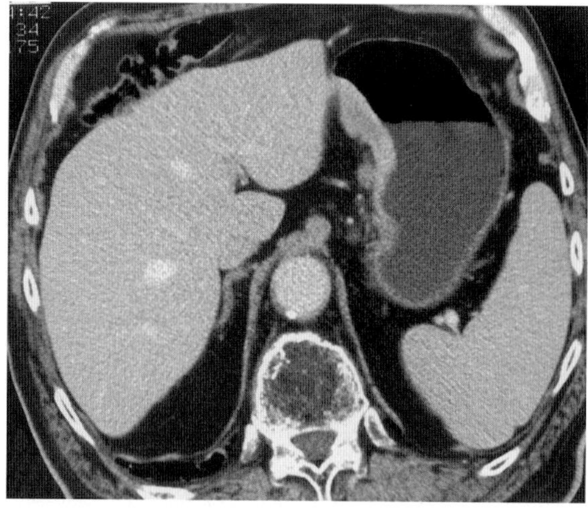

Fig. 10.22A, B. Normal esophageal hiatus. The esophagus passes through a gap between the two diaphragmatic crura (**A**), which join together at a lower level, where they limit the crural space (**B**)

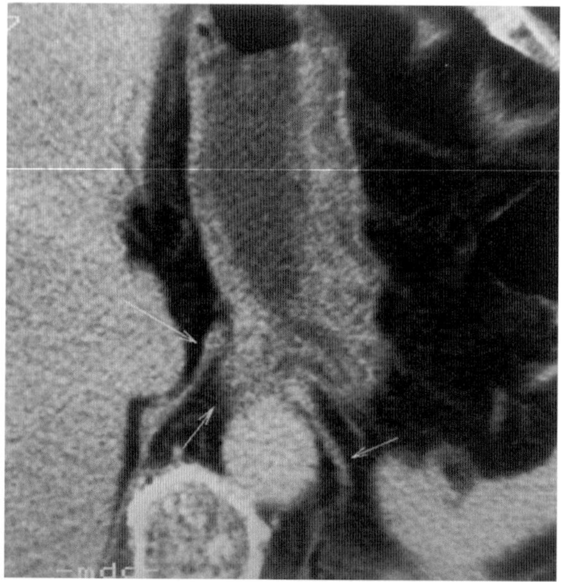

Fig. 10.23. Normal esophageal hiatus and gastroesophageal junction

10.1.5 Inguinal Herniae

Inguinal herniae protrude through the anterior abdominal wall above the pubis. According to their passage through the internal, median or external inguinal fossae, they can be classified into:

1) Internal oblique or supravesical
2) Median or direct
3) External oblique

The internal oblique inguinal hernia protrudes from the internal inguinal fossa between the urachus and the atretic umbilical artery; after crossing the rectus abdominis muscle, it extends obliquely and inward up to the front of the pubis.

The median inguinal hernia originates from the median umbilical fossa, between the cord of the atretic umbilical artery and the inferior epigastric vessels; after a short extension, it reaches the superficial inguinal ring and protrudes in front of the pubis. There is a wide communication between its sac and the peritoneal cavity. It may pull on the fundus of the urinary bladder, which is intimately joined to the overhanging peritoneum.

The external oblique inguinal hernia is the most frequent (90%) type of inguinal hernia; it originates from the lateral umbilical fossa outside the inferior epigastric vessels. In men, it penetrates the inguinal canal, where it is located near the spermatic cord, along its extension downward as far as the scrotum. This type of hernia is favored by the persistence of the vaginal process of the peritoneal sac, which accompanies the descent of the testis. In normal conditions, this process is obliterated at birth.

In women, in contrast, such a hernia extends along the round ligament of the uterus to the labium majus pudendi.

CT shows external oblique inguinal herniae along the anterior pelvic wall. Initially, they are located on

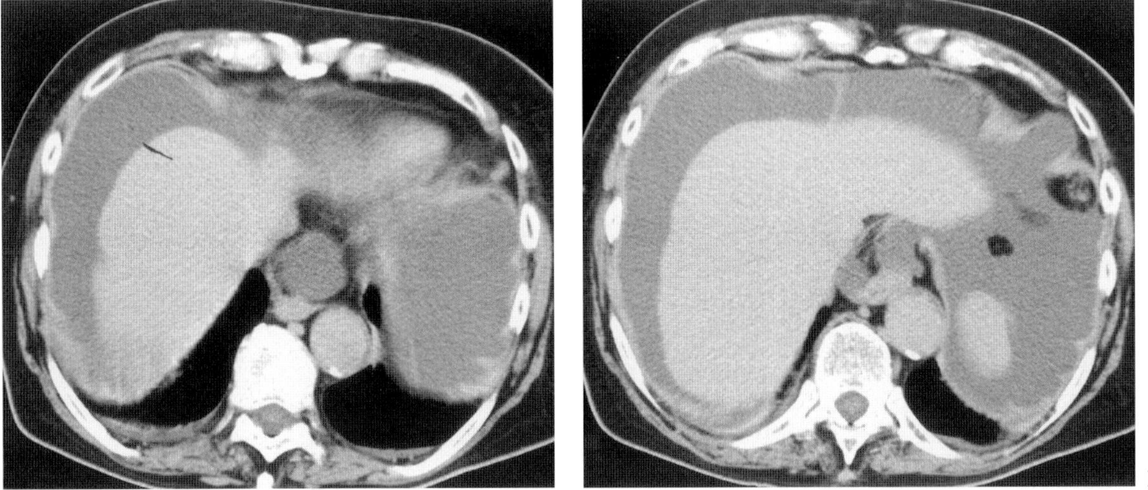

Fig. 10.24A, B. Small hiatal hernia in the presence of ascites. The hernial sac only contains ascitic fluid, which shows the continuation of the sac in the peritoneal cavity

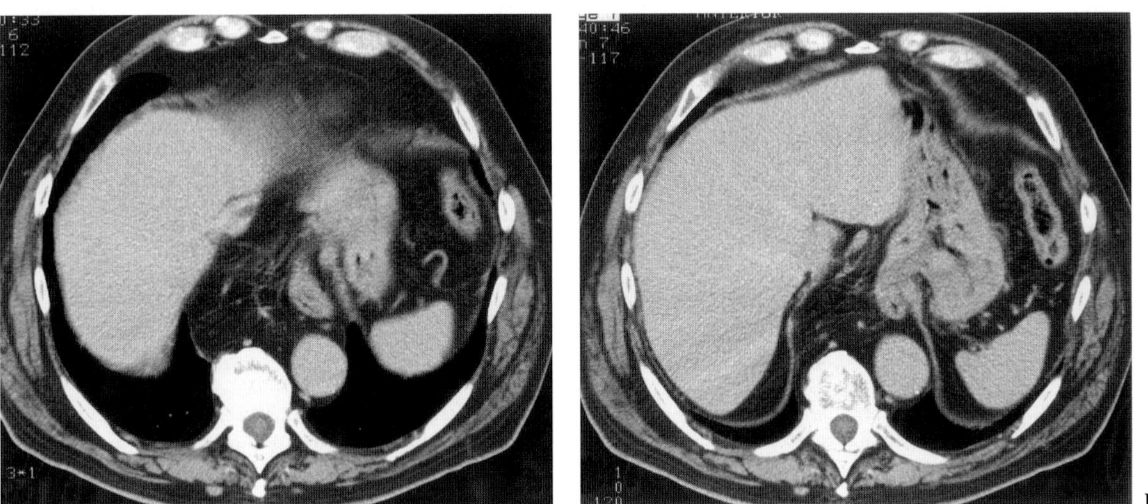

Fig. 10.25A, B. Hiatal hernia. Wide hiatus with open diaphragmatic crura. The omentum and the abdominal fat with their relative vessels are protruding into the posterior mediastinum

the sides of the inferior epigastric vessels, then they extend in front of the pelvic wall and the pubis in the underlying planes, and finally enter the scrotum in men or the labium majus pudendi in women. Preperitoneal or omental adipose tissue alone (Fig. 10.17) or together with hollow viscera: ileum (Fig. 10.18), colon, sigmoid (Fig. 10.18) and urinary bladder may be contained by the hernia. The elements of the spermatic cord (vessels and deferents) are pushed outward and backward by the hernial sac (Fig. 10.19).

In the presence of ascites, the fluid may penetrate the hernial sac through the communication between the peritoneal cavity and a pervious vaginal process (Fig. 10.19).

10.1.6 Crural Herniae

Crural herniae penetrate the femoral canal, pushing the preperitoneal fat, the septum cruralis and the adi-

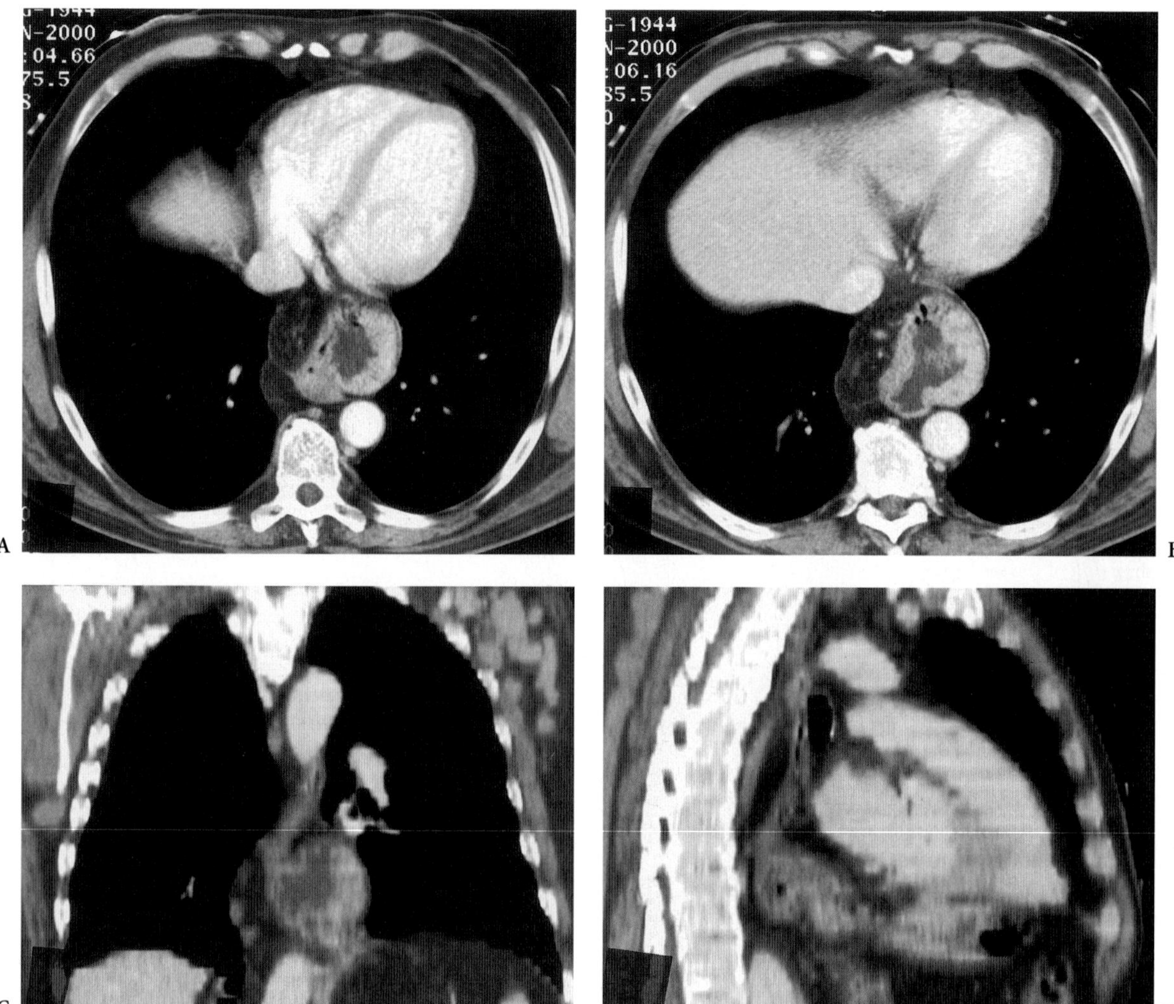

Fig. 10.26A–D. Sliding hiatal hernia with fundus ventriculi and supradiaphragmatic gastroesophageal junction. **A, B** Axial sections; **C** coronal and **D** sagittal reconstructions. Supradiaphragmatic posterosuperior entrance of the esophagus in the herniated fundus ventriculi

Fig. 10.27A–H. Paraesophageal hiatal hernia. Voluminous hernia in the posterior mediastinum extending up to below the carina, through an exceptionally wide hiatus. The esophagus (*E*) can be followed up to the level of the diaphragm; some segments contain air, whereas other tracts are collapsed. The corpus ventriculi is located to the left of the hernial sac, whereas the antrum extends transversely under the carina. The herniated duodenum (*D*) extends vertically from above downward on the right and in front of the stomach up to below the diaphragm, where it again takes up its normal anatomical position at the level of the hepatic artery. The fundus ventriculi remains under the diaphragm

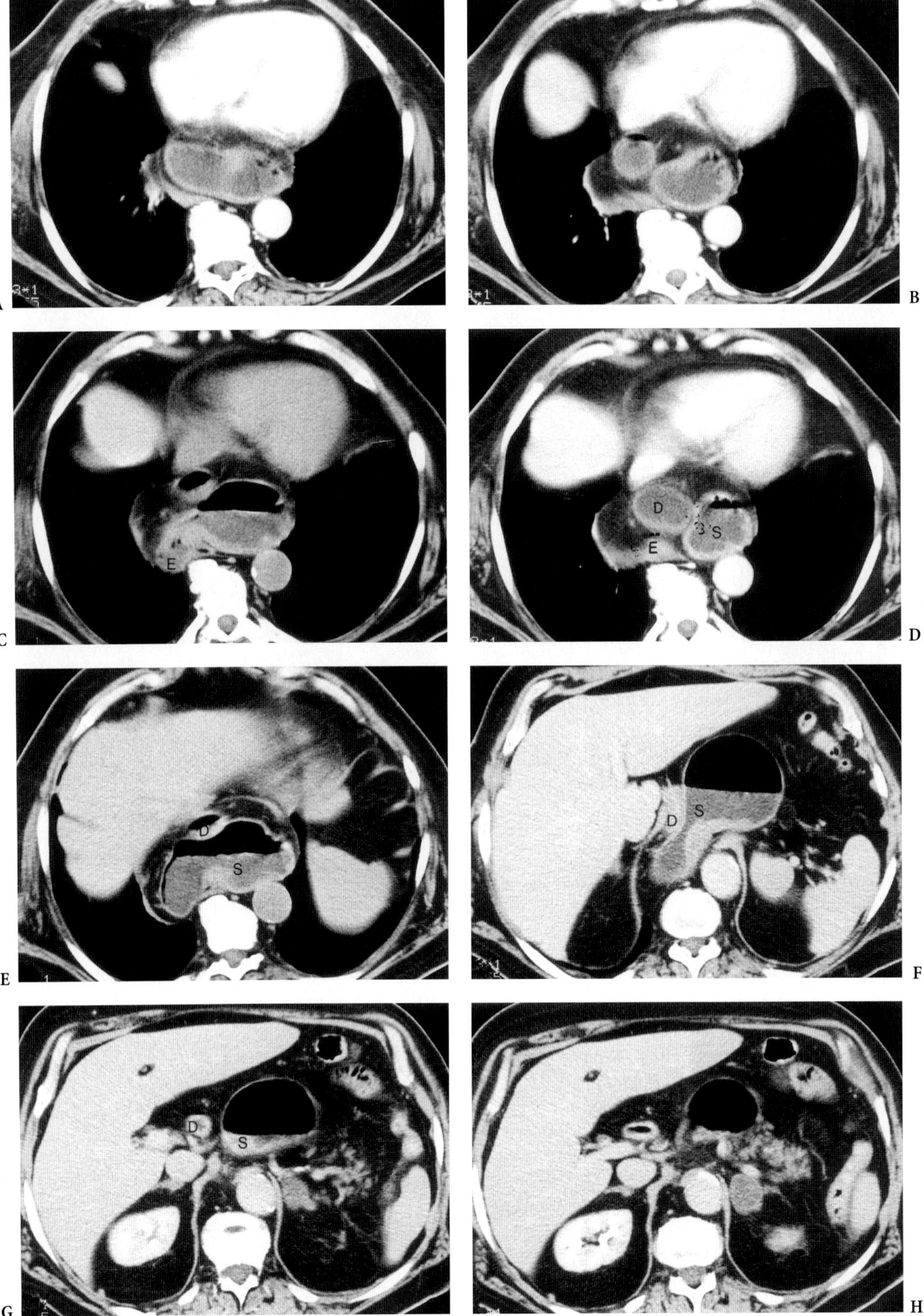
A
B
C
E
D
D
S
E
D
E
D
S
D
S
F
G
D
S
H

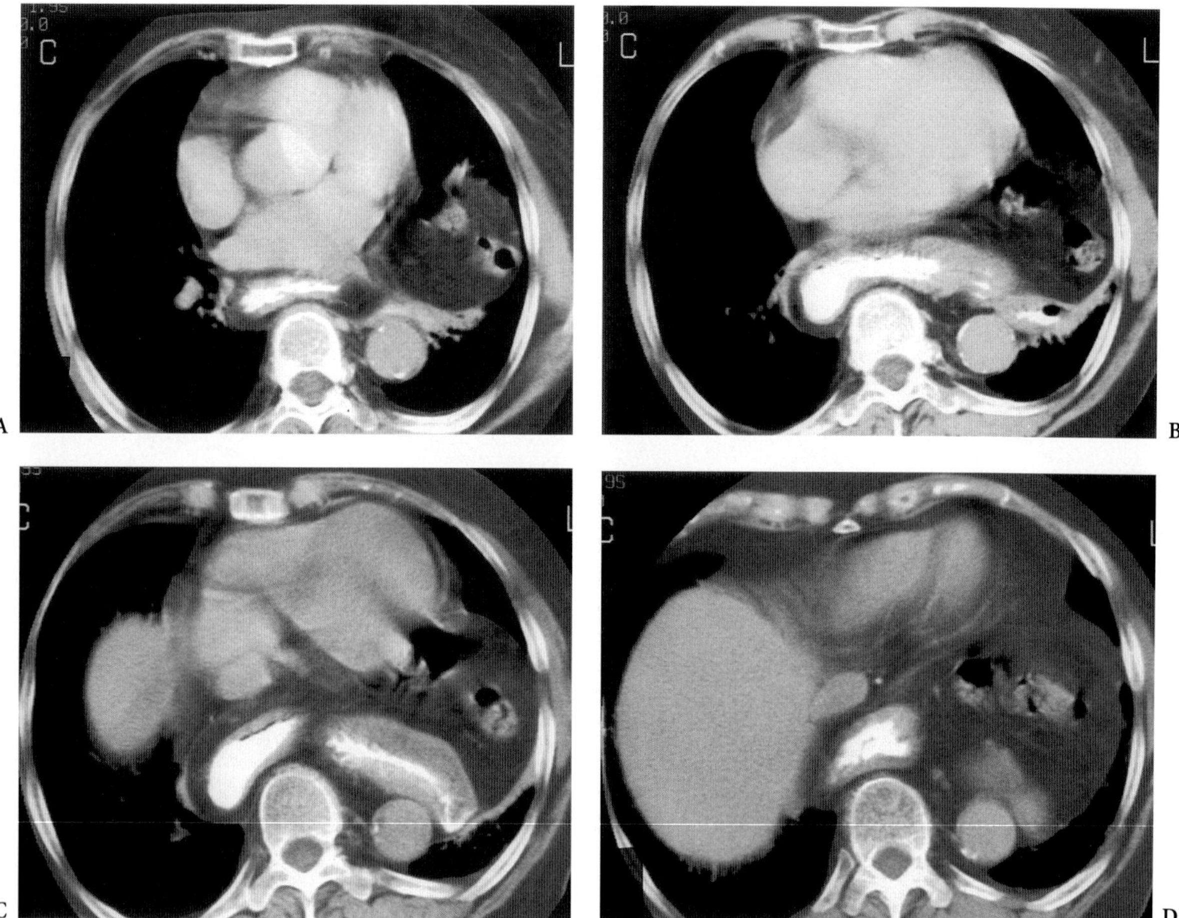

Fig. 10.28A–D. Hiatal and left diaphragmatic hernia. Through a wide diaphragmatic hernial porta, the fundus and corpus ventriculi have slid into the mediastinum and the antrum with the colonic splenic flexure, into the left thoracic cavity. In the absence of any restraint exerted by the left diaphragmatic crus, the aorta has moved outward and backward

pose tissue outward and extending into the sheath of the femoral vessels. Preperitoneal fat, omentum, peritoneum, ileal loops and; exceptionally, the appendix, the cecum, the adnexa uteri and a portion of the urinary bladder may be contained by the hernia. It is not unusual for the clinical diagnosis to be difficult, because of the deep anatomical location of these herniae, which are covered by thick adipose tissue, and also because of their insidious development.

On CT, the femoral canal corresponds to the space occupied by adipose tissue and the femoral vein and artery, between the oval image of the iliopsoas muscle outside and the oblique band of the ileopectineus muscle inside; anteriorly, it is limited by the horizontal line of the ligament of Fallopius and by the superficial leaf of the fascia lata. In this space, the hernial sac protrudes adjacent to the femoral artery and vein (Fig. 10.21).

10.2 Diaphragmatic Herniae

Diaphragmatic herniae are classified into:

1) Esophageal hiatus
2) Morgagni-Larrey
3) Bochdalek
4) Traumatic

10.2.1 Esophageal Hiatus Herniae

An esophageal hiatus is located on the median line above and in front of the arch formed by the diaphragmatic crura, which are the anterior limit of the canal crossed by the aorta, the azygos and hemi-

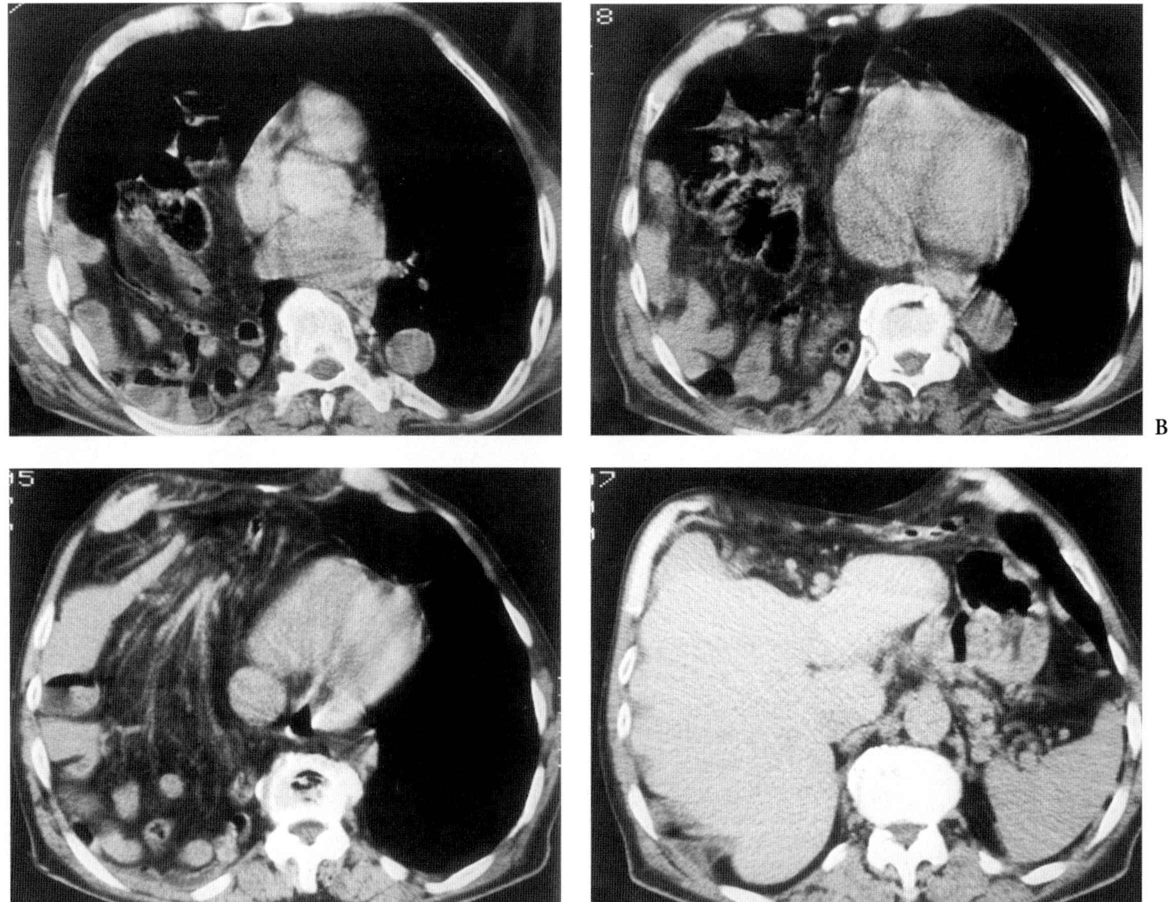

Fig. 10.29A–D. Morgagni's hernia. The ileal loops and the right colon have slid upward through a wide anterior diaphragmatic breach (*D*); they first extended in the front and then above the diaphragm up to the level of the posterior wall of the thoracic cavity. Fan-like disposition of the mesenteric vessels from the front backward, and from the hernial porta toward the sac. The liver remains in its anatomical position, being fixed by the coronary ligament

azygos veins, the thoracic duct, and the nerves. The width of the hiatus is very variable; it is limited by the muscular bundles of the diaphragmatic crus and is crossed by the esophagus.

In normal conditions, CT always clearly shows the esophagus at the level of the hiatus. The esophagus appears to be round or, when it contains air, circular in the supradiaphragmatic tract, and tubular where it crosses the hiatus obliquely, extending to the left and forward to reach the gastroesophageal junction (Figs. 10.22, 10.23). A layer of adipose tissue varying in thickness may surround the esophageal image.

Herniae protruding through the hiatus are constituted by the dislocation into the posterior mediastinum of the preperitoneal adipose tissue alone or together with a more or less conspicuous portion of the stomach, the gastroesophageal junction being above or below the diaphragm.

These herniae include:

- Sliding herniae with esophagus of normal length: the distal esophagus and the proximal portion of the stomach with the gastroesophageal junction are shifted upward because of an abnormally wide hiatus and hypoplasia or senile involution of the phrenoesophageal membrane of Bertelli.
- Sliding herniae attributable to a short or shortened esophagus: the fundus ventriculi and the cardia are displaced above the diaphragm.
- Paraesophageal herniae: the fundus ventriculi is shifted above the diaphragm at the sides of the esophagus; together with the gastroesophageal junction the esophagus remains in the abdomen, fixed by the phrenoesophageal membrane of Bertelli.

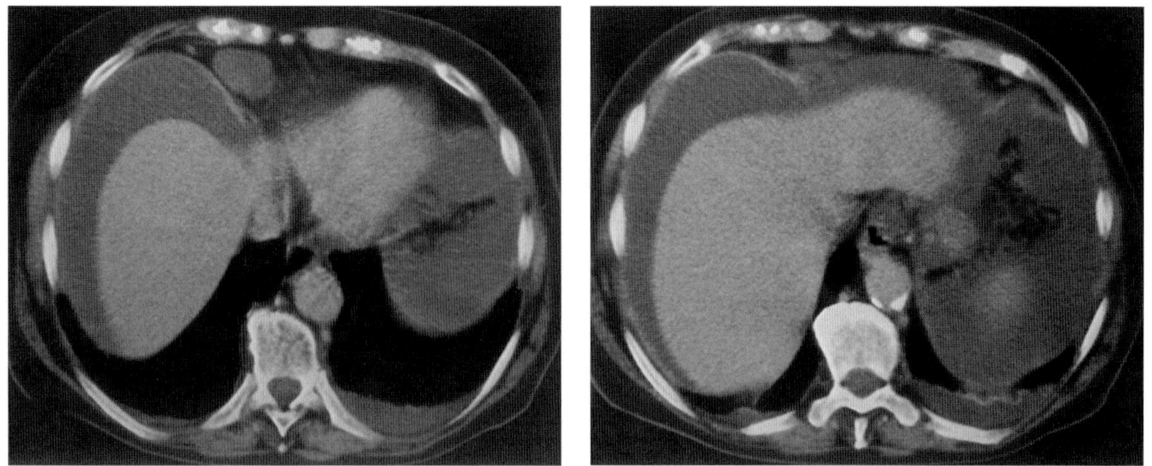

Fig. 10.30A–D. Small Morgagni's hernia in the presence of ascites. Ascitic fluid fills the hernial sac through the communication with the peritoneal cavity

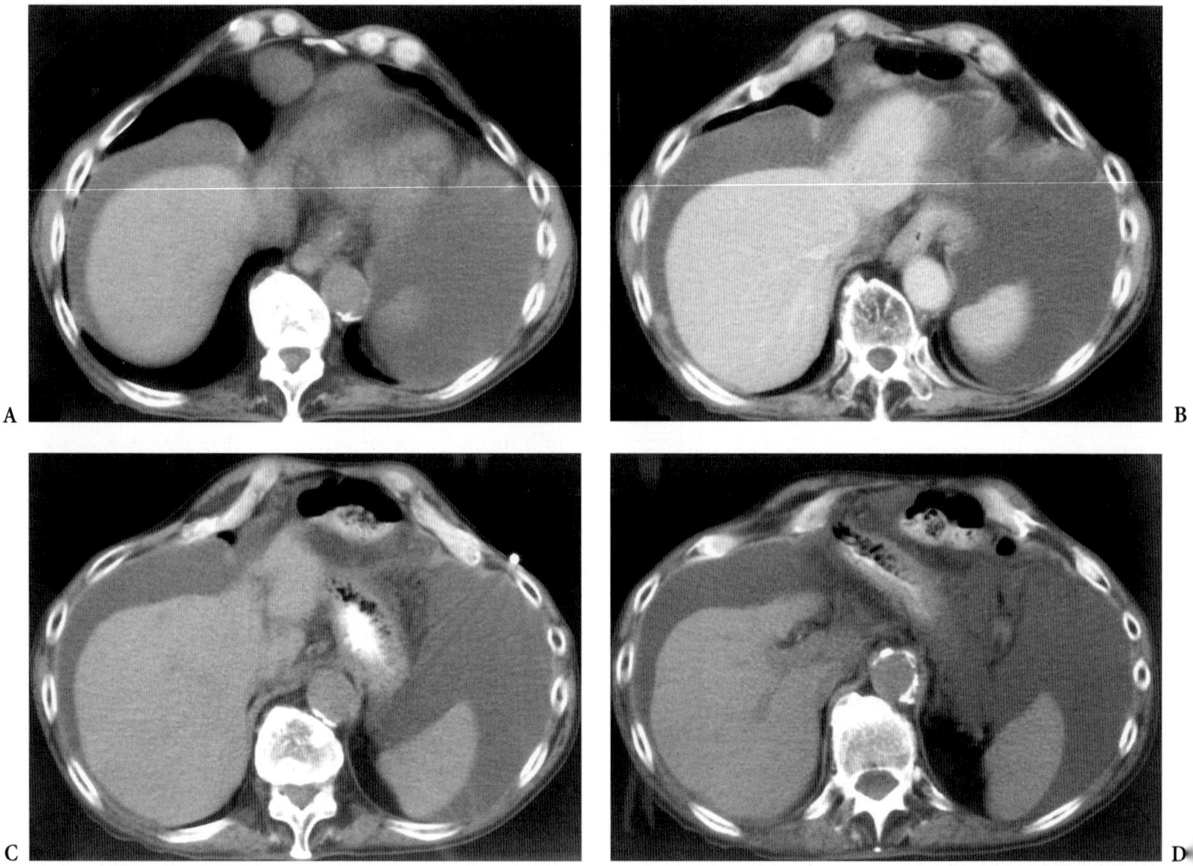

Fig. 10.31A–D. Morgagni's hernia in the presence of ascites. Hernial sac expanded by the ascitic fluid and containing the transverse colon

CT clearly shows not only the hernial porta in the form of an enlarged hiatus, which is limited by the hypoplastic muscular bundles of the diaphragm at the sides, but also the herniated structures. When these are only adipose tissue of preperitoneal or omental origin, they appear as a small mass with fat density, which is most frequently located on the right side and in front of the esophagus (Fig. 10.25).

When a section of the stomach also protrudes into the posterior mediastinum above the diaphragm (within the space that should be occupied by the esophagus alone), the hollow viscus generally appears to be expanded by air or shows an air-fluid level (Figs. 10.25, 10.26). Oral introduction of water or of a radiopaque contrast medium expands the herniated part, which may then become more evident.

The introduction of a radiopaque tube into the esophagus or a reconstruction makes it possible to distinguish a sliding hernia from a paraesophageal one. In the former case, both cardia and esophagus (whose length is normal) are located above the diaphragm after sliding into the posterior mediastinum through a wide hiatus also containing adipose tissue (Fig. 10.26); in the latter case, we must follow the esophagus beyond the diaphragm, where it reaches the cardia located in its normal position. In contrast, the herniated stomach penetrates the hiatal canal, extending laterally, usually on the right side or in front of the esophagus (Fig. 10.27).

The presence of ascites in the peritoneum shows even small evaginations of the peritoneal cavity through the esophageal hiatus (Fig. 10.24).

10.2.2 Morgagni-Larrey's Herniae

These herniae protrude through the retrosternal Morgagni-Larrey's foramen, which is wider than normal owing to a natural weakness of the sternocostal muscular bundles. They usually contain the omentum and the transverse colon, and occasionally the stomach and the small bowel, surrounded by their peritoneal sac; on the other hand, they may only contain preperitoneal adipose tissue without a sac. In most cases, these herniae are asymptomatic.

When the hernia is constituted only by the omentum, it is shown by CT as a fat-density mass and structure at the level of the right (Morgagni's hernia) or the left (Larrey's hernia) anterior costophrenic angle. Its continuation into the preperitoneal fat and through the gap in the diaphragmatic wall is characteristic.

When the peritoneal hernial sac also contains the colon (Fig. 10.29–10.31), the stomach, or the ileal loops (Fig. 10.29), the presence of air or radiopaque contrast medium and the continuity of the viscus and its vessels under the diaphragm make diagnosis easy. In the presence of ascites, the hernial sac may be expanded by the peritoneal fluid (Figs. 10.30–10.31).

10.2.3 Bochdalek's Herniae

These herniae protrude through a posterolateral foramen of the diaphragm, the lumbocostal trigone of Bochdalek, because there is no closure of the pleuropulmonary hiatus. This abnormality may vary in width, extending to partial agenesis of the diaphragm.

Such herniae are most common in neonates and must be differentiated from those observed in adults.

In the neonatal age group, such herniae are conspicuous in size and may contain the liver on the right and the small bowel, the colon, and more rarely the stomach and the spleen, on the left. From a clinical point of view, the patients show symptoms of cardiorespiratory failure consequent on pulmonary collapse and cardiomediastinal displacement caused by the hernial mass. These herniae are easily diagnosed on simple direct radiography of the thorax, because it shows gas-expanded intestinal loops (not uncommonly with air-fluid levels) sliding into the thoracic cavity. After administration of contrast medium orally or as an enema it is possible to distinguish the herniated viscera, the site and the width of the hernial porta. A CT examination is superfluous in these cases.

In adults, these herniae are usually small, resulting solely from hypoplasia of the lumbocostal muscular bundles surrounding Bochdalek's foramen. They are usually asymptomatic and are occasionally discovered as supradiaphragmatic laterovertebral masses on radiological examination of the thorax. CT is always useful for a correct diagnosis of the nature and the characteristics of the lesion: the extent of the diaphragmatic defect, the hernial sac and its fatty, visceral or omental content. The diaphragmatic aperture is always easily visible; it varies in width and may also involve a diaphragmatic crus, constituting a wide communication with the aortic canal; this canal is also a communication between the thoracic cavity and the retroperitoneal space (Figs. 10.32–10.34).

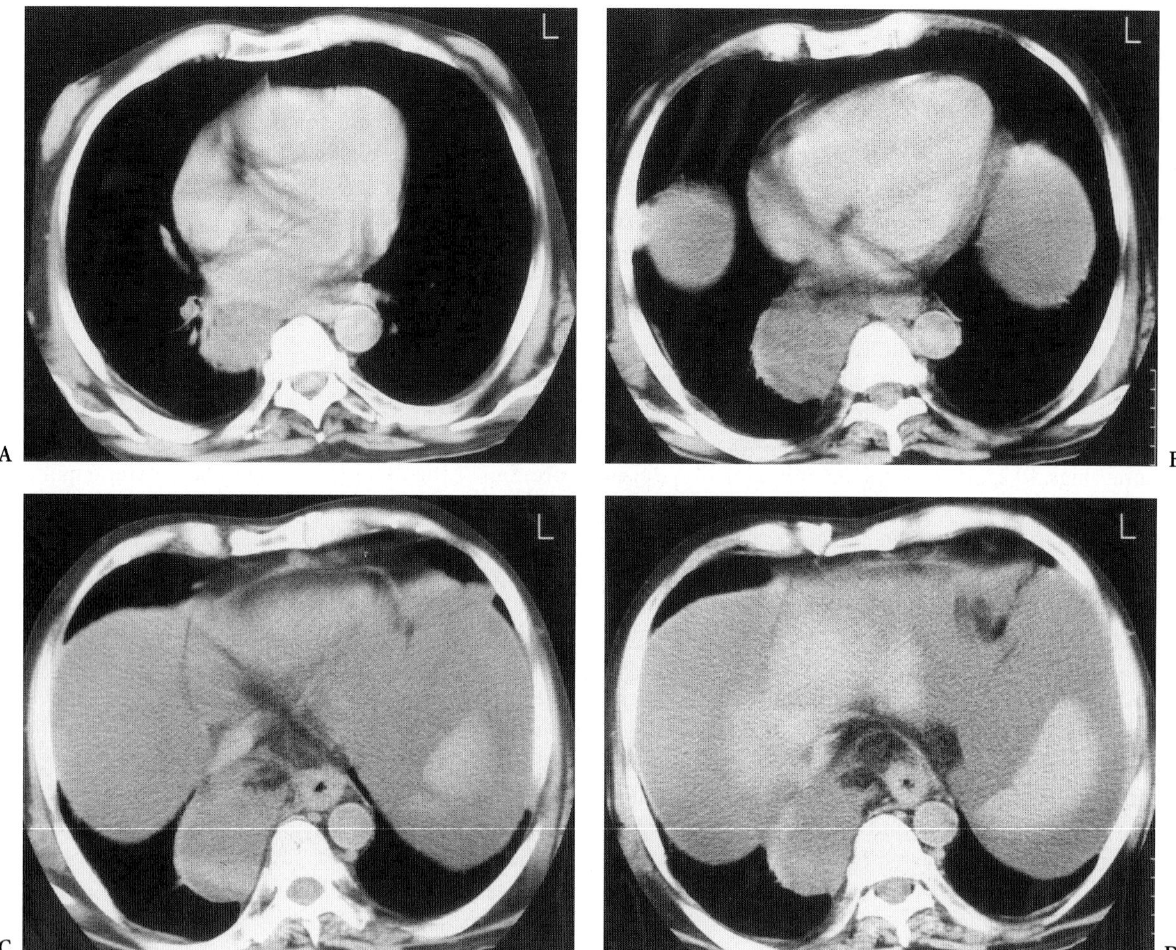

Fig. 10.32A–C. Right Bochdalek's hernia in the presence of ascites. Paravertebral hernial sac distended by ascitic fluid protruding up to the level of the pulmonary hilum and in direct communication with the peritoneal cavity

10.2.4 Traumatic Diaphragmatic Herniae

These herniae are closely associated with the width and the site of the diaphragmatic break produced by the trauma and may contain the omentum with or without abdominal viscera. The CT aspect changes according to the hernial content (Fig. 10.35).

10.3 Internal Herniae

Internal herniae are caused by the protrusion of one or more intestinal loops into an anatomical or abnormal aperture, such as the paraduodenal fossae, Winslow's foramen, the paracecal fossa, or the sigmoidal fossa inside the abdominal cavity.

They are clinically silent and often recover spontaneously, but they can sometimes, cause vague epigastric or periumbilical pain, and occasionally intestinal subobstruction.

In order to help physicians in recognizing internal herniae on CT examination, Meyers (1988) and Ghahremani (1994) underlined some common elements:

1) Abnormal position or orientation of an intestinal loop in a region where a hernia may occur (e.g., the lesser sac)
2) Increased density and encapsulation of ileal loops inside the peritoneal cavity
3) Dilated air-fluid-filled loops before the hernia and/or stasis of contrast medium
4) Fixed site of the herniated loops, with no change in position over time

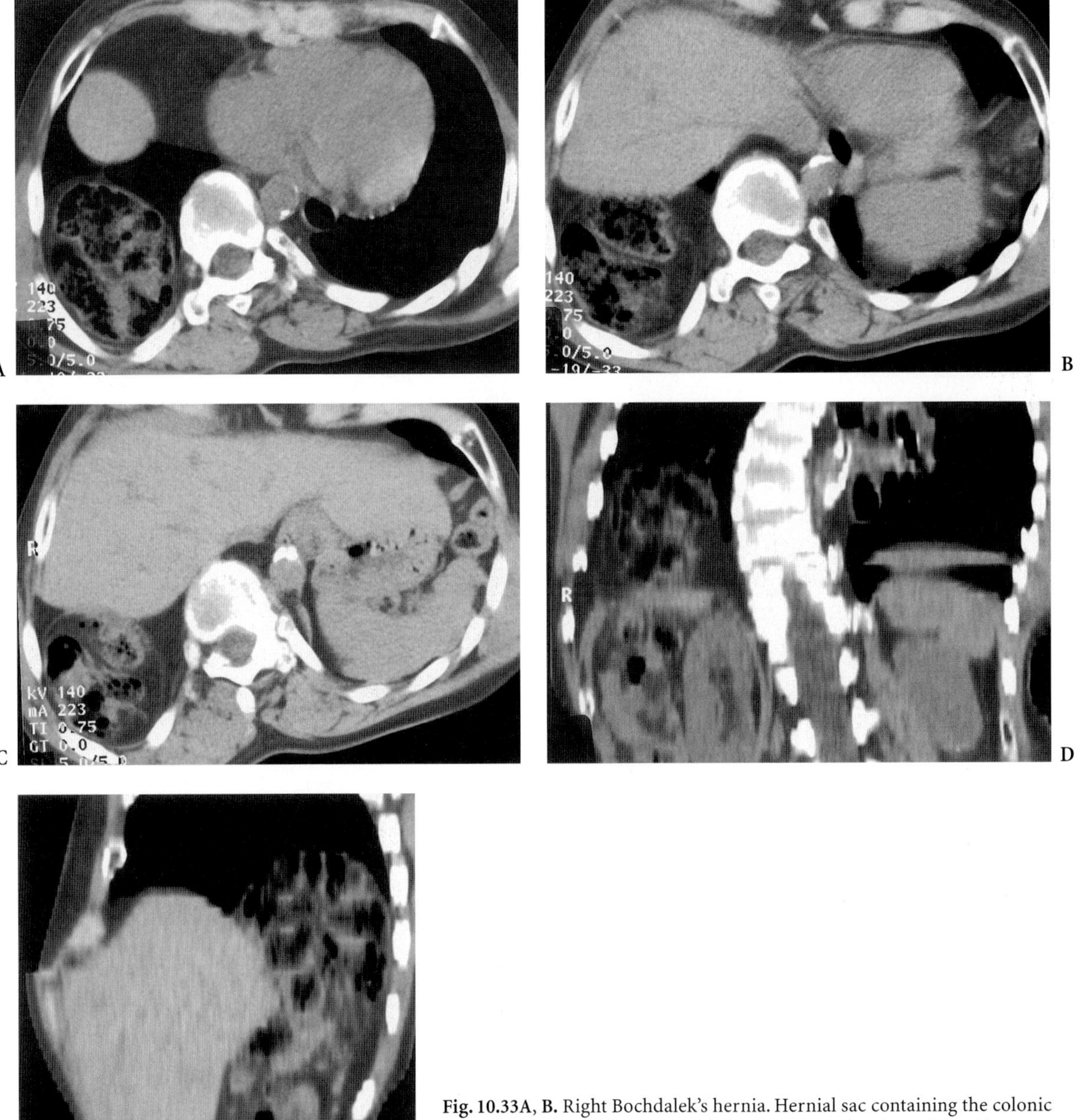

Fig. 10.33A, B. Right Bochdalek's hernia. Hernial sac containing the colonic hepatic flexure, which penetrated the thoracic cavity through a wide retrohepatic Bochdalek's foramen

10.3.1 Paraduodenal or Mesocolic Herniae

Right and left paraduodenal herniae are the most common internal herniae; they are caused by abnormalities of growth, associated with incomplete intestinal rotation around the superior mesenteric artery. These herniae are characterized by incarceration of small bowel loops in the mesocolon, before its complete fixation. In other words, they are jejunal herniae, whose hernial sac is formed by the mesocolon. These herniae occur more commonly on the left side (3:1 ratio).

A paraduodenal or left mesocolic hernia is caused by penetration of the first jejunal loop in Landzert's paraduodenal fossa through a lacuna of the transverse mesocolon or the descending mesocolon, next to the splenic flexure. The afferent jejunal loop penetrates the sac from behind as the continuation of the duodenum and extends toward the left and down-

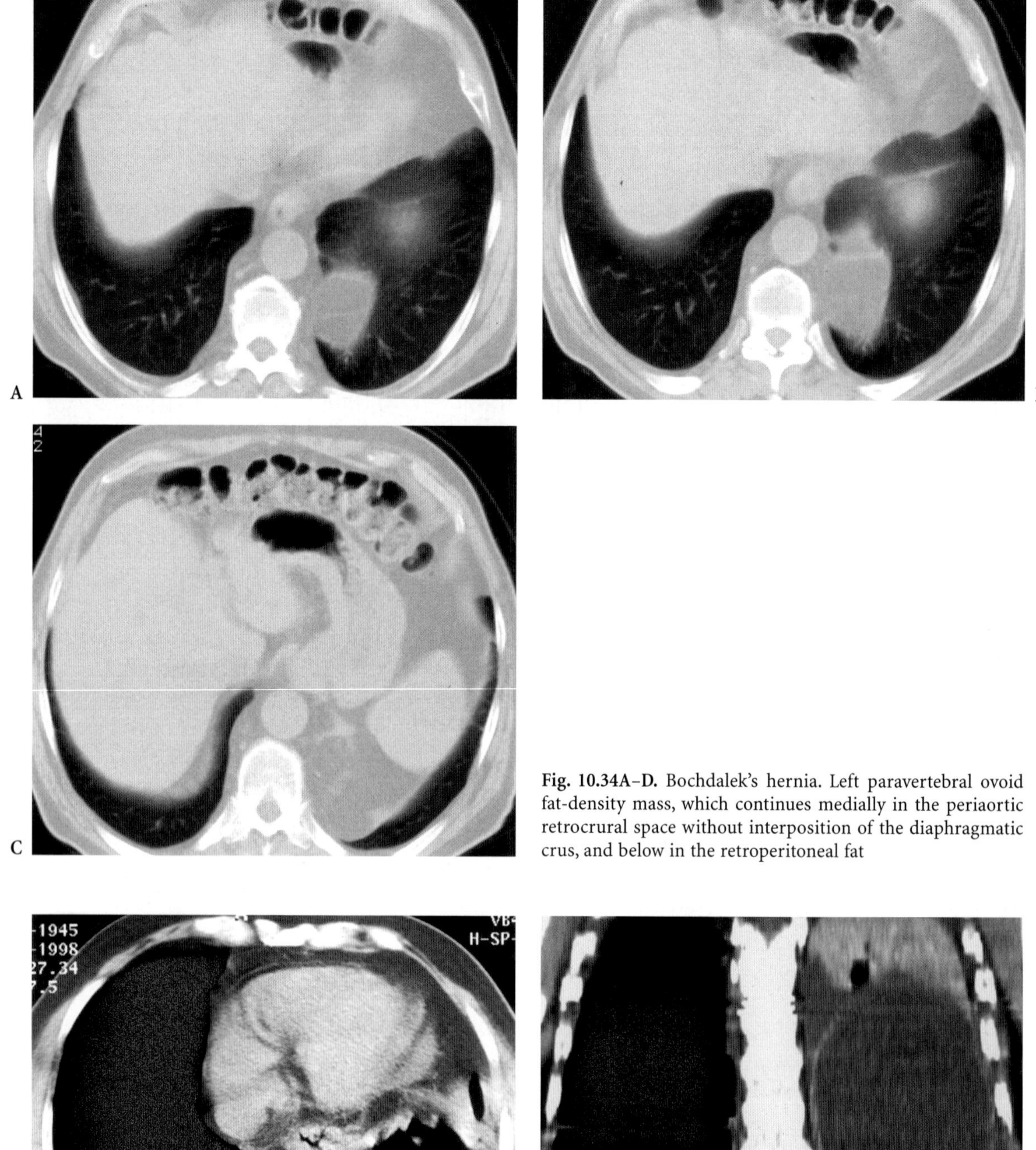

Fig. 10.34A–D. Bochdalek's hernia. Left paravertebral ovoid fat-density mass, which continues medially in the periaortic retrocrural space without interposition of the diaphragmatic crus, and below in the retroperitoneal fat

Fig. 10.35A, B. Traumatic diaphragmatic hernia. A wide portion of the stomach expanded by an abundant amount of fluid has herniated into the thoracic cavity through a wide radial diaphragmatic breach extending from the tendinous center up to the esophagus

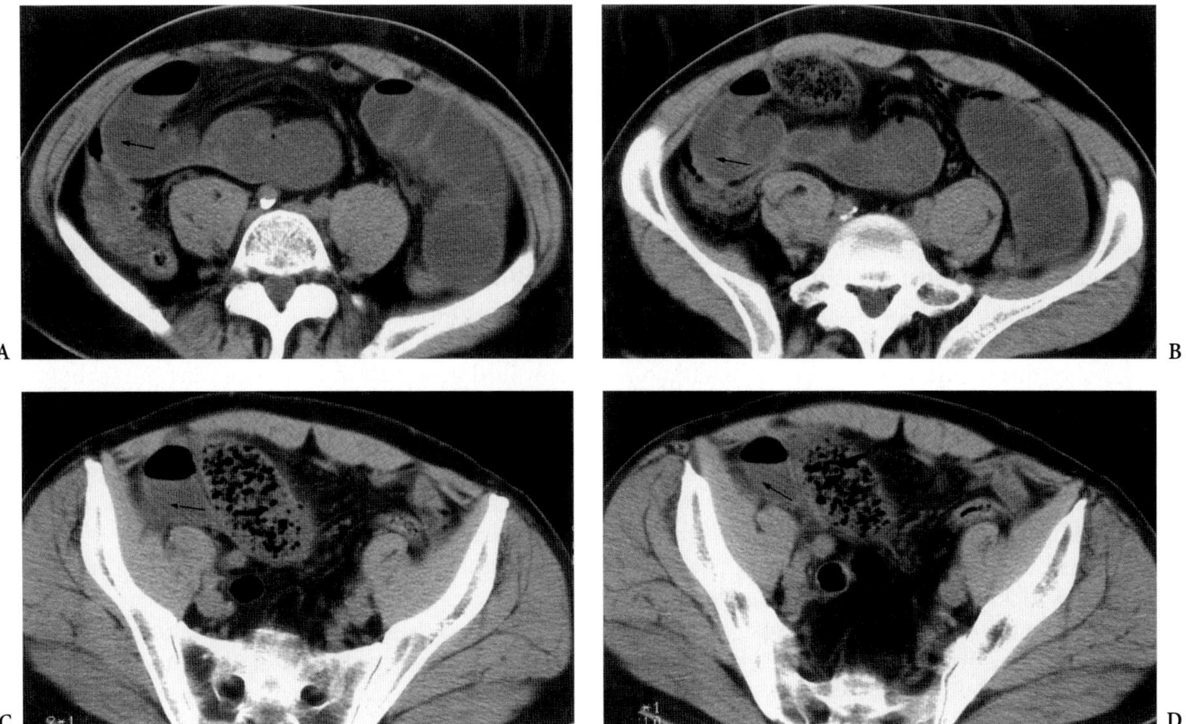

Fig. 10.36. Paracecal hernia with intestinal obstruction. Ileal loop herniated (*arrow*) through a defect of the mesentery outside the cecum, which is pushed medially. The ileal loops preceding the incarcerated hernia are expanded and show air-fluid levels

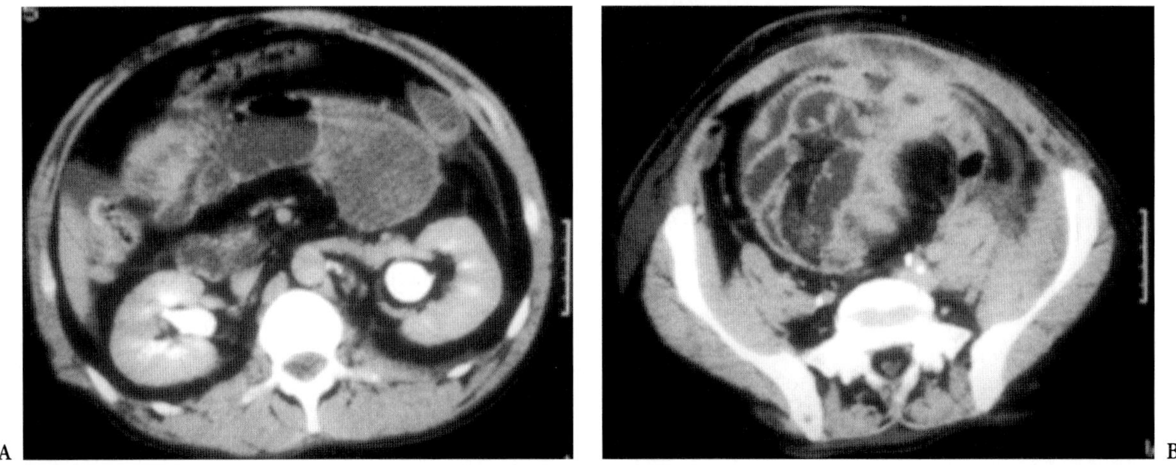

Fig. 10.37. Intersigmoidal hernia containing the whole of the small bowel. Expanded ileal loops with air-fluid levels grouped in the hypogastrium. The sigmoid is displaced upward and to the right

ward, outside the descending colon and the splenic flexure, which are dislocated medially. The efferent loop emerges at a distal point, which is often much lower than the site of the afferent loop.

A radiological examination of the digestive tract may correctly indicate the position and disposition of the jejunal loops. These are densely grouped and fixed in the left hypochondrium, and displace the stomach and the colonic splenic flexure medially. A direct continuation of the duodenum toward the left side, without the angle of Treitz' s flexure, is characteristic of this hernia. At the point of penetration of the hernia, a short stretch of the jejunum is slightly narrowed. The efferent loop is located at a much lower site than the afferent loop.

CT shows the hernia as a sac with sharp limits and very thin walls, containing an ovoid mass made up of dilated and grouped jejunal loops. These loops protrude backward and laterally, extending behind and outside the colon, and are in close contact with the anterior pararenal fascia in the left paraduodenal space. At the point of penetration into the sac, the jejunal loop shows a ring-like narrowness.

The jejunal vessels have a characteristic orientation: they extend along the hernial loops, behind the inferior mesenteric vessels and the left colic vessels, and in front of the hernial sac (Ghahremani 1994).

A paraduodenal or right mesocolic hernia is formed by the protrusion of a group of jejunoileal loops into Waldayer's mesentericoparietal fossa through a defect in the ascending mesocolon or the right half of the transverse mesocolon. Such herniae extend just in front of the parietal peritoneum, outside the second duodenal portion behind the superior mesenteric artery.

Examination of the digestive tube makes it possible to recognize this hernia from the arrangement of the proximal jejunal loops on the right side under the second duodenal portion. These loops appear to be grouped and heaped up as in the mesenterium commune, except for the normal location of the right colon and its extension outside the ileal loops.

CT scans show the jejunoileal loops, with their respective arterial and venous vessels of the superior mesenteric stalk, densely grouped and extending on the right side of the abdomen, outside and under the second duodenal portion. In addition, the jejunal branches of the superior mesenteric artery and vein extend toward the right rather than the left side and are located behind the main trunks.

10.3.2 Herniae of Winslow's Foramen or of the Lesser Sac

Herniae of the lesser sac usually protrude through the foramen of Winslow, and exceptionally through the fissure of the gastrohepatic ligament or that of the transverse mesocolon. They are favored by abnormalities in development (Winslow's foramen wider than normal, abnormal mobility of the ileocolic loops owing to long or lax mesenteries) and are provoked by a sudden increase in the intraabdominal pressure (traumas, parturition, weight lifting).

In most cases (60–70%), the loops of the small bowel, and occasionally the cecum, the ascending or the transverse colon, the gallbladder and the omentum, herniate into the omental bursa.

Clinical symptoms are characterized by progressively increasing epigastric pain and occur acutely.

CT allows recognition and localization of the hernial porta between the portal vein and the inferior vena cava, and the sac with the herniated loops extending between the stomach and the pancreas, medially to the liver in the site of the lesser sac. The bowel loops before the hernia are always expanded. We can establish exactly which intestinal segment has herniated after administration of a radiopaque contrast medium by mouth.

10.3.3 Paracecal Herniae

Paracecal herniae occur when one or more ileal loops penetrate through a defect of the mesocecum into the right paracecal fossa, with the cecum in a medial position relative to these loops. They are the consequence of abnormalities in development owing to stopped rotation of the ileal loops when these are located behind the cecum. These herniae frequently cause intestinal obstruction.

A direct radiography and a barium enema may be enough to show the sliding of the herniated ileal loops outside the cecum and the air-fluid-filled ileal loops before the hernia.

CT (Fig. 10.36) clearly shows the abnormal position of the herniated loop outside the cecum (that is pushed medially), the air-fluid-filled ileal loops preceding the herniated tract, and the collapse of the colon and the sigmoid.

10.3.4 Intersigmoidal Herniae

Intersigmoidal herniae protrude into the hypogastrium through a fissure in one or both the mesosigmoidal leaves with sliding of a portion of the jejunum or of the ileum, or the total small intestine, from above downward and from right to left.

The most common clinical manifestation of such herniae is acute intestinal obstruction directly resulting from incarceration of the herniated segment.

Up to now, these herniae have been studied only radiographically following barium enema, which shows retrograde filling of the herniated ileal loops incarcerated between the sigmoidal loops (MEYERS 1988; GHAHREMANI 1994). CT shows a hypogastric circumscribed ovoid mass of grouped air-fluid-filled ileal loops pushing the sigmoid upward and to the right (Fig. 10.37).

Bibliography

Bach DB, Satin R, Palayew M, et al (1984) Herniation and strangulation of the gallbladder through the foramen of Winslow. AJR Am J Roentgenol 142:541–542
Baker ME, Weinerth JL, Andriani RT, Cohan RH, Dunnick NR (1987) Lumbar hernia: diagnosis by CT. AJR Am J Roentgenol 148:565–567
Baker ME, Ungerlaider R, Cooper C, Dunnick NR (1988) Computed tomography of a traumatic, diaphragmatic, Richter's hernia: findings mimicking an abscess. J Comput Assist Tomogr 12:42–44
Balthazar EJ, Subramanyam BR, Megibow A (1984) Spigelian hernia: CT and ultrasonography diagnosis. Gastrointest Radiol 9:81–84
Bergonzi M, Bonfioli C, Motta F, Urani A, Colago MF (1996) Ernie di Spigelio complicate: quadri con tomografia computerizzata. Descrizione di 2 casi. Radiol Med 92:822–823
Caltagirone G, Bianchi G, Lo Bello G, Ponzio S, Tramontano S (1995) Ernia crurale recidiva. Impiego della TC nella valutazione preoperatoria: due casi. Radiol Med 92:820–821
Cubillo E (1983) Obturator hernia diagnosed by computed tomography. AJR Am J Roentgenol 140:735–736
Day DL, Drake DG, Leonard AS, Letourneau JG (1988) CT findings in left paraduodenal herniae. Gastrointest Radiol 13:27–29
Donnelly LF, Rencken IO, De Lorimier AA, Gooding CA (1996) Left paraduodenal hernia leading to ileal obstruction. Pediatr Radiol 26:534–536
Ekberg O, Kullenberg K (1988) Direct diverticular inguinal hernia. Acta Radiol Diagn 29:57–60
Ekberg O, Nordblom I, Fork FT, et al (1985) Herniography of femoral, obturator and perineal hernias. Rofo Fortschr Geb Rontgenstr Neuen Bildgeb Verfahr 143:193–199
Fagelman D, Caridi JG (1984) CT diagnosis of hernia of Morgagni. Gastrointest Radiol 9:153–155
Faro SH, Racette CD, Lally JF, et al (1990) Traumatic lumbar hernia: CT diagnosis. AJR Am J Roentgenol 154:757–759
Fish AE, Brodey PA (1981) Computed tomography of the anterior abdominal wall: normal anatomy and pathology. J Comput Assist Tomogr 5:728–733
Gale ME (1985) Bochdalek hernia: prevalence and CT characteristics. Radiology 156:449–452
Gallone L (1986) Ernie dei visceri addominali. In: Gallone L (ed) Patologia chirurgica. Ambrosiana, Milan
Gharemani GG (1994) Abdominal and pelvic hernias. In: Gore RM, Levine MS, Laufer I (eds) Textbook of gastrointestinal radiology. Saunders, Philadelphia
Ghahremani GG, Gore RM (1989) CT diagnosis of postoperative abdominal complications. Radiol Clin North Am 27:797–804
Ghahremani GG, Meyers MA (1981) Iatrogenic abdominal hernias. In: Meyers MA, Ghahremani GG (eds) Iatrogenic gastrointestinal complications. Springer, New York Berlin Heidelberg
Ghahremani GG, Michael AS (1991) Sciatic hernia with incarcerated ileum: CT and radiographic diagnosis. Gastrointest Radiol 16:120–122
Ghahremani GG, Jemenez MA, Rosenfeld M, et al (1987) CT diagnosis of occult incisional hernias. AJR Am J Roentgenol 148:139–142
Goldberger LE, Berk RN (1980)Cecal herniation into the lesser sac. Gastrointest Radiol 5:169–172
Gossios KJ, Tatsis CK, Lykouri A, Constantopoulos SH (1991) Omental herniation through the foramen of Morgagni. Diagnosis with chest computed tomography. Chest 100:1469–1470
Hahn Pedersen J, Bojsen Moller F, Rosenklint A (1989) Functional closure of the femoral canal revealed by computed tomographic scanning. Br J Surg 76:1195–1197
Hahn Pedersen J, Lund L, Hansen Hojhus J, et al (1994) Evaluation of direct and indirect inguinal hernia by computed tomography. Br J Surg 81:569–572
Harkin WP (1982) Computed tomographic diagnosis of internal hernia. Radiology 143:736–737
Hoeffel JC, Zimberger J, Pocard B, Hoeffel C (1992) Demonstration by computed tomography of a case of internal small bowel herniation. Br J Radiol 65:1045–1046
Hojer AM, Rygaard H, Jess P (1997) CT in the diagnosis of abdominal wall hernias: preliminary study. Eur Radiol 7:1416
Hosaka S, Yoshii S, Takano K, Iwasaki M, Kamiya K, Matsukawa T, Ueno A (1991) A case of Morgagni's hernia: availability of CT scan, ultrasonography, and trans-abdominal surgical approach. Kyobu-Geka 44:503–506
Kane VG, Silverstein GS (1986) CT demonstration of hernia through an iliac crest defect. J Comput Assist Tomogr 10:432–434
Lawdahl RB, Moss CN, Van Dyke JA (1986) Inferior lumbar (Petit's) hernia. AJR Am J Roentgenol 147:744–745
Lee MJ, Breathnach E (1990) CT and MRI findings in paraoesophageal omental herniation. Clin Radiol 42:207–209
Lewin JR (1981) Femoral hernia with upward extension into abdominal wall: CT diagnosis. AJR Am J Roentgenol 136:206–207
Lubat E, Gordon RB, Birnbaum BA, et al (1990) CT diagnosis of posterior perineal hernia. AJR Am J Roentgenol 154:761–762
Luedke M, Scholz FJ, Larsen CR (1988) Computed tomographic evaluation of Spigelian hernia. Comput Med Imaging Graph 12:123–129

Megibow AJ, Wagner AG (1983) Case report: obturator hernia. J Comput Assist Tomogr 7:350–352
Meyers MA (1988) Internal abdominal hernias. In: Meyers MA (ed) Dynamic radiology of the abdomen. Normal and pathologic anatomy. Springer, New York Berlin Heidelberg
Meziane MA, Fishman EK, Siegelman SS (1983) Computed tomography of obturator foramen hernia. Gastrointest Radiol 8:375–377
Pandolfo I, Blandino M, Gaeta M, et al (1986) CT findings in palpable lesions of the anterior abdominal wall. J Comput Assist Tomogr 10:629–633
Papierniak KJ, Wittenstein B, Bartizal JF, Wielgolewski JW, Love L (1983) Diagnosis of Spiegelian hernia by computed tomography. Arch Surg 118:109–110
Passas V, Karavias D, Grilias D, Birbas A (1986) Computed tomography of left paraduodenal hernia. J Comput Assist Tomogr 10:542–543
Peters JC, Reinertson JS, Polansky SM, et al (1988) CT demonstration of traumatic ventral hernia. J Comput Assist Tomogr 12:710–711
Pyatt RS, Alona BR (1982) Spigelian hernia. J Comput Assist Tomogr 6:643–645
Rossi G, Orsi P, Montanari M (1996) Valutazione dell'ernia di Spigelio mediante tomografia computerizzata. Osservazione su due casi. Radiol Med 91:658–660
Salomonowitz E, Frick MP, Sommer G, et al (1983) Symptomatic inguinal hernia: association with intraabdominal mass lesions. Gastrointest Radiol 8:371–374
Schuster MR, Tu RK, Scanlan KA (1992) Caecal herniation through the foramen of Winslow: diagnosis by computed tomography. Br J Radiol 65:1047–1048
Shenouda NF, Hyams BB, Rosenbloom MB (1990) Evaluation of Spigelian hernia by CT. J Comput Assist Tomogr 14:777–778
Tamura A, Murakami K, Sato K, Komatsu H, Uoneda R, Takahash (1988) A case of intrathoracic omental herniation through the esophageal hiatus. Nippon Kyobu Shikkan Gakkai Zasshi 26:1010–1104
Tran TL, Pitt PCC (1989) Hernia through the foramen of Winslow. A report of two cases with emphasis on plain film interpretation. Clin Radiol 40:264–266
Tran TL, Regan F, Al Kutoubi NA (1991) Computed tomography of lesser sac hernia through the gastrohepatic omentum. Br J Radiol 64:372–374
Warshauer DM, Mauro MA (1992) CT diagnosis of paraduodenal hernia. Gastrointest Radiol 17:13–15
Wechsler RL, Kurtz AB, Needleman L, et al (1989) Cross-sectional imaging of abdominal wall hernias. AJR Am J Roentgenol 153:517–521
Wojasek DA, Codner MA, Nowak EJ (1991) CT diagnosis of cecal herniation through the foramen of Winslow. Gastrointest Radiol 16:77–79
Zarvan NP, Lee FT, Yandow DR et al (1995) Abdominal hernias: CT findings. AJR Am J Roentgenol 164:1391–1395

11 Cysts

CONTENTS

A cyst (from the Greek κιστισ or κιστη = cyst) is a pathologic formation consisting of a closed cavity with its own wall of definite epithelium or anomalous tissue, which usually contains fluid or other materials. Cysts are classified according to etiological or histopathological criteria. We will follow the latter convention, as this corresponds more closely to the CT findings (Table 11.1).

11.1 True Cysts

True cysts (embryonal or benign neoplastic cysts) are spherical or oval, uni- or multilocular structures containing fluid. The walls are thin or very thin, with uniform thickness and a smooth surface without calcifications. These cysts displace the intestinal loops and the other organs and abdominopelvic structures without infiltrating them or merging intimately with them. They include enteric cysts, enteric duplications, cystic lymphangiomas and cystic mesotheliomas. CT provides an excellent opportunity to evaluate the different kinds of true cysts, whose common characteristics are represented by the sharply limited round or oval uni- or multilocular mass, with a thin or sometimes imperceptible wall and homogeneous low-density content ranging from –20 to +20 HU (Figs. 11.1–11.6). After contrast medium injection, no attenuation changes are observed in cysts, except in the case of enteric duplications, whose wall and internal septa may become slightly more opaque. Negative densitometric values indicate a lipidic chylous content; in contrast, high values (60–80 HU) are the expression of a recent intracavitary hemorrhage.

11.1.1 Enteric

Enteric cysts (Figs. 11.1–11.4) can be uni- or multilocular with serous content and walls made up of a single layer of enteric epithelium without muscular support; they adhere to the intestinal wall and/or to the mesentery. These cysts are asymptomatic and are occasionally found during diagnostic tests.

On CT, they appear as cystic unilocular or septate structures with extremely thin walls, a sharp profile and a fluid content with water density (zero to +10 HU). No densitometric changes occur after contrast medium injection.

11.1.2 Enteric Duplication

Enteric duplication cysts are characterized by a wall made up of intestinal mucosa and by two layers of smooth muscular tissue with neural elements and a blood supply. Usually unilocular, but sometimes subdivided by thin septa and containing a serous, chylous or hemorrhagic fluid, they adhere to the intestinal walls and grow in the mesentery or in the mesocolon, reaching conspicuous dimensions (up to 10–15 cm in diameter). In children between 5 and 10 years of age they come to clinical attention because of pain and/or the development of an abdominal palpable mass.

Table 11.1. Pathologic and CT appearances of cystic and cyst-like formations (A appendix, P peritoneum, C enh contrast enhancement, S single, Me mesentery, PP preperitoneal, C calcified, M multiple, O omentum, EP extraperitoneal)

	Pathology			CT						
Formation	Internal surface	Wall	Content	Location	Wall thickness	C enh	Septa	Density	Inclusions	No.
True cysts										
Enteric	Epithelium	Connective	Serous	Me	Thin	No	No/yes	0/+20		S
Enteric duplication	Epithelium, endothelium	Muscle	Serous, chylous	Me	Thin	Yes	No/yes	–20/+20		S
Cystic lymphangioma	Endothelium	Connective	Serous, chylous	Me	Very thin	No	Yes	0/+20		S
Cystic mesothelioma	Mesothelium	Connective	Serous	P	Very thin	No	No/yes	0/+20		S
Ovarian cyst										
Pseudocysts										
Hematic		Fibrous	Blood	P/M	Thick/perhaps C	No	NO	0/+60		S/M
Purulent		Fibrous	Pus	P/Me	Thick	Yes	NO	20/+50		S/M
Pancreatic		Fibrous	Pancreatic secretion	P	Thick	Yes	NO	15.+40		S/M
Cerebrospinal fluid	Mesothelium	Peritoneum	CSF	P	Thin	No	NO	0/+30		S/M
Serous	Mesothelium	Peritoneum	Serous	P	Thin	No	NO	0/+30		S/M
Lymphatic	Endothelium	Connective	Lymph	P/EP	Thin	No	NO	0/+20		S/M
Parasitic cysts										
Echinococcus	Proligerous membrane	Fibrous	Hydatic fluid Daughter cysts Debris	P	Thin/thick/C	No	NO	5/+50	Daughter cysts Debris	S/M
Dysembryogenetic tumors										
Dermoid cyst	Epithelium		Fat, sebum, hair	Me	Thin/thick/C	No	NO	–100/+300	Fat, sebum, hair	S
Teratomas			Multiple tissue types	Me				–100/+300	Bone, teeth, fat	S
Urachal cyst	Urothelium	Fibromuscular	urea	PP	Thick	Yes/no	NO	0/+20		
Cyst-like formations										
Ascites located in	Mesothelium	P	Serous	P	Thin	No	NO	0/+20		S/M
A Mucocele	Mucosa	A wall	Mucus	A	Thin/thick/C	Yes/no	NO	–15/+30		S
Gossypiboma	Granulomatous	Fibrous	Gauze	Me/O	Thick uniform	Yes	No	20/+30	Serpiginous, wheel-like	S
Leiomyoma, leiomyosarcoma	Tumoral	Tumoral	Necrotic	P/O	Thick nonuniform	Yes	No	0/+50		S/M
Pseudomyxoma	Mesothelium	Peritoneum	Mucin	P	Thin/thick	Yes	Yes	0/+30		M
Necrotic metastases	Tumoral	Tumoral	Necrotic	P	Thick nonuniform	Yes/no	No	20/+50		S/M
Necrotic lymphomas	Tumoral	Tumoral	Necrotic	Me	Thick, nonuniform	No	No	20/+50		S/M
Caseous TB	Granulomatous	Capsule	Caseous	Me	Thin/thick	No	No	0/+50		S/M

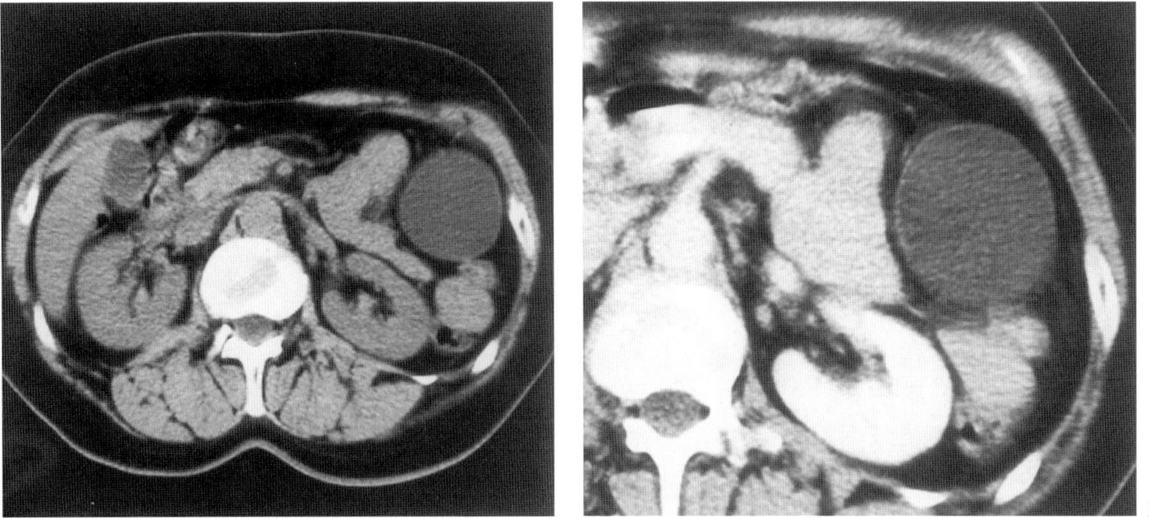

Fig. 11.1A, B. Mesenteric cyst. Spherical mass with water-density content and a thin well-defined wall arising from the junction of the mesentery with the left mesocolon

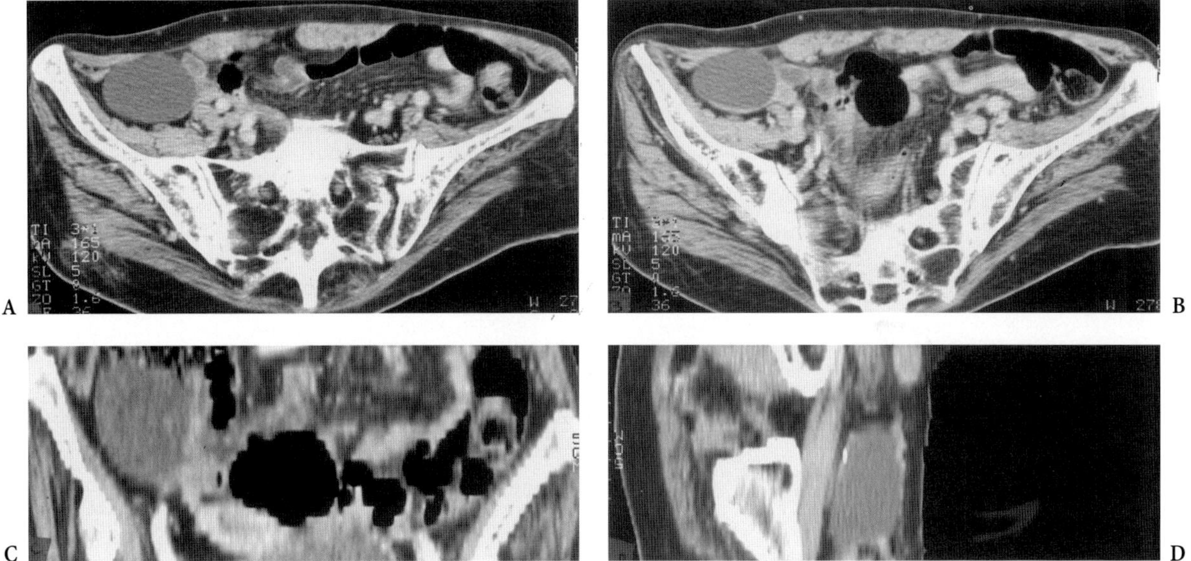

Fig. 11.2A–D. Mesenteric cyst. The cyst is located in the right iliac fossa, where it connects closely with the wall of a ileal loop

At CT, these cysts, often already quite large when first discovered, appear as unilocular cystic structures with a thin but always visible and uniformly thick wall, which enhances slightly with the contrast medium. The attenuation values of the fluid inside the cysts change according to its characteristics: negative (≤20 HU) when it is chylous, water density (0 to +20 HU) if it is serous. In the case of recent hemorrhage it may reach elevated values (>+60 HU). Sometimes thin intraluminal septa can be seen. The close adhesion of these cysts to the intestinal wall is a characteristic feature.

11.1.3 Cystic Lymphangioma

Cystic lymphangioma (Figs. 11.5, 11.6) is a benign congenital tumor of the lymphatic vessels, characterized by abnormal growth of lymphatic tissue without communication with the lymphatic system; it may also be secondary to obliteration and subsequent expansion of the lymphatic vessels.

Macroscopically, these cysts have a multilocular appearance, thin walls, thin intracavitary septa of endothelial tissue and a serous or chylous fluid con-

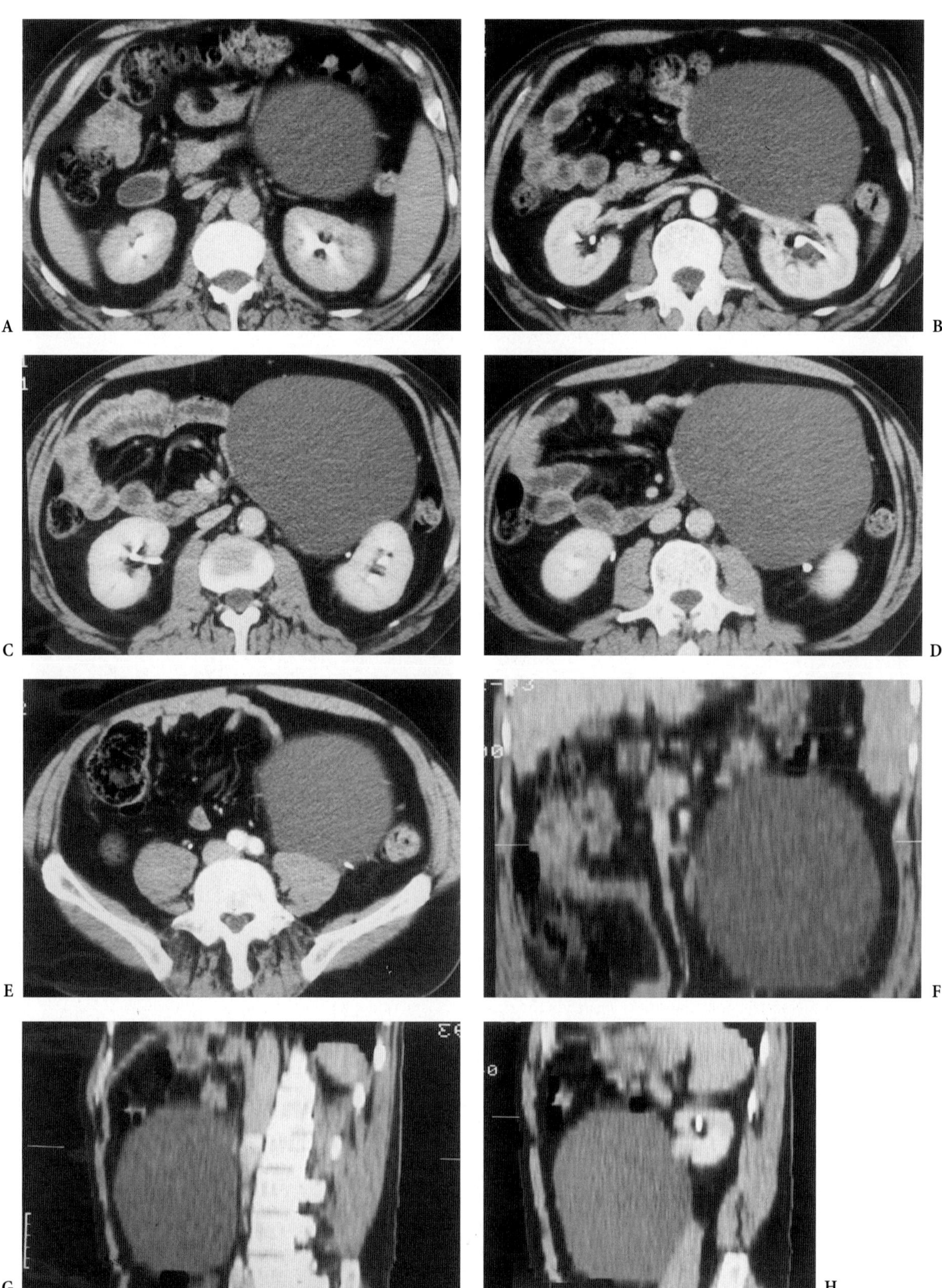

Fig. 11.3A–H. Mesenteric root cyst. The cyst pushes the jejunoileal loops and the mesenteric vessels toward the right side (**A–E**) and the transverse colon upward (**A**). Anteriorly, it takes up contact with the omentum, where the punctiform images of the vessels are recognizable. Furthermore, it compresses the left renal vein (**B**) from the front backwards. The descending colon extends posterolaterally to the cyst. The coronal (**F**), sagittal (**G**) and oblique (**H**) reconstructions contribute to correct localization of the cyst

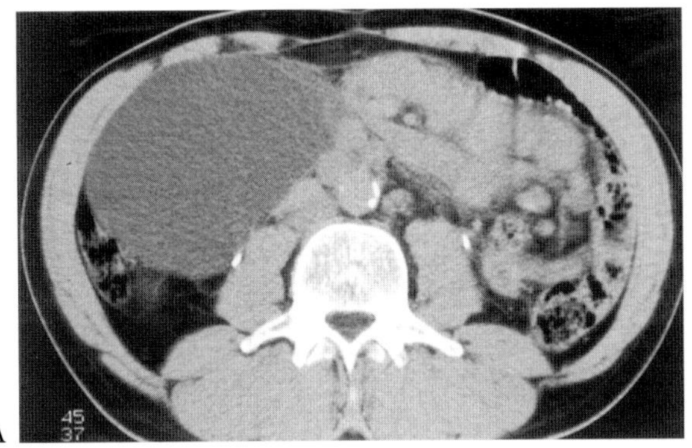

A

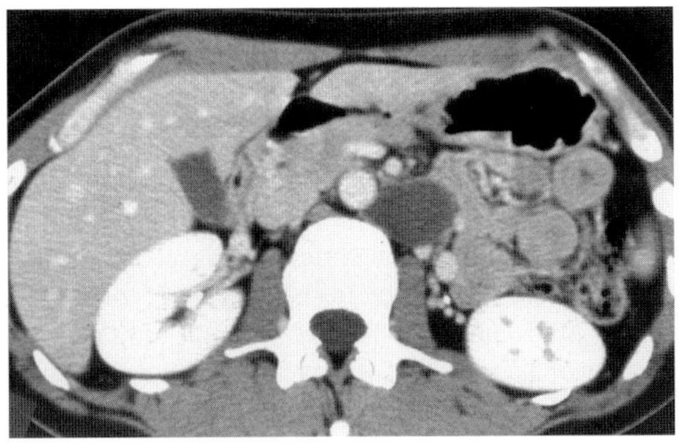

B

Fig. 11.4. Mesocolic cyst. The cyst pushes the ascending colon backward and outward, and the ileal hank and the enlarged mesenteric lymph nodes toward the left side. Patient affected by lymphoma

Fig. 11.5. Cystic lymphangioma. Ovoid mass with a thin wall and homogeneous water-density content located in the left para-aortic site

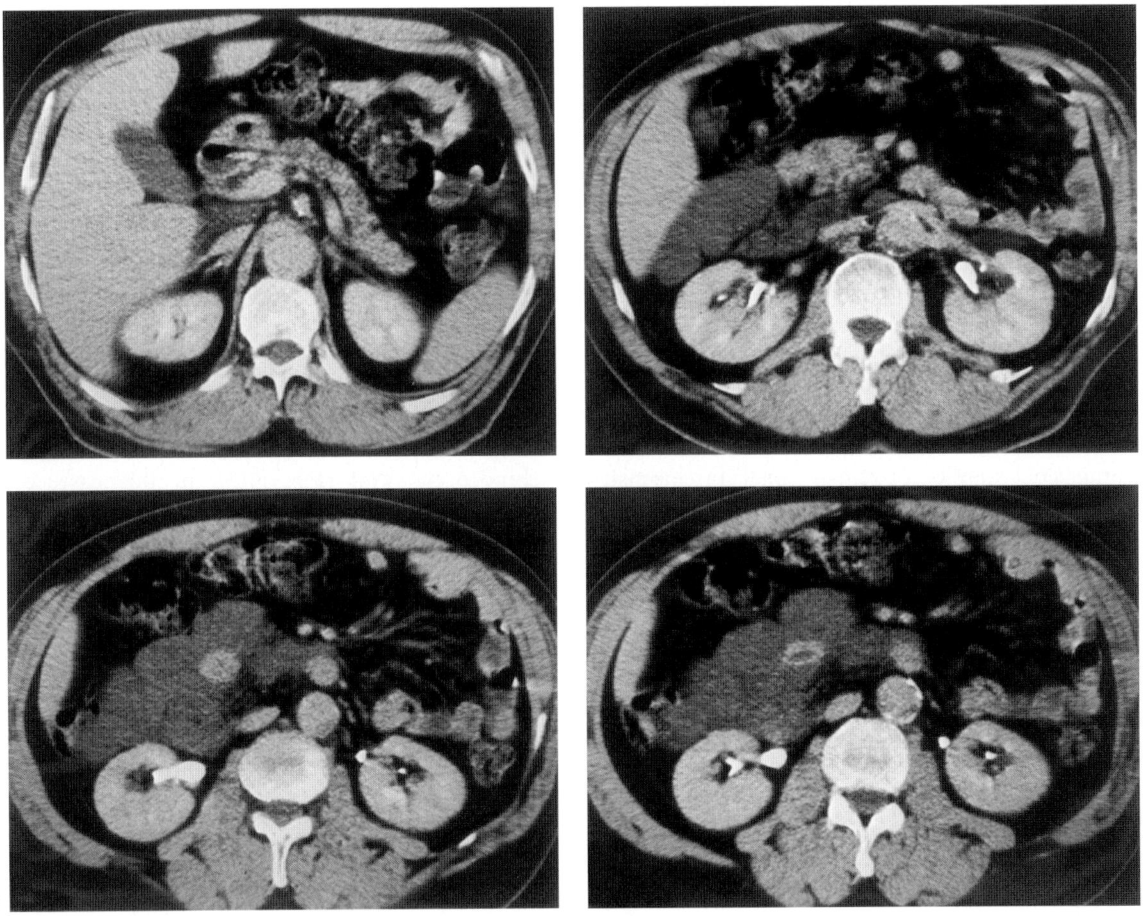

A B C D

Fig. 11.6A–D. Cystic lymphangioma. Water-density homogeneous thin-walled expansive process extending into the intra- and extraperitoneal spaces. In the peritoneal cavity it is located around the ileal loops and penetrates the vestibulum of the lesser sac (A). In the retroperitoneum, it occupies the anterior pararenal space

tent. They are variable in size, reaching 5–6 cm in diameter, and grow in the mesentery, the mesocolon, or the omentum.

A cystic lymphangioma is usually discovered in childhood following the clinical observation of an abdominal swelling and a painless palpable mobile and elastic mass with a smooth surface. Sometimes, inflammatory or necrotic-hemorrhagic complications may cause acute abdominal pain; only in exceptional cases does it develop invasive characteristics. Treatment is surgical removal, perhaps with associated intestinal resection.

CT shows a mass that is sharply defined, usually voluminous, round and multilocular, with a thin, often imperceptible wall and homogeneous fluid content. If the fluid is chylous its attenuation values are negative; if it is serous, its values are the same as those for water; in the case of inflammatory or hemorrhagic complications more elevated values are reached. Occasionally, the chylous types show a characteristic "level" of negative-adipose density. Usually, the contrast medium does not produce any significant change, but occasionally the wall or the septa are enhanced.

11.1.4 Cystic Mesothelioma

Cystic mesothelioma is a rare neoformation that originates from the mesothelial cells lining the peritoneum. It has a thin wall constituted by a single layer of flat or cubic mesothelial cells, without atypia or mitotic divisions, and a serous content. It develops inside the peritoneum, mostly in the pelvic cavity. Its dimensions may be extremely small; in contrast, it may grow up to occupy a wide part of the peritoneal cavity. Middle-aged women are the group most frequently affected by cystic mesothelioma. In 27%–50% of cases it relapses (O'Neal 1989). In exceptional cases it is malignant, but it does not produce metastases.

Clinical symptoms, such as moderate abdominal pain, are reported only when a cystic mesothelioma reaches significantly large dimensions and produces compressive phenomena; acute pain is caused by torsion, rupture or hemorrhagic complications.

The CT appearance reflects the anatomopathological characteristics of the neoformation: a uni- or multilocular spherical mass with thin wall, sharp profile and a water-density homogeneous content (0+20 HU).The wall density does not change after contrast medium injection, but when the structure is multilocular the thin internal septa may enhance. The benign and the rare malignant forms are identical in appearance.

11.2 Pseudocysts

11.2.1 Hematic, Purulent, Pancreatic

The pseudocysts are encapsulated collections left behind after inflammatory processes (Figs. 11.7, 11.9), traumas, surgical operations and hemorrhages (Figs. 5.24, 11.8). They have a thick wall and a purulent, hematic, necrotic, serous or mixed content or are filled with pancreatic juice. They are uni- or, more rarely, multilocular and are found in mesenteric, mesocolic or omental sites, where they may reach conspicuous dimensions with a diameter greater than 20 cm.

In contrast to true cysts, pseudocysts are preceded by significant clinical-anamnestic manifestations and are accompanied by a complex of symptoms, which are sometimes relevant (ache, acute pain, fever, signs of compression owing to expansion, palpable mass).

CT shows these lesions as spherical or ovoid masses with a thick wall and a profile that may be sharp or shaded. They are uni- or multilocular and contain fluids ranging in density from 0 (serous) to + 60 HU (in recent hemorrhagic collections). Contrast medium injection produces a consistent increase in density of the wall, extending to the pericystic tissues in the case of infections (Figs. 11.7, 11.9).

The wall of long-lasting pseudocysts is not only thick, but also calcified and may simulate an echinococcus cyst (Fig. 11.7). In this case, the anamnestic data and the biological tests are sufficient to establish the correct diagnosis.

11.2.2 Cerebrospinal Fluid

Cerebrospinal fluid pseudocysts may develop in the peritoneum in patients with ventriculoperitoneal shunts, as a result of adhesions next to the opening of the catheter.

CT shows the collections of cerebrospinal fluid as cyst-like structures filled with a homogeneous water-density content (0/+20 HU); the wall is thin when it is made up of peritoneum only, whereas it is thicker and contrast enhanced if it is surrounded by a reactive capsule.

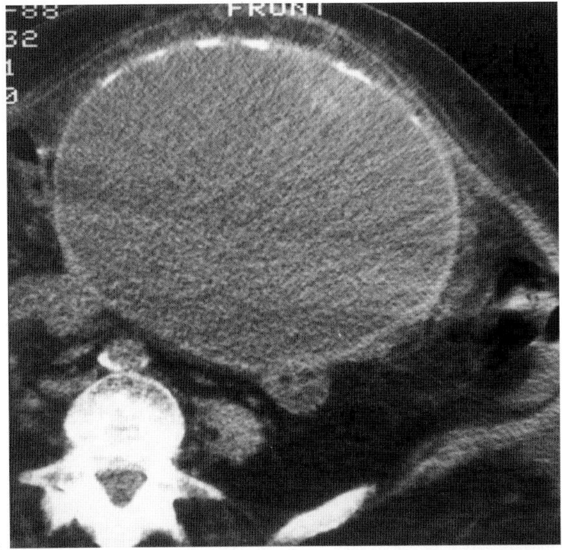
A

11.2.3 Serous

For information on serous pseudocysts the reader is referred to section 5.7 in Chapter 5: Fluid Collections)

11.2.4 Lymphatic

For information on lymphatic pseudocysts the reader is referred to section 5.6 in Chapter 5: Fluid Collections)

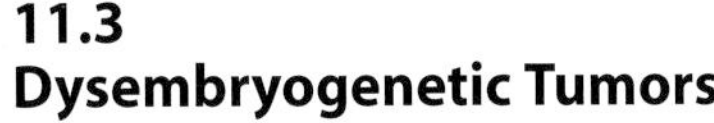

11.3 Dysembryogenetic Tumors

11.3.1 Dermoid Cysts and Teratomas

Dysembryogenetic tumors include dermoid cysts, which are made up exclusively of ectodermal tissues and teratomas, which contain derivatives of the three germ layers:

- Dermoid cysts are spherical, with a thin epithelial wall, and contain fat, sebum and hair. They are prevalent in women. In most cases they are asymptomatic and are occasionally discovered during radiographic or ultrasonographic examinations.
- Teratomas may have a cystic appearance with a fluid content (serous, sebaceous, colloidal, gelatinous or proteic) or may appear as a well-limited solid spherical mass with a smooth or nodular surface and a multitissular structure with a prevalent fat component; however, they may also contain bones, teeth and other tissues.

  In most cases, teratomas take benign well-differentiated forms, but in 10% of cases, mostly in elderly subjects, they are made up of malignant immature undifferentiated cells.

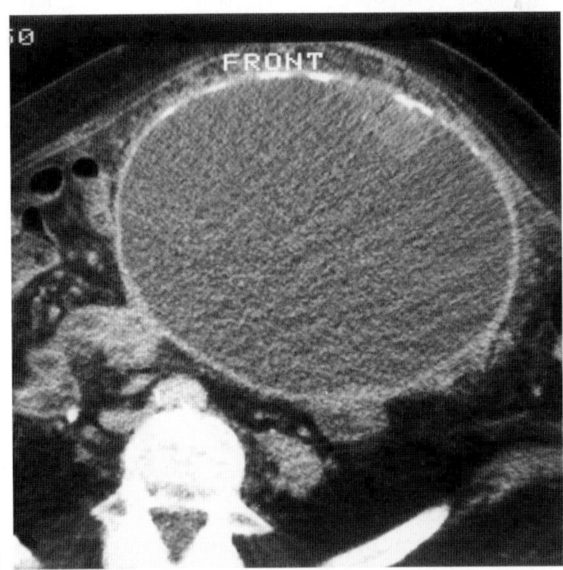

B

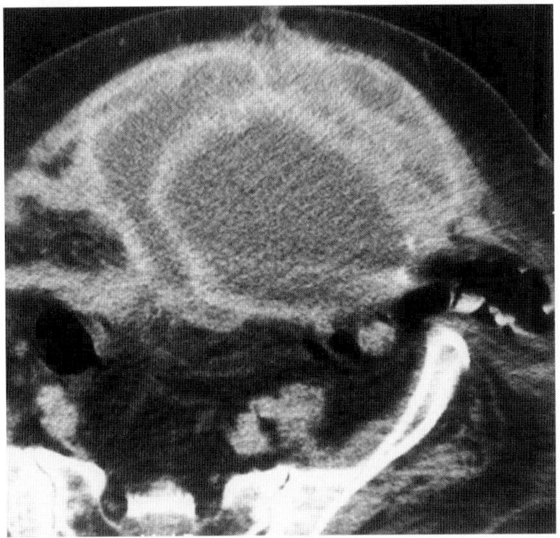
C

Fig. 11.7A–C. Suppurated omental pseudocyst. Ovoid cystic mass with dense and partially calcified wall and thick septations strikingly enhanced after i.v. contrast medium injection (C), containing dense fluid (25–36 HU) and some inclusions adhering to the wall. The anterior position of the cyst suggests the omental location, and the shaded surrounding fat a perifocal extension of the infection

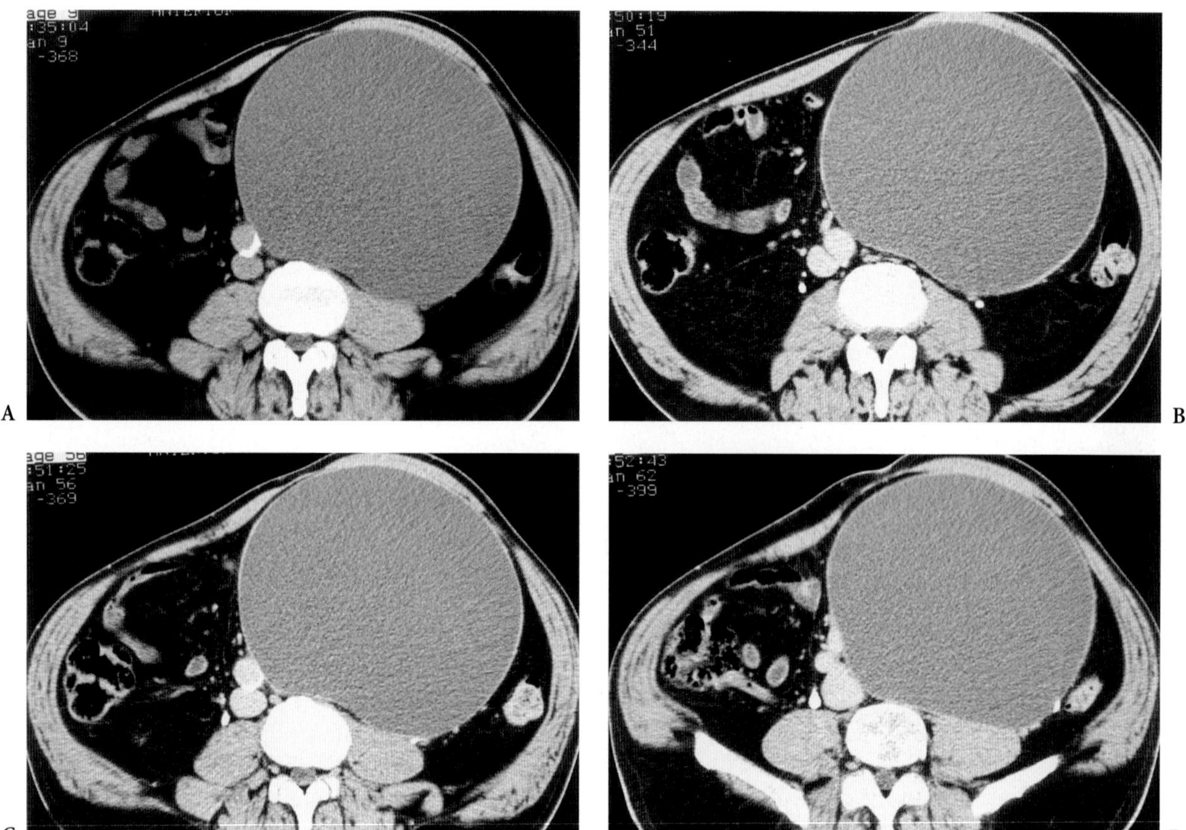

Fig. 11.8A–D. Hemorrhagic pseudocyst. The pseudocyst originates from the retroperitoneum and extends into the mesentery. It adheres to the aorta, the spine and the lateral wall of the left iliac artery, which is pushed upwards and is dissociated from the homonymous vein. The left ureter is pushed outward by the cystic mass. Characteristic appearances are represented by the higher density than that of water (30 HU) of the pseudocyst's content and by the thick, dense and uniform wall

The CT appearance reflects the structure and variety of their components, with the common characteristic of a well-limited mass with a very sharp profile that does not infiltrate the adjacent tissues (Figs. 11.10–10.13).

Dermoid cysts are typically seen as spherical masses with thin walls, and their content is very variable in density and disposition. Among other components, fat and sebum are recognizable because of their negative attenuation values, whereas serum is shown by its water density. Sometimes a fat-fluid level is present.

A characteristic finding is Rokitansky's dermoid plug (Fig. 11.12), a solid structure containing calcifications, which is inserted in the cystic wall and protrudes into the cavity or outwards.

The cystic teratoma appears as an approximately spherical mass with smooth contours, a polymorphous structure and variable attenuation values, ranging from the negative value of the adipose component to the hyperdense ones of bones and teeth. A fat-fluid level may also be observed, which means that the sebum, being lighter and having negative values, is located in the upper part, separated by a horizontal interface from the underlying water-density serous fluid (Fig. 11.11, 11.13).

Usually, cystic teratoma can easily be correctly diagnosed because of its multistructural appearance, with the negative values of fat and sebum, the elevated value of calcifications, and the sharp profile of the mass evident.

The main diagnostic problem concerns the differentiation between benign and malignant types. The differential elements are the sharp profile without signs of infiltration of the surrounding tissues and the cystic appearance in the case of benign teratomas, and the solid structure with shaded contour and eventual metastases to the lymph nodes (Fig. 11.13) or liver in the case of malignant teratomas. Nevertheless, all teratomas should be entirely removed because histological mistakes are possible.

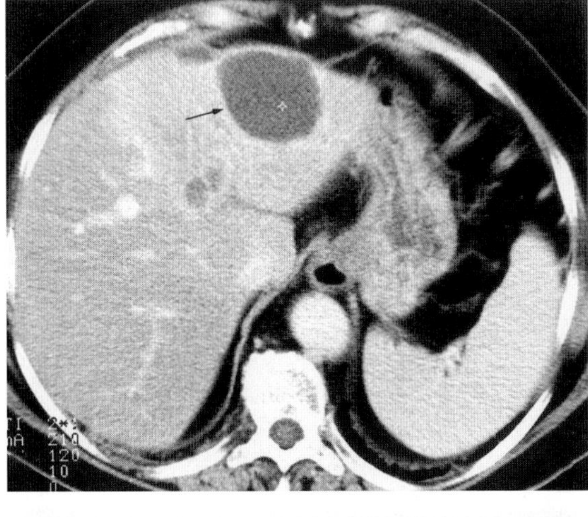

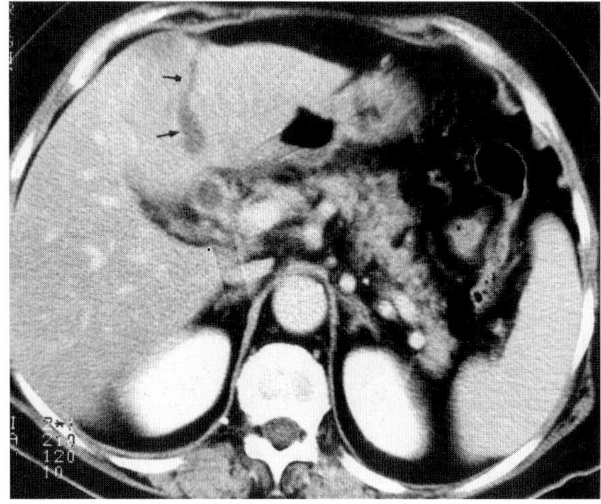

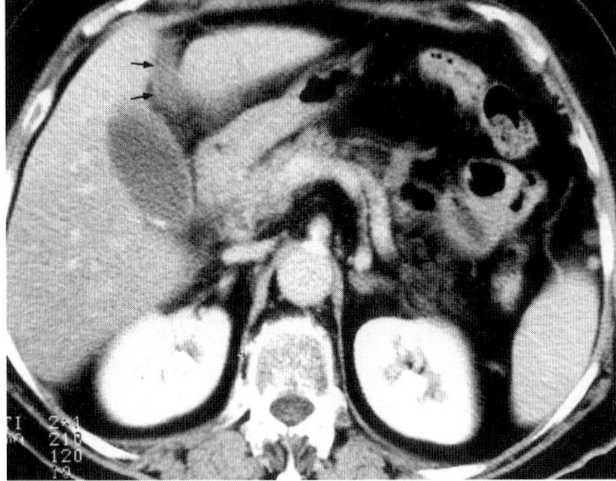

Fig. 11.9A–C. Postpancreatitic pseudocyst. The pseudocyst is located in the longitudinal fissure of the liver and along the extension of the round ligament; it shows thick, and after contrast hyperdense, walls because of a reactive inflammatory process

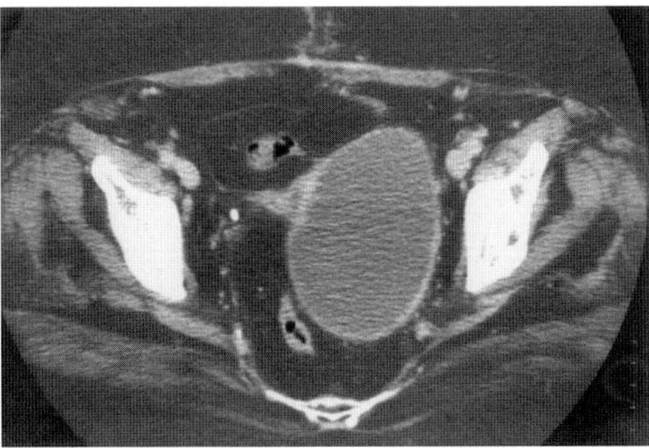

Fig. 11.10. Dermoid cyst with sebaceous content. Hypodense ovoid mass with a uniform and well-defined wall.. Their content seems to be homogeneous, but its attenuation values ranges from –38 to +48 HU, suggesting the nature of the cyst

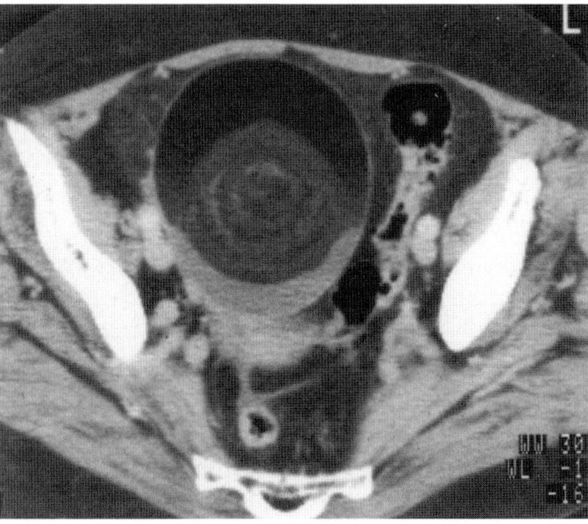

Fig. 11.11. Cystic teratoma. Polystructured spherical mass limited by a well-defined uniform wall and containing fat-fluid level and a hair ball

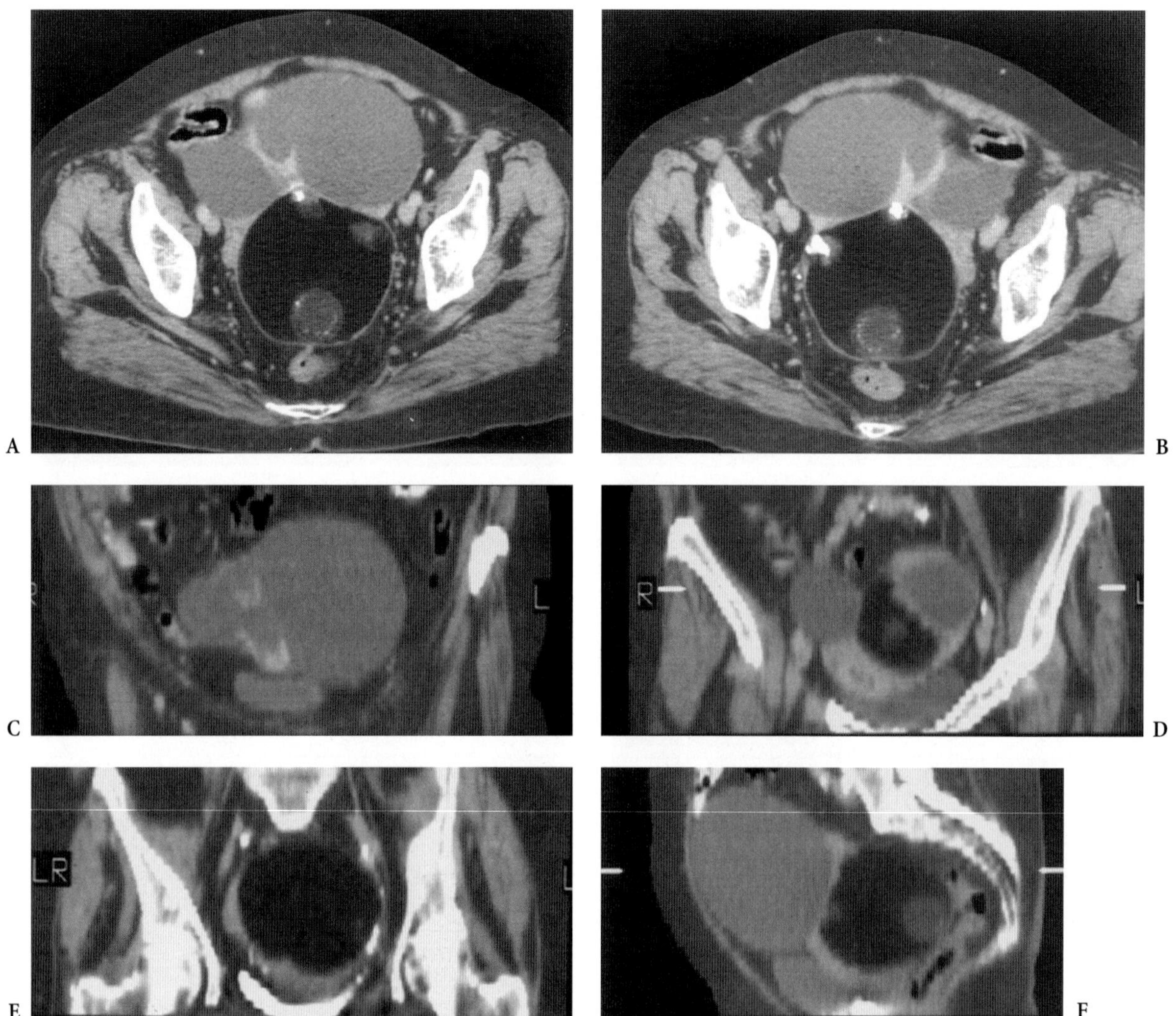

Fig. 11.12A–F. Dermoid cyst. Spherical thick-walled mass with fatty content (—95 HU) including a small water-density spherical mass. On the left side, the partially calcified Rokitansky's dermoid plug protrudes into the cavity. Two ovarian cysts with the characteristic water-density content and thin wall are adhering to the teratoma anteriorly. **C–E** Coronal reconstructions: **C** anterior, **D** median, and **E** posterior plane; **F** Median sagittal reconstruction

11.3.2 Urachal

Cyst of the urachus or allantoic cyst is due to postnatal persistence of the intermediate tract of the urachus, where a very slowly accumulating collection develops. The cyst does not communicate with the umbilicus or the urinary bladder.

It appears as a spherical structure (whose walls are made up of urothelium and fibromuscular tissue) containing a clear citrine fluid in which urea is present.

Usually, this cyst is asymptomatic and is occasionally discovered as an incidental finding during diagnostic tests (echography, CT) carried out to study other pathologies or becomes evident because of a concomitant inflammation or tumoral degeneration.

CT shows characteristic features, such as the position of the cyst (along the median line, anteriorly, between the linea alba and the parietal peritoneum), the round cystic appearance, the parahydric density (0/+20 HU) and the thick and easily visible walls (Fig. 11.14).

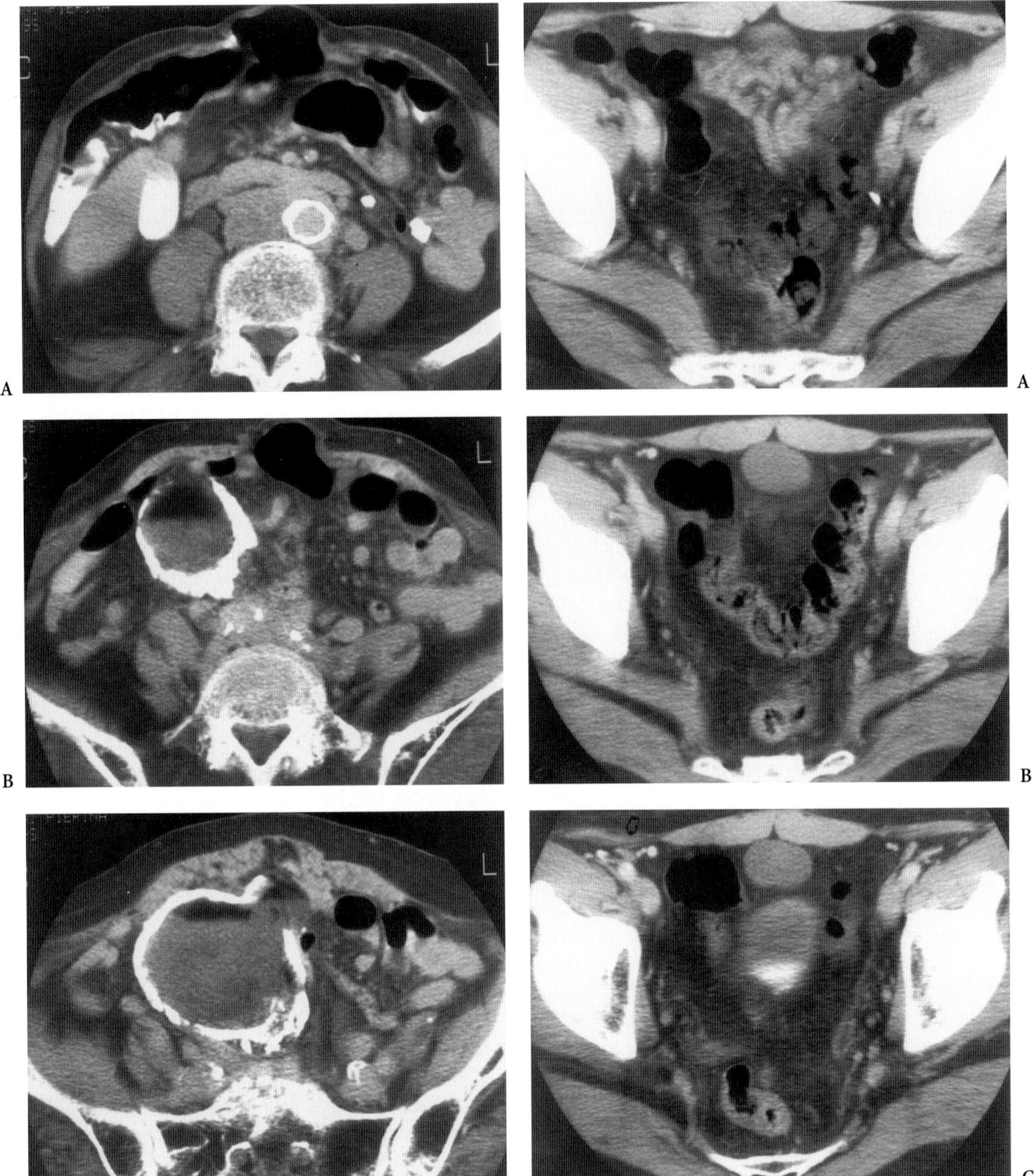

Fig. 11.13A–C. Malignant cystic teratoma with retroperitoneal lymph nodal metastases. Ovoid mass with thick and calcified walls and fat-fluid level inside. **A** Enlarged lumboaortic lymph nodes

Fig. 11.14A–C. Urachal cyst. Small ovoid well-defined mass with water-density content located anteriorly along the median line, between the umbilicus and the urinary bladder

11.4 Parasitic Cysts: Echinococcosis

Echinococcosis is an endemic parasitic disease caused by the larval stage of the tapeworm *Echinococcus granulosus*, which gives origin to a hydatid cyst constituted by an external cuticular membrane, an intermediate proligerous membrane, and an internal hydatic fluid.

The external cuticular membrane is a fragile, stratified, 1- to 2-mm-thick protective lamina, which allows the passage of nutritional substances, but not of pathogenic microorganisms.

The marginal or proligerous membrane is as thick as a cell and shows a granular appearance. It represents the living parasite that generates the scolices. The daughter cysts develop inside the marginal membrane and are seen as small globes adhering to the wall or floating in the hydatic fluid. The marginal membrane continuously secretes a crystalline and colorless fluid, which is a transudate containing proteins and sodium chloride. The constant increase in intracystic pressure produces progressive enlargement of the cyst. Besides the daughter cysts, the fluid also contains sedimentary layers that are called hydatic sand and the hooks.

Frequently (in more than 40% of cases) the wall of the cyst may undergo a variably extensive degree of calcification because of scarce trophism, whereas the endocystium may be detached from the pericystium, or may rupture, with partial or total outflow of the fluid and death of the cyst.

The hydatic cyst is not commonly found in the peritoneum (only 5 cases have been described in the literature); this localization is secondary to the rupture of hepatic or splenic cysts with spread of daughter cysts into the peritoneal cavity, where they tend to localize in the lowest parts: the pouch of Douglas and the paravesical spaces. The absence of tissues limiting expansion in these sites allows rapid growth, depending to the adjacent structures.

At CT examination, the peritoneal hydatic cyst has the same appearance as those located in other sites (liver, spleen): spherical shape, a thin wall in recent forms, a thicker wall after evolution. The calcification of the wall is frequently observed in other sites, whereas it is less frequent in the peritoneum, because of the rapid and easy growth of the cyst and the absence of reactions of the limiting peritoneum. Generally, the content of the cyst (water, proteins, NaCl) is homogeneous and shows parahydric absorption values (2/+14 HU); it becomes dense and nonhomogeneous in the presence of debris and free scolices.

The daughter cysts extend in a crown-like shape along its internal surface. They are seen as small globes, whose content shows lower attenuation values than the mother cyst. This condition produces a multilocular appearance, resembling the rays of a wheel or a honeycomb. Occasionally, smaller cysts may be seen inside the daughter cysts.

In the case of recent death of the cyst, the detachment of the endocystium from the pericystium may become evident as a thin line crossing the cavity.

The CT appearance may be atypical: for example, unilocular cysts with a thin wall without calcifications and containing a homogeneous fluid, whose density is low, closely resemble cysts of a different origin. In contrast, in the typical forms the CT appearance is pathognomonic and reliably allows correct diagnosis of echinococcus cyst. When doubts persist, the use of immunodiagnostic tests becomes necessary, especially if the patient comes from an area where echinococcosis is endemic.

11.5 Cyst-like Structures: Mucocele of the Appendix

The mucocele is a rare lesion caused by the accumulation of a mucinous substance in the appendix, stretching it. It has a cyst-like appearance.

It develops after a stenosis of the appendiceal lumen next to the cecum, which in most cases is due to scarring, inflammatory processes, coproliths or appendiceal carcinoid. A slow accumulation of the secretory products of the intense muciparous activity of the epithelium mucosae lining the appendix fills the cavity with a gelatinous substance, swelling the appendix, which becomes a sac with its wall reduced to a thin membrane.

If the mucocele ruptures, its mucinous content spreads into the peritoneal cavity forming a pseudomyxoma (see Chapter 13).

The lesion may be silent or characterized by chronic pain and the evidence of a palpable mass in the right iliac fossa.

Radiologic barium examination shows a round transparent mass in the fundus of the cecum as a filling defect; the mass has a very sharp profile and moves together with the cecum. The wall is often partially or totally calcified.

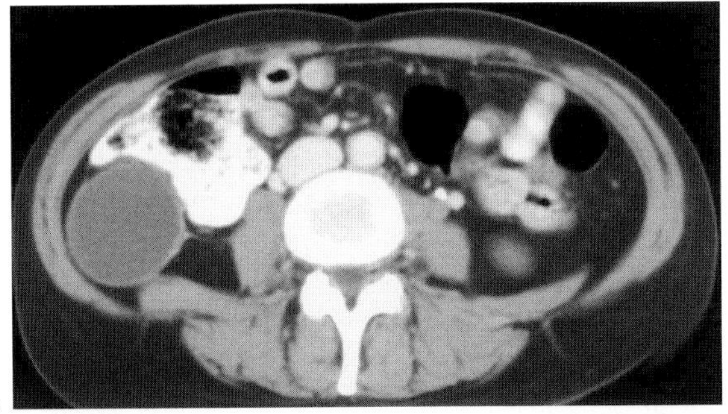
A

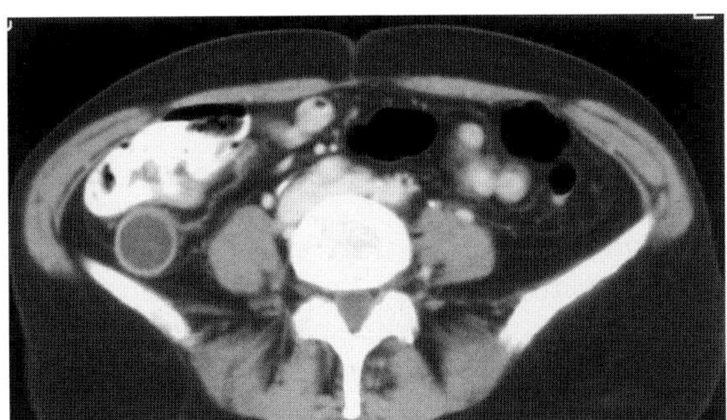
B

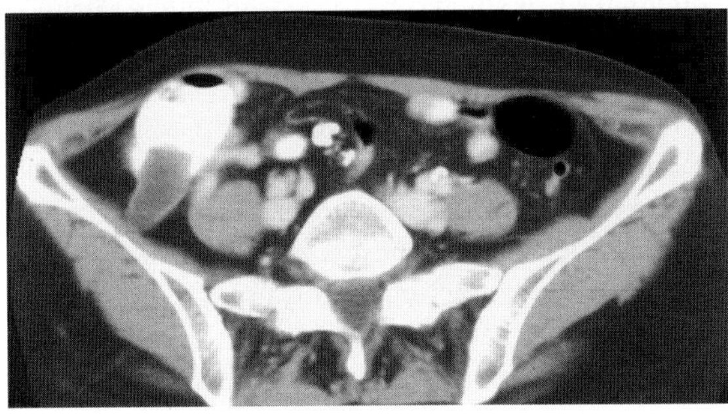
C

Fig. 11.15A–C. Appendiceal mucocele. Spherical well-capsulated cystic mass with smooth regular profile and low-attenuation contents, which is causing an impression in the fundus of the cecum at the point of the appendiceal insertion. A small mesentery surrounds this formation (**A**)

CT (Fig. 11.15) shows the mucocele as a cyst-like small spherical or ovoid mass with sharp contours. Its density varies from the negative value of adipose tissue to that of soft tissues; however, in most cases it has the attenuation values of water. The mass is limited by a wall of variable thickness, which is sometimes calcified and assumes close contact with the fundus of the cecum; its development often seems to be intraluminal.

The site and the close relationships with the cecum provide the opportunity to distinguish mucoceles from true cysts and pseudocysts.

11.6 Diagnostic Role of CT

Our presentation indicates that CT can recognize cysts, providing information on their morphological characteristics, position and extension; it also clarifies the relationships of the cysts with the contiguous abdominal structures.

Furthermore, CT makes it possible to:

a) Distinguish among different true cysts in some cases
b) Distinguish true cysts from pseudocysts
c) Differentiate true cysts from cyst-like structures of other origins
d) Establish whether the origin is mesenteric or mesocolic

a) Distinction Among Different True Cysts. Differential diagnosis among the various types of true cysts is only possible when negative densitometric values indicate a chylous nature of the content or when the wall becomes slightly denser after contrast medium, as in enteric duplication cysts.

b) Distinction Between True Cysts and Pseudocysts. The distinction between true cysts and pseudocysts is based mainly on the shape of the wall: it is thin in true cysts, whereas it is thick and made denser by contrast medium in the pseudocysts. The evaluation of the density of the cystic content usually shows parahydric or negative values in true cysts and higher values in pseudocysts.

Saccate ascitic collections may resemble true cysts, especially when they are located in the lesser sac, where they assume a retrogastric ovoid shape. The position, the orientation, the limits constituted by the peritoneum, and the concomitant presence of other peritoneal collections or ascites-producing diseases (cirrhosis, tumors) usually allow easy differential diagnosis.

The characteristics of the various types of pseudocyst are not substantially different; the only specific features are the presence of a high-density content, which suggests a recent hemorrhage, and sudden contrast enhancement of the wall and of the pericystic fat, which indicates a suppurative character (Fig. 11.7).

c) Differential Diagnosis of True Cysts Against Cyst-like Structures of Other Origins. Differential diagnosis among true cysts also includes dermoid cysts, echinococcus cysts, gossypibomas, leiomyomas, leiomyosarcomas, and colliquative lymph nodes.

In contrast to true cysts, dermoid cysts have a thick wall that is partially or completely calcified and shows negative values (adipose tissue and sebum).

Hydatic cysts cannot be distinguished from true cysts when their wall is thin and their content is fluid and homogeneous. In contrast, they can be classified if they have a thick wall and/or there are daughter cysts inside them. The calcification of the wall is not different from that observed in teratomas either when it appears as a thin circle or when it has the appearance of a curvilinear peripheral thick plaque; however, the different content frequently provides the possibility of an easy differential diagnosis.

Gossypiboma can be distinguished from all other cystic structures when it contains a mass with slightly higher than water density (20–30 HU), where more opaque and often calcified serpiginous lines stand out. In the absence of these serpiginous lines, a gossypiboma can simulate a true cyst, even though its content shows a higher density. It is almost impossible to distinguish a gossypiboma with a thick wall, which is made opaque intensely and for a long time by contrast medium and shows a para-suprafluid content, from pseudocysts that are suppurative in nature, because of the postsurgical development of both pathologies.

Encysted hematomas may have cyst-like appearances, which are often not distinguishable from those of a true cyst. The wall is thicker and often partially calcified; previous surgical operations or traumas suggest the presence of a hematoma.

Leiomyoma and intestinal leiomyosarcoma can have a cyst-like appearance caused by stromal degeneration or tumoral necrosis. They cannot be distinguished either on CT or macroscopically from true cysts, and a histological examination may be the only way of reaching a correct identification (Volk et al. 1983).

d) Determination of Mesenteric vs Other Origin of Cysts. A mesenteric origin of cysts and the differentiation of mesenteric cysts from cysts of different origins (mesocolon, mesosigmoid, ovary) can be established by considering the positions of these cysts relative to the intestinal loops, the ligaments, the mesenteries and the vessels (Figs. 11.1–11.3).

Mesenteric cysts originate from the deep abdominal planes and tend to localize in a sagittal direction, extending toward the anterior abdominal wall. The ileal loops are displaced forward and to the sides and form a ring or a semicircle around the cysts. The last loop is not dissociated from the other ileal loops and extends along the anterior face of the cyst. The cecum is pushed downward. The sigmoid maintains its normal position.

Cysts of the mesocolon are in close contact with the colon within the mesocolon transparency and are limited medially by the loops of the small intestine (Fig. 11.4).

Cysts of the sigmoid mesocolon displace the sigmoid upward and forward; the cysts are limited by the arcuate orientation of the viscus (with an arch turned downwards and backwards) and assume close contact with the sigmoid at various points inside the mesentery, without the interposition of adipose tissue, in contrast to the situation in the case of ovarian cysts, which must be distinguished from mesosigmoidal cysts.

The large-volume ovarian cysts (Figs. 11.16–11.19) that develop upward in the abdominal cavity may resemble mesocolic, mesenteric or mesosigmoidal cysts. They may be distinguished by considering their pelvic origin, their close contact with a broad ligament and their development in anterior planes. The ileal loops are lifted and extend with an arch-like disposition above, to the sides of and behind (never in front of or under) the cyst, with the concavity facing downward.

The relative positions of the ovarian cysts and the sigmoid are important in recognition of the origin of the cyst. In cysts located on the right (Fig. 11.16) the sigmoid is overtaken by the cyst penetrating under and in front of the viscus, which is pushed toward the left and backward. In cysts located on the left (Figs. 11.17, 11.18) the sigmoid is pushed contralaterally and upward around the cyst, forming an arch open to the left and below.

In the differential diagnosis against mesenteric cysts, we must remember that in adult women almost all cysts developing in the pelvis, in the hypogastrium, and in the mesogastrium in anterior planes are ovarian cysts and that cysts of different origins are extremely rare.

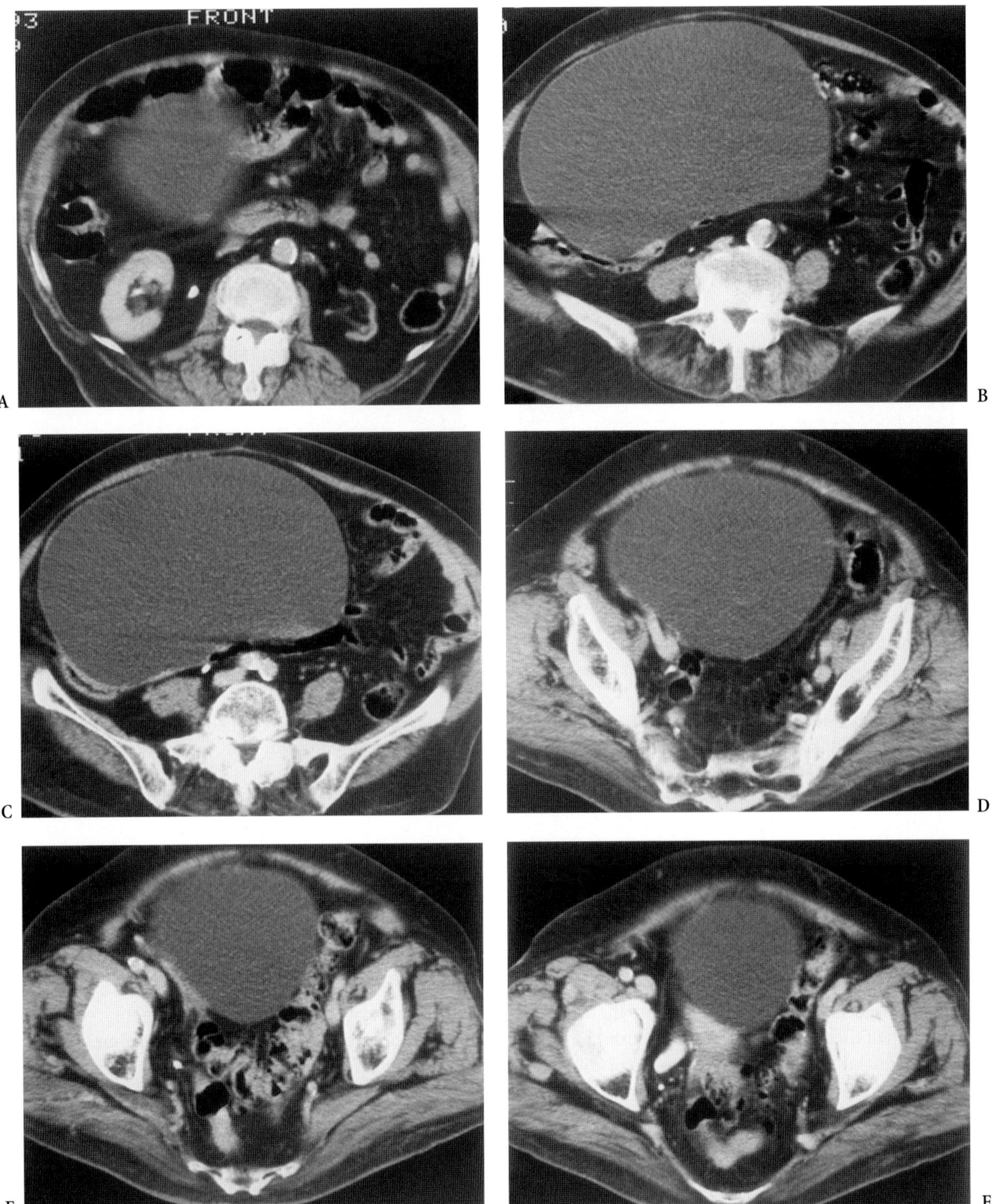

Fig. 11.16A–F. Right ovarian cyst. Ovoid mass with pelvic and abdominal development. It shows a very thin wall, a sharp profile and a homogeneous content with water attenuation values (**A**). This structure displaces the sigmoid toward the left side (**E**, **F**) and pushes the small bowel loops upward (**A–C**). On the right, it extends in front of the cecum and of the last ileal loop (**B**, **C**). Only a very thin transparent interstice of adipose tissue remains between the mass located in the peritoneal cavity and the anterior abdominal wall. It is closely related with the fundus uteri and the right broad ligament (**E**, **F**). At a higher level, the cyst is limited by the transverse colon and its mesentery (**A**)

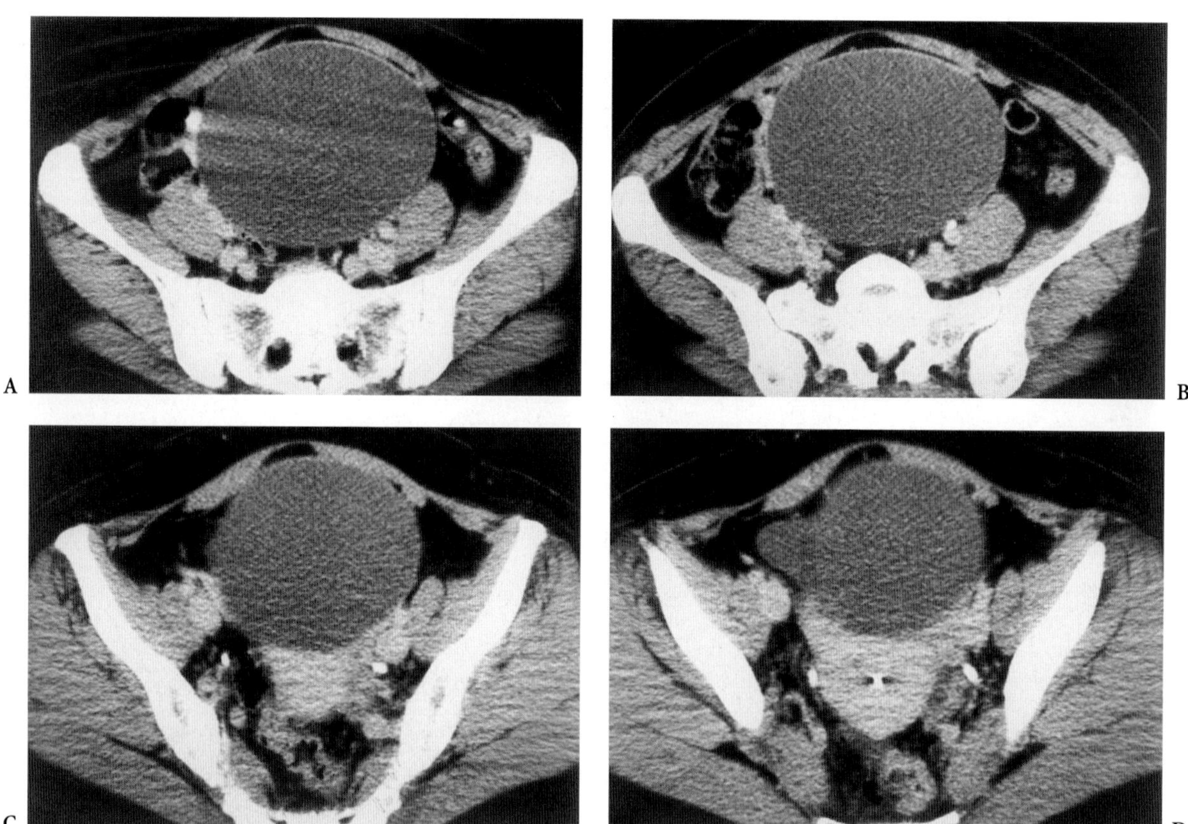

Fig. 11.17A–D. Left ovarian cyst. The cyst shows close contacts with the anterior wall of the uterus and the broad ligaments; it extends upward toward the hypogastrium, displacing the rectum and the sigmoid toward the right. These viscera form a semicircle limiting the cyst

Extraperitoneal cysts that may simulate a mesenteric cyst are renal or pancreatic in origin. The renal cysts are more easily recognizable, even when they develop forward up to envelop the pancreas and the splenic vessels anteriorly, because of the close relationship of these cysts with the organ from which they originate and because of the presence of the anterior pararenal fascia by which they are limited (Fig. 11.20).

In the case of pancreatic pseudocysts, there is also a tendency to be doubtful about their origin, nature and generating organ, because they extend upward and forward into the transverse mesocolon and into the gastrosplenic and gastrocolic ligaments. The most significant signs in the characterization of these cysts are the prevalent development in the pancreatic compartment with the involvement (even partial) of this organ and the persistence of a cleavage plane between stomach and cyst.

Fig. 11.18A–C. Left ovarian cystoadenocarcinoma. The origin of the neoplasm from the left ovary is indicated by the displacement of the sigmoid toward the right side. The broad ligaments and the uterus take a close contact with the mass, forming a semicircle that limits the mass posteriorly. The retroperitoneal tissues and structures show no alterations

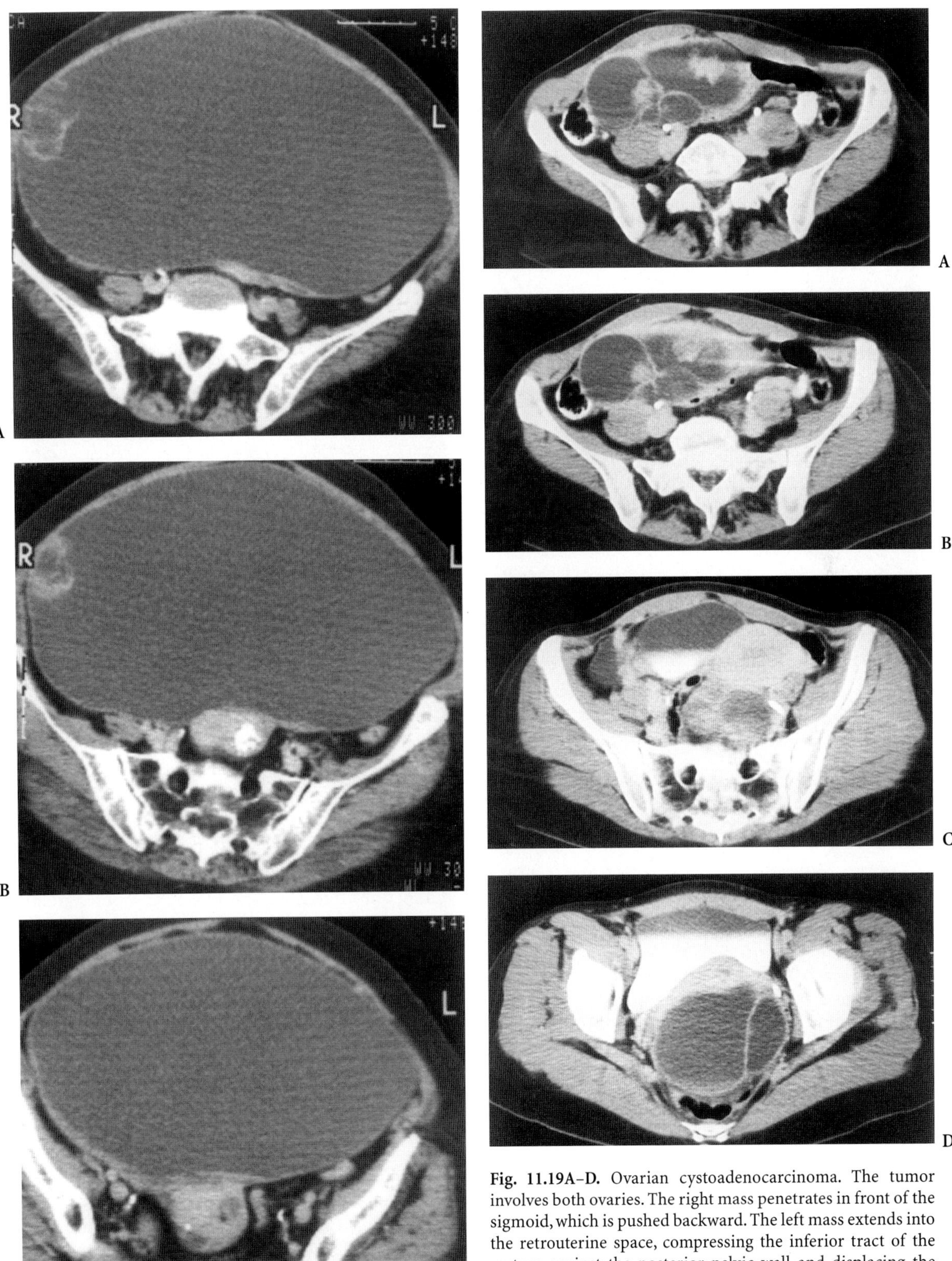

Fig. 11.19A–D. Ovarian cystoadenocarcinoma. The tumor involves both ovaries. The right mass penetrates in front of the sigmoid, which is pushed backward. The left mass extends into the retrouterine space, compressing the inferior tract of the rectum against the posterior pelvic wall and displacing the upper half of the rectum and the sigmoid toward the right

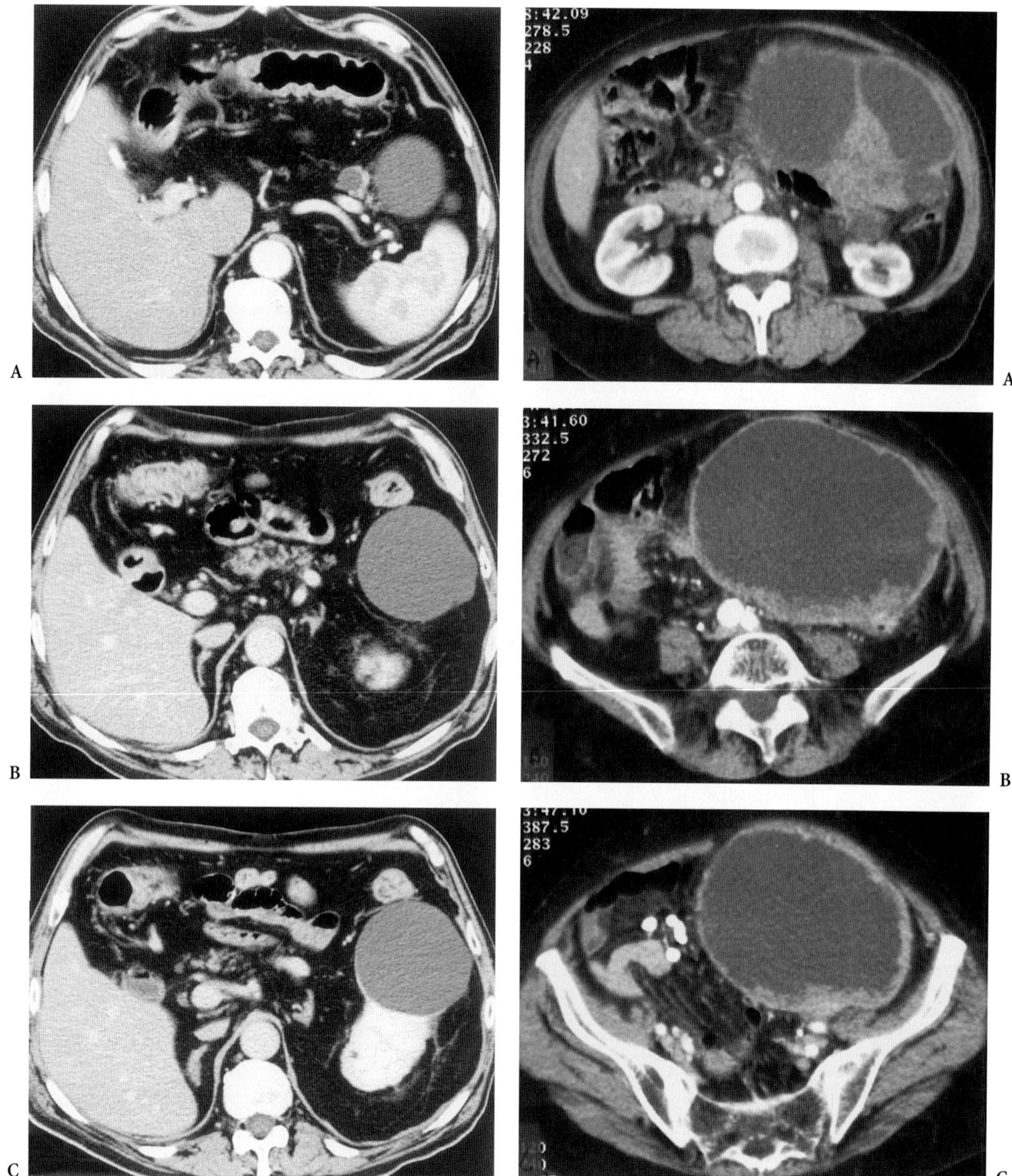

Fig. 11.20A–C. Renal cyst with anterior development in front of the pancreas and the splenic vessels

Fig.11.21. Ovarian carcinoma metastasis. Large intraperitoneal similcystic mass with thick, nonuniform and enhancing wall, and with internal septa. The mass displaces the sigmoid to the right and the descending colon downward

Bibliography

Cysts

Agha FP, Francis IR, Simms SM (1983) Cystic lymphangioma of the colon. AJR Am J Roentgenol 141:709–710

Baldrati L, Brunetti L, Rocchi A, et al (1989) Calcificazioni di cisti peritoneali in un paziente in emodialisi periodica. Radiol Med 78:402–403

Berry M, Monneins F, Delafolie A, et al (1987) Lymphangiomatose péritonéale kystique diffuse. Etude clinique, echographique et tomodensitométrique au long cours. A propos d'un cas. J Radiol 68: 199–203

Bernardino ME, Jing BS, Wallace S (1979) Computed tomography diagnosis of mesenteric masses. AJR Am J Roentgenol 132:33–35

Bruneton JN, Benattar E, Drouillard J, et al (1987) Kystes du mésentère de l'adulte. J Radiol 68:687–691

Buonomo C, Griscom NT (1991) Pediatric case of the day. Cystic lymphangioma (omental cyst). Radiographics 11:1146–1148

Canty MD, Williams J, Volpe RJ, Yunan E (1990) Benign cystic mesothelioma in a male. Am J Gastroenterol 85:311–315

Chou YH, Tiu CM, Lui WY, et al (1991) Mesenteric and omental cysts: an ultrasonographic and clinical study of 15 patients. Gastrointest Radiol 16:311

Contino A, Salzano A, Radice L, Montemurro D, Amendola G, Romano G, Ragozzino A, Smaltino F (1988) La diagnostica per immagini nello studio delle cisti mesenteriali. Proceedings of the XXXIIIrd National Congress of SIRM, Rome. Monduzzi, Bologna

Cornaglia-Ferraris P, Perlino GF et al (1982) Cystic lymphangioma of the spleen, report of CT scan findings. Pediatr Radiol 90:94–95

Cutillo DP, Swayne LC, Cucco J, Dougan H (1989) CT and MR imaging in cystic abdominal lymphangiomatosis. J Comput Assist Tomogr 13:534–536

Cyna-Gorse F, Frija J, Yana C, Ollier P, Laval-Jeantet M (1989) From lymphangioma to lymphangiomatosis. A propos of 10 cases. J Radiol 70:381–387

Geer LL, Mittelstaedt CA, Staab EV, Gaisie G (1984) Mesenteric cyst: sonographic appearance with CT correlation. Pediatr Radiol 14:102–104

Gyves Ray K, Hernandez RJ, Hillemeier AC (1990) Pseudoascites: unusual presentation of omental cyst. Pediatr Radiol 20:560–561

Hamrick-Turner JE, Chiechi MV, Abbitt PL, Ros PR (1992) Neoplastic and inflammatory processes of the peritoneum, omentum, and mesentery: diagnosis with CT. Radiographics 12:1051

Haney PJ, Whitley NO (1984) CT of benign cystic abdominal masses in children. AJR Am J Roentgenol 142:1279–1281

Hasan AKH, Sinclair DJ (1993) Case report: calcification in benign cystic peritoneal mesothelioma. Clin Radiol 48:66

Hatten MT, Hamrick-Turner JE, Smith DB (1996) Mesenteric cystic lymphangioma: radiologic appearance mimicking cystic teratoma. Pediatr. Radiol 26:458–460

Hjermstad BH, Sobin LH (1987) Mesenteric and omental cysts: Histologic classification with imaging correlation. Radiology 164:327

Katsube Y, Mukai K, Silverberg SG (1982) Cystic mesothelioma of the peritoneum: a report of five cases and a review of the literature. Cancer 50:1615–1622

Kozakewich H, Colodny A, Goldstein DP (1988) Peritoneal inclusion cysts: ovarian fluid in peritoneal adhesions. Radiology 169:189

Krahe T, Schneider B, Schmidt C (1985) Zystisches Lymphangiom des Omentum majus. Rofo Fortschr Geb Rontgenstr Neuen Bildgeb Verfahr 143:476–478

Leonidas JC, Brill PW, Bhan I et al (1987) Cystic retroperitoneal lymphangioma in infants and children. Radiology 127:203–208

Li YP, Guico R, Parikh S, et al (1992) Cystic mesothelioma of the retroperitoneum. J Clin Ultrasound 20:65

Liessi G, Sandini F, Spaliviero B (1989) Linfangiomi cistici dell'addome. Rilievi TC e US. Radiol Med 78:204–209

Lopez C, Miralles M, Muñoz A, Borruel S, Peral L, del Pozo G, Martinez A (1993) Paediatric intraperitoneal cystic masses: 10 years' follow-up. Eur Radiol 3:311–315

Lucaya J, Herrera M, Espax RM, Boix J (1978) Mesenteric and omental cysts in children: report of eight cases and review of the literature. Ann Radiol 21:161–172

O'Neal JD, Ros PR, Storm BL, Buck JL, Wilkinson EJ (1989) Cystic mesothelioma of the peritoneum. Radiology 170:333–337

Phillips GWL, Senapati A, Young AE (1988) Chylolymphatic mesenteric cyst: a diagnostic appearance on computed tomography. Br J Radiol 61:413

Rifkin MD, Kurtz AB, Pasto ME (1983) Mesenteric chylous (lymph containing) cysts. Gastrointest Radiol 8:267–269

Ros PR, Olmsted WW, Moser RP, Dachman AH, Hjermstad BH, Sobin LH (1987) Mesenteric and omental cysts: histologic classification with imaging correlation. Radiology 164:327–332

Schnarkowski P, Friedrich JM, Muller M, Limmer J (1991) The radiological detection of mesenteric chylous cysts. Rofo Fortschr Geb Rontgenstr Neuen Bildgeb Verfahr 155:284–285

Silvestre de Sacy V, Keilani K, Duron JJ, Vayre P (1992) Lymphangioma of the mesentery. A rare cause of acute abdominal pain syndrome in adults. J Chir (Paris) 129:78–80

Skaake P, Hueber KH (1983) Computed tomography of cystic ovarian teratomas with gravity dependent layering. J Comput Assist Tomogr 7:837

Stevens SK, Nino Murcia M, Bloom R, et al (1989) Mesenteric cyst with atypical computed tomography appearance. Clin Imaging 13:119

Thomas AMK, Leung A, Lynn J (1985) Abdominal cystic lymphangiomatosis: report of a case and review of the literature. Br J Radiol 58:467–469

Volk BA, Scholmerich J, Farthmann E, Gerok W, Wenz W (1983) Leiomyoblastoma of the stomach – a case report on ultrasonographic differential diagnosis of cystic lesions in the abdomen. Hepatogastroenterology 30:33–35

Dermoid Cysts – Cystic Teratomas

Bowen B, Ros PR, McCarthy MJ, Olmsted WW, Hjermstad BM (1987) Gastrointestinal teratomas: CT and US appearance with pathologic correlation. Radiology 162:431–433

Buy JN, Bazot M, Ghossain M, Sciot C, Hugol D, Bigot JM, Truc JB, Poitout PH, Vadrot D, Ecoiffier J (1989a) Appearance

tomodensitométrique des kistes dermoïdes de l'ovaire. J Radiol 70:103–109
Buy JN, Ghossain MA, Moss AA, Bazot M, Doucet M, Hugol D, Truc JB, Poitout P, Ecoiffier J (1989b) Cystic teratoma of the ovary: CT detection. Radiology 171:697
Cawley KM, Mahoney PD, Wilmot MD, Longrace TL (1983) Clinical image. Ovarian dermoid: unusual CT presentation. J Comput Assist Tomogr 7:1116–1117
Cederlung CG, Karlsson S, Nyman U (1981) Computer tomography of dermoid cysts. Acta Radiol (Diagn) 22:435–439
Feldberg MAM, Van Waes PFGM, Hendriks MJ (1984) Direct multiplanar CT findings in cystic teratoma of the ovary. J Comput Assist Tomogr 8:1131–1135
Friedman AC, Payatt RS, Hartman DS, Downey EF, Olson BO (1982) CT of benign cystic teratoma. AJR Am J Roentgenol 138:659–665
Prieto ML, Casanova A, Delgado J, et al (1989) Cystic teratoma of the mesentery. Pediatr Radiol 19:439
Ralls PW, Hartman B, White W, et al (1987) Computed tomography of benign cystic teratoma of the omentum. J Comput Assist Tomogr 11:548–549
Skaane P, Huebener KH (1983) Computed tomography of cystic ovarian teratomas with gravity-dependent layering. J Comput Assist Tomogr 7:837–841
Skaane P, Klott KJ (1981) Fat-fluid level in a cystic ovarian teratoma. J Comput Assist Tomogr 5:577–579
Weinstein BJ, Lenkey JL, Williams S (1979) Ultrasound and CT demonstration of a benign cystic teratoma arising from the retroperitoneum. AJR Am J Roentgenol 133:936–938
Wjamg SH, Lee KS, Kim PN, Bae WK, Lee BH (1990) Omental teratoma in an adult: a case report. Gastrointest Radiol 15:301–2

Echinococcus Cysts

Abignoly AM, de Belsunce M, Saoi JP, et al (1984) A propos d'un cas d'hydatidose intrapéritonéale diagnostiquée par la tomodensitométrie. Ann Radiol 27:34–36
Di Palma A, Ettorre GC, Scapati C (1991) Ruolo della tomografia computerizzata nella diagnosi della malattia idatidea. Radiol Med 82:430–436
Kalovidouris A, Pissiotis C, Pontifex G, et al (1986) CT characterization of multivesicular hydatid cysts. J Comput Assist Tomogr 10:428–431
Kotoulas G, Gouliamos A, Kalovidouris A, Vlabos L, Papavasiliou C (1990) Computed tomographic localization of pelvic hydatid disease. Eur J Radiol 11:38–41
Munzer D (1991) New perspectives in the diagnosis of *Echinococcus* disease. J Clin Gastroenterol 13:415–423
Taneja K, Gothi R, Kumar K, et al (1990) Peritoneal Echinococcus multilocularis infection: CT appearance. J Comput Assist Tomogr 14:493–494
Von Sinner WN (1990) Ultrasound, CT and MRI of ruptured and disseminated hydatid cysts. Eur J Radiol 11:31–37

12 Primary Tumors

CONTENTS

Tumors of the peritoneum, the omentum and the subperitoneal spaces originate from the various tissues that constitute these structures: coelomic epithelium, mesothelium, fibrous connective tissue, adipose tissue, muscular tissue, hematic vessels, lymphatic tissue, nerves, and embryonal tissue.

These primary neoplasm are rare, whereas metastatic abnormalities arising from abdominal, prevalently intestinal and ovarian, tumors are more common. Therefore, when a neoplastic mass is shown by the CT at the peritoneal or omental level a secondary tumor must be suspected as the most probably correct interpretation; only when no primary tumor is discovered can the possibility that it is a primary form be considered. In this connection, we must point out that primary ovarian tumors may be not recognized on CT examination, because they may be small and masked by intestinal loops sinking into the pelvis and swelled by gas and fluids. Similarly, asymptomatic intestinal tumors may be not discovered because the CT technique used may be inadequate.

In the present treatment we will use the most common classification, which has been made according to rigorous histopathological criteria (Table 12.1).

12.1 Coelomic Epithelium

12.1.1 Papillary Serous Tumors of the Peritoneum

Papillary serous tumors of the peritoneum are very rare. They were identified by Swerdlow in 1959; only recently they have been recognized as an autonomous pathologic entity. They arise from the pluripotent cells of the peritoneal serosa. Their anatomo-histological characteristics are homologous to those of the corresponding ovarian tumors. They can be correctly classified only when their ultrastructure is examined by electron microscopy or when immunohistochemical methods are used.

Two theories have been proposed to explain this analogy. The first theory suggests that the tumor originates from the malignant degeneration of nests of ovarian cells left in the peritoneum during the

Table 12.1. Primary tumors of the peritoneum, omentum and mesenteries

Tissue	Benign	Malignant
EPITHELIAL		
Coelomic epithelium	Papillary serous cystadenoma	Papillary serous cystadenocarcinoma
MESOTHELIAL		
Mesothelium	Cystic mesothelioma	Malignant mesothelioma
Fetal mesothelium	Multicystic mesothelioma	Desmoplastic small round cell tumor
MESENCHYMAL		
Fibrotic structures	Desmoid	Fibrosarcoma
	Fibroma	Malignant histiocytoma
Lipomatous tissue	Lipoma	Liposarcoma
	Lipoblastoma-lipoblastomatosis	
	Pseudotumoral lipomatosis	
	Infiltrating lipomatosis	
Smooth muscle	Leiomyoma	Leiomyosarcoma
	Leiomyomatosis	Leiomyosarcomatosis
Striated muscle	Rhabdomyoma	Rhabdomyosarcoma
Blood vessels	Hemangioma	Hemangiosarcoma
	Benign hemangio-endothelioma	Malignant hemangio-endothelioma
	Hemangiopericytoma	Malignant hemangiopericytoma
		Kaposi's sarcoma
Lymphatic vessels	Lymphangioma	Lymphangiosarcoma
		Lymphangioendothelioma
Undifferentiated tissue		Malignant mesenchymoma
LYMPHATIC		
Lymphatic cells		Lymphoma
		Chronic lymphatic leukemia
NERVOUS		
Sheaths of peripheral nerves	Neurinoma	Neurosarcoma
	Neurofibroma	Neurofibrosarcoma
	Neurofibromatosis	
Nervous ganglia	Ganglioneuroma	Ganglioneuroblastoma
Neuroendocrine chromaffin cells		Carcinoid
EMBRYONAL		
Embryonal cells	Dermoid cysts	Malignant teratoma
	Cystic Teratoma	

process of embryonal gonadal migration. The second supposes that the analogies between the two entities are due to the common origin of the ovarian epithelium and the peritoneum from the mesoderm, which has a muellerian potential.

These tumors are very rare; we have distinguished them in micropapillary serous cystic tumors and papillary serous solid carcinomas.

The micropapillary cystic tumors fall into three classes:

- Benign micropapillary serous cystic tumors (serous cystadenomas)
- Micropapillary serous cystic tumors with a low potential malignancy (borderline serous cystadenomas)
- Malignant micropapillary serous cystic tumors (cystadenocarcinomas)

Macroscopically, benign or borderline micropapillary serous cystic tumors appear as cyst-like ovoid masses with a smooth surface and a uni- or multilocular structure; their walls and septa are thin, and the content is a serous and clear fluid. Cystadenocarcinomas appear as peritoneal or omental unique or multiple masses with a cystic or prevalently cystic structure.

The benign and the borderline forms are often asymptomatic, whereas the malignant types cause abdominal pain, anorexia and abdominal tumescence.

No cases of papillary serous cystadenomas studied with CT have been reported in the literature.

Borderline papillary serous cystadenomas (MARRUCCI et al. 1992) appear as intraperitoneal ovoid structures with sharp margins; basal and postcontrast examinations show them as hypodense masses.

The papillary serous cystadenocarcinomas appear as peritoneal masses with a mixed structure, whose prevalent component is cystic. They have thick walls and postcontrast hyperdense solid areas with associated multiple small cyst-like localizations, which are scattered in the peritoneal cavity above and below the mesocolon and in the omentum (Fig. 12.1).

Papillary serous solid carcinomas are similar to ovarian tumors in their biological and clinical manifestations and in their solid metastases or peritoneal carcinosis; they also have the same favorable response to cisplatin treatment.

The CT findings when these tumors are present are described as large nonhomogeneous solid peritoneal and omental masses (Stafford-Johnson et al. 1998; Furukawa et al. 1999), sometimes calcified (Stafford-Johnson et al. 1998), or massive ascites with fine enhancing surface nodularity in the parietal peritoneum and marked omental caking suggestive of peritoneal carcinosis (Chopra et al. 2000).

Practically, the CT aspect of one of these tumors is similar to that of a peritoneal carcinosis or a malignant mesothelioma. However, the presence of normal-sized ovaries and the absence of an identifiable malignant tumor should suggest the possibility of a papillary serous peritoneal tumor (Stafford-Johnson et al. 1998; Chopra et al. 2000), and a high CA125 level in the serum makes it possible to distinguish it from mesotheliomas and from nonovarian peritoneal carcinomatosis. A laparoscopy or an exploratory laparotomy with biopsy specimens taken for ultrastructural and immunohistochemical investigations is useful to establish the definitive diagnosis. The US or CT negativity of the ovarian involvement does not exclude the presence of an ovarian neoplasm.

CT is also useful in therapeutic programs including the surgical reduction of the tumor and the intravenous or intraperitoneal perfusion chemotherapy.

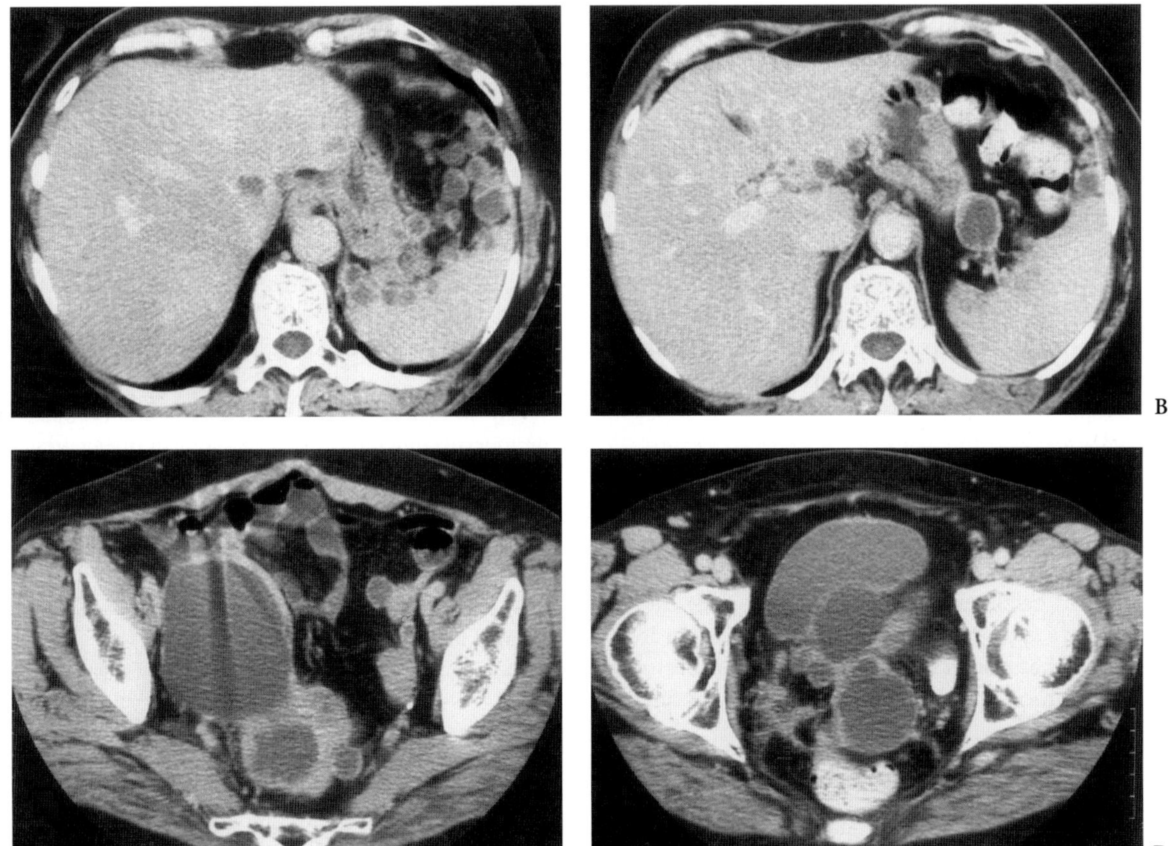

Fig. 12.1A–D. Peritoneal micropapillary serous cystadenocarcinoma. Multiple confluent peritoneal cyst-like nodules with thick and postcontrast hyperdense wall in the hypogastrium and in the pelvis; they are in bunches at the perisplenic and gastrocolic levels (**A**). Isolated nodule in the gastrosplenic ligament (**B**)

12.2 Mesothelium

12.2.1 Cystic Mesothelioma

In keeping with histopathological criteria, cystic mesothelioma is usually included under the cystic forms, and it has therefore been discussed in the chapter on Cysts (chapter 11).

12.2.2 Multicystic Mesothelioma

Peritoneal multicystic mesothelioma is a rare benign tumor of mesothelial origin. It has only recently been recognized and clearly defined as an autonomous entity, ultrastructural and immunohistochemical studies having distinguished this form from malignant mesothelioma, cystic lymphangioma and mucinous adenocarcinoma, with all of which it has been erroneously confused in the past.

Peritoneal multicystic mesotheliomas usually affect adult women and become evident after a long period of clinical latency, with vague abdominal or pelvic pains, malaise, abdominal distension, nausea and vomiting. Macroscopically and on CT scans it is characterized by numerous cystic structures varying in size from a few millimeters to several centimeters, each limited by a thin wall and with a serous, clear and transparent fluid inside, which are distributed along the wall of the parietal and visceral peritoneum. These structures may merge into an agglomeration with the appearance of a mass.

12.2.3 Malignant Mesothelioma

Malignant mesothelioma arises from the pluripotent cells of the serous membranes of the body cavity. It is a rare tumor, but is constantly increasing in frequency because of the industrial use of asbestos; the pleural form is closely correlated with the direct or indirect inhalation of asbestos fibers as a result of environmental pollution. Links with other serous localizations (peritoneal, pericardial or vaginal) are still not clear; the mechanism underlying the tumoral effect of asbestos is also unknown.

Mesotheliomas become manifest after a long period of latency (20 years for pleural localizations, between 40 and 45 years for the peritoneal type) from the initial exposure to asbestos. They can also be correlated with the kind and duration of the exposure. Mesotheliomas are located prevalently in the pleura, whilst in 12–20% of cases the tumor involves the peritoneal serosa. In 30–40% of peritoneal cases it has a double localization: pleural and peritoneal.

From a histological point of view, the mesothelioma is classified as epithelial (solid or tubopapillary), fibrosarcomatoid or mixed (epithelial and sarcomatoid).

The epithelial form is the most frequent; it develops rapidly, infiltrating the peritoneum and forming small nodules that are spread over its surface. The peritoneal invasion becomes progressively wider, involving the mesentery, the omentum, and the intestinal walls.

The sarcomatoid type appears as a solid encapsulated mass that preferentially extends into the omentum without infiltrating or involving the mesentery.

The mixed epithelial and sarcomatoid type has the characteristics of both types.

Initially, the clinical signs of this tumor are nonspecific, such as aching, abdominal distension, and malaise; later, increasing abdominal cramps, weight loss, intestinal subocclusion, ascites and palpable swellings become evident.

Mesothelioma has an unfavorable prognosis and leads to death within 1 year after diagnosis. However, surgical treatment with excision of the mass and intensive radiochemotherapies have made it possible to obtain complete, albeit temporary, remissions of the disease and to extend patients' survival by 18–78 months (Antman et al. 1985; Ledermann et al. 1987).

The CT aspect of the mesothelioma is related to the macroscopic and histopathological ones (Ros et al. 1991) (Table 12.2).

Table 12.2. CT findings of the malignant mesothelioma. (Modified from Ros 1991)

Epithelial form	Ascites Thickening of the parietal and visceral peritoneum and mesentery Nodular peritoneal dissemination Infiltration and thickening of the omentum
Sarcomatoid form	Well-defined mass in the omentum and in the mesentery Ascites
Mixed form	Peritoneal and mesenteric thickening Solid mass Ascites

Initially, the only sign of the epithelial type of this tumor (Figs. 12.2–12.4, 12.6) is ascites limited to one or a few spaces or spread into the whole cavity. After a short time, thickening of the parietal and visceral peritoneum becomes evident, with increasingly numerous and extensive nodules and plaques on its surface.

Mesenteric extension is seen as linear or sinuous images around the vessels and the subperitoneal adipose cellular tissue. The thickness of these images is not uniform; they have a radiated, fan-like, stellate, or railway track-like shape and converge toward the mesenteric root: these aspects do not change even when the patient is in a recumbent position (Fig. 12.6) (WHITLEY et al. 1982a, b).

In the advanced forms, when the parietal peritoneum is extensively infiltrated, a circumferential "shell-like" thickening of the total internal surface of the abdominal cavity (Fig. 12.6) becomes evident. Furthermore, the nodules that are in contact with the stomach or the intestinal loops make the profile of these viscera spiny because of a desmoplastic reaction (Ros et al. 1991).

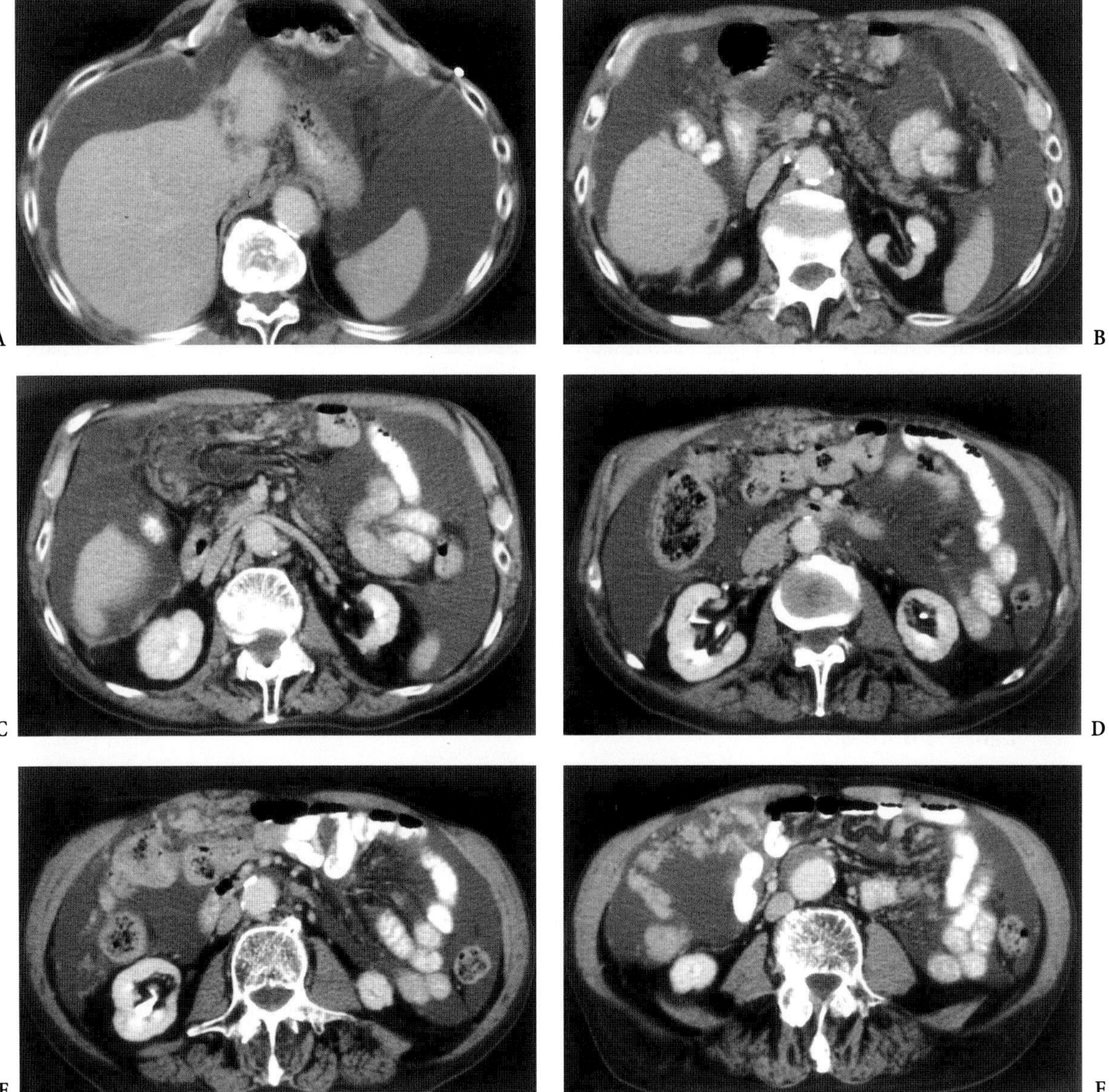

Fig. 12.2A–F. Malignant epithelial mesothelioma. Typical findings: extensive ascites, multiple small nodules, lines or plaques on the parietal peritoneum and increased thickness of the omentum with micronodules

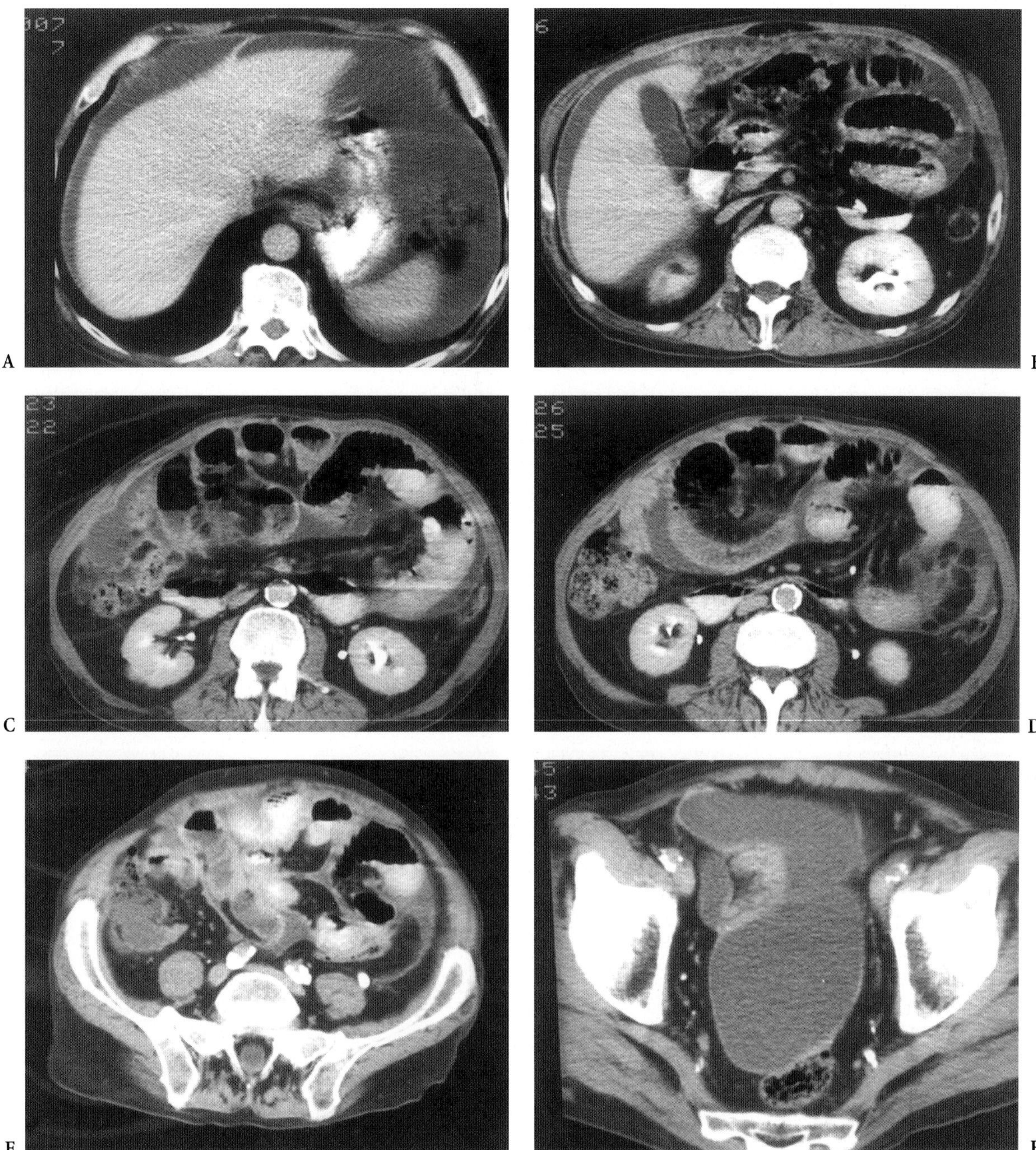

Fig. 12.3A–F. Malignant epithelial mesothelioma. Extensive ascites, diffuse thickening of the supra- (**B**, **C**) and submesocolic (**C**–**E**) and pelvic (**F**) peritoneum. The infiltrated omentum is denser and thicker on the *right* (**B**–**D**)

An omental localization (Figs. 12.2, 12.3, 12.6) is indicated by increased thickening and density or by a reticular or spongy aspect.

In contrast, the sarcomatoid type (Fig. 12.5) appears as one or more than one well encapsulated solid masses, sometimes containing calcifications. After i.v. contrast agent injection peripheral enhancement appears, whereas the colliquative cystic-like central parts remain hypodense. The contours separating areas of different density are always shaded and irregular. This type is preferentially located in the omentum, where it may produce a thick transversal omental caking mass interposed between the anterior abdominal wall and the intestinal loops, which are pushed backward.

The mixed types show the CT characters of both histological types: epithelial and sarcomatoid.

12.2.4 Desmoplastic Small Round Cell

The desmoplastic small round cell tumor is a rare malignant tumor of the peritoneum; it is only recently that it was identified with immunohistochemical techniques and recognized as an autonomous pathologic entity. It must be distinguished from neoplasms with analogous characteristics, with which it has been confused hitherto – atypical small cell tumors, mesotheliomas, carcinomas, carcinoids, germinal cell tumors – and newly classed in the category of tumors originating from the fetal mesothelium. It occurs predominantly in adolescent boys or young adult males.

Macroscopically, it is seen as a voluminous well-defined peritoneal or omental mass with a smooth surface and necrotic areas inside; it is constantly associated with peritoneal dissemination. It generally in such a way as to dislocate without infiltrating the adjacent tissues and produces hematic metastases or metastases to the lymph nodes only later. It is frequently located in the pelvic retrovesical space.

Histologically,it is characterized by nests of small round cells with numerous mitoses, which are densely packed in a thick desmoplastic stroma.

The presence of atypical clinic manifestations does not suggest a desmoplastic tumor. It can be that only vague abdominal or pelvic pain or discomfort and a palpable mass may be present.

Few cases of CT studies of this tumor have been reported in the literature (Outwater et al. 1992; Varma et al. 1992; Dao and Dachman. 1995; N'Dri et al. 1998; Pickhardt et al. 1999)

On CT the desmoplastic small cell tumor appears in the early stage as a well-defined lobulated solid mass with mild nonhomogeneous enhancement and low-density necrotic-hemorrhagic areas and, sometimes, punctate calcifications inside, frequently localized between the bladder and the rectum (Fig. 12.7). Later in the course, low-density necrotic-hemorrhagic intratumoral areas ascites with small multiple intraperitoneal nodular implants and hepatic capsule scalloping appear, together with omental localizations and lymphoadenomegalies and hematogenous metastases.

In the early stage the suspicion of a small round cell tumor may be raised when a mass is seated inside the peritoneum, well limited from the serosa, located in the pelvis between the bladder and the rectum, and has punctate calcifications inside, and the patient concerned is young, especially a male patient.

The differential diagnosis includes only the abdominal tumors of young men, such as lymphoma and neurosarcoma. Lymphomas are not generally located in the peritoneum, but develop in the sub- or retroperitoneal lymph nodes. Neurosarcomas are frequently associated with neurofibromatosis. In the advanced stages the CT findings mimic other pathologic conditions, such as peritoneal carcinomatosis and lymphomatosis.

12.3 Fibrous Tissue

CT examination may show fibrous tissue and tumors as hyperdense relative to muscle and solid viscera, both before and after i.v. contrast medium injection (Rubenstein et al. 1986). In the precontrast CT the hyperdensity is due to the high attenuation of the collagen within this tissue, whereas the marked contrast enhancement reflects the rich capillary network of the fibrocollagenous tissue (Rubenstein et al. 1986).

12.3.1 Fibroma and Fibrosarcoma

Both fibroma and fibrosarcoma are tumors that arise from the peritoneal, omental and mesenteric fibrous structures.

Histologically they appear to be composed of knotted bundles of spindled fibroblasts that are closely packed with scant intervening collagen. Frequent mitoses and marked pleomorphism characterize fibrosarcomas.

Macroscopically, these tumors are seen as ovoid or spherical encapsulated solid masses with a smooth, shiny, silvery white surface and pearly-gray cut surfaces on cross section.

Their growth is slow and expansive; only occasionally do such tumors infiltrate the adjacent tissues.

Both fibroma and fibrosarcoma have the CT characteristics of precontrast attenuation values equal to or slightly higher than those of muscular tissue and becoming markedly opaque after contrast injection. The lower contrast enhancement sometimes observed in the central area probably depends on the presence of mature fibrous tissue lacking central capillaries, whereas the peripheral hyperdensity might be due to a more active, and thus more highly vascularized, tissue (Rubenstein et al. 1986).

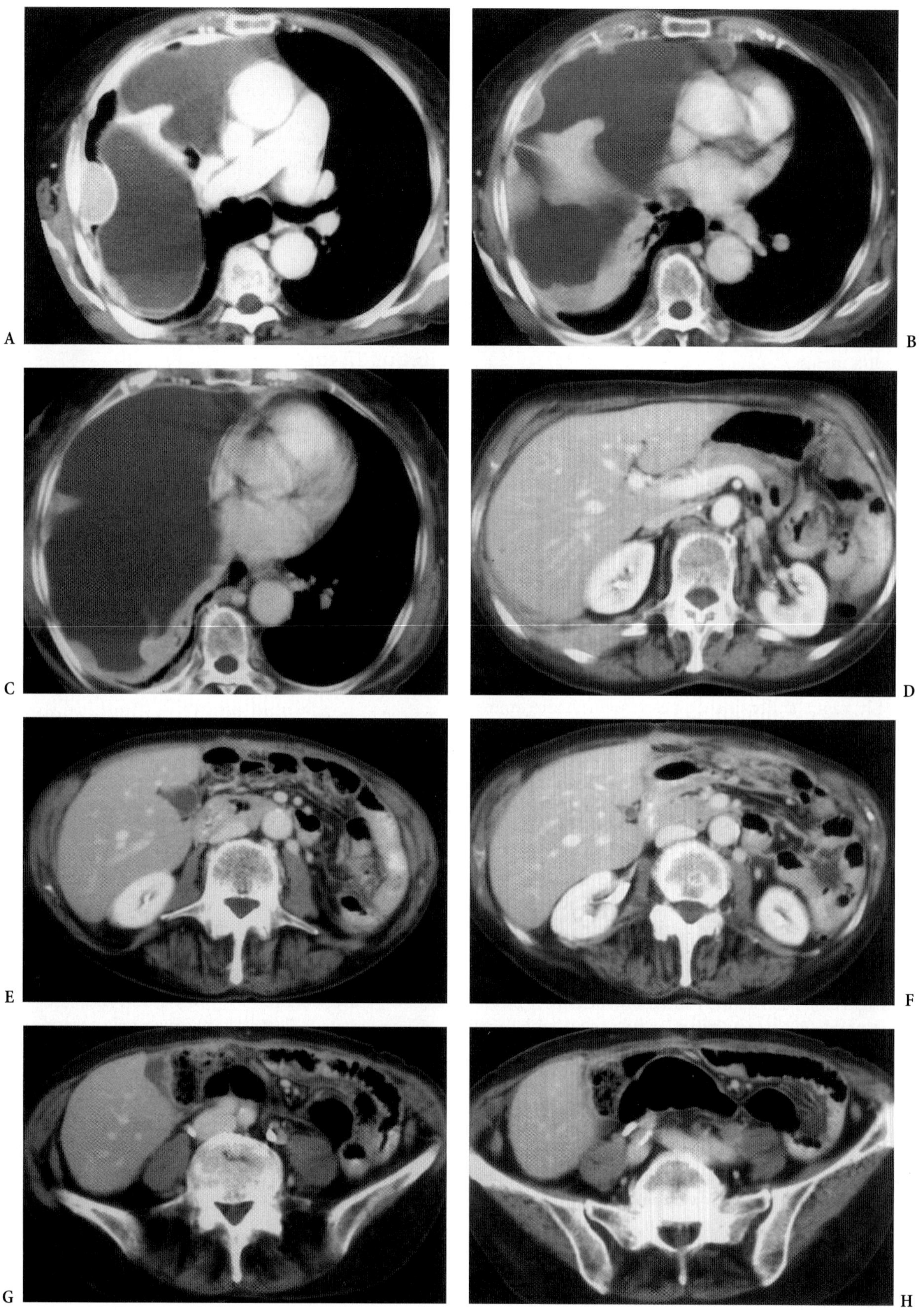
A
B
C
D
E
F
G
H

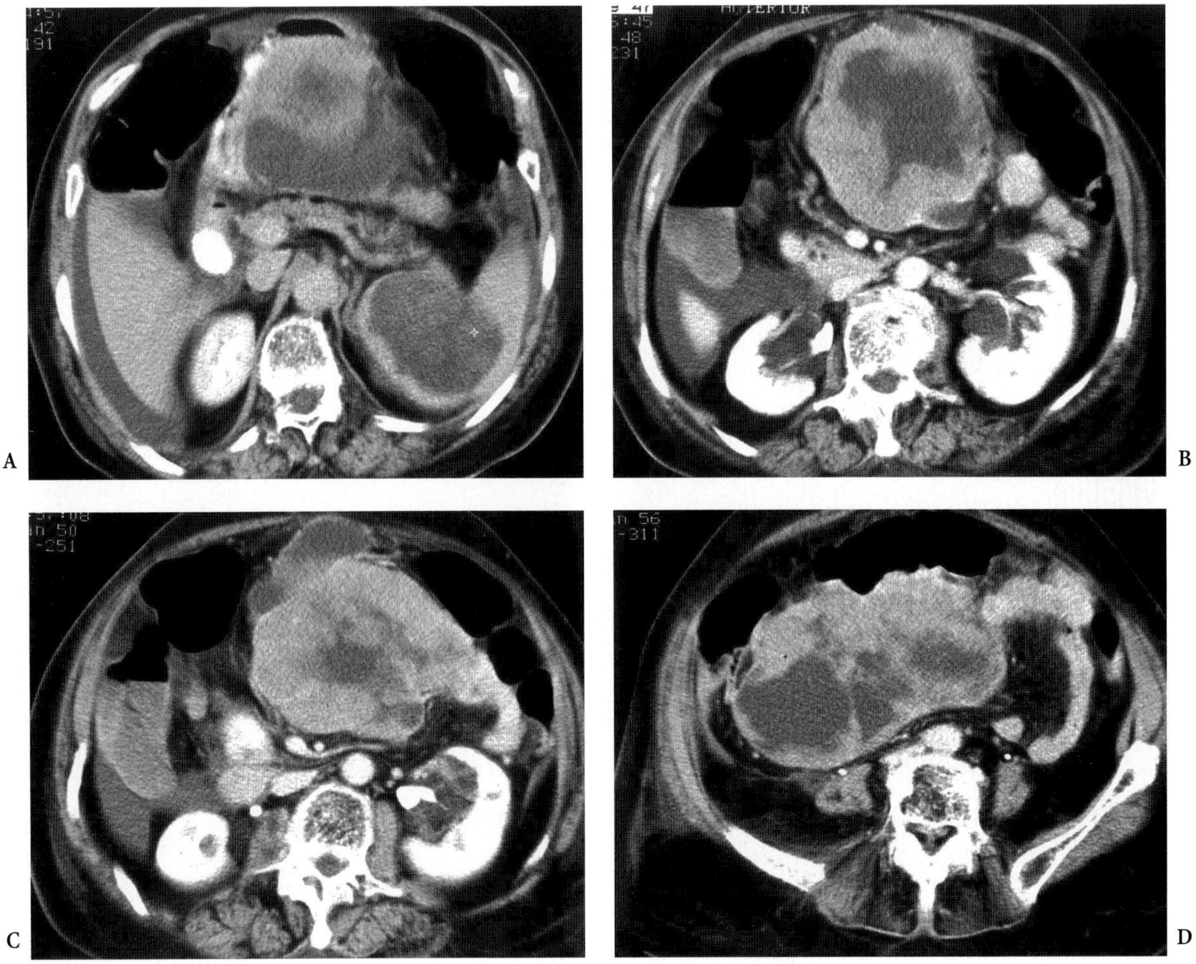

Fig. 12.5A–D. Malignant sarcomatoid mesothelioma. Voluminous bosselated mass, with low-density and cyst-like colliquative areas, which comes in close contact with the posterior wall of the stomach and of the transverse colon. The retroperitoneal and mesenteric planes are well delineated behind the mass by adipose tissue, where the splenic vein, the pancreas (**A**) and the superior mesenteric vessels with their right and left branches (**B, C**) stand out. Splenic nodular metastasis (**A**). Modest ascites

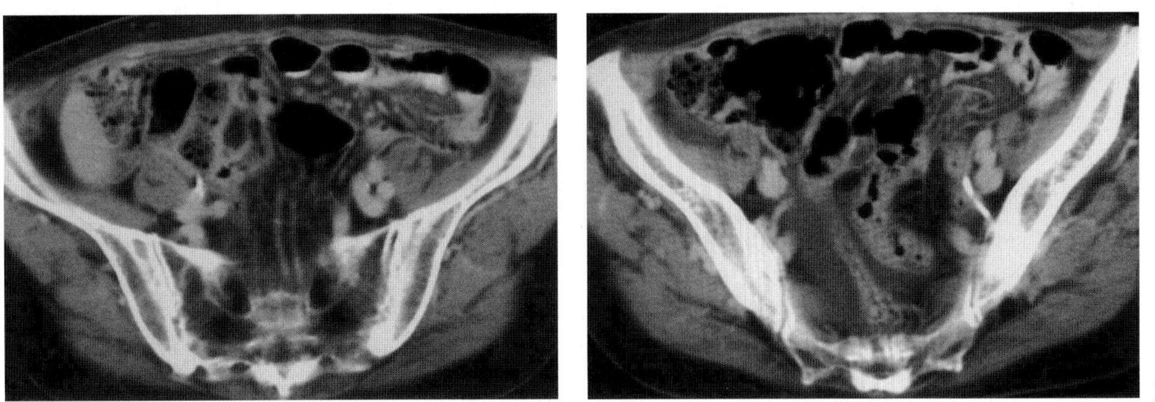

Fig. 12.4A–J. Malignant epithelial mesothelioma with pleural and peritoneal localization. Classic aspect at the pleural level with nodules, masses and effusion (**A–C**). At the peritoneal level, the signs of localization are milder: mild effusion in the pelvic peritoneal spaces (**J**), thickening of the peritoneum, the gastrocolic ligament, the transverse mesocolon next to the colon (**E**), the mesentery (**F–H**) and the sigmoid mesocolon (**I**).Omental infiltration (**D–G**)

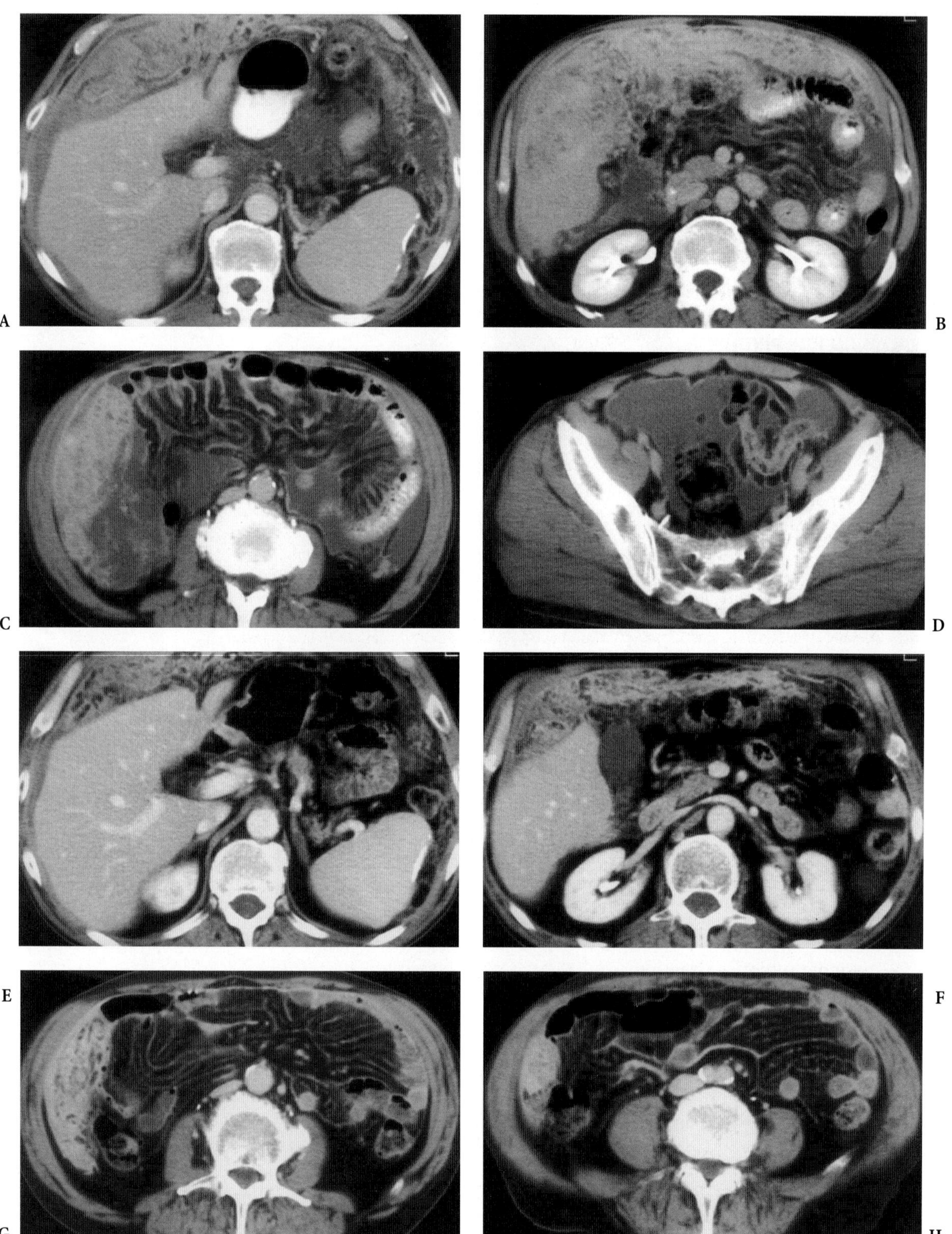

Fig. 12.6A–H. Malignant epithelial mesothelioma. A conspicuous increase in circumferential thickness and density of the antero-superior peritoneum and the omentum appears as a thick transversal plaque pushing the liver and the hollow viscera (**A, D**) backward. Infiltration of the mesenteric peritoneum showing a "railway track"-like shape around the perivascular adipose tissue (**C**). Ascites spreading over the total peritoneal cavity. Follow-up control performed 1 year after therapy (**E–H**): the ascitic effusion has been completely reabsorbed and the perivascular mesenteric peritoneum has become thinner, even though it is denser and shows a sharp profile. The anterior mass appears to have a reduced thickness and extension

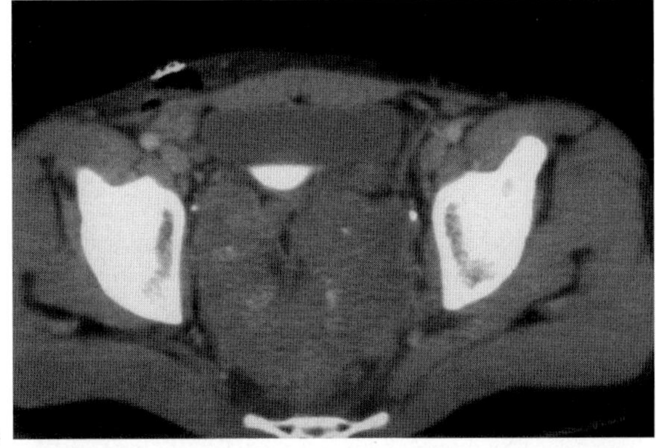

A

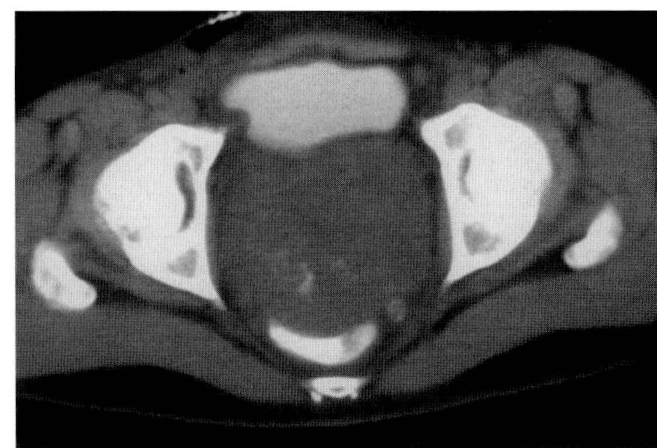

B

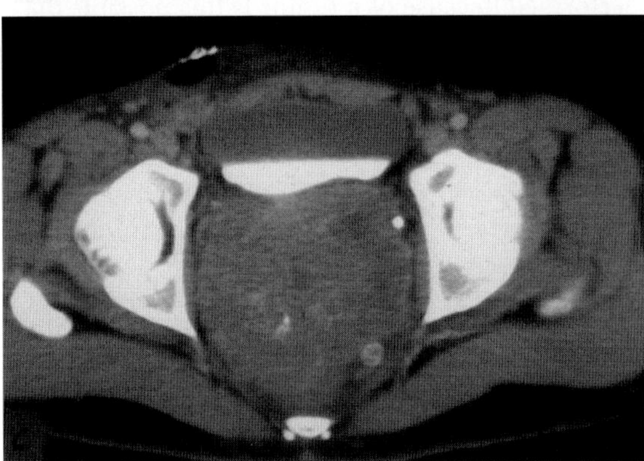

C

Fig. 12.7. Desmoplastic small round cell tumor. Well-defined intraperitoneal dense nonhomogeneous mass with punctate calcifications and hypodense necrotic areas inside. Slight nonuniform contrast enhancement

CT cannot allow a distinction between benign and malignant fibromatous tumors or between these and other neoplasms.

12.3.2 Desmoid

The desmoid tumor is a well-differentiated fibroblastic proliferation of the fibrous tissue of the mesenterium, omentum and abdominal wall in subjects with a genetic disposition to the hyperproduction of fibrous tissue. Most desmoid tumors occur in young female subjects with Gardner's syndrome after proctocolectomy. It can develop as an isolated and limited or as a locally aggressive, expansive process.

Macroscopically, the expansive form appears as a homogeneous solid mass with a smooth surface, displacing the adjacent tissues without infiltrating them. In this case, the desmoid tumor grows slowly without producing subjective symptoms and becomes manifest only when it has reached conspicuous dimensions.

In contrast, the invasive form appears to be aggressive in the site where it is located, because of its tendency to infiltrate the mesenteric, omental and peritoneal structures, the adjacent organs and the abdominal wall. This type also grows slowly, and even though it has no histopathologically malignant characteristics and does not metastasize, the tumor frequently relapses if it is not completely excised by surgery.

Different CT aspects correspond to the two forms of this tumor:

1) The expansive form appears as a well-limited mass with a smooth profile, which displaces the adjacent structures without infiltration. It has a solid structure; its density is equal to that of the muscular tissue and increases sharply after contrast medium (Figs. 12.8, 12.9).
2) The invasive form appears as a poorly defined solid mass with a density equal to that of the muscular tissue. It involves and infiltrates the mesentery, the omentum, and the adjacent organs. Contrast medium induces an increase in the density of the neoplastic tissue, which varies in degree.

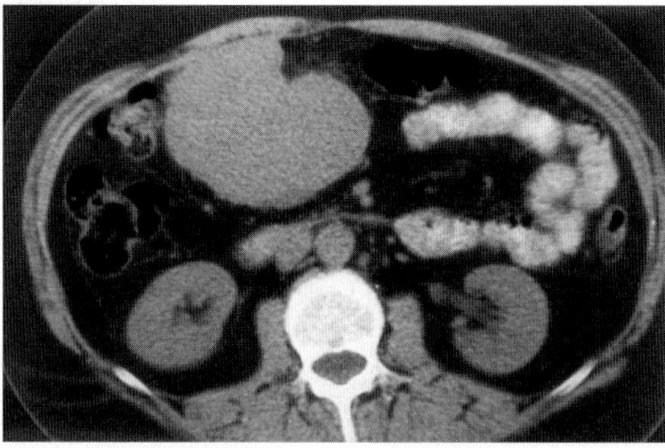

Fig. 12.8. Desmoid tumor. Bosselated homogeneous solid mass with smooth profile, well limited by omental and mesenteric fat

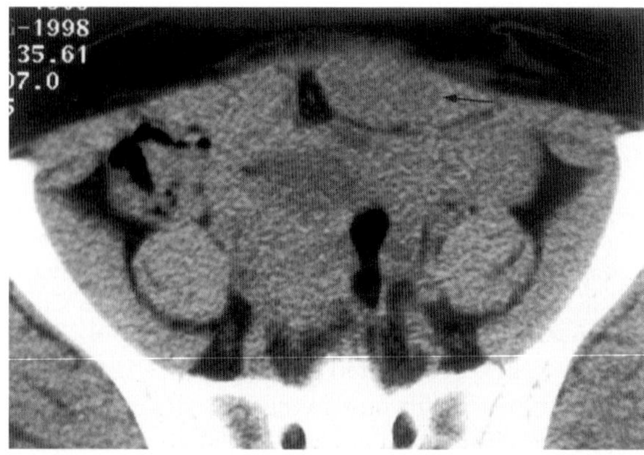

A

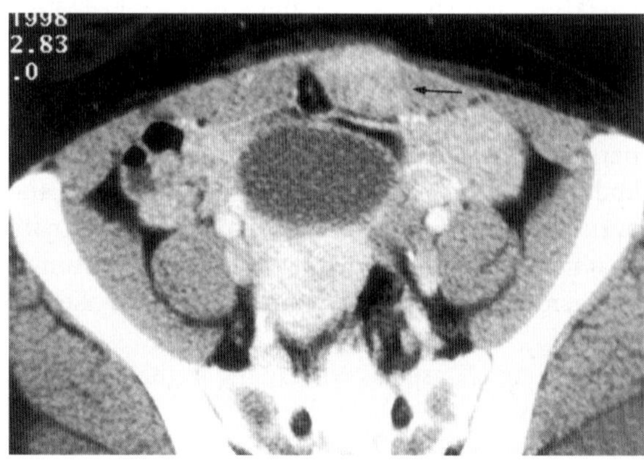

B

Fig. 12.9. Desmoid tumor. Slightly hypodense homogeneous mass with sharp limits (**A**), intensely absorbing the contrast medium (**B**). It is located in the left rectus abdominis muscle (*arrows*)

The appearance of the expansive form (sharp contours without signs of infiltration of the adjacent tissue, absence of hypodense areas possibly because of necrotic-hemorrhagic degeneration, elevated contrast enhancement, absence of metastases in lymph nodes or liver) suggests the benign nature of the lesion and makes it possible to distinguish it from other expansive processes with similar morphological characters (neurinomas, neurofibromas, leiomyomas) whose density is not intensely increased by the contrast medium.

Conversely, when the abdominal structures located in the site of a surgical incision made for resection of a previous tumor appear to be infiltrated, a relapse of the tumor is usually expected, without consideration of the possibility of a desmoplastic tumor. Only when the patient is affected by Gardner's syndrome or the surgical operation was not performed because of a tumor is this possible diagnosis usually considered.

Like all young fibrous tissues, the desmoplastic tumor is sensitive to radiotherapy; if such treatment is carried out before surgery it may reduce the extension and severity of the infiltration and make it possible to perform an operation that might otherwise be considered impossible.

12.3.3 Malignant Histiocytoma

Malignant fibrous histiocytoma is a sarcomatous tumor that is typically seen in elderly subjects (50–60 years old); it arises from histiocytes that have changed their shape, assuming a fibroblast-like aspect. It is particularly frequent in the soft tissue of the limbs, being rare in peritoneal and subperitoneal sites.

Microscopically it presents a pleiomorphic aspect with sheets of histiocyte-like cells, bundles of fibroblastic spindle cells, and malignant giant and foam cells.

Macroscopically, it is seen as a spherical mass with necrotic areas inside, which are often wide. As the tumor grows it invades or involves the adjacent viscera, to the extent of producing a stenosis or an intestinal obstruction.

This tumor becomes clinically evident in a late phase, when it is already well developed and extending as a painless mass; sometimes it is accompanied by vague abdominal aches or by gastrointestinal disturbances. It does not metastasize to the liver until late in the course, although it tends to relapse early.

CT shows if as a poorly defined solid mass (Fig. 12.10) that often contains low-density necrotic areas and sometimes calcifications; it tends to involve the contiguous structures and viscera. The contrast medium increases the density of the solid component, producing irregular spots with persistent peripheral enhancement.

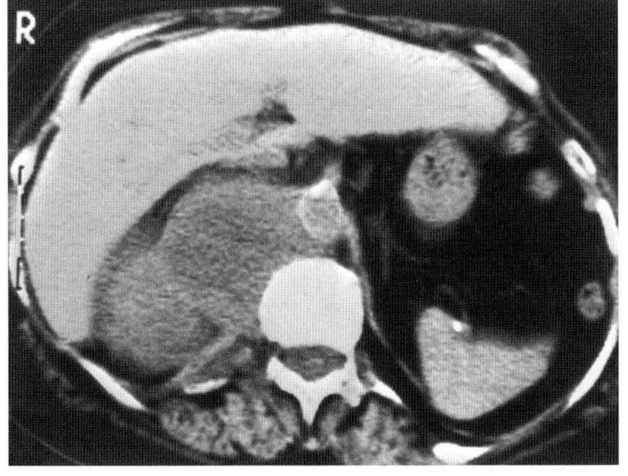

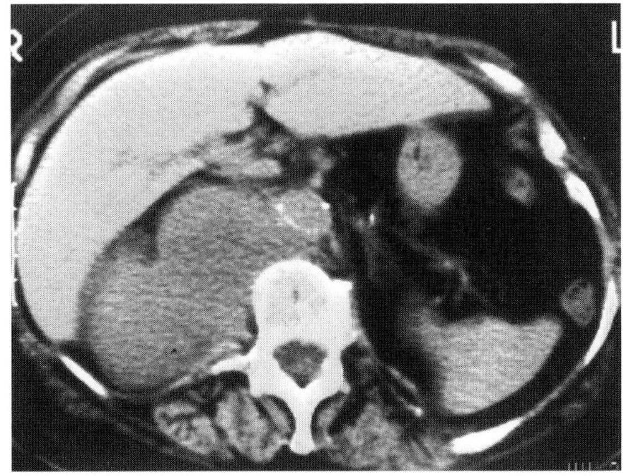

Fig. 12.10A, B. Malignant histiocytoma. Bilobate retroperitoneal mass with central hypodense areas; it is in very close contact with the spinal column and the posterior renal fascia and is adhering to the aorta.

CT is unable to distinguish this form from the other peritoneal sarcomas, and it can thus only establish the extension of the tumor and the involvement of contiguous organs, where present, and provide early recognition of relapses.

12.4 Fatty Tissue

Lipomatous tumors are the most frequent primary mesenchymal neoplasms in the abdomen. Even though they are prevalently located in the retroperitoneum and involve the subperitoneal spaces only secondarily, they do sometimes arise from the mesentery or the omentum.

The identification of adipose tissue or of a relevant lipidic component inside the mass is one of the most significant parameters that can be used to identify the tumor; furthermore, a correct diagnosis of the nature of the expansive process is often possible when the site and other morphostructural characteristics are taken into account.

This points to CT as the method of choice for tissue characterization of this pathology, because it makes it possible to measure the negative densitometric values typical of fat (–80/–150 HU) by electronic methods and to localize the tumor exactly with its axial vision.

12.4.1 Lipoma

The lipoma is an encapsulated benign tumor made up of well-differentiated adipocytes separated by thin bundles of fibrous connective tissue. In most cases, it is clinically silent, and it may therefore grow to large dimensions without producing disturbances.

The lipoma has the typical CT aspect (Fig. 12.11) of a sharply marginated mass made up of fat-density tissue, which is sometimes crossed by thin fibrous linear denser streaks and limited by a thin capsule of higher attenuation, which is not always visible, with no signs of local invasions, and associated with simple dislocations of adjacent structures or organs.

12.4.2 Liposarcoma

Liposarcomas are malignant tumors originating from adipose tissue. They are characterized by different histological subtypes, which are classified according to their more aggressive component into: lipogenic, myxoid and pleiomorphous.

- Lipogenic or well-differentiated liposarcomas are prevalently made up of lipoblasts with a high lipoid content and a low level of malignancy. They grow slowly and often displace the adjacent tissues without infiltrations; occasionally, these tumors metastasize.

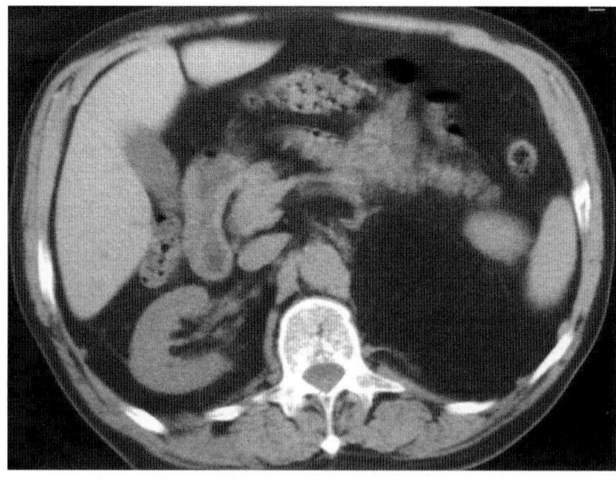
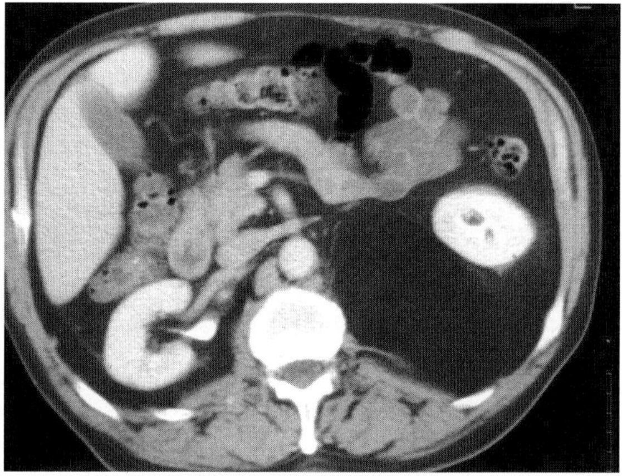

Fig. 12.11A, B. Lipoma. Homogeneous mass with fat density (-70/-120 HU) well limited by a very thin capsule located in the left renal compartment between the anterior and posterior leaves of the renal fascia

- Myxoid liposarcomas are made up of abundant mucinous connective tissue and a scant lipoid content; they have an intermediate level of malignancy.
- Pleiomorphous liposarcomas are characterized by a high level of cellular pleiomorphism and reduced lipidic and mucinous components. These tumors show the highest level of malignancy; they undergo rapid development with invasion of the contiguous tissues and metastasis.

The various CT appearances of the liposarcomas reflect their lipidic, mucinous, fibrous and cellular components. Some authors (Waligore et al. 1981; Caprio et al. 1987; Ferrozzi et al. 1990; Kim et al. 1996) have suggested a correlation between CT findings and histological subtypes, according to the predominant attenuation values: fat density (-120/ -80 HU) for the lipogenic form, intermediate and soft tissue attenuation (0/+40) for the myxoid type, and higher values for the pleiomorphous form. Since the aspect of liposarcomas is often not homogeneous, the highest values must be used for their classification.

To classify and evaluate the aggressivity of the liposarcoma the shape of the borders and the contrast enhancement should also be considered. The borders are sharp in the lipogenic liposarcoma and poorly defined in the pleiomorphous type. The contrast enhancement is absent in the lipogenic type, subtle in myxoid liposarcoma, and more intense in the pleiomorphic type.

These tumors show the common aspect of a mass that is often voluminous and can be uni- or multinodular containing fat-density tissue.

- A well differentiated lipogenic liposarcoma (Fig. 12.12, 11.13) has an ovoid form and a homogeneous structure. Its attenuation values are close to those of adipose tissue, even though they are slightly higher than body fat values. It is crossed

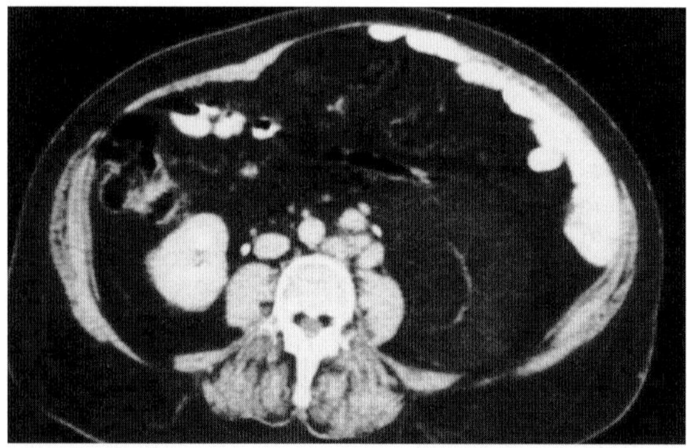
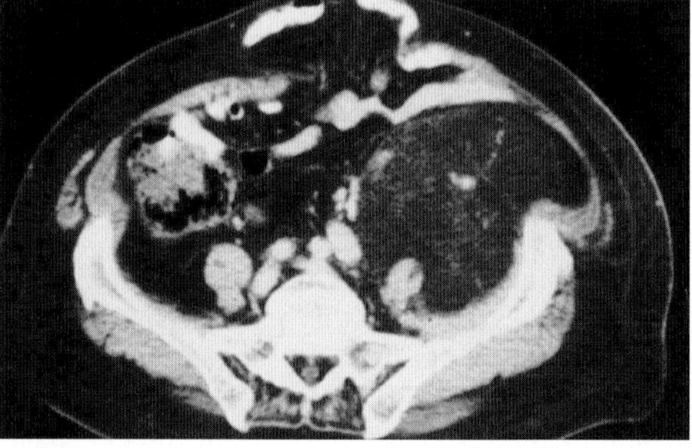

Fig. 12.12A, B. Lipogenic liposarcoma. Ovoid retroperitoneal mass extending in the renal compartment (**A**) and in the iliac fossa (**B**), surrounded by a thin capsule with a very sharp profile. It is characterized by negative attenuation values, which are slightly higher than those of the abdominal fat, and by a disorderly net of thin vessels

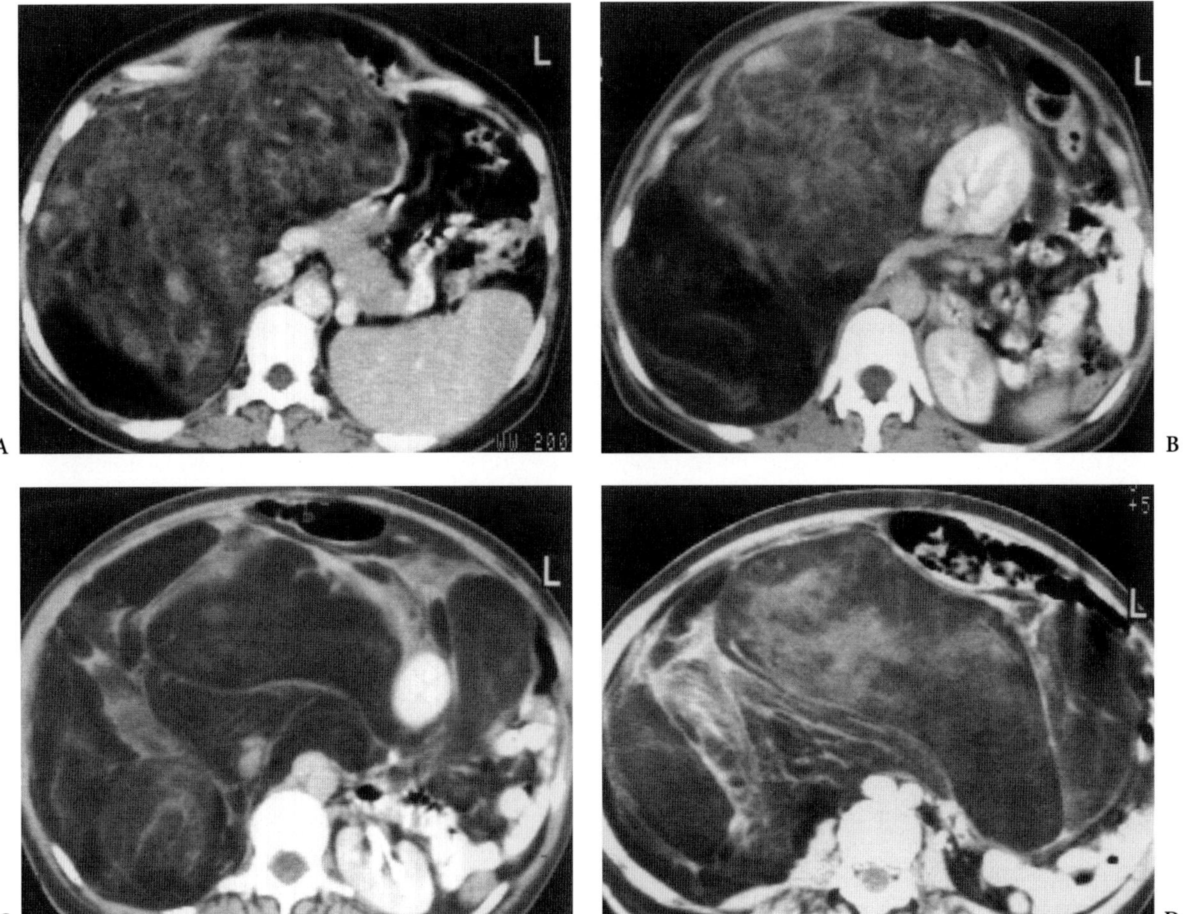

Fig. 12.13A–D. Well-differentiated lipogenic liposarcoma. The mass originates from the right perirenal space and is well limited and roughly lobular. It is constituted by multiple converging structures prevalently made of a fat-density tissue blending with water and soft-tissue attenuation areas and surrounded by a thick capsule. The right kidney and the bowel loops are displaced on the left side

and subdivided into lobules (Fig. 12.13) by a network with reticula varying in width and thickness and is surrounded by a thin capsule. The lipoma-like subtype is the same in appearance and density (equal to that of the mesenteric and retroperitoneal fat) as the lipoma. It is a relatively benign tumor with slow growth, which does not infiltrate and rarely metastasizes (Kim et al. 1996).

- Myxoid liposarcoma (Figs. 12.14, 12.15) appears as a well-defined mass with polycyclic contours and a mixed structure including fat, muscular tissue and parahydric attenuation values. Occasionally it may have a homogeneous cyst-like aspect before contrast injection, and it shows graduated reticular contrast enhancement in the solid components (Kim et al. 1996).
- A pleiomorphous liposarcoma (Figs. 12.16, 12.17) appears as a mass made up of nodules of variable width and density (most of them show elevated attenuation values, with a further significant increment after injection of contrast medium). The contours of the mass are usually indefinite because of their tendency to infiltrate the adjacent tissues.

In CT diagnosis of liposarcomas, electronic measurement of a negative density is a fundamental element in characterization of the tumor, especially when the simultaneous presence of various tissues does not allow immediate visual identification of the adipose component.

In most cases, small transparent areas with the density of fat can be recognized in the mass and allow characterization of the tumor. However, in the types with a prevalent myxomatous component, in the ple-iomorphous forms, and in all the varieties with complex histotype, identification of the pathog-

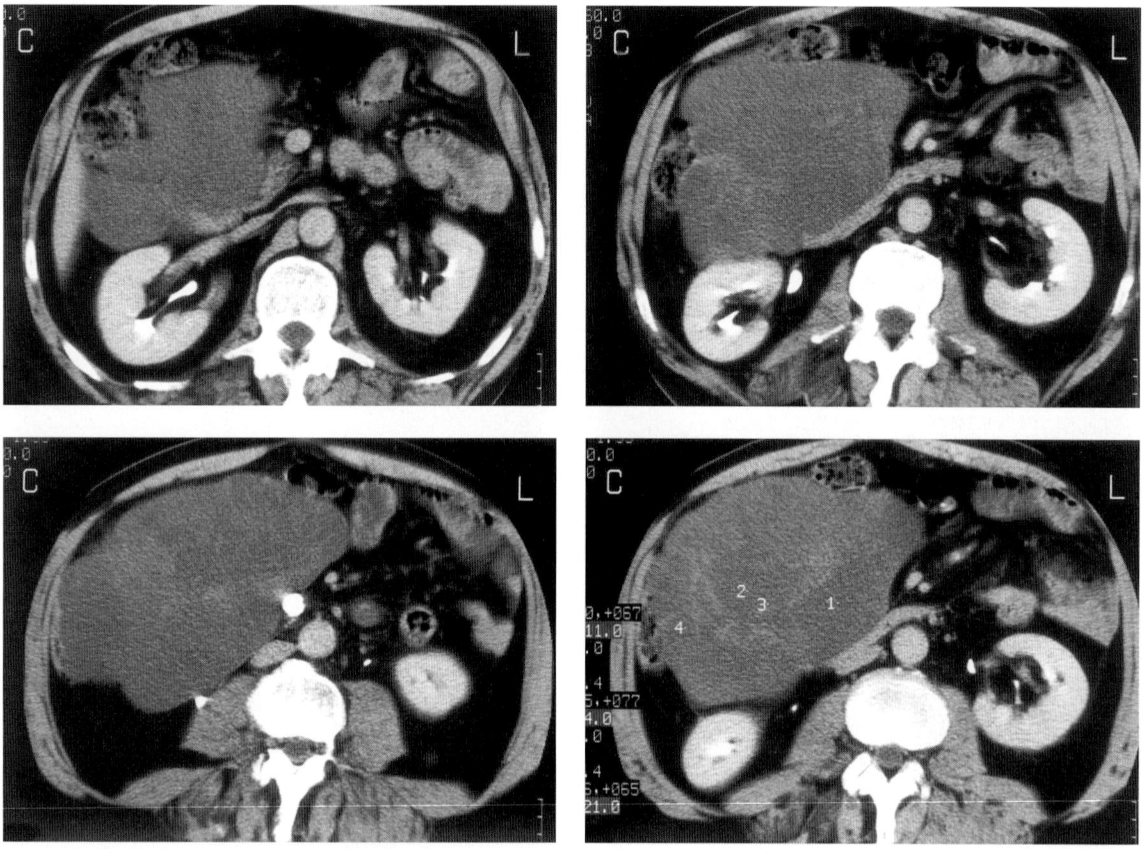

A B

C D

Fig. 12.14A–D. Myxoid liposarcoma. The mass shows an intramesenteric development with myxomatous, near-water-density, fatty areas and denser stromal areas (**D**); it displaces the second duodenal portion and the inferior vena cava (**B**) backwards. The mass adheres closely to the ascending colon and the hepatic colonic flexure, which is pushed laterally and is compressed against the abdominal wall

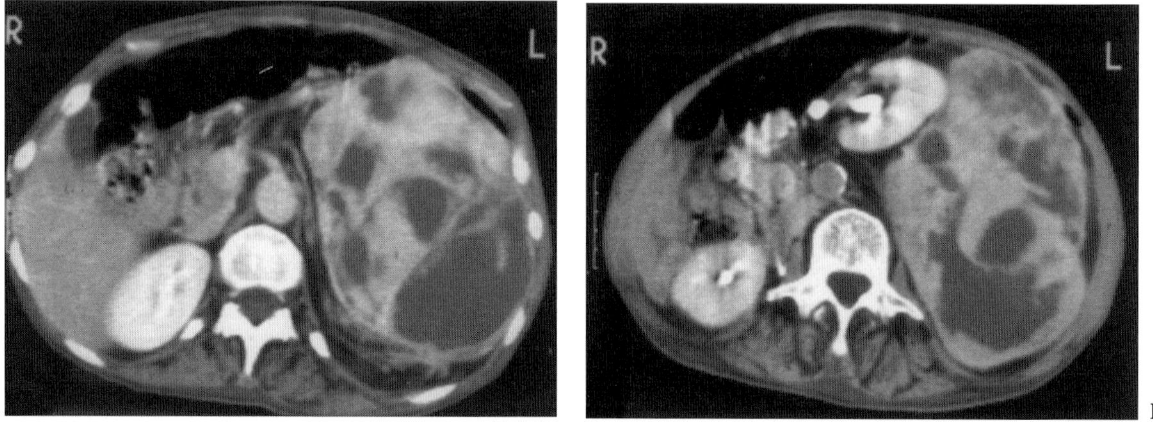

A B

Fig. 12.15A, B. Myxoid liposarcoma with a scarce lipomatous content. Huge mass originating from adipose tissue of the left perirenal compartment and pushing the kidney forward. The neoplasm has a polymorphous aspect with solid and fluid components. The lipomatous component is undetectable at CT, because it is masked by the predominant presence of other tissues and by colliquative-necrotic phenomena

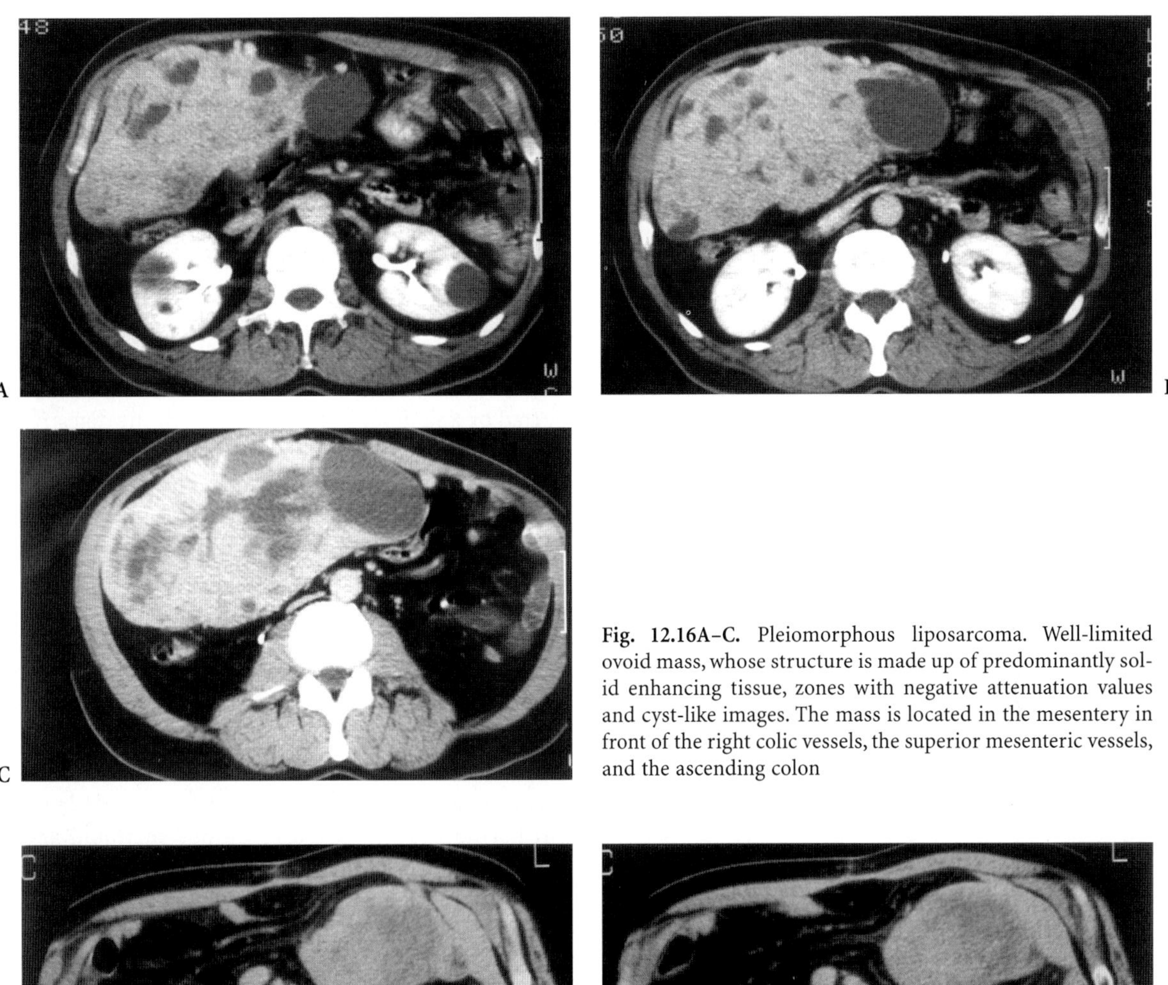

Fig. 12.16A–C. Pleiomorphous liposarcoma. Well-limited ovoid mass, whose structure is made up of predominantly solid enhancing tissue, zones with negative attenuation values and cyst-like images. The mass is located in the mesentery in front of the right colic vessels, the superior mesenteric vessels, and the ascending colon

Fig. 12.17A, B. Pleiomorphous liposarcoma of the mesentery. Well-defined ovoid mesenteric mass located in front of the jejunal vessels. The tumor has a solid structure, with postcontrast enhancement in the periphery and with near-water-density central areas. The adipose component is limited by a small peripheral zone

nomonic negative densities for tissue characterization may sometimes be impossible even with electronic measurements, because of the dominant character of other tissues, the presence of hemorrhagic complications, or necrotic-colliquative regressive phenomena that completely mask the lipomatous component of the tumor. In these cases, CT representation is aspecific and re-sembles that of other tumors of mesenchymal origin.

In contrast, in the well-differentiated forms with a prevalent lipogenic component identification of the adipose nature of the tumor is immediate, but the diagnostic problems encountered are those of the differentiation between benign and malignant forms. In fact, even though in the typically malignant forms the classic parameters of atypia (values higher than those of the subcutaneous fat, areas with tissue density absorbing the contrast medium, absence of a capsule, infiltrating characters, etc.) clarify all the diagnostic problems, in the highly differentiated malignant tumors with homogeneous structure the distinction between a benign and a malignant nature may sometimes, albeit rarely, remain uncertain.

12.4.3 Lipoblastoma

The lipoblastoma is a very rare benign tumor of the embryonal adipose cells, which is typical for infancy and early childhood (90% of cases appear before the third year of life) and preadolescence.

Macroscopically, it is seen in two forms: one is an encapsulated mass (lipoblastoma), while the other is infiltrating, diffuse and multicentric (lipoblastomatosis) (Fisher et al. 1981; Schulman et al. 1992).

Like the other adipose tumors, lipoblastoma and lipoblastomatosis are preferentially located in the limbs, the trunk, the mediastinum and the retroperitoneum. They are rarely observed in the peritoneum and in the mesentery; in fact, only seven cases have been described in the literature (Fisher et al. 1981; Schulman et al. 1992).

Histologically, the lipoblastoma is constituted by lobules of immature adipose tissue separated by thin septa of a highly vascularized fibrous connective tissue surrounding a mass of myxoid tissue.

Clinically, the lipoblastoma is a rapidly growing mass with well-defined limits and a smooth surface; it is mobile and asymptomatic.

On CT examination, a lipoblastoma appears as a mass that is generally voluminous and shows the typical negative density of adipose tissue (–80 HU or lower); it is subdivided by septa, contains denser areas of myxoid tissue, and is peripherally well limited by a thin capsule with a very sharp profile. The density of the mass does not change after contrast medium administration.

According to Friedman et al. (1981), the CT appearance of lipoblastomatosis is similar to that of lipoblastoma, except for the multicentric diffusion.

Generally, in view of the adipose consistency of the tumor and its benign characters (capsule and very sharp, smooth profile) there are no diagnostic problems on CT examination. Furthermore, the age of the patient is a sufficient criterion to exclude a liposarcoma.

12.4.4 Pseudotumoral Lipomatosis

Pseudotumoral lipomatosis is an excessive, localized or diffuse, accumulation of normal adipose tissue among the mesenteric folds in the omentum, frequently associated with a concomitant increase in the amount of adipose tissue in the retroperitoneum or in the pelvis of obese subjects or of patients affected by Cushing's syndrome or being treated with steroids.

Clinically, it may appear as an abdominal mass that resembles a tumor. This suspicion may be supported by a radiological examination of the digestive tract showing displacement, distortion or compression of hollow viscera (stomach pushed forward, enlarged duodenal C-shaped curvature, lowered Treitz's loop, loops of the small intestine separated by nodular structures, thinner and laterally compressed rectum).

Lipomatosis is easily recognizable on CT (Figs. 12.18, 12.19) because of the characteristic negative density of the pseudomasses of adipose tissue that push forward the ileal loops, making impressions in them that divide them, and surround the superior mesenteric vessels at the mesenteric level. Furthermore, at the pelvic level they surround and narrow the sigmoid (Fig. 12.18) and the rectum.

In the omental locations, the adipose tissue extends in an arcuate orientation in front of the colon and the ileal loops, which are detached from the anterior abdominal wall; within the mass, the punctiform images of the omental vessels stand out (Fig. 12.19).

12.4.5 Infiltrating Lipomatosis

Infiltrating lipomatosis is a rare disease characterized by diffuse proliferation of normal adipose tissue that has the tendency to infiltrate tissues progressively, even though it is histologically benign; therefore, it constitutes a potential threat to life. It resembles pseudotumoral lipomatosis except for the tendency to infiltrate and involve the organs instead of simply displacing them. After surgical excision, it tends to relapse (Waligore et al. 1981).

CT shows a focal accumulation (pseudomass) of homogeneous adipose tissue subdivided by septa that displaces, compresses, deforms and infiltrates the abdominal structures; its density does not increase after contrast medium administration.

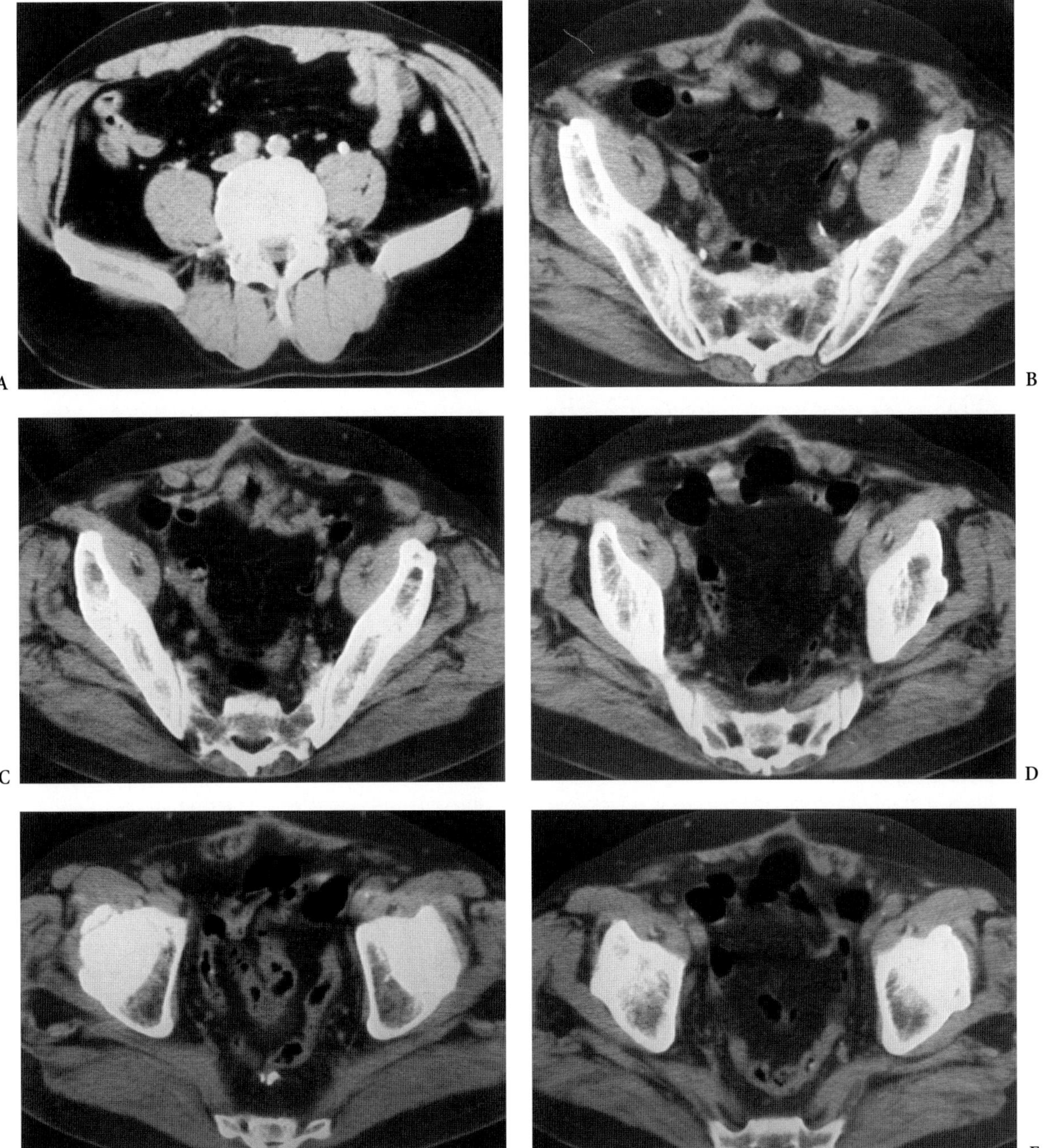

Fig. 12.18A–F. Pseudotumoral lipomatosis of the mesentery and the sigmoid mesocolon. Accumulation of adipose tissue in the mesentery and in the sigmoid mesocolon, compressing and dividing the ileal loops and pushing the sigmoid downward. Typical characters are represented by the negative attenuation of the adipose tissue, the regular distribution of the mesenteric and sigmoidal vessels (even though they are separated) and the marks on the ileal loops without signs of infiltration

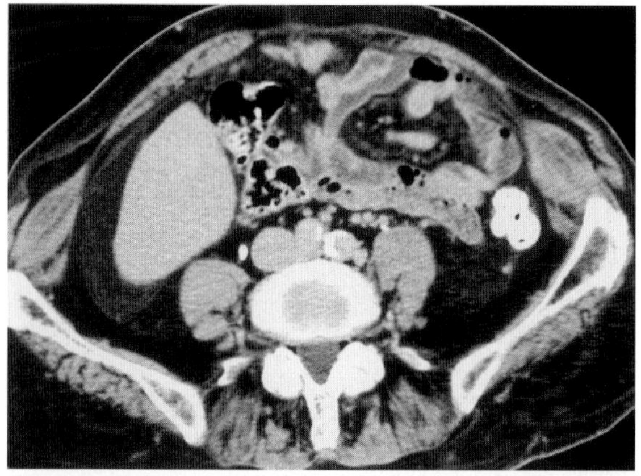
A

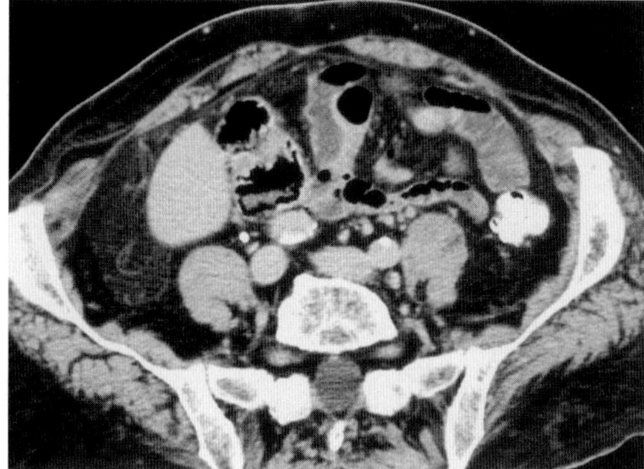
B

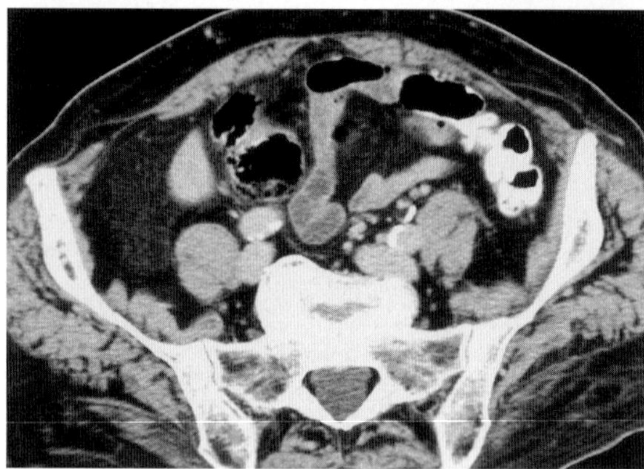
C

Fig. 12.19A–C. Omental lipomatosis. Greatly developed omental adipose tissue slightly increased in density on the right side, with thin strands and small vascular spots inside

12.5 Smooth Muscle Tissue

12.5.1 Leiomyoma

The leiomyoma is a benign tumor of smooth muscle fibers, most frequently arising from the walls of the alimentary tract, particularly the stomach, and occasionally from the peritoneum, the mesentery, and the omentum.

Macroscopically, the leiomyoma generally appears as a voluminous well-encapsulated solid mass constituted by muscular tissue and collagen, with a lobulated smooth surface.

Clinically, it becomes evident only when it reaches conspicuous dimensions with vague abdominal pains or intestinal hemorrhage.

CT usually shows a solid spherical or ovoid mass with a sharp profile, homogeneous structure and uniform density both before and after contrast medium injection.

However, there is sometimes a wide central area of necrosis in a leiomyoma, whose attenuation is similar to that observed in the sarcomatous forms (Fig. 12.20). This phenomenon is probably attributable to the reduced central vascularization of the largest tumors.

12.5.2 Disseminated Peritoneal Leiomyomatosis

Disseminated peritoneal leiomyomatosis is a very rare disease exclusively observed in women in the late part of the reproductive period who have had previous pregnancies and have taken oral contraceptives for long periods. It is characterized by the development of numerous nodules of normal smooth muscular tissue spread over the entire peritoneal cavity.

It is thought to originate from metaplasia of the submesothelial multipotent mesenchymal cells after excessive endogenous and/or exogenous stimulation with female gonadal steroids, particularly estrogens and progesterone. Disseminated peritoneal leiomyomatosis is generally benign, but it does sometimes degenerate.

The CT aspect is characterized by numerous small solid nodules, with a homogeneous structure and

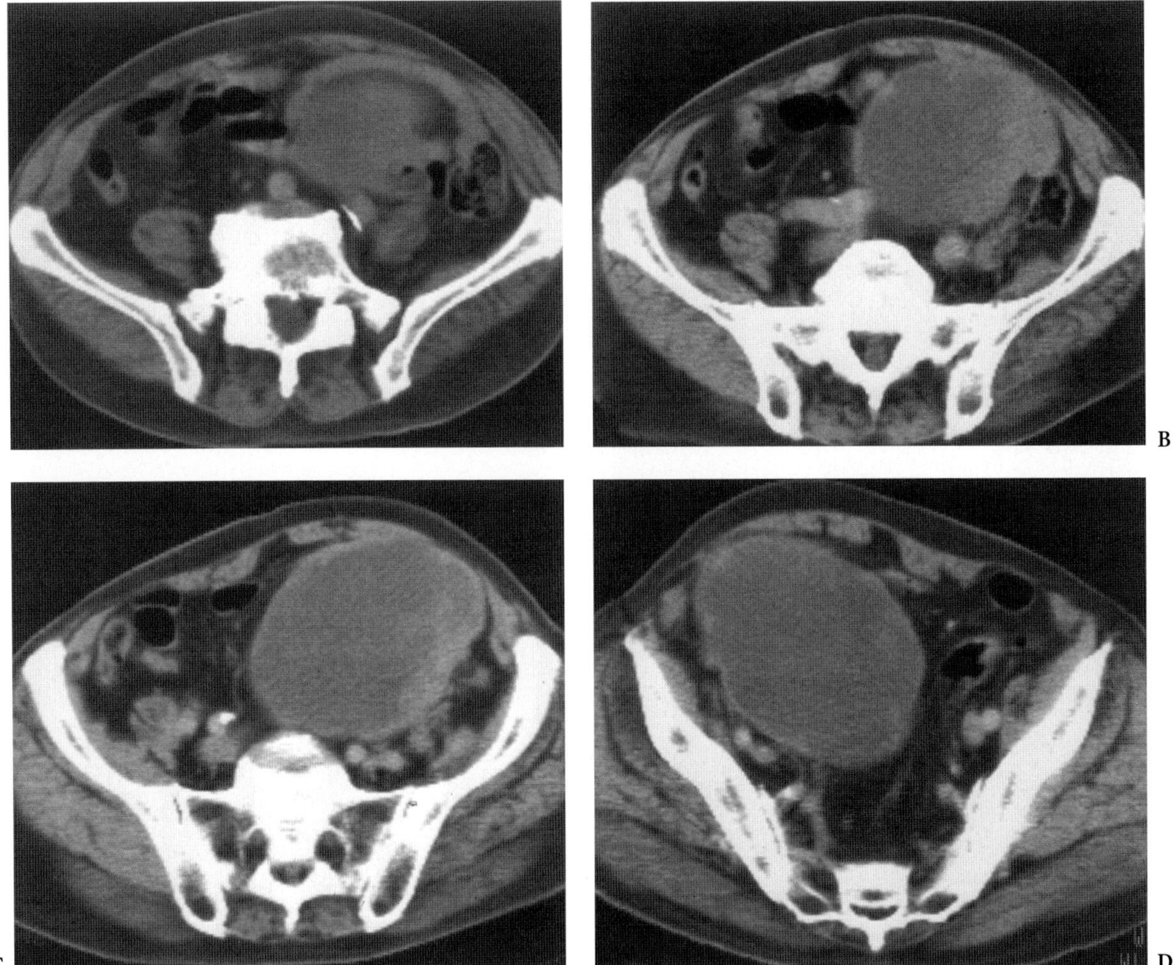

Fig. 12.20A–D. Mesenteric leiomyoma. Large well-defined ovoid mass in the right iliac fossa. It is peripherally solid, showing a contrast-enhancing wall and a wide hypodense central necrotic area

smooth profile, which are spread throughout the omentum and in the parietal and visceral peritoneum and which become uniformly opaque after injection of contrast medium.

12.5.3 Leiomyosarcoma and Leiomyosarcomatosis

Leiomyosarcoma is a malignant tumor of the smooth muscular tissue that originates predominantly from the digestive tube (in 90% of cases from the stomach) and occasionally from the uterus, ovaries, retroperitoneum, subperitoneal structures, peritoneum, and omentum. At the intestinal level, the neoplasm is characterized by exophytic growth in the adipose cellular tissue of the ligaments, which detaches and parts the peritoneal leaflets. It also has a characteristic tendency to develop masses that are sometimes conspicuous and often contain wide necrotic areas with a cyst-like appearance. In the course of its extension, the leiomyosarcoma may penetrate the peritoneum, spreading over the cavity (leiomyosarcomatosis) as happens in the case of carcinosis; leiomyosarcomatosis is differentiated from this latter disease by the development of single or multiple nodules with the characteristic central hypodense area and by the absence of ascites.

Furthermore, leiomyosarcoma frequently metastasizes to the liver via the hematic pathway (75% of cases); its localizations are also characterized by central necrosis and by the tendency to grow rapidly and to become voluminous. In contrast, it does not spread via the lymphatic pathway and thus does not produce lymph node metastases.

Two properties that are peculiar to peritoneal and mesenteric leiomyosarcomas are their manner of

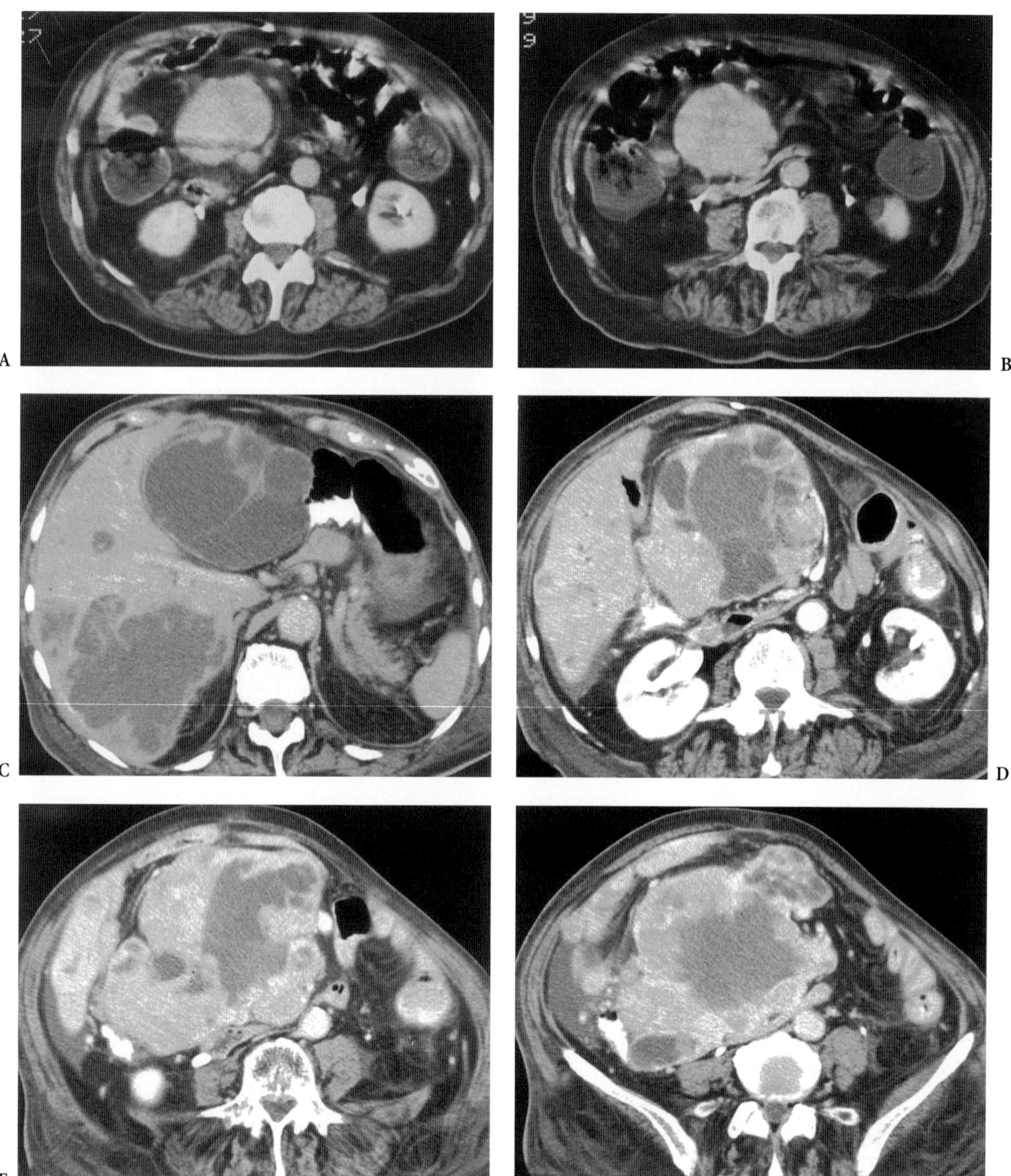

Fig. 12.21A–F. Mesenteric leiomyosarcoma. **A, B** Solid mass with a well-defined profile and a homogeneous structure resembling that of a leiomyoma in the transparency of the mesentery, without direct relationships with the intestinal loops. **C–F** Evolution of the neoplasm. After 16 months: typical aspect of the leiomyosarcoma: bosselated, solid and striking contrast enhancing mass that contains wide cyst-like areas .It widely occupies the central part of the abdominal cavity between the stomach and the liver at a high level (**C**); at a low level, it extends up to the border with the pelvis (**F**). Concomitant ascites (**E, F**) and hepatic metastases, which show the same structure as the primary neoplasm (**C**). The mesenteric planes in front of the pancreas, the duodenum, the mesenteric vessels and the retroperitoneal fat are preserved

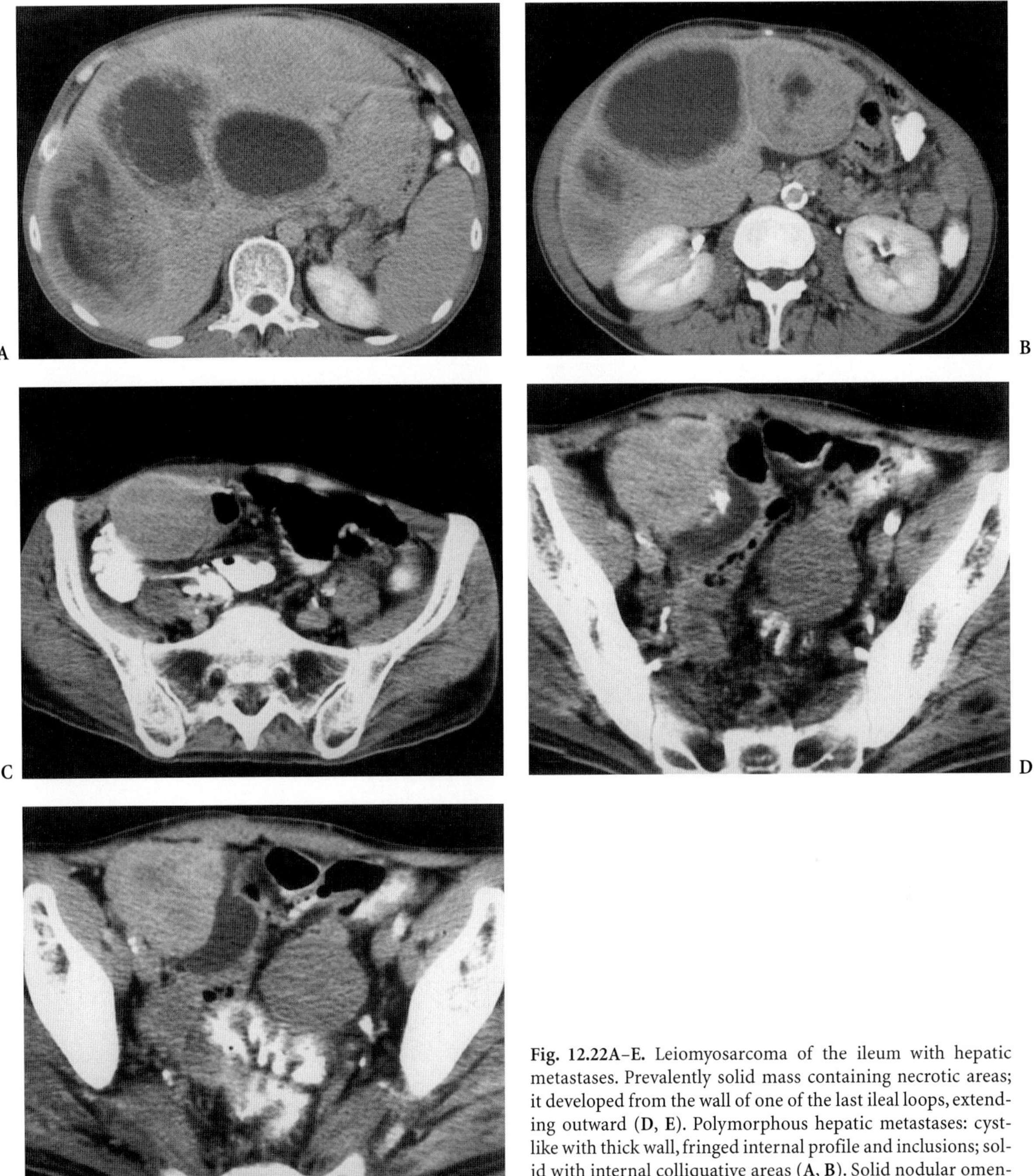

Fig. 12.22A–E. Leiomyosarcoma of the ileum with hepatic metastases. Prevalently solid mass containing necrotic areas; it developed from the wall of one of the last ileal loops, extending outward (**D, E**). Polymorphous hepatic metastases: cyst-like with thick wall, fringed internal profile and inclusions; solid with internal colliquative areas (**A, B**). Solid nodular omental (**C**) and mesosigmoidal (**D, E**) metastases

growing without infiltrating the adjacent tissues and their displacement of only the intestinal loops.

The primary tumor (Figs. 12.21–12.23) shows the characteristic CT aspect of a mass that is mostly voluminous (diameter >5 cm) and solid with central areas of low attenuation. Their aspect is partly cyst-like and partly irregular, resembling a "geographic map." The tumoral mass always has a sharp external profile, even though it is sometimes curled and bosselated; after contrast medium administration the density of the solid component increases rapidly and intensely.

Leiomyosarcomas originating from the stomach and from the ileum involve the intestinal wall only marginally, because they extend predominantly outward, tending to displace the contiguous viscera

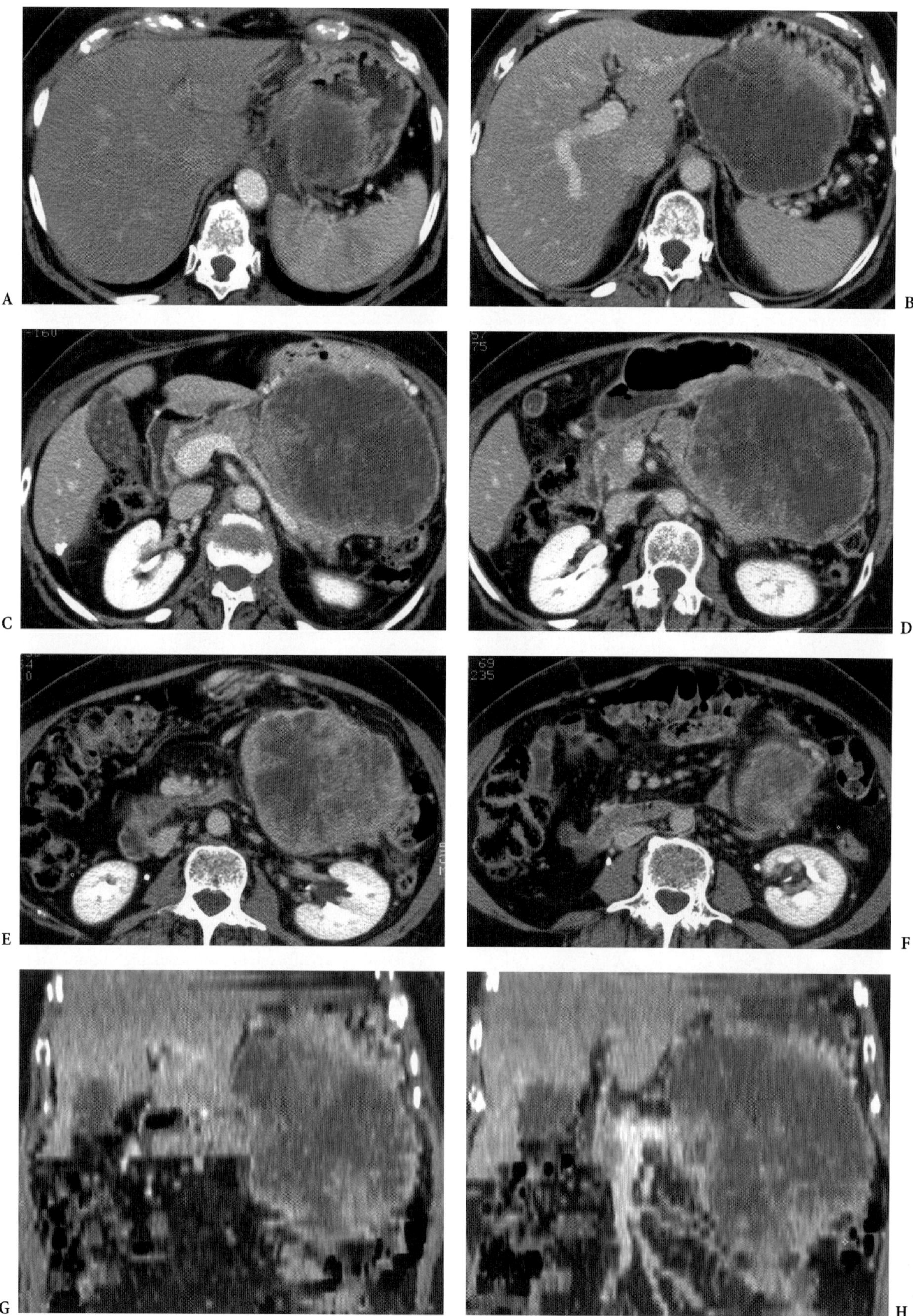

Fig. 12.23A–J

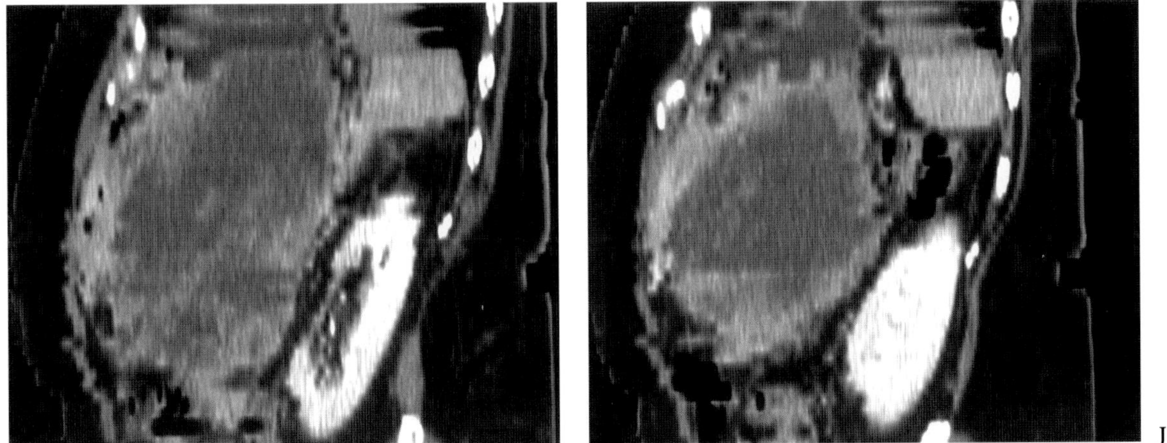

Fig. 12.23A–J. Gastric leiomyosarcoma. Huge ovoid mass, characterized by a solid peripheral component that is irregularly thick and appears hyperdense after contrast, and a wide central necrotic-hemorrhagic area. It is located in the lesser sac in front of the pancreas and the splenic vessels in close contacts with the posterior gastric wall. **G, H** Coronal reconstructions; **I, J** sagittal reconstructions

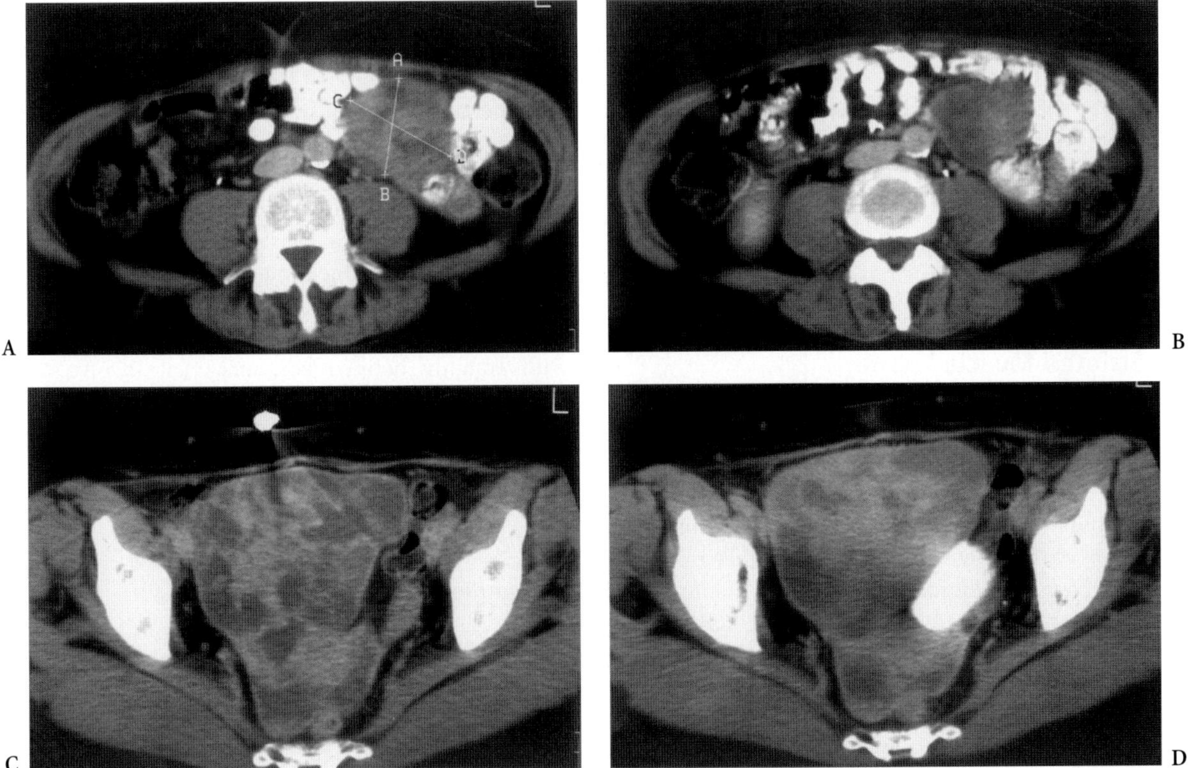

Fig. 12.24A–D. Abdominopelvic peritoneal leiomyosarcomatosis. Masses with a sharp profile and a mixed structure (solid with wide cyst-like hypodense areas), limited by a thin dense capsule. The mesenteric mass is limited by the ileal loops at the sides and by the retroperitoneal adipose tissue at the back (**A, B**), whereas the pelvic mass (**C, D**) displaces the sigmoid and the vesical dome toward the left side. At this level, the peritoneal location of the neoplasm is recognizable by its disposition in the supravesical space, in the right paravesical recess and in the pouch of Douglas, limited all around by the thin line of the peritoneum and surrounded by the transparency of the extraperitoneal adipose cellular

without infiltrating them. The intestinal origin of these neoplasms is shown by their close relationship with the visceral walls, even though (conversely) these may be secondarily involved by a tumor originating from the mesentery or the peritoneum. In fact, the extraintestinal origin may be recognized only when the tumor is small dimensions and is not linked with the adjacent intestinal walls, from which it is separated by adipose tissue, except in being sited adjacent to them.

Even though a nonhomogeneous appearance with central necrotic areas is generally characteristic of malignant types, it cannot always be stated that benign tumors correspond to neoplasms with pre- and postcontrast homogeneity of structure.

According to CHOI et al (1990), the level of malignancy of peritoneal leiomyosarcomas can be correlated with the central attenuation value of the tumoral mass: it is low when there are no hypodense areas and high in the presence of wide hypodense areas. Our personal opinion is at odds with this theory, because in our patients we have observed highly malignant peritoneal leiomyosarcomas with homogeneous aspects (Fig. 12.21) and benign forms (leiomyomas) with wide hypodense central areas of necrosis (Fig. 12.20).

CT shows the peritoneal dissemination of the leiomyosarcoma (leiomyosarcomatosis) (Fig. 12.24) as multiple nodules or masses with well-delimited central hypodense areas that look like primary neoplasms.

12.6 Striated Muscle Tissue

12.6.1 Rhabdomyosarcoma

Rhabdomyosarcoma is a rather rare malignant tumor of the striated muscular tissue that grows rapidly. Four histological types can be distinguished: pleiomorphous, embryonal, botryoid and alveolar; however, only the alveolar form sometimes localizes at abdominal level.

Like all other sarcomas of the soft tissues, rhabdomyosarcoma has the macroscopic appearance of a mass that is very variable in size, consistency and presence of invasive characters and necrotic areas; the mass is surrounded by a pseudocapsule made up of an increased density of the most external layers of tumoral cells, which tend to infiltrate the adjacent tissues.

CT (Fig. 12.25) shows a cyst-like ovoid mass limited by a thick capsule, from which multinodular vegetations and thin shoots project inward; after contrast medium these structures become hyperdense, whereas the density of the liquid component does not change.

During childhood, rhabdomyosarcoma spreads solid masses or nodules widely over the peritoneum; these structures become hyperdense after contrast medium. They show pseudomyxomatous aspects and are associated with ascites and an omental plaque (CHUNG et al. 1998).

12.7 Blood Vessels

12.7.1 Hemangioendothelioma

Hemangioendothelioma is a rare tumor originating from the endothelial cells of the capillaries and is usually observed in the skin and in soft tissues. It can be benign or malignant. It is formed by a rich and active proliferation of capillaries covered by endothelial cells and by perivascular cords and rather voluminous accumulations of fusiform, round or ovoid cells. It is an expansive tumor and grows slowly. In exceptional cases it can be found at the peritoneal and omental level: only one case of malignant hemangioendothelioma studied by CT (SHIN-LIN et al. 1995) has been reported in the literature; it is described as multiple converging nodular lesions, with roughly defined contours, that involve the omentum and are characterized by intense and homogeneous contrast enhancement; these features suggest vascular lesions.

12.7.2 Hemangiopericytoma

Hemangiopericytoma is a rare tumor that arises from the contractile cells (Zinnerman's pericytes) surrounding the capillary and postcapillary venules. It is often observed in the limbs, the retroperitoneum, the uterus, the mediastinum and the rhinopharynx; in exceptional cases it is found in the omentum (BERTOLOTTO et al. 1996).

Hemangiopericytoma has the macroscopic appearance of a pseudoencapsulated bosselated mass; it is generally very voluminous at the time of

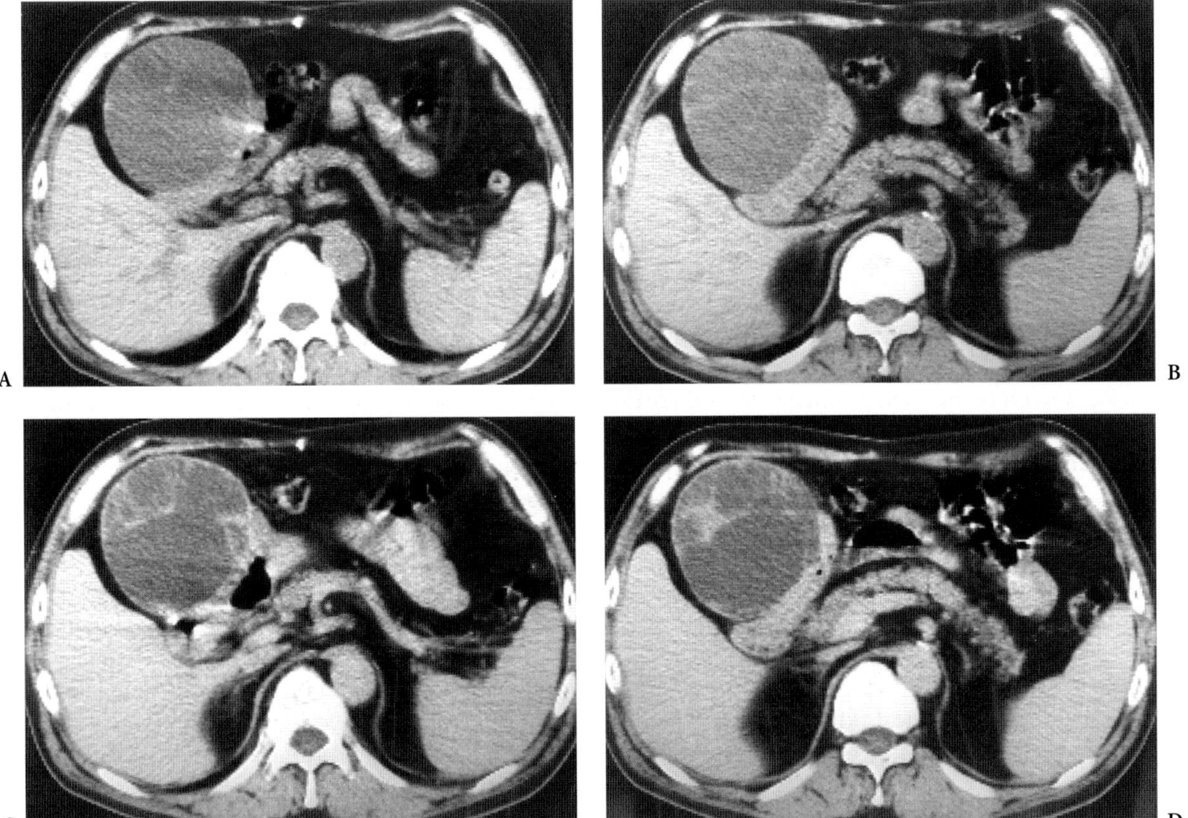

Fig. 12.25A–D. Alveolar rhabdomyosarcoma. Intraligamental cyst-like formation limited by a thick capsule, with thin septations and small nodule inside (**A**, **B**), the capsule becoming hyperdense after i.v. contrast medium injection (**C**, **D**)

its discovery and contains wide necrotic-hemorrhagic areas. It is richly vascularized and easily bleeds. At the abdominal level, the hemangiopericytoma tends to displace the intestinal loops, but it sometimes infiltrates them after adhesion.

Histologically, it is made up of dense perivascular cells that are round, fusiform or polygonal and have different dimensions, embedded in layers of collagen of variable thickness.

Even after histological examinations, it is impossible to establish whether the hemangiopericytoma is benign or malignant. The presence of pulmonary or osteal metastases and the frequent relapse after excision are the only signs definitely indicating malignancy (Goldman et al. 1988; Bertolotto et al. 1996).

Usually hemangiopericytomas are asymptomatic, and only in a late phase do they sometimes cause compressive symptoms or invade the adjacent organs.

CT shows this tumor as a mass that is generally already voluminous. It has well-defined contours and a solid structure with cyst-like areas and nonconstant speckled calcifications inside. The fact that the solid areas become hyperopaque after contrast is the most distinctive feature of this tumor.

From a diagnostic point of view, hemangiopericytoma must be differentiated from the other hypervascularized tumors, such as hemangioendothelioma, carcinoid and Kaposi's sarcoma. The hemangiopericytoma has a homogeneous structure without cyst-like areas or spicular calcifications inside, while the carcinoid has radiate contours and typical clinical manifestations and Kaposi's sarcoma is present most frequently in patients with AIDS.

12.7.3 Kaposi's Sarcoma

Kaposi's sarcoma is a malignant tumor with a vascular structure, which is generally located in the hand or foot. It slowly extends to the mucosa of the digestive tract and to the mesenteric lymph nodes. The pathogenesis of the disease is unknown; in the past it was uncommon, whereas it is now most frequently observed in the advanced phases of AIDS.

From a structural point of view, it consists of multiple purpuric granulomatous nodules with an angiomatous character, which are made of newly formed capillaries, dilated vessels and plaques and contain atypical immature cells of variable shape and hyperchromic nuclei.

On abdominal CT, the tumoral lesions are characterized by elevated postcontrast hyperdensity at the level of both the small mesenteric lymph nodes and the parenchymas.

When patients know to have AIDS show these typical focal hyperdense manifestations, the presence of this sarcoma must be assumed.

12.8 Lymphatic Tissue

12.8.1 Hodgkin's and Non-Hodgkin's Lymphoma

Lymphomas are malignant neoplasms arising from cells of the lymphoid tissue. They are classified into two forms: non-Hodgkin's lymphoma (NHL) and Hodgkin's lymphoma (Hodgkin's disease; HD), which have a common origin but show different clinical, biological and evolutive characters and different localizations.

In fact, HD preferentially affects the mediastinal lymph nodes (65–70% of cases), grows in contiguous sites and has better chances of healing (76%).

NHL has a multifocal origin, with statistically significant localizations at the abdominal level that are both lymph nodal (retro- and subperitoneal) and extra-lymph nodal (spleen, liver, kidneys, bowel and pancreas); it tends to invade and infiltrate the perinodal tissues, the peritoneum, the subperitoneal spaces and the fasciae.

CT has an important primary role in the discovery of the nodal and extranodal lymphomatous localizations, in staging of the disease, in evaluation of the effects of the therapy and in the follow-up carried out to detect early signs of any relapse of the disease.

CT appearances. This description will be limited to the primary intestinal lymphomatous alterations, the celiacomesenteric lymph nodal localizations, the infiltrations of the peritoneum, the subperitoneal cellular tissue of the mesenteries, the ligaments and the fasciae, and the localizations in the retroperitoneum and in the parenchymatous organs are excluded because these topics are beyond the scope of this text.

The intestinal localizations usually produce a conspicuous circumferential and uniform thickening of the walls around a lumen that is expanded in most cases, and rarely narrowed (Fig. 12.26–12.29). I this, these tumors differ from carcinomas and Crohn's disease, in which the wall is irregularly thickened and the lumen is narrowed.

Less frequently, an intestinal lymphoma appears as a solid, homogeneous, bosselated spherical mass with a sharp profile that is enclosing or compressing one or more intestinal loops without narrowing the lumen (Fig. 12.32).

The lymph nodes affected by the lymphoma appear as small roundish nodular masses, in most cases multiple; they have a diameter greater than 2 cm and are homogeneous with sharp contours. Generally, these structures are well distinguishable from each other along the lymphatic pathways (Figs. 12.27, 12.30, 12.32) or they appear as a single spherical mass owing to the fusion of more lymph nodes (Figs. 12.27, 12.32, 12.34); finally, they may form conglomerates that largely occupy the subperitoneal spaces instead of adipose tissue and extend on the sides of the vessels that they enclose (Figs. 12.31–12.33).

At the mesenteric level, the lymph nodes show a characteristic "sandwich"-like disposition in front and behind the vascular axis (Figs. 12.26, 12.30, 12.32, 12.35); at the back, a transparent cleavage plane constituted by the anterior pararenal adipose tissue is always present and separates the mesenteric from the lumboaortic lymph nodes.

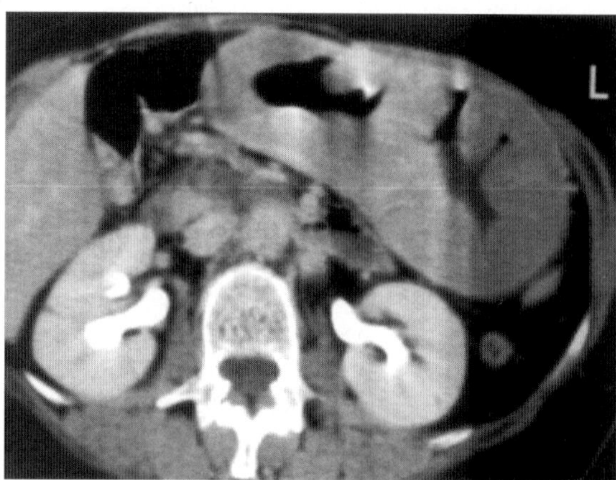

Fig. 12.26. Gastric non-Hodgkin's lymphoma. Wall of the stomach markedly and widely thickening, with very sharp external profile and normal perigastric fat

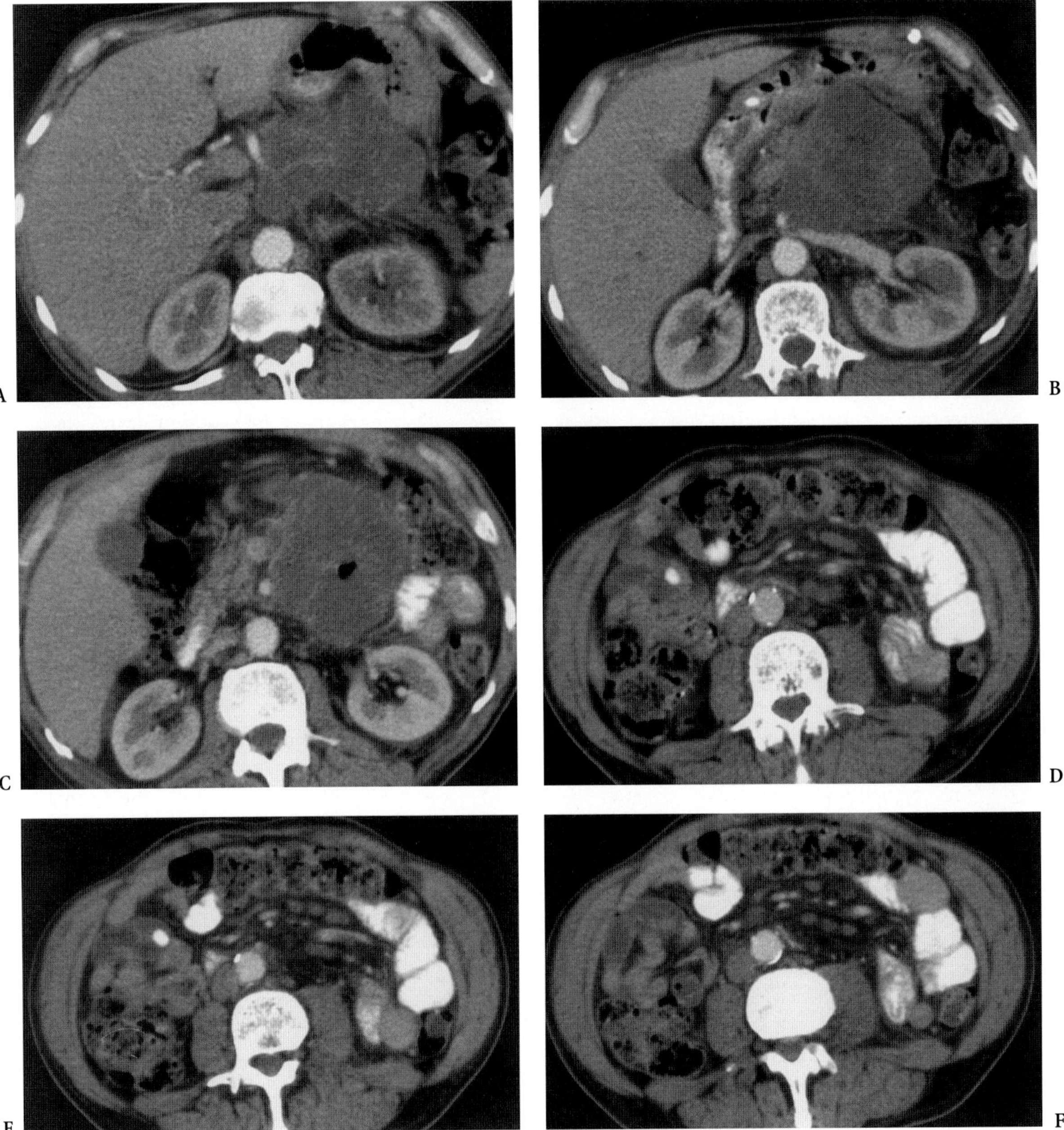

Fig. 12.27A–F. Duodenojejunal non-Hodgkin's lymphoma with celiaco-mesenteric lymph nodal involvement. The intestinal lymphomatous mass constitutes a thick ring around the visceral lumen (**C**). The celiac and splenopancreatic lymph nodes are enlarged and blended, constituting a unique mass that includes the homonymous vessels (**A**, **B**). In the underlying planes, the enlarged lymph nodes extend in a "sandwich"-like shape in the front and behind the superior mesenteric vessels and their jejunoileal branches (**D–F**). Two additional enlarged isolate lymph nodes are located along the extension of the left colic vessels (**E**, **F**) and in the omentum (**F**)

Both isolated and conglomerate lymph nodes have attenuation values equal to those of the muscular tissue (40–60 HU) and increasing slightly after contrast medium in most cases (+20 HU). After chemotherapy, rare calcifications and colliquative areas are observed.

In contrast to other pathologies affecting lymph nodes, infiltration of the structures next to the subperitoneal lymph nodal localizations is frequently observed; it is characterized by thickening, sometimes marked, of the peritoneum (Figs. 12.29, 12.30, 12.32, 12.34, 12.35) and the lateroconal and anterior

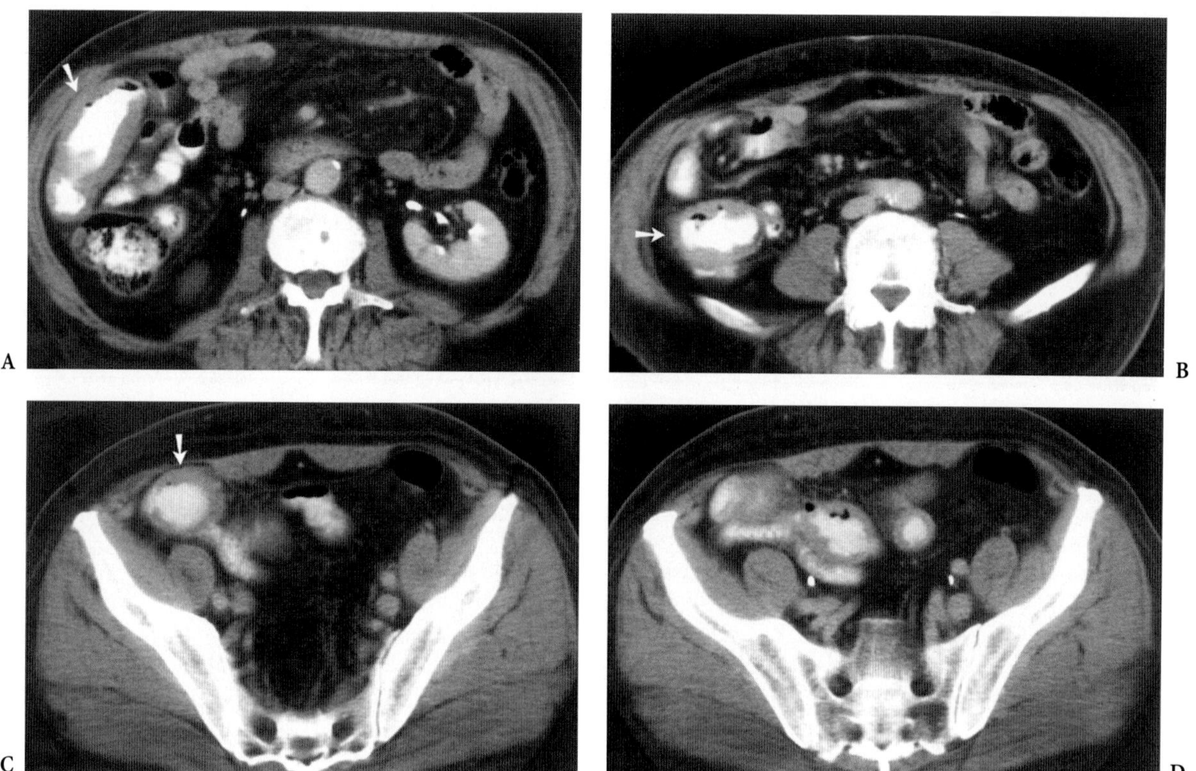

Fig. 12.28A–D. Ileal non-Hodgkin's lymphoma. Uniform thickening of the ileal wall with distension of the lumen (*arrows*)

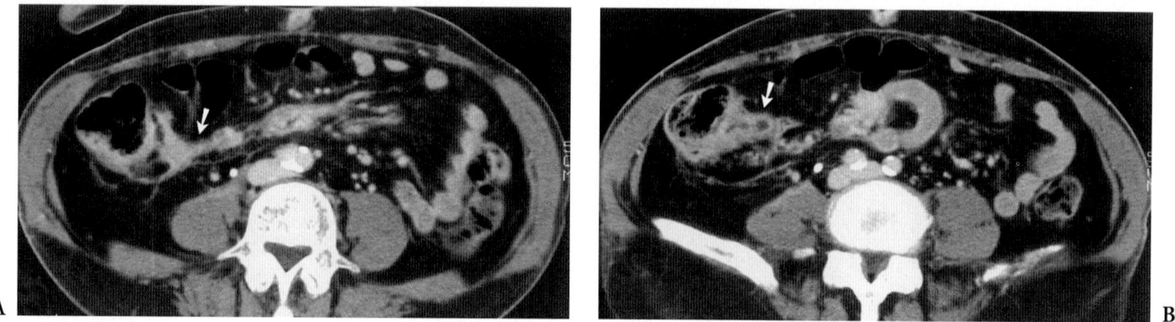

Fig. 12.29A, B. Distal ileal non-Hodgkin's lymphoma with mesenteric infiltration. Thickening of the wall of the last ileal loop (*arrows*), the ileocolic perivascular cellular and the adjacent posterior peritoneum

Fig. 12.31A,B. Non-Hodgkin's lymphoma. Characteristic "sandwich"-like aspect of the enlarged mesenteric lymph nodes in front and behind the homonymous vessels ▷

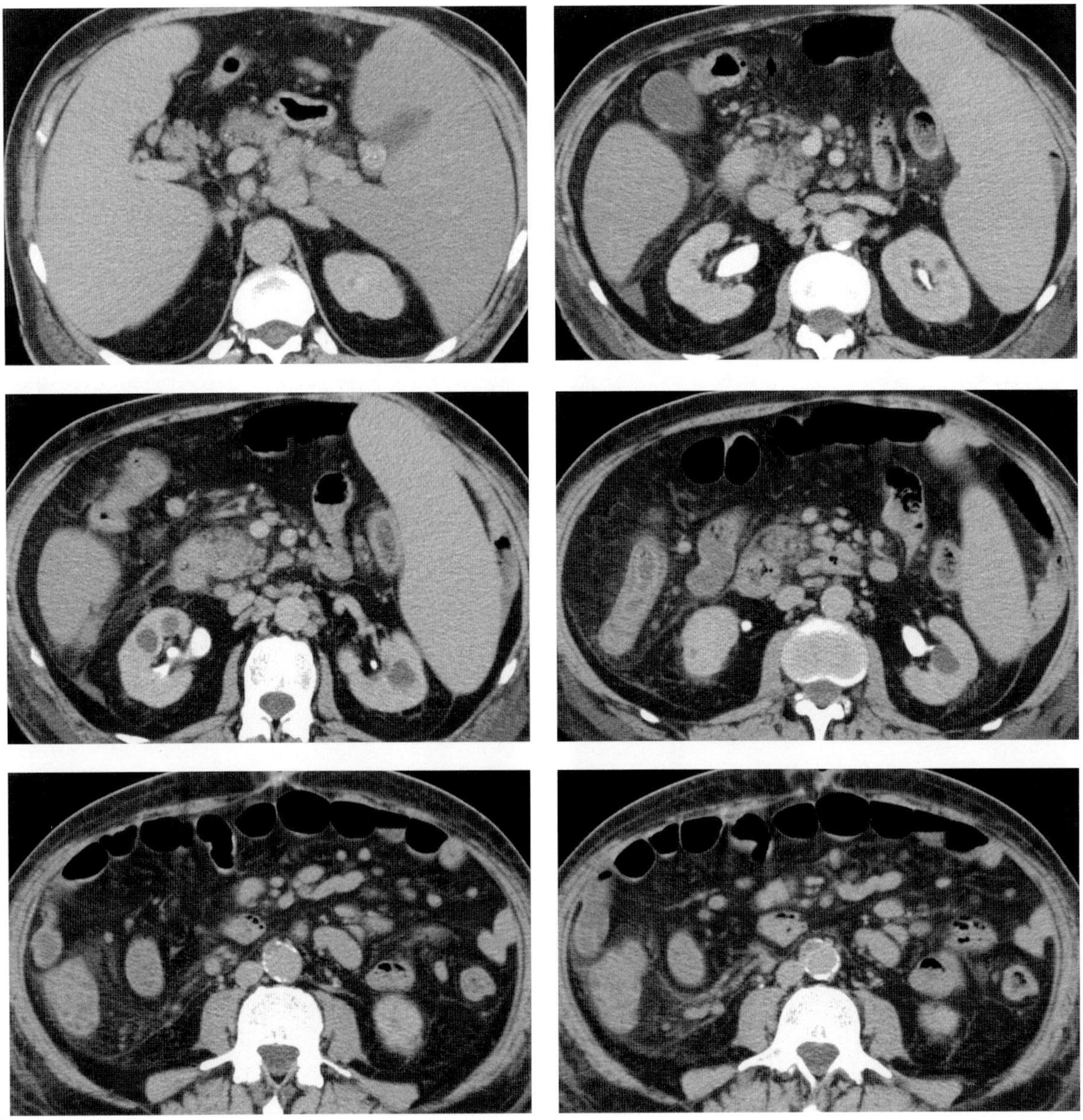

A B

C D

E F

Fig. 12.30A–F. Non-Hodgkin's lymphoma. Nonconverging, enlarged lymph nodes. Involvement of almost all the supramesocolic [hepatic (**A**), splenic (**A**), pancreaticoduodenal (**B**), pancreatic (**C**), celiac (**A**)], intra- and submesocolic [superior mesenteric (**B–D**), jejunal (**D**), ileal (**E**, **F**) and left colic (**F**)) lymph nodes. Infiltration of the peritoneum, the anterior renal and lateroconal fasciae on the right side (**B**-F), the transverse mesocolon and the mesentery (D-F). Splenomegaly

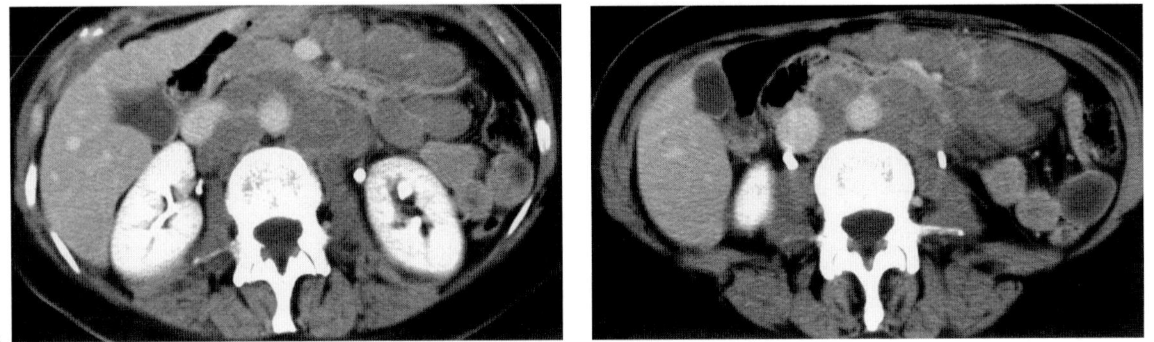

A B

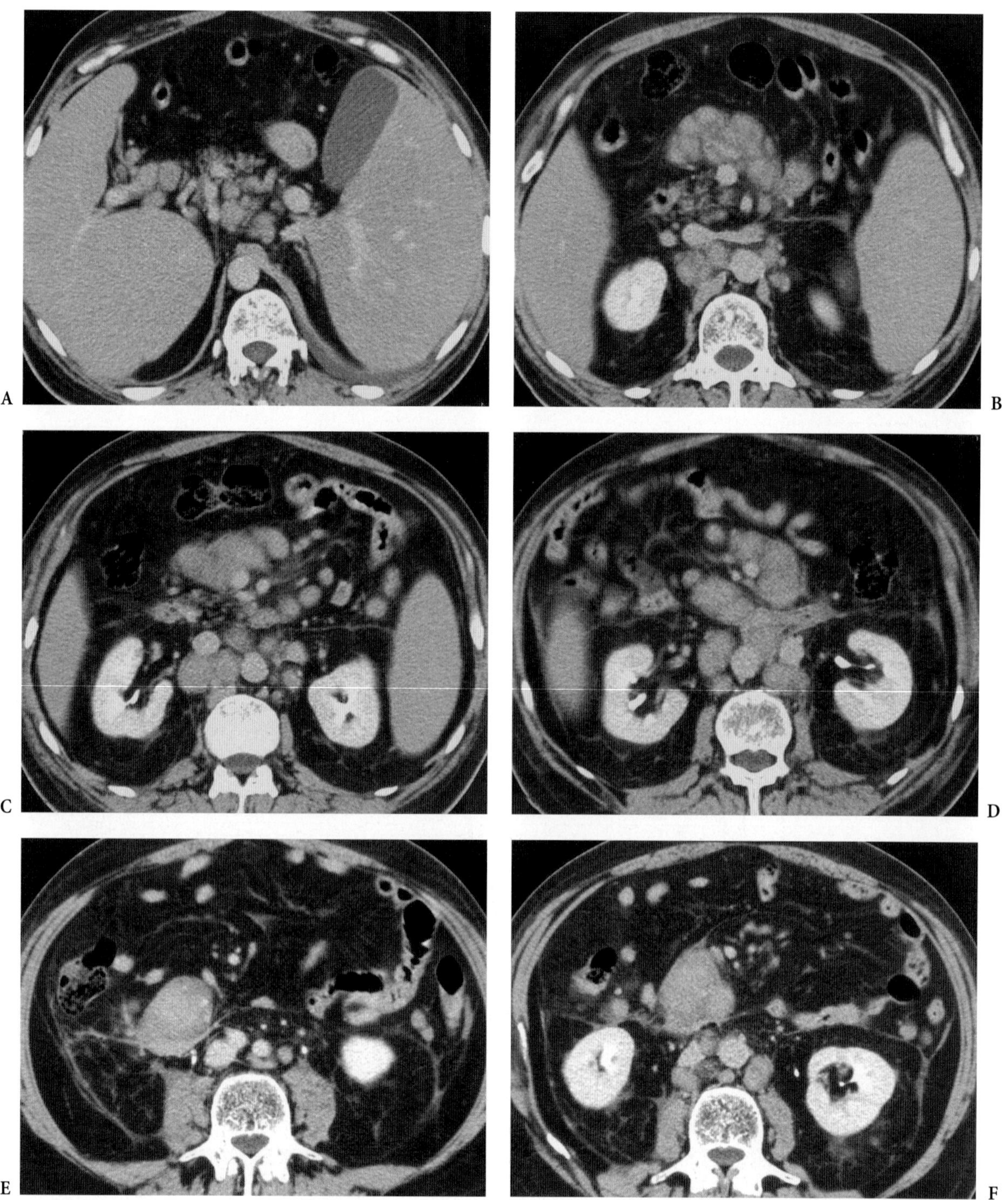

Fig. 12.32A–J. Non-Hodgkin's lymphoma. Besides splenomegaly and retroperitoneal lymphadenomegaly, mesenteric lymph nodal polylocalization can be observed, characterized by isolate adenomegalies and converging in large masses. Voluminous lymph nodal and intestinal mass including and compressing the ileocecal region (**G, H**). Around the mass, the adipose cellular is shaded and the peritoneum is thickening with intracavitary fluid (J ▷

renal fasciae (Figs. 12.30, 12.35), and by an increased density of the subperitoneal cellular tissue (Figs. 12.32, 12.35). The peritoneal involvement may cause ascites (Fig. 12.32, 12.34).

Sometimes, the mesenteric lymph nodal masses cause a block of the circulation in the lymphatics flowing from the intestinal walls with consequent dilatation of the afferent collectors, which are seen on CT as dense serpiginous lines within the mesenteric and omental cellular (Fig. 12.33).

When the therapy is successful, the lymph nodes and the lymphomatous areas (Fig. 12.36) progressively decrease in size to less than 1 cm or disappear. During treatment, a hypodense colliquative area may develop in the central part of the lymph nodes.

The residual lymph nodes may show a median-high density, particularly after radiotherapy.

Sometimes, lymph nodes or masses with diameters greater than 1 cm may persist after treatment, raising diagnostic and therapeutic problems about the persistence of the disease, which may be clarified by a CT-guided needle biopsy. However, since biopsies are not easily performed, because lymph nodes contained into the ligaments are mobile, and the results of the biopsy are reliable only when they are positive (negative results always raise the suspicion that the active area of the lesion has not been examined), CT monitoring is often needed to evaluate the persistence of the disease. When no changes are observed for longer than 6 months, a pathological significance may be excluded, especially in the absence of clinical and biological manifestations.

Of course, CT monitoring makes it possible to detect enlargements of lymph nodes or peritoneal and/or subperitoneal infiltrations in the case of relapse of the disease.

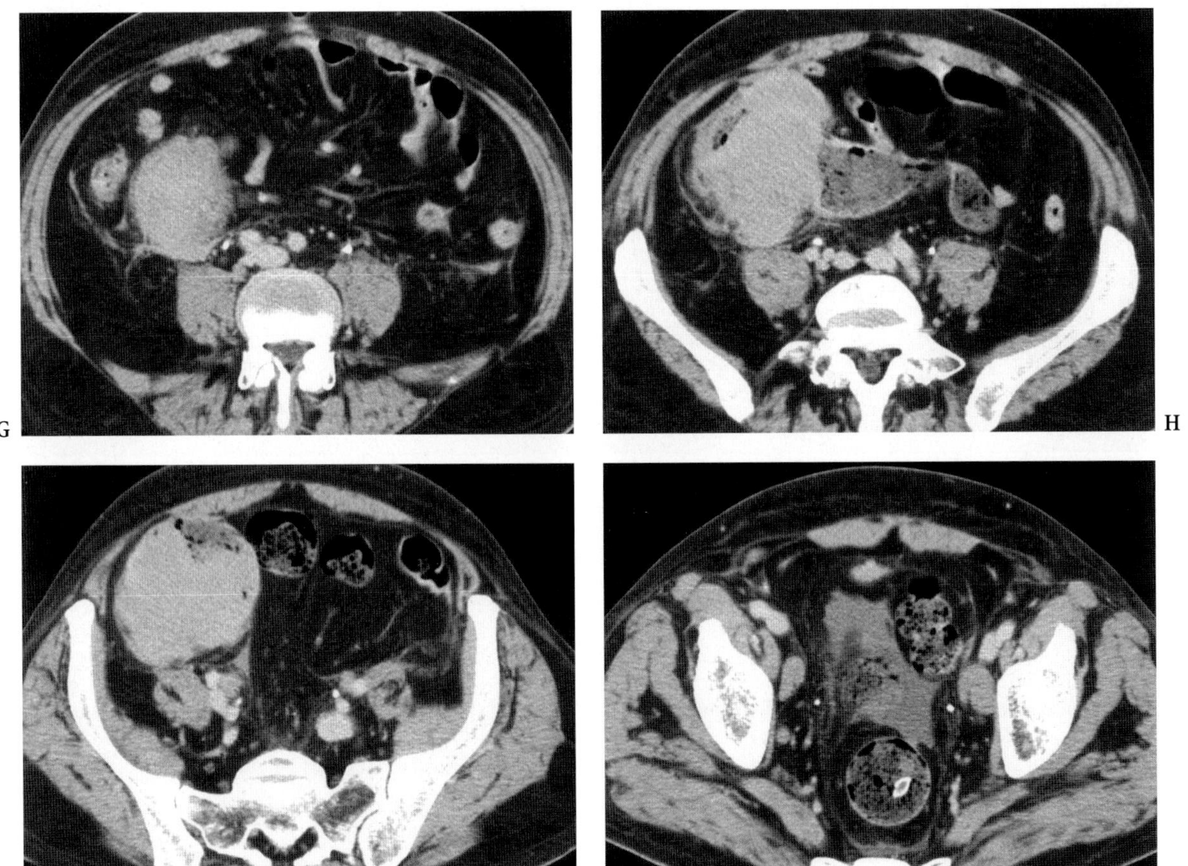

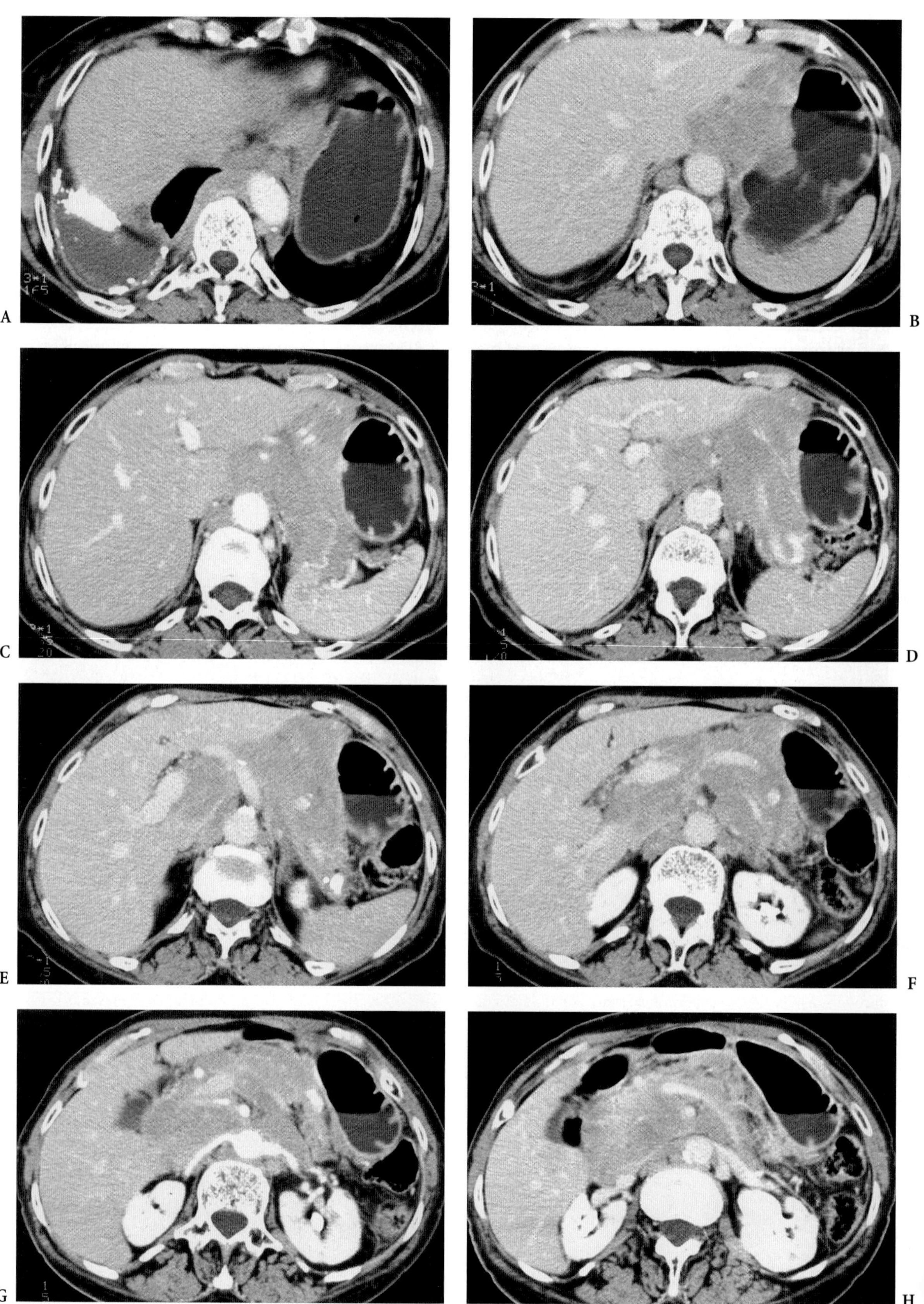
A
B
C
D
E
F
G
H

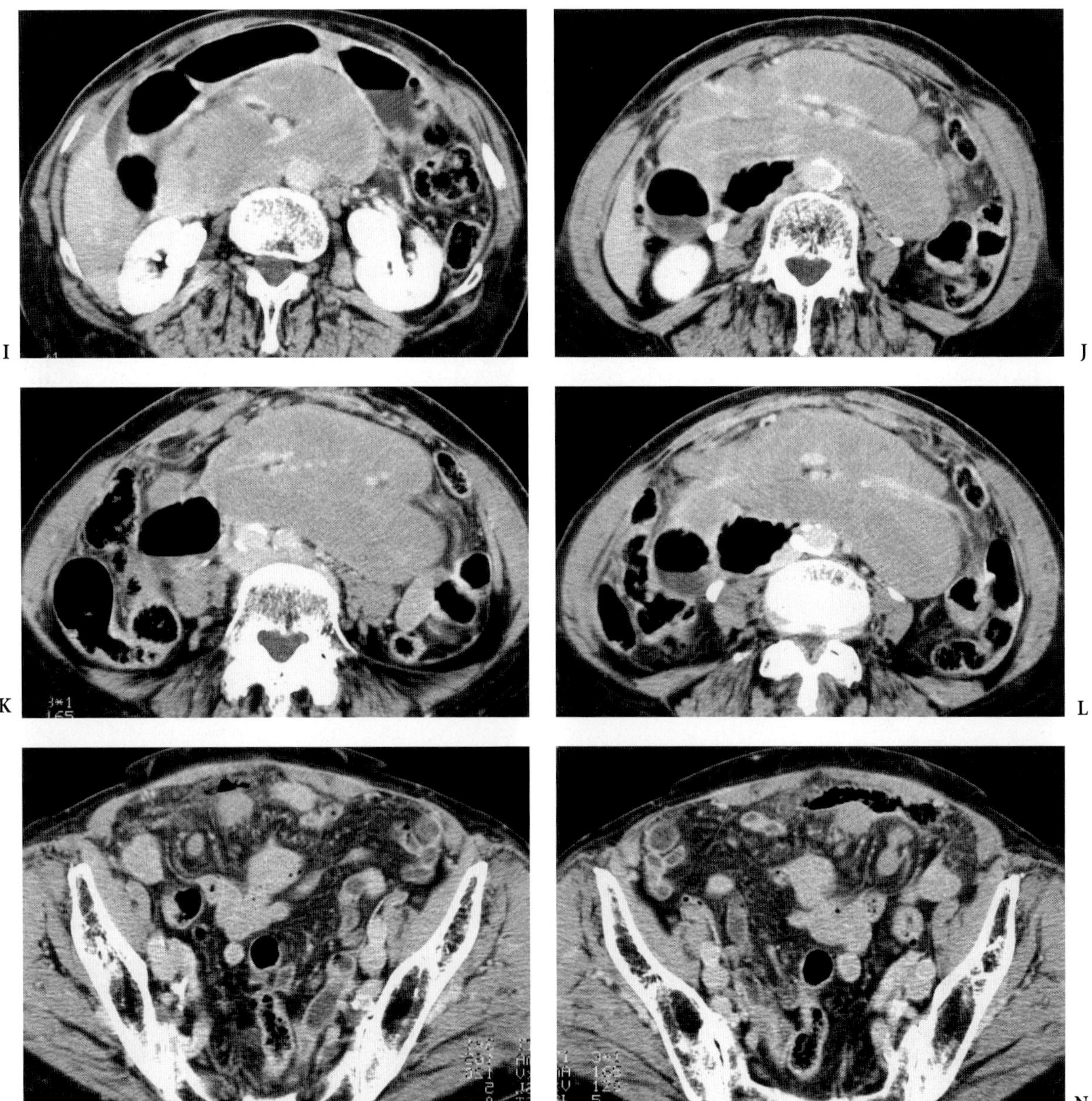

Fig. 12.33A–N. Non-Hodgkin's lymphoma. Enlarged lymph nodes converging in a mass, which widely occupies the supramesocolic and mesenteric subperitoneal spaces on the sides of the vessels. "Sandwich"-like aspect of the superior mesenteric localizations (**J–L**). Dense serpiginous network at the pelvic level of the lymphatic vessels coming from the intestinal loops that are expanded as a result of mesenteric lymphatic blockade (**M, N**)

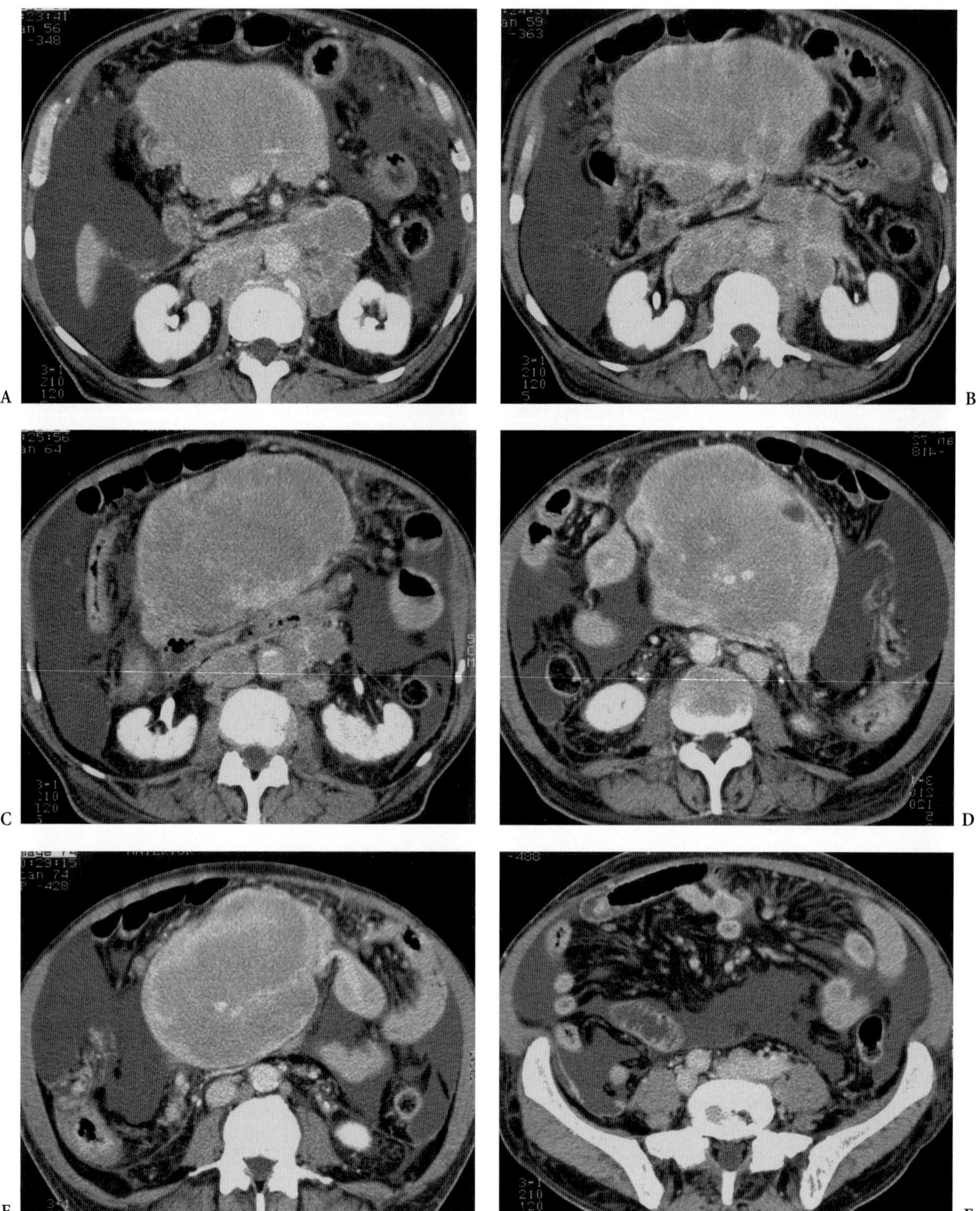

Fig. 12.34A–F. Non-Hodgkin's lymphoma. Voluminous mesenteric lymph nodal mass on the median line, in front of the trunks of the superior mesenteric vessels. Thickening of the parietal and mesenteric peritoneum (**F**) with ascites

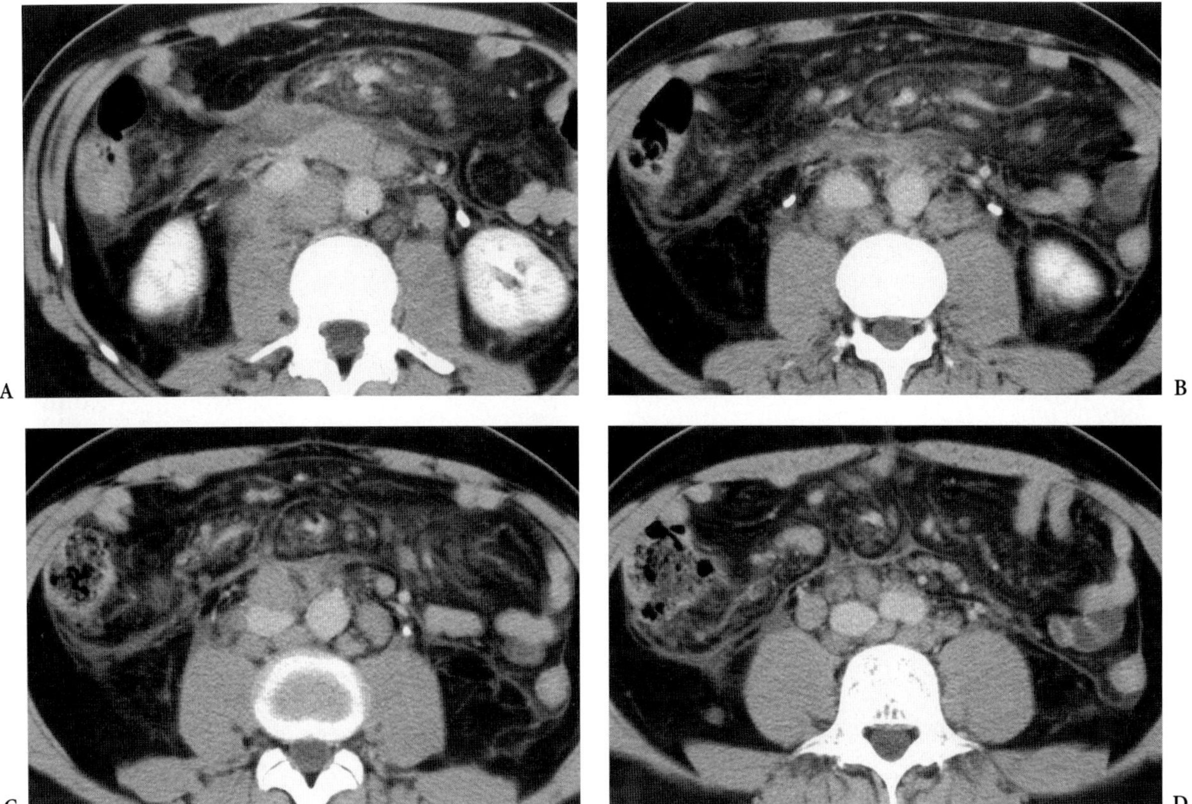

Fig. 12.35A–D. Non-Hodgkin's lymphoma. Mesenteric and retroperitoneal lymph nodal localization with perifocal infiltration of the perivascular adipose cellular, the posterior peritoneum, and the lateroconal and anterior renal fasciae on the right

12.8.2 Chronic Lymphatic Leukemia

Chronic lymphatic leukemia is a neoplasm of the lymphatic system that is due to activation of P lymphocytes, which accumulate in the bone marrow, the lymph nodes, the blood and the spleen. In most cases, it is characterized by polyadenomegaly, splenomegaly, and lymphatic leukocytosis with a prevalence of mature lymphocytes.

The lymphoadenomegalies affect all the superficial lymph nodal stations, with an asymmetrical development, and the deep (paraaortic and abdominal) ones. The lymph nodes appear to be enlarged, but never in a conspicuous manner, and they preserve their individuality, with no tendency to converge or adhere to the adjacent tissues. The spleen never shows age-appropriate dimensions.

In the initial phase, which sometimes last for years, the symptomatology is mostly unclear, , characterized by asthenia, anorexia, vague malaise, lymphocytosis, and anemia; thereafter, attenuated cutaneous nodules or enlarged superficial lymph nodes and splenomegaly develop.

Also on CT examination, the enlarged lymph nodes (Figs. 12.37, 12.38) are seen to maintain their individuality, even when they reach conspicuous dimensions. Furthermore, in contrast to lymphomas, they do not show signs of infiltration of the peritoneum, the subperitoneal spaces and the fasciae and they are not associated with ascites. Polyadenopathy is almost always accompanied by slight splenomegaly.

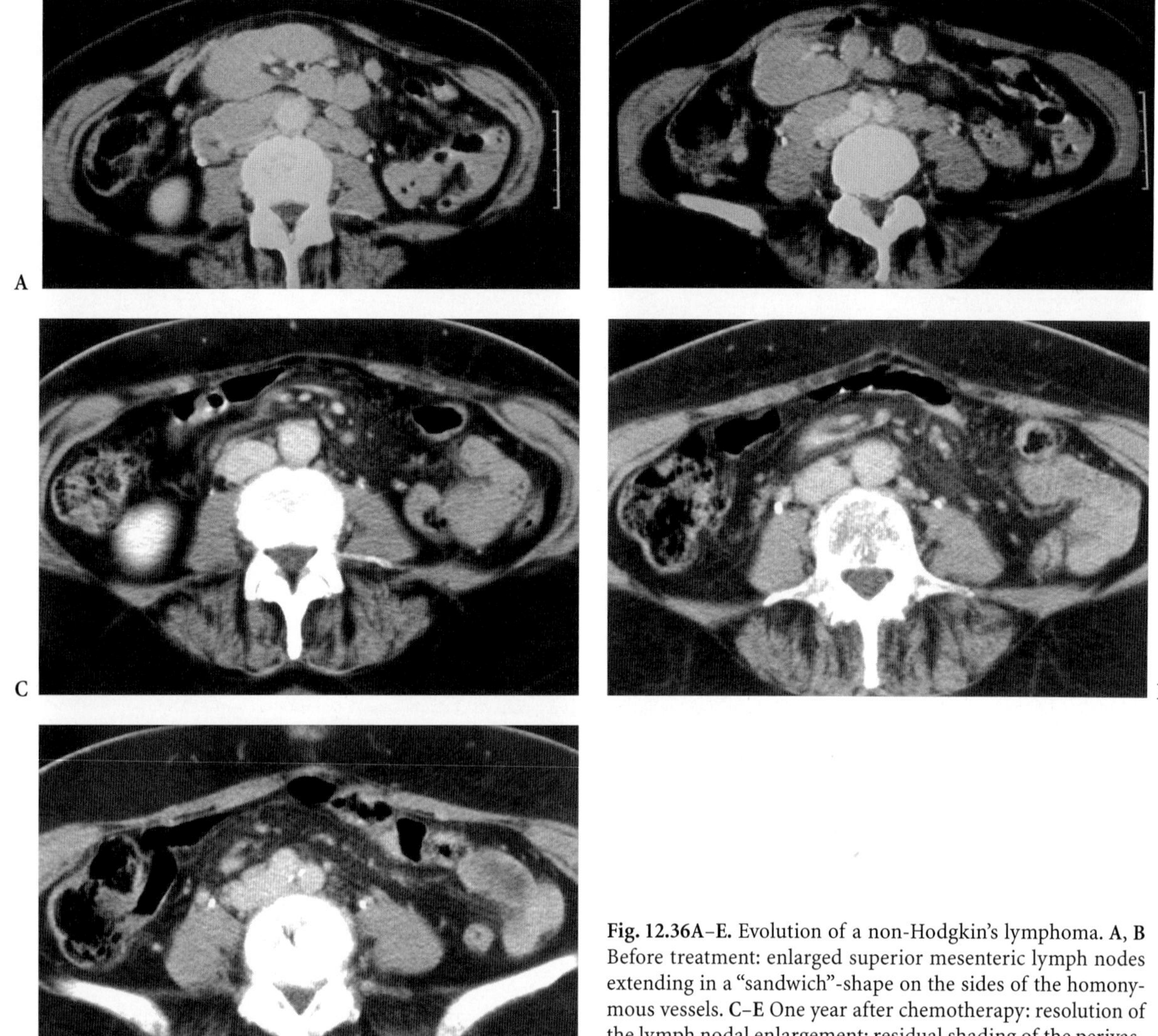

Fig. 12.36A–E. Evolution of a non-Hodgkin's lymphoma. **A, B** Before treatment: enlarged superior mesenteric lymph nodes extending in a "sandwich"-shape on the sides of the homonymous vessels. **C–E** One year after chemotherapy: resolution of the lymph nodal enlargement; residual shading of the perivascular cellular with thin serpiginous images without pathological significance

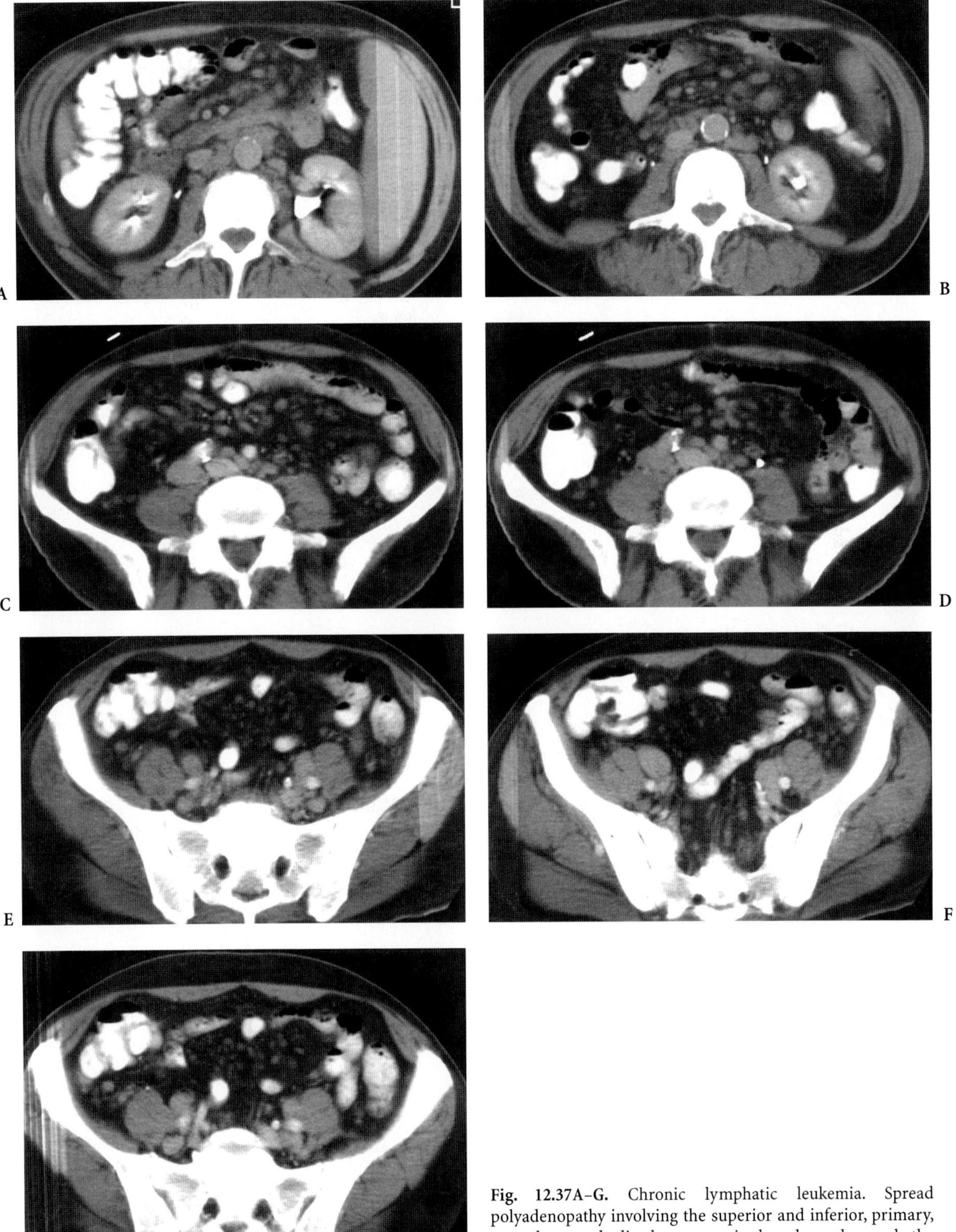

Fig. 12.37A–G. Chronic lymphatic leukemia. Spread polyadenopathy involving the superior and inferior, primary, secondary and distal mesenteric lymph nodes and the retroperitoneal lymph nodes. Splenomegaly

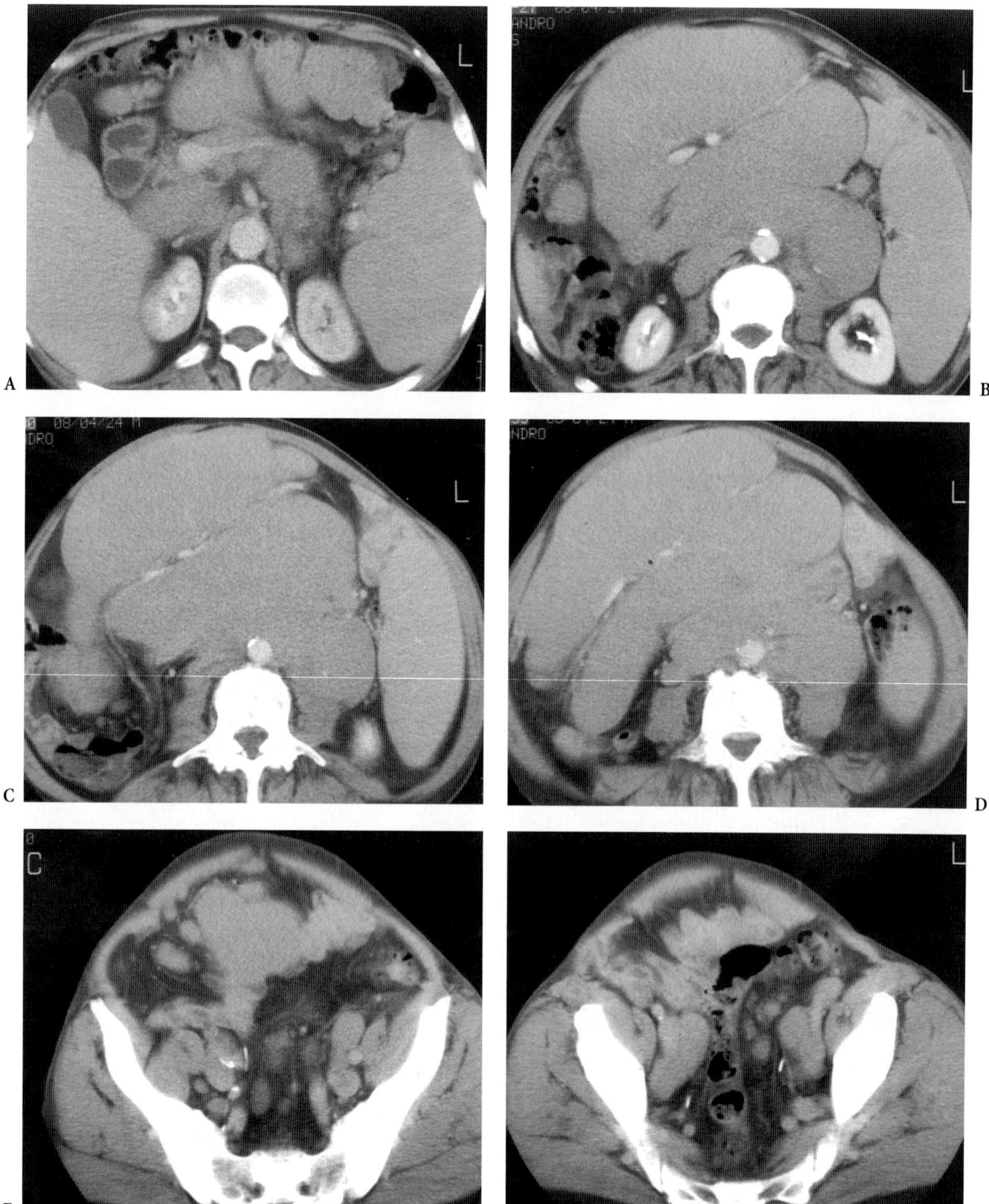

Fig. 12.38A–D. Chronic lymphatic leukemia. Conspicuous volumetric increment of almost all the subperitoneal submesocolic, lumboaortic, iliac and inguinal lymph nodes

12.9 Nervous System

Tumors of the nervous system may originate from the sheaths of the peripheral nerves extending in the subperitoneal spaces or from the enterochromaffin cells of the bowel (neuroendocrine tumors).

12.9.1 Neurinoma

The neurinoma (schwannoma or neurilemmoma) is a benign tumor that arises from the sheaths of the peripheral nervous trunks and grows slowly, displacing the adjacent organs and structures. Few cases have been observed in the peritoneum (McDonnell et al 1990), in the lesser omentum (Sakai et al. 1988; Kodama et al. 1989; Lee et al. 1992), in the greater omentum (Bankier et al. 1996), and in the mesentery (Di Franco et al. 1995).

Macroscopically it appears as a well-encapsulated ovoid swelling of a visceral nerve, with a smooth surface and a solid structure containing central areas of cystic degeneration. It causes clinical symptoms, such as abdominal pain, only when it reaches conspicuous dimensions.

At CT examination the neurinoma (Fig. 12.39) appears as a sharply limited ovoid mass with a thin or thick wall, containing tissues with low values of absorption (20–30 HU) and multiple cyst-like areas (0–10 HU). The contrast medium increases the density of the solid component (up to 60–80 HU) without changing that of the fluid component.

The low density of a part of the tumor is due to its composition: Schwann cells with high lipidic content, hypocellular areas adjacent to areas that are rich in cells and collagen, and finally, xanthomatous formations and cystic degeneration (Cohen et al. 1986). Because of these nonhomogeneous attenuation values, this tumor cannot be distinguished from those with malignant evolution (malignant neurinoma, leiomyosarcoma, etc.).

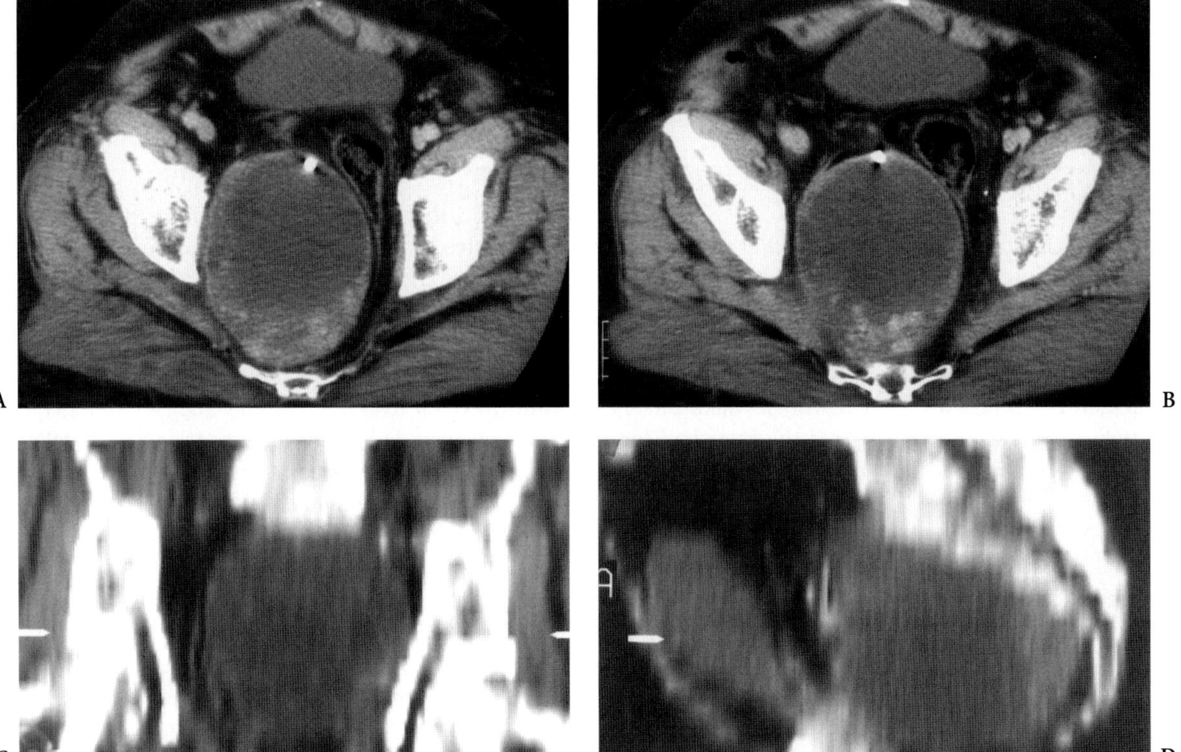

Fig. 12.39A–D. Neurinoma. Presacral ovoid mass limited by a thick capsule. It has a water-density content with multiple nodular formations with internal isolate microcalcifications protruding. These structures become hyperdense after contrast medium and have the appearance of a festoon

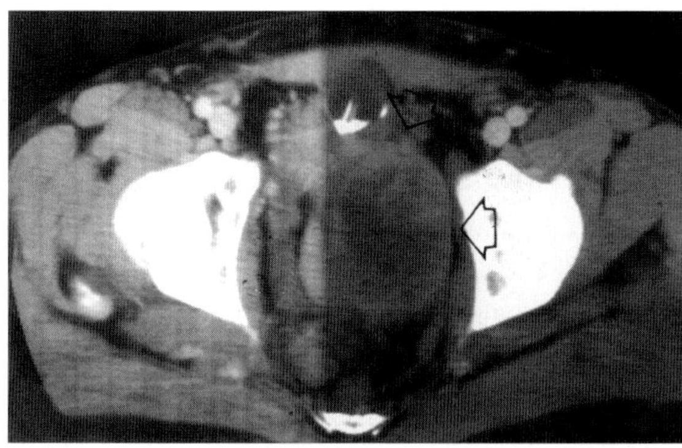

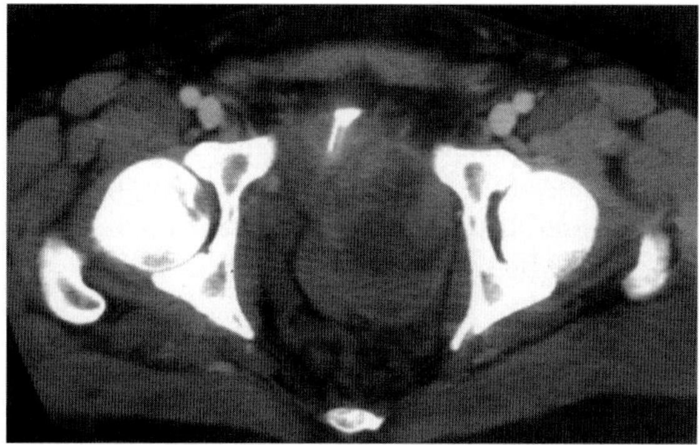

Fig. 12.40A, B. Neurofibrosarcoma in a patient with neurofibromatosis. Ovoid mass with mixed structure and irregular profile, infiltrating the urinary bladder and the pelvic adipose tissue

12.9.2 Neurofibroma

Neurofibroma is a benign tumor made up of Schwann cells and fibroblasts, which originates from the neurilemmal sheath of the peripheral nerves and, in contrast to neurinoma, includes and infiltrates the nerve.

It is extremely rare at the peritoneal, omental or mesenteric level, where it grows slowly, displacing the adjacent organs and structures. It becomes clinically evident as a palpable abdominal swelling only after reaching conspicuous dimensions.

Macroscopically, it appears as a bosselated and encapsulated voluminous mass, whose structure is partly solid and partly altered by cyst-like degeneration.

The CT appearance resembles that of the neurinoma, that is, a voluminous mass with regular contours and prevalently liquid content (10–20 HU), which is limited by a thick wall from which nodular structures protrude inward. The density of these structures increases after contrast medium. The mass displaces and compresses the intestinal loops without infiltration.

12.9.3 Malignant Peripheral Nerve Sheath

Various terms are applied to malignant neural neoplasm – neurofibrosarcoma, malignant schwannoma, malignant neurilemmoma, neurogenic sarcoma – which develops in most cases from degeneration of neurofibromas in patients with neurofibromatosis after a long period of latency and just occasionally from normal nerves. They cause pain, peripheral neurological deficits or compressive disturbances.

Macroscopically they appear as large masses with infiltrating characters, and are not easily separable from the adjacent tissues; necrotic areas are present inside the mass.

At CT examination, they appear as large masses, greater that 3.5 cm, with a nonhomogeneous structure. Low attenuation areas (30 H.U.) are visible within a solid contrast enhancing mass that shows a poorly defined profile with infiltrating characters (Fig. 12.40,12.41).

12.9.4 Neurofibromatosis

Neurofibromatosis is one of the commonest chronic progressive disorders of the neuroectodermic and mesodermic tissues; it is due to dominant autosomic hereditary transmission or to spontaneous mutation. Neurofibromatosis is subdivided into a peripheral form or type 1 neurofibromatosis (NF1, also known as Von Recklinghausen's disease) and a central form, or type 2 neurofibromatosis (NF2, or bilateral acoustic neurofibromatosis).

Type 1 neurofibromatosis is characterized by multiple neurofibromas, by plexiform neurofibromatosis, and by "white coffee" punctiform cutaneous spots.

Neurofibromas are benign tumors made up of Schwann cells and fibroblasts of the neurilemmal sheath of peripheral nerves, which develop as multiple nodules along the extension of the nerves.

Plexiform neurofibromatosis is characterized by an anomalous proliferation of Schwann cells of the sheaths of peripheral nerves, which induces a thickening of the nerves, sometimes conspicuous. It is preferentially located in paraspinal retroperitoneal

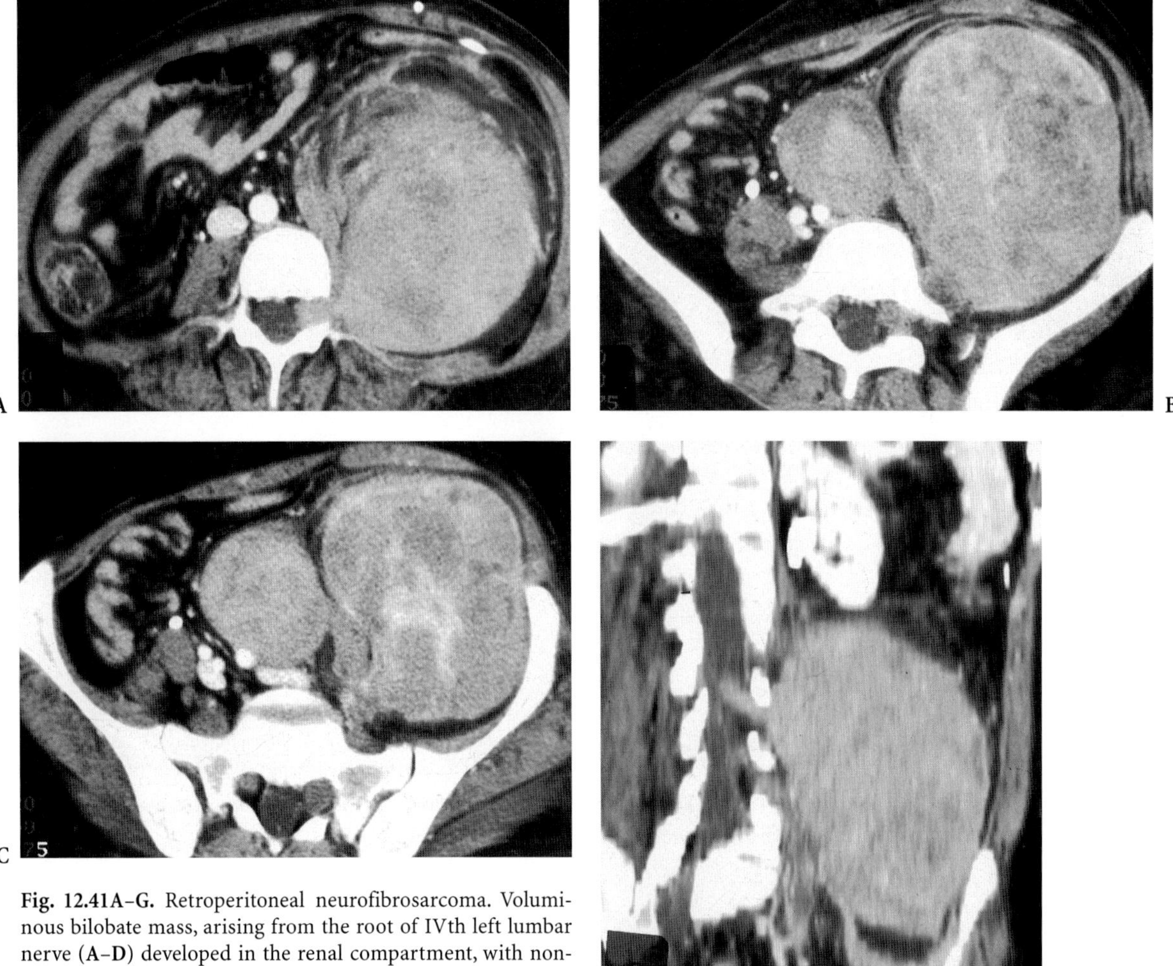

Fig. 12.41A–G. Retroperitoneal neurofibrosarcoma. Voluminous bilobate mass, arising from the root of IVth left lumbar nerve (**A–D**) developed in the renal compartment, with nonhomogeneous appearance owing to low-density areas within a solid contrast-enhancing structure

sites on both sides of the column, with symmetrical involvement of the lumbosacral plexus. It may extend forward with tortuous digitiform prolongations along the nervous branches.

NF1 is asymptomatic except in advanced phases, when a neurofibroma may remain incarcerated at the level of the nervous roots in the conjugation foramina or when it adopts a sarcomatous character.

In association with the primary and typical manifestations of NF1 (neurofibromas and cutaneous spots) osteal dysplasias (of the sphenoid alae: pseudoarthrosis, kyphosis and/or scoliosis) and lesions in the central (macrocephaly with hydrocephalus due to corticocerebral dysplasia, optic glioma) and peripheral (pheochromocytomas) nervous system may be observed.

Neurofibromas have a marked predisposition to sarcomatous degeneration.

On CT examination, neurofibromas appear as homogeneous nodules of variable dimensions with a smooth profile, which are preferentially located at the roots of the nervous trunks. They show low attenuation values (20–25 HU); after contrast medium, their density homogeneously increases up to 30–50 HU. When the contrast medium is administered rapidly, in early scans one can easily observe an opaque central area that is quickly followed by homogenization of the nodule.

Sarcomatous degeneration is heralded by asymmetry in size and low-attenuation areas in a higher enhancing density mass (Bass et al. 1994).

Plexiform neurofibromatosis is shown by CT (Figs. 4.89–4.92, 12.42) as symmetrical, bilateral, paraspinal, multilobular masses with a homogeneous structure and low attenuation (20–40 HU), which expand along the nervous roots, involving the

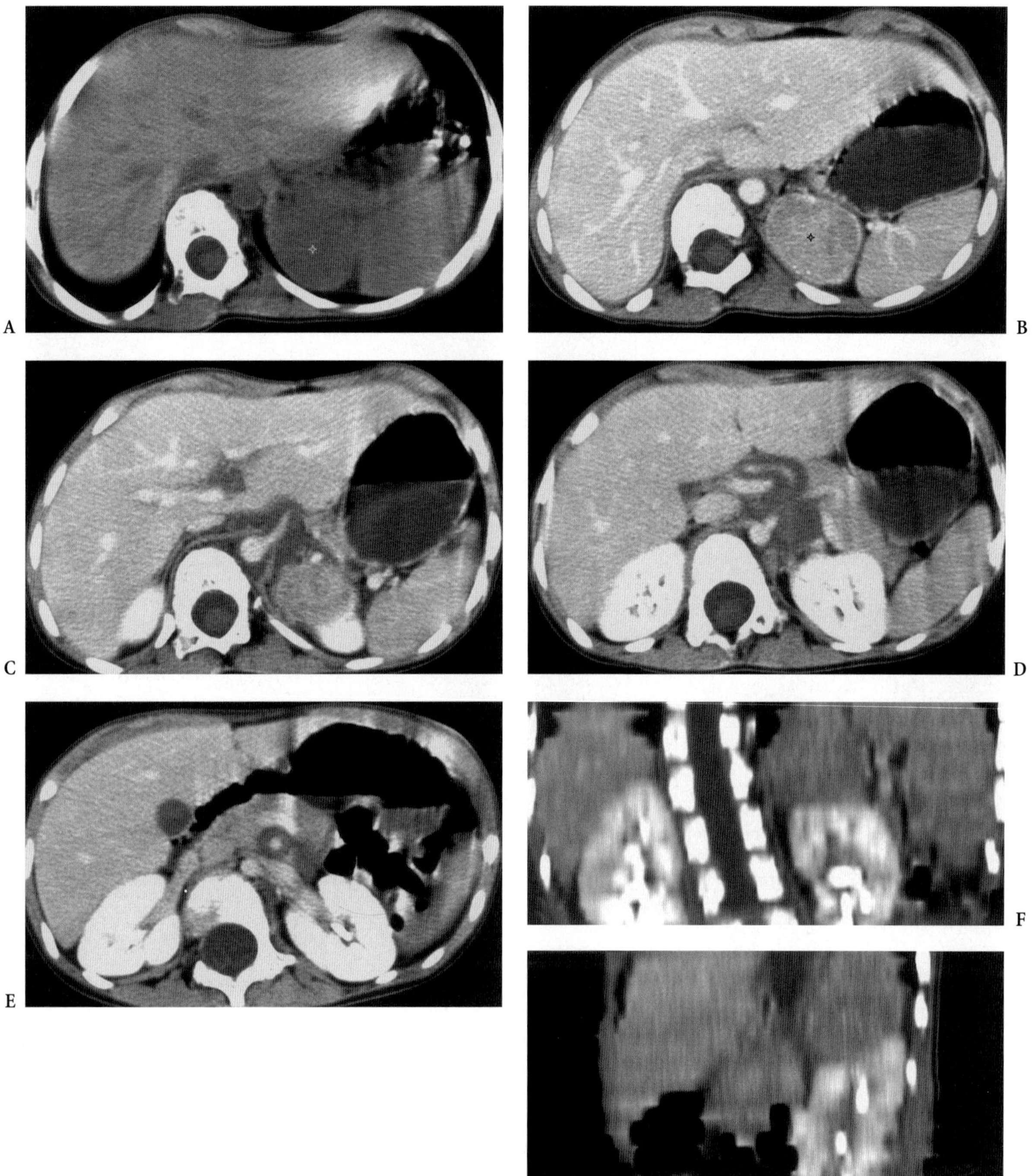

Fig. 12.42A–H. Celiaco-mesenteric and retroperitoneal neurofibromatosis associated with a pheochromocytoma of the left adrenal gland. The greater and lesser splanchnic nerves (**C**), the celiac trunk (**C**), the hepatic, splenic (**D**) and superior mesenteric (**E**) nerves are bigger and slightly denser than water (30 HU).Homogeneous low-attenuation ovoid mass of the left adrenal gland (**A**); after contrast medium, its peripheral part becomes intensely opaque, delineating a pseudocapsule, whereas the internal part becomes less opaque (**B**): pheochromocytoma. Coronal (**F**) and sagittal (**G**) reconstructions

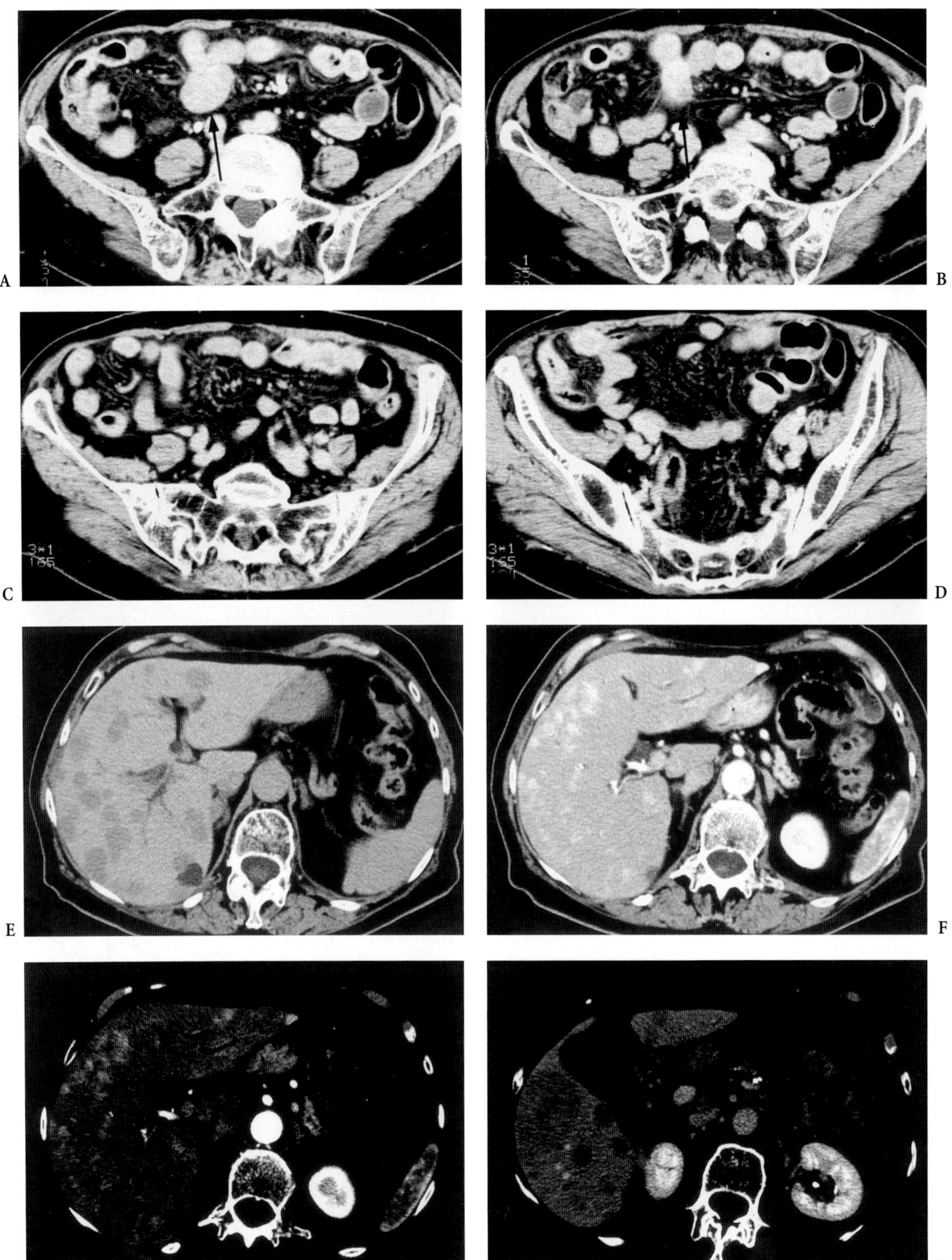

Fig. 12.43A–F. Ileal carcinoid with mesenteric infiltration and hepatic metastases. **A, B** Ileal ovoid solid contrast enhancing nodule, with radiated linear strands in the mesentery. Low-attenuating intrahepatic metastatic nodules (**E**), which become hyperdense during the arterial phase after bolus contrast medium administration (**F, G**) and again hypodense during the portal phase (**H**)

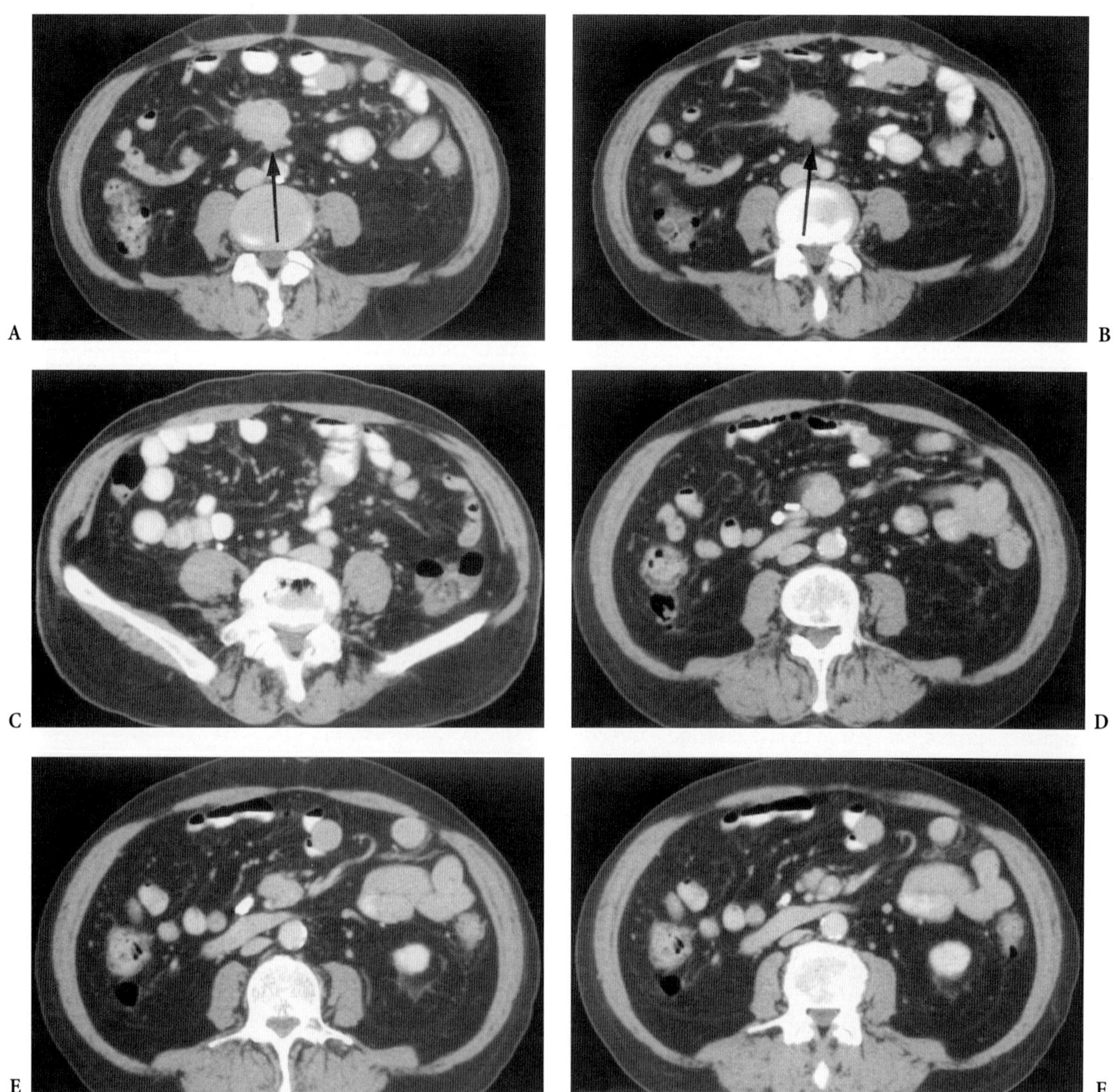

Fig. 12.44. Ileal carcinoid with mesenteric development and lymph nodal metastases. Small homogeneous nodular mass (**A**, **B**) with curled and frayed contours projecting thin radiated shoots toward the mesentery (**A**, **B**). The mass takes origin in an ileal loop (*arrow*) (**C**). Superior mesenteric lymph nodal metastases which are partly calcified (**CD–E**)

celiac and mesenteric plexus and their peripheral branches, and infiltrating the vascular structures. The low attenuation of the perineural plexiform proliferations has been variously attributed to entrapment and inclusion of the perineural adipose tissue, to the high content of lipids of mucinous matrix or to cystic degeneration (Mirich et al. 1989).

In most cases the CT aspects of the plexiform neurofibromatosis are typical and allow a specific diagnosis (Bass et al. 1994).

12.9.5 Carcinoids

Intestinal carcinoids are neuroendocrine tumors arising from enterochromaffin cells, with peculiar histological and biochemical characteristics. The carcinoids of the appendix (which is the most frequent: about 50% of cases), the stomach and the colon originate from EC cells, which secrete histamine, ^{5}H-tryptophan and ACTH; they grow slowly and are asymptomatic for a long time, remaining within the viscus without producing characteristic clinical signs or secondary spread.

The ileal carcinoids originate from EC, EC1, EC2 and ECN cells, which produce serotonin and 5-H-try-ptamine; they grow stealthily and become clinically ev-ident with the typical "carcinoid syndrome." This is characterized by diarrhea, abdominal cramps, periodic cutaneous flushes, intermittent obstructions, and sudden blood pressure loss. These symptoms appear after the tumor has metastasized to the liver, and thus, the vasoactive tumoral secretions are no longer metabolized by the liver and pass into the systemic circulation.

The diagnosis of carcinoid is based on laboratory tests: assay of 5-HIAA in urine, 5HT in total blood and serotonin in the serum; stimulation tests with catecholamines or alcohol, which induce vasomotor disturbances and increments in blood pressure.

Intestinal carcinoids grow slowly, involving both mucosa and submucosa inside, protruding in the lumen with a polypoid aspect, and extending into the muscular layer, the serosa and the mesenteric cellular outside. At this level, the serotonergic activity provokes an intense desmoplastic reaction, with conspicuous development of fibrous tissue around the tumor and the formation of a solid mass containing both the primary neoplasm and the fibrous reaction, which may result in kinking or obstruction of the adjacent small bowel loops.

CT is requested for discovery and localization of the primary tumor and any secondaries.

CT scans show the carcinoid (Figs. 12.43, 12.44) as a unifocal solid mass that is highly enhanced after contrast medium. Linear radiate prolongations extend toward the mesentery, which seems to be attracted by the mass. It is not rare for small stripped or coarse dense calcifications to be observed inside the neoplasm. However, this characteristic CT aspect becomes evident only when the tumor has extended beyond the muscular layer and the intestinal serosa, causing a mesenteric desmoplastic reaction.

The concomitant presence of hepatic metastases is almost constant. In the precontrast scans metastases appear hypodense or isodense relative to the surrounding liver. In the arterial phase, during contrast agent injection the metastases become hyperdense, whereas in the portal phase the contrast enhancement is poorer (Sako et al. 1982; De Santis et al. 1996). Mesenteric adenomegalies are detected at presentation in 35% of patients (Picus et al. 1984).

Less frequently, only observe linear striations extending in rays from the intestinal wall toward the mesentery are observed, or thickening of the intestinal wall. When these specific features or the clinical and laboratory elements supporting the diagnosis of the nature of the tumor are not found, the carcinoid cannot be differentiated from a retractile nodular mesenteritis, except for the characteristic hyperdensity after contrast medium.

12.10 Embryonal Tissue

According to histopathological criteria, dermoid cysts and cystic teratomas are classed under cystic forms. They have therefore been discussed in the appropriate chapter (see chapter 11).

Bibliography

Primary Peritoneal, Subperitoneal and Omental Tumors

Berezin A, Seltzer SE (1984) Differential diagnosis of huge abdominal masses visualized on CT scans. Comput Radiol 8:95–99

Bernardino ME, Jing BS, Wallace S (1979) Computed tomography diagnosis of mesenteric masses. AJR Am J Roentgenol 132:33–36

Bollaert A, Bremer A, Grivegnee A, De Graef J, Sernagor M, Louis O (1983) Apport de la tomodensitométrie en pathologie abdominale pelvienne. Radiologie 3:29–37

Cooper C, Jeffrey RB, Silverman PM, Federle MP, Chun GH (1986) Computed tomography of omental pathology. J Comput Assist Tomogr 10:62–66

Dalla Palma L (1989) Il retroperitoneo. Diagnositica per immagini. LINT, Trieste

De Maria M (1988) La TC nello studio della patologia primitiva del mesentere. Acta Med Mediterr 4:203–207

Haaga JK, Alfidi RJ (1976) Precise biopsy localization by computed tomography. Radiology 118:603–607

Hamrick-Turner JE, Chiechi MV, Abbit PL, Ros PR (1992) Neoplastic and inflammatory processes of the peritoneum, omentum, and mesentery: diagnosis with CT. Radiographics 12:1051–1068

Jeffrey RB (1983) Computed tomography of the peritoneal cavity and mesentery. In: Moss AA, Gamsu G, Genant H (eds) Computed tomography of the body. Saunders, Philadelphia, pp 955–986

Pistolesi GF, Procacci C, Caudana C, Bergamo Andreis IA, Manera V, Recla M, Grasso G, Florio C (1984) CT criteria of the differential diagnosis in primary retroperitoneal masses. Eur J Radiol 4:127–138

Silverman PM, Baker ME, Cooper C, Kelvin FM (1987) Computed tomography of mesenteric disease. Radiographics 7:309–320

Whitley NO (1986) Mesenteric disease. In: Mayers MA (ed) Computed tomography of the gastrointestinal tract including the peritoneal cavity and mesentery. Springer, New York Berlin Heidelberg, pp 139–178

Whitley NO, Bohlman ME, Baker LP (1982a) CT patterns of mesenteric disease. J Comput Assist Tomogr 6:490–496

Whitley NO, Bohlman ME, Baker LP, Whitley J (1982b) CT patterns of mesenteric disease. Radiographics 2:208

Micropapillary Serous Tumors

Altaras MM, Aviram P, Rohen I, Cordoba M, Weiss E, Beyth Y (1991) Primary peritoneal papillary serous adenocarcinoma: clinical and management aspects. Gynecol Oncol 40:230–236

Bell DA, Scully RE (1990) Serous borderline tumors of the peritoneum. Am J Surg Pathol 14:230–239

Bloss JD, Liao S, Buller RE, et al (1993) Extraovarian peritoneal serous papillary carcinoma: a case-control retrospective comparison to papillary adenocarcinoma of the ovary. Gynecol Oncol 50:347–351

Boldorini R, Cristina S (1992) Primary papillary serous tumor of the peritoneum: report of a case. Patologica 84:403–409

Chopra S, Laurie LR, Chintipalli KN, Valente PT, Dodd GD III (2000) Primary papillary serous carcinoma of the peritoneum: CT – pathologic correlation. J Comput Assist Tomogr 24:395–399

Furukawa T, Ueda J, Takahashi S, et al (1999) Peritoneal serous papillary carcinoma: radiological appearance. Abdom Imaging 24:78–81

Ikuma K, Yamada K, Yamasaki H, Takemura T (1992) Serous surface papillary carcinoma of the peritoneum: a case report. Nippon Sanka Fujinka Gakkai Zasshi 44:877–880

Kannerstein M, Churg J, McCaughey WT, Hill DP (1977) Papillary tumors of the peritoneum in women: mesothelioma or papillary carcinoma. Am J Obstet Gynecol 127:306–314

Marrucci A, Boraschi P, Viacava P (1992) Cistoadenoma sieroso extragonadico "borderline" del peritoneo. Descrizione di un caso. Radiol Med 84:815–817

Raju U, Fine G, Greenwald KA, et al (1989) Primary papillary serous neoplasia of the peritoneum: a clinicopathological and ultrastructural study of eight cases. Hum Pathol 20:426–436

Stafford-Johnson DB, Bree RL, Francis JR, Korobkin M (1998) CT appearance of papillary serous carcinoma of the peritoneum. AJR Am J Roentgenol 171:687–689

Swerdlow M (1959) Mesothelioma of the pelvic peritoneum resembling papillary cystoadenoma of the ovary. Am J Obstet Gynecol 77:197–200

Mesotheliomas

Antman K II, Osteen RT, Klegar KL, et al (1985) Early peritoneal mesothelioma: a treatable malignancy. Lancet I:977–981

Bernardino ME, Jing BS, Wallace S (1979) Computed tomography diagnosis of mesenteric masses. AJR Am J Roentgenol 132:33–36

Bighi S, Lupi L, Limone CL (1988) Ruolo diagnostico di US e TC nella diagnosi di mesotelioma peritoneale: descrizione di un caso. Arcisp, S Anna, pp 173–178

Boccalatte M, Giusti S, Torelli L (1993) Aspetti con tomografia computerizzata del mesotelioma maligno peritoneale. Presentazione di due casi. Radiol Med 85:496–499

Brenner DE, Whitley NO, Goldstein WZ, Aisner J (1981) Computed tomographic demonstration of peritoneal mesothelioma. Lancet I:939–940

Bruno C, De Santis M, Comba P, et al (1990) Mortality in malignant tumors of the peritoneum in Italy: search for correlations with exposure to asbestos. Epidemiol Prev 12:39–47

Cooper CC, Jeffrey RB Jr, Silverman PM, Federle MP, Chun GH (1986) Computed tomography of omental pathology. J Comput Assist Tomogr 10:62–66

Cozzi G, Bellomi M, Frigerio LF, Ostinelli C, Marchiano A, Patrillo R et al (1989) Double contrast barium enema combined with noninvasive imaging in peritoneal mesothelioma. Acta Radiol 30:21–24

Dach J, Patel N, Patel S, Petasnick J (1980) Peritoneal mesothelioma: CT sonography and gallium-67 scan. AJR Am J Roentgenol 135:614–616

Fukuda T, Hayashi K, Mori M, Ashizawa K, Isomoto I, Nagayoshi K, Uetani M, Mori H (1991) Radiologic manifestations of peritoneal mesothelioma. Nippon Igaku Hoshasen Gakkai Zasshi 51:643–648

Granke DS, Ellis JH, Richmond BD (1987) CT findings of hypervascular malignant peritoneal mesothelioma. Comput Radiol 11:91–94

Guest PJ, Reznek RH, Selleslag D, Geraghty R, Slevin M (1992) Peritoneal mesothelioma – the role of computed tomography in diagnosis and follow-up. Clin Radiol 45:79–84

Gupta S, Gupta RK, Gurial RB, et al (1992) Peritoneal mesothelioma simulating pseudomyxoma peritonei on CT and sonography. Gastrointest Radiol 17:129–131

Hamrick-Turner JE, Chiechi MV, Abbitt PL, Ros PR (1992) Neoplastic and inflammatory processes of the peritoneum, omentum, and mesentery: diagnosis with CT. Radiographics 12:1051–1068

Katsabe Y, Mukai K, Silverberg SG (1982) Cystic mesothelioma of the peritoneum: a report of five cases and a review of the literature. Cancer 50:1615–1622

Lederman GS, Recht A, Herman T, Osteen R, Corson J, Antman KN (1987) Long-term survival in peritoneal mesothelioma. Cancer 59:1882–1886

Levitt RG, Sagel SS, Stanley RJ (1978) Detection of neoplastic involvement of the mesentery and omentum by computed tomography. AJR Am J Roentgenol 131:835–838

Lowell FA, Cranston PE (1990) Well differentiated papillary mesothelioma of the peritoneum. AJR Am J Roentgenol 155:1245–1246

O'Neal JD, Ros PR, Storm BL, Buck JL, Wilkinson EJ (1989) Cystic mesothelioma of the peritoneum. Radiology 170:333–337

Preidler KW, Steiner H, Szolar D, Kern R (1994) Cystic appearance of a malignant peritoneal mesothelioma by ultrasonography and computed tomography: a case report. Eur J Radiol 18:137–139

Raptopoulos V (1985) Peritoneal mesothelioma. CRC Crit Rev Diagn Imaging 24:293

Reuter K, Raptopoulos V, Reale F, et al (1983) Diagnosis of peritoneal mesothelioma: computed tomography, sonography, and fine needle aspiration biopsy. AJR Am J Roentgenol 140:1189–1194

Ros PR, Yusehok TJ, Buck JL, Shekitka KM, Kaude JV (1991) Peritoneal mesothelioma: radiologic appearances correlated with histology. Acta Radiol 32:355–358

Sans N, Cnudde F, Cnudde F, Chevallier J, Mathieu S, Giron J, Railhac JJ (1993) Une tumeur peritoneale rare: le mesotheliome malin. A propos d'un cas et revue de la littérature. Ann Radiol 36:118–124

Smith TR (1994) Malignant peritoneal mesothelioma: marked variability of CT findings. Abdom Imaging 19:27–29

Steffen HM, Wambach G, Hoffmann A, Jaursch-Hancke C, Kaufmann W (1989) Diagnosis and therapy of malignant peritoneal mesothelioma. J Med Klin [15] 84:469–473

Whitley NO, Bohlman ME, Baker LP (1982a) CT patterns of mesenteric disease. J Comput Assist Tomogr 6:490–496

Whitley NO, Brenner DE, Antman KH, Grant D, Aisner J (1982b) CT of peritoneal mesothelioma: analysis of eight cases. AJR Am J Roentgenol 138:531–535

Yeh HC, Chahinian AP (1980) Ultrasonography and computed tomography of peritoneal mesothelioma. Radiology 135:705–712

Desmoplastic Small Round Cell Tumor

Dao H-NV, Dachman AH (1995) CT findings of regression in intraabdominal desmoplastic small-cell tumor. Clin Imaging 19:244–245

N'Dri K, Aguéhoundé C, Konan A, Ouattara ND, Abby CB (1998) Tumeur desmoplastique intra-abdominal à petites celles rondes: aspect échographiques et tomodensitométriques. À propos d'un cas. J Radiol 79: 1506–1508

Outwater E, Schiebler ML, Brooks JJ (1992) Intrabdominal desmoplastic small cell tumor: CT findings in five cases. J Comput Assist Tomogr 16: 429–432

Pickhardt PJ, Fisher AJ, Balfe DM, Dehner LP, Huettner PC (1999) Desmoplastic small round cell tumor of the abdomen: radiologic-histopathologic correlation. Radiology 210:633–638

Varma DG, McDaniel K, Ordonez NG, Granfield CA, Charnsangavej C, Wallace S (1992) Primary malignant small round cell tumor of the abdomen: CT findings in five cases. AJR Am J Roentgenol 158:1031–1034

Fibrous

Desmoid, Fibroma and Fibrosarcomas

Baron RL, Lee JKT (1981) Mesenteric desmoid tumors: sonographic and computed tomographic appearance. Radiology 140:777–779

Brooks AP, Reznek RH, Nugent K, Farmer KC, Thomson JP (1994) CT appearances of desmoid tumours in familial adenomatous polyposis: further observations. Clin Radiol 49:601–607

Campbell AN, Chan HSL, Daneman A, et al (1983) Aggressive fibromatosis in childhood, tomographic findings in three patients. J Comput Assist Tomogr 7:109–113

Capra S, Casoni S, Busetti L, Cominotti A (1996) Tumore desmoide intraddominale in paziente operata per carcinoma del retto: descrizione di un caso. Radiol Med. 92:141–142

Casillas J, Sais GJ, Greve JL, Iparraguirre MC, Morillo G (1991) Imaging of intra and extraabdominal desmoid tumors. Radiographics 11:959–968

Corbel L, Souissi M, Chrétien Y, Dufour B (1992) La tumeur desmoïde du mésentère. Une cause exceptionnelle d'obstruction urétérale. J Radiol 73:669–672

Einstein DM, Tagliabue JR, Desai RK (1991) Abdominal desmoids: CT findings in 25 patients. AJR Am J Roentgenol 157:275–279

Francis IR, Dorovini-Zis K, Glazer GM, et al (1986)The fibromatosis: CT pathologic correlation. AJR Am J Roentgenol 147:1063–1066

Greget M, Veillon F, Meyer C, Tongio J, Imler M (1994) Tumeur desmoide dans le cadre du syndrome de Gardner. A propos d'un cas evalué en echographie, TDM et IRM. J Radiol 75:199–202

Imana FJ, Nasr A, Aguilera C, Zalcman M, Struyven J (1991) Tumeur desmoide et syndrome de Gardner. J Belge Radiol 74:301–302

Ito T, Nakahara H, Ikeda M, Kuranishi F, Ogawa Y, Kuroda Y, Watanabe K (1990) Intra abdominal mesenteric desmoid tumor. South Med J 83:330–331

Janzen DL (1991) Residents corner. Answer to case of the month. Desmoid tumours of the mesentery and abdominal wall in Gardner's syndrome. Can Assoc Radiol J 42:64–65

Kawashima A, Goldman SM, Fishman EK, Kuhlman JE, Onitsuka H, Fukuya T, Masuda K (1994) CT of intraabdominal desmoid tumors: is the tumor different in patients with Gardner's disease? AJR Am J Roentgenol 162:339–342

Magid D, Fishman EK, Jones B, Hoover HC, Feinstein R, Siegelman SS (1984) Desmoid tumors in Gardner's syndrome: use of computed tomography. AJR Am J Roentgenol 142:1141–1145

Outwater E, Schiebler ML, Brooks JJ (1992) Intraabdominal desmoplastic small cell tumor: CT and MR findings. J Comput Assist Tomogr 16:429–432

Paksoy Y, Sahin M, Açikgozoglu S, Odev K, Omeroglu E (1998) Omental fibroma: CT and US findings. Eur Radiol 8: 1422–1424

Potente G, Osti M, Torriero F, Scattoni Padovan F, Maurizi Enrici R (1993) Tumore desmoide della parete addominale anteriore. Radiol Med 85:142–143

Richaud J, Carette MF, Boudghene F, Lebreton C, Izrael V, Bigot JM (1989) Desmoid tumors of the mesentery in Gardner's syndrome. Value of x-ray computed tomography. J Radiol 70:711–715

Rubenstein WA, Gray G, Auh YH et al (1986) CT of fibrous tissue and tumors with sonographic correlation. AJR Am J Roentgenol 147:1067–1074

Schopp D, Dinkel E, Mappes HJ, Hoffmann E (1989) Aggressive abdominal fibromatosis: the place of diagnostic imaging. Rofo Fortschr Geb Rontgenstr Nuklearmed 151:536–541

Unemoto S, Makuuchi H, Amemiya T, Yamaguchi H, Oka S, Owada T, Koizumi K (1991) Intra abdominal desmoid tumors in familial polyposis coli: a case report of tumor regression by prednisolone therapy. Dis Colon Rectum 34:89–93

Wegner H, Fleige B, Dieckmann KP (1994) Mesenteric desmoid tumor 19 years after radiation therapy for testicular seminoma. Urol Int 53:48–49

Histiocytoma

Bruneton JN, Drouillard J, Rogopoulos A, Laurent F, Normand F, Balu-Maestro C, Monticelli J (1988) Extraretroperitoneal abdominal malignant fibrous histiocytoma. Gastrointest Radiol 13:299–305

Contran RM, Stocker JT (1985) Malignant fibrous histiocytoma of the liver. A case report. Am J Gastroenterol 80:813–815

Duchat A, Landel JF, Villand J, et al (1985) Hystiocytome fibreux malin du mésentère. Aspects echographiques et scanographiques. J Radiol 66:241–244

Meis JM, Enzinger FM (1992) Inflammatory fibrosarcoma of the mesentery and retroperitoneum: a tumor closely simulating inflammatory pseudotumor. Radiology 184:292

Paling MR, Hyams DM (1982)Computed tomography in malignant fibrous histiocytoma. J Comput Assist Tomogr 6:785–788

Ros PR, Viamonte M Jr, Rywlin AM (1984) Malignant fibrous histiocytoma: mesenchymal tumor of ubiquitous origin. AJR Am J Roentgenol 142:753–759

Lipomatous

Bernardino ME, Jing BS, Wallace S (1979) Computed tomographic diagnosis of mesenteric masses. AJR Am J Roentgenol 132:33–36

Caprio F, Cerioni M, Giacomuzzi G, Amoroso L, Lanza R (1987) Possibilità di tipizzazione dei liposarcomi con TC. Radiol Med 74:221–224

Cohen WN, Seidelmann FE, Bryan PJ (1977) Computed tomography of localized adipose deposits presenting as tumor masses. AJR Am J Roentgenol 128:1007–1011

Dalla Palma L, Pozzi Mucelli R, Ricci C (1986) Ecografia e tomografia computerizzata nella diagnostica addominale. Radiol Med 72:795

Dalla Palma L (1989) Il retroperitoneo. Diagnostica per immagini. LINT, Trieste

Denath FM (1988) Intraperitoneal lipoblastoma. Semin Roentgenol 23:241–242

De Santos LA, Ginaldi S, Wallae S (1981) Computed tomography in liposarcoma. Cancer 47:46

Dooms GC, Hricak H, Sollitto RA, Higgins CB (1985) Lipomatous tumors with fatty component: MR imaging potential and comparison of MR and CT results. Radiology 157:479

Eresue J, Philippe JC, Casenave P, Laurent F, Grenier N, Simon JM, Drouillard J, Tavernier J (1984) La tomodensitométrie des lipomes et liposarcomes abdominaux de l'adulte. J Radiol 65:145

Ferrozzi F, Ferrozzi G, Draghi F, Rossi A (1990) La tomografia computerizzata nella tipizzazione delle neoplasie a componente adiposa: possibilità e limiti. Boll Soc Med Chir PC 14:82–89

Fisher MF, Fletcher BD, Dahms BB, Haller JO, Friedman AP (1981) Abdominal lipoblastomosis: radiographic, echographic and computed tomographic findings. Radiology 138:593–596

Friedman AC, Hartman DS, Sherman J, Laulin EM, Goldman SM (1981) Computed tomography of abdominal fatty masses. Radiology 139:415–429

Fultz PJ, Hampton WR, Skucas J, Sickel JZ (1993) Differential diagnosis of fat-containing lesion with abdominal and pelvic CT. Radiographics 13:1265–1280

Gerson ES, Gerzel SG, Robbins AH (1977) CT confirmation of pelvic lipomatosis. Two cases. AJR Am J Roentgenol 129:338–340

Gupta DK, Rohatgi M, Rao PS (1988) Mesenteric lipoma. Indian Pediatr 25:1007–1009

Kim T, Murakami T, Di H, et al (1996) CT and MR imaging of abdominal liposarcoma. AJR Am J Roentgenol 166:829–833

Lewis VL, Shaffer HA, Williamson BRJ (1982) Pseudotumoral lipomatosis of the abdomen. J Comput Assist Tomogr 6:79–82

Pistolesi GF, Procacci C, Caudana R, Bergamo Andreis IA, Manera V, Recla M, Grasso G, Florio C (1984) CT criteria of the differential diagnosis in primary retroperitoneal masses. Eur J Radiol 4:127–138

Rossi A, Ferrozzi F, Rossi G, Tosi C, Rossi L (1987) Integrazione ECO-TAC nella caratterizzazione tissutale dell'angiomiolipoma renale. Radiol Med 74:42–48

Schulman H, Barki Y, Hertzanu Y (1992) Case report: mesenteric lipoblastoma. Clin Radiol 46:57–58

Waligore MP, Stephens DH, Soule EH, McLeod RA (1981) Lipomatous tumor of the abdominal cavity: CT appearance and pathologic correlation. AJR Am J Roentgenol 137:539–545

Yannopoulus K, Stout AP (1963) Primary solid tumors of the mesentery. Cancer 16:914–927

Muscle Tissue

Smooth Muscle Tissue

Abulafia O, Angel C, Sherer DM, Fultz PJ, Bonfiglio TA, DuBeshter B (1993) Computed tomography of leiomyomatosis peritonealis disseminata with malignant transformation. Am J Obstet Gynecol 169:52–54

Alaniz Sanchez A, Castaneda Delgado Y (1994) Leiomiomatosis peritoneal diseminada con degeneracion maligna. Informe de un caso. Ginecol Obstet Mex 62:336–340

Choi BI, Lee WJ, Chi JG, et al (1990) CT manifestations of peritoneal leiomyosarcomatosis. AJR Am J Roentgenol 155:799

Kruczynski D, Merz E, Beck T, Bahlmann F, Wilkens C, Weber G, Macchiella D, Knapstein PG (1994) Minimalinvasive Therapie bei peritonealer Leiomyomatose. Ein Fallbericht über die diagnostische und therapeutische Problematik. Geburtshilfe Frauenheilkd 54:181–183

Lee JT, Kim MJ, Yoo HS, Suh HJ, Jeong HJ (1991)Primary leiomyosarcoma of the greater omentum: CT findings. J Comput Assist Tomogr 15:92–94

McLeod AJ, Zornoza J, Shirkhoda A (1984) Leiomyosarcoma: Computed tomographic findings. Radiology 152:133–136

Nguyen GK (1993) Disseminated leiomyomatosis peritonealis. Report of a case in a postmenopausal woman. Can J Surg 36:46–48

O'Brien JG, Allen JE, Queen TA (1986) Leiomyoma of the omentum in a child. J Pediatr Surg 21:981–982

Souda K, Shiramitzu T, Oka N, Tsumura H, Miyamoto Y (1984) Primary leiomyosarcoma of lesser sac. Jpn J Surg 14:505–509

Tsurumi H, Okada S, Koshino Y, Oyama M, Higaki H, Shimokawa K, Uamauchi O, Moriwaki H, Muto Y (1991) A case of leiomyoblastoma (epithelioid leiomyosarcoma) of the greater omentum. Gastroenterol Jpn 26:370–375

Villanueva A, Perez C, Sabate JM, Llauger J, Monill JM (1993) CT manifestations of peritoneal leiomyosarcomatosis. Eur J Radiol 17:166–169

Striated Muscle Tissue

Chung CJ, Bui V, Fordham LA, Hill J, Bulas D (1998) Malignant intraperitoneal neoplasm of childhood. Pediatr Radiol 28: 317–321

Chung L, Fordham L, Little S, Rayder S, Nimkin K, Kleinman PK, Watson I (1998) Intraperitoneal rhabdomyosarcoma in children: incidence and imaging characteristic on CT. AJR Am J Roentgenol 170:1385–1387

Blood Vessels

Hemangioendothelioma

Shin-Lin Shih, Jin-Cherng Sheu, Be-Fong Chen, Yei-Chang MA (1995) Malignant hemangioendothelioma presenting as omental masses in a child. J Pediatr Surg 30:118–119

Hemangiopericytoma

Alpern MB, Thorsen MK, Kellman GM, Pojunas K, Lawson TL (1986) CT appearance of hemangiopericytoma. J Comput Assist Tomogr 10:264–267

Bertolotto M, Cittadini G Jr, Crespi G, Perrone C, Pastorino R (1996) Hemangiopericytoma of the greater omentum: Us and CT appearance. Eur Radiol 6:454–456

Goldman SM, Davidson AJ, Neal J (1988) Retroperitoneal and pelvic hemangiopericytomas: clinical, radiologic, and pathologic correlation. Radiology 168:13–17

Hamrick-Turner JE, Chiechi MV, Abbit PL, Ros PR (1992) Neoplastic and inflammatory processes of the peritoneum, omentum, and mesentery: diagnosis with CT. Radiographics 12:1051–1068

Lorigan JG, David CL, Evans HL, Wallace S (1989) The clinical and radiologic manifestations of hemangiopericytoma. AJR Am J Roentgenol 153:345–349

Weekes RG, McLeod RA, Reiman HM, Pritchard DJ (1985) CT of soft-tissue neoplasms. AJR Am J Roentgenol 144:355–360

Yoo RE, Sunwoo YC, Markivee CR (1986) Male pelvic hemangiopericytoma on computed tomography. J Comput Assist Tomogr 10:73–76

Lymphatic Tissue

Blackledge G, Best JJK, Crowther D, Isherwood I (1980) Computed tomography (CT) in the staging of patients with Hodgkin's disease: a report of 136 patients. Clin Radiol 31:143–147

Brady LW, Asbell O (1980) Malignant lymphoma of the gastrointestinal tract. Radiology 137:291–298

Breiman RS, Castellino RA, Harrell GS, Marshall WH, Glatstein E, Kaplan HS (1978)CT pathologic correlations in Hodgkin's disease and non-Hodgkin's lymphoma. Radiology 126:159–166

Burgener FA, Hamlin DJ (1981) Histiocytic lymphoma of the abdomen: radiographic spectrum. AJR Am J Roentgenol 137:337–342

Buy JN, Moss AA (1982) Computed tomography of gastric lymphoma. AJR Am J Roentgenol 138:859–865

Castellino RA (1986) Hodgkin disease: practical concepts for the diagnostic radiologist. Radiology 159:305–310

Castellino RA, Cheng J (1989) Post-treatment calcification of mesenteric non-Hodgkin lymphoma: CT findings. J Comput Assist Tomogr 13:64

Castellino RA, Marglin S (1982) Imaging of the abdominal and pelvic lymph nodes: lymphography or computed tomography. Invest Radiol 17:433–443

Crowley KS, Don G, Gibson GE, et al (1982) Primary gastrointestinal lymphoma. A clinico-pathologic study of 28 cases. Aust NZ J Med 12:135–142

Dalla Palma L (1989) Il retroperitoneo. Diagnostica per immagini. LINT, Trieste

Ellert J, Kreel L (1980) The role of computed tomography in the initial staging and subsequent management of the lymphomas. J Comput Assist Tomogr 4:368

Goodman P, Raval B (1989) Omental cakes in American Burkitt lymphoma. Computed tomography demonstration. Clin Imaging 13:117–118

Harell GS, Breiman RS, Glatstein EJ, Marshall WH, Castellino RA (1977) Computed tomography of the abdomen in the malignant lymphomas. Radiol Clin North Am 15:391

Lee JKT, Stanley RJ, Sagel SS, Levitt RG (1978) Accuracy of computed tomography in detecting intraabdominal and pelvic adenopathy in lymphoma. AJR Am J Roentgenol 131:311–315

Lewis E, Bernardino ME, Salvador PG, Cabanillas FF, Barnes PA, Thomas JL (1982) Post-therapy CT detected mass in lymphoma patients: is it viable tissue? J Comput Assist Tomogr 6:792–795

Lynch MA, Cho KC, Jeffrey RB, Alterman DD, Federle MP (1988) CT of peritoneal lymphomatosis. AJR Am J Roentgenol 151:713–715

Megibow AJ, Balthazar EJ, Naidich DP, Bosniak MA (1983) Computed tomography of gastrointestinal lymphoma. AJR Am J Roentgenol 141:541–547

Mueller PR, Ferrucci JT Jr, Harbin WP, Kirkpatrick RH, Simeone JF, Wittenberg J (1980) Appearance of lymphomatous involvement of the mesentery by ultrasonography and body computed tomography: the "sandwich sing". Radiology 134:467–473

Neumann CH, Robert NJ, Camellas G, Rosenthal D (1983) Computed tomography of the abdomen and pelvis in non-Hodgkin lymphoma. J Comput Assist Tomogr 7:846–850

Pera A, Capek M, Shirkoda A (1987) Lymphangiography and CT in the follow-up of patients with lymphoma. Radiology 164:631–633

Pombo E, Rodriguez E, Caruncho MV, Villalva C, Crespo C (1994) CT attenuation values and enhancing characteristics of thoracoabdominal lymphomatous adenopathies. J Comput Assist Tomogr 18:59–62

Rahmouni A, Divine M, Lavaud A, Hayoun C, Reyes F, Vasile N (1993) Rôle de la tomodensitométrie dans le suivi évolutif de la maladie de Hodgkin. J Radiol 74:99–103

Schaner EG, Head GL, Doppman JL, Young RC (1977) Computed tomography in the diagnosis, staging, and management of abdominal lymphoma. J Comput Assist Tomogr 1:176–180

Van Krieken JHJM, Otter R, Hermans H, et al (1990) Malignant lymphoma of the gastrointestinal tract and mesentery: a clinico-pathologic study of the significance of histologic classification. Radiology 174:898

Zornoza J, Cabanillas FF, Altoff TM, Ordonez N, Cohen MA (1981) Percutaneous needle biopsy in abdominal lymphoma. AJR Am J Roentgenol 136:97–103

Nervous System

Neurinoma, Neurosarcoma, Neurofibroma, Neurofibrosarcoma, Neurofibrosarcomatosis

Bankier AA, Stanek C, Hubsch P (1996) Benign solitary schwannoma of the greater omentum: rare case of acute intraperitoneal bleeding diagnosis by CT. Clin Radiol 51:517–518

Bass IC, Korobkin M, Francis IR, Ellis JM, Coman RM (1994) Retroperitoneal plexiform neurofibromas: CT findings. AJR Am J Roentgenol 153:617–620

Biondetti PR, Vigo D, Fiore D, Faveri D, Ravasini R, Benedetti L (1983) CT appearance of generalized von Recklinghausen neurofibromatosis. J Comput Assist Tomogr 7:886–869

Breidahl WH, Khangure MS (1991) MRI of lumbar and sacral plexus nerve sheath tumors. Australas Radiol 35:140

Burk DL, Brunberg JA, Kanal E, Latchaw RE, Wolf GL (1987) Spinal and paraspinal neurofibromatosis: surface coil MR imaging at 1.5 T. Radiology 162:797–801

Cammarota T, Mecozzi B, Sarno A, Becchis G, Fava C (1993) Neurofibromatosi di von Recklinghausen. Descrizione di un caso caratterizzato da estese localizzazioni toraciche e addominali. Radiol Med 85:117–119

Cerofolini E, Landi A, De Santos G, Maiorana A, Canossi G, Romagnoli R (1991) MR of benign peripheral nerve sheath tumors. J Comput Assist Tomogr 15:593–597

Cohen LM, Schwartz AM, Rockoff SD (1986) Benign schwannomas: pathologic basis for CT inhomogeneities. AJR Am J Roentgenol 147:141–143

Coleman BG, Arger PH, Dalinka MK, Obringer AC, Raney BR, Meadows AT (1983) CT of sarcomatous degeneration in neurofibromatosis. AJR Am J Roentgenol 140:383–387

Daneman A, Mancer K, Sonley M (1983) CT appearances of thickened nerves in neurofibromatosis. AJR Am J Roentgenol 141:899–900

Day DL, Allan BT (1985a) Pediatric case of the day. AJR Am J Roentgenol 144:1296–1302

Day DL, Allan BT (1985b) Plexiform neurofibroma in neurofibromatosis. AJR Am J Roentgenol 144:1300–1302

Dietemann JL, Sick H, Wolfram-Gabel R, Cruz da Silva R, Kontke JG, Wackenheim A (1987) Anatomy and computed tomography of the normal lumbosacral plexus. Neuroradiology 29:58–68

Di Franco SA, Trovatello AB, Broggi B, Di Franco F (1995) Il neurofibroma del mesentere: descrizione di un caso. Acta Chir Mediterr 11:9

Gebarski KS, Gebarski SS, Glazer GM, Samuels BI, Francis IR (1986) The lumbosacral plexus: anatomic radiologic-pathologic correlation using CT. Radiographics 6:401–425

Gierada DS, Erickson SJ, Haughto VM, Estkowski LD, Nowichki BH (1993) MR imaging of the sacral plexus: normal findings. AJR Am J Roentgenol 160:1059–1065

Gossios KJ, Guy RL (1993) Case report: imaging of widespread plexiform neurofibromatosis. Clin Radiol 47:211–213

Hammond JA, Driedger AA (1978) Detection of malignant change in neurofibromatosis (von Recklinghausen's disease) by gallium-67 scanning. Can Med Assoc J 119:352–353

Kalff V, Shapiro B, Lloyd R, et al (1982) The spectrum of pheochromocytoma in hypertensive patients with neurofibromatosis. Arch Intern Med 142:2092

Kodama A, Sakamoto K, Hase M, Yonezawa K, Sako M, Kono M, Miura J, Furumoto M (1989) Neurilemmoma of lesser omentum. Rinsho Hoshasen 34:1417–1420

Kumar AJ, Kuhajda P, Martinez CR, Fishman EK, Jezic DV, Siegelman SS (1983) Computed tomography of extracranial nerve sheath tumors with pathological correlation. J Comput Assist Tomogr 7:857–863

Lederman SM, Martin EC, Laffey KT, Lefkowitch JH (1987) Hepatic neurofibromatosis, malignant schwannoma, and angiosarcoma in von Recklinghausen's disease. Gastroenterology 92:234–239

Lee K, Ono K, Suzuki K, Yamamoto Y, Miyagawa M, Okuyama T, Ishiwata H, Kano M, Tsubaki K, Ishizuka H, et al (1992) A case of neurinoma arising from the lesser omentum in differentiating from primary hepatic cancer. Nippon Shokakibyo Gabbai Zasshi 89:538–541

Levine E, Huntrakoon M, Wetzel LH (1987) Malignant nerve-sheath neoplasms in neurofibromatosis: distinction from benign tumors by using imaging techniques. AJR Am J Roentgenol 149:1059–1064

McDonnell CH III, McLeod M, Baker ME (1990) Primary peritoneal neuroblastoma: computed tomography findings. Clin Imaging 14:41–44

Mirich DR, Gray RR, Grosman H (1989) Abdominal plexiform neurofibromatosis simulating pseudomyxoma peritonei on computed tomography. J Comput Assist Tomogr 13:709–711

Paling MR (1984) Plexiform neurofibroma of the pelvis in neurofibromatosis: CT findings. J Comput Assist Tomogr 8:476–478

Png MA, Teh HS, Poh WT (1995) Angiosarcoma in a patient with von Reckinghausen's disease. Clin Radiol 51:521–523

Reinbold WD, Wimmer B, Adler CP, Genant HK (1987) Radiologic findings in peripheral neurilemmoma. Eur J Radiol 7:268–273

Rodriguez E, Pombo F, Rodriguez I, Vasquez-Iglesias JL, Galed I, et al (1993) Diffuse intrahepatic periportal plexiform neurofibroma. Eur J Radiol 16:151–156

Ros PR, Eshaghi N (1991) Plexiform neurofibroma of the pelvis: CT and MRI findings. Magn Reson Imaging 9:463–465

Sakai F, Sone S, Yanagisawa S, Ishii Z (1988) Schwannoma of the lesser omentum. Eur J Radiol 8:113–114

Shu HN, Mirowitz SA, Wippolo FJ (1993) Neurofibromatosis. MR imaging findings involving the head and spine. AJR Am J Roentgenol 160:159–164

Suh JS, Abenoza P, Galloway HR, Everson LI, Griffiths HJ (1992) Peripheral (extracranial) nerve tumors: correlation of MR imaging and histologic findings. Radiology 183:341

Varma DGK, Moulopoulos A, et al (1992) MR imaging of extracranial nerve sheath tumors. J Comput Assist Tomogr 16:448

Carcinoid

Adolph JM, Kimming BN, Georgi P, et al (1987) Carcinoid tumors: CT and I-131 meta-iodo-benzylguanidine scintigraphy. Radiology 164:199–203

Andersson T, Eriksson B, Hemmingsson A, Lindgren PG, Oberg K (1987) Angiography, computed tomography, magnetic resonance imaging and ultrasonography in detection of liver metastases from endocrine gastrointestinal tumours. Acta Radiol 28:535–539

Balthazar EJ (1978) Carcinoid tumors of the alimentary tract. Gastrointest Radiol 3:47–56

Bressler PL, Alpern MB, Glazer GM, et al (1987) Hypervascular hepatic metastases: CT evaluation. Radiology 162:49–53

Buck JL, Sobin LH (1990) Carcinoids of the gastrointestinal tract. Radiographics 10:1081–1095

Chopier-Richaud J, Quahes N, Breittmayer F, Lotz JP, Bigor JM (1993) Tumeurs carcinoïdes digestives. J Radiol 74:279–282

Cirillo LC, Maurano A, Miniero E, Chef GM, Di Palma R, Iovino P, Orabona P (1992) Su di un raro caso di disseminazione secondaria da carcinoide intestinale. Ital Curr Radiol 11:107–112

Cockey BM, Fishman EK, Jones B, Siegelman SS (1985) Computed tomography of abdominal carcinoid tumor. J Comput Assist Tomogr 9:38–42

De Santis M, Santini D, Alborino S, Carubbi F, Romagnoli R (1996) Metastasi epatiche da carcinoide: semeiotica per immagini. Radiol Med 92:594–599

Dudiak KM, Johnson CD, Stephens DH (1989) Primary tumors of the small intestine. CT evaluation. AJR Am J Roentgenol 152:995–998

Falaschi F, Boraschi P, Battolla L, Braccini G, Salvadori R, Bagnolesi P (1993) Diagnosi con tomografia computerizzata del carcinoide dell'intestino tenue. Radiol Med 86:472–477

Gould M, Johnson RJ (1986) Computed tomography of abdominal carcinoid tumor. Br J Radiol 59:881–885

Halvorsen RA, Wilkinson RH, Feldman JM (1987) Carcinoid liver metastases: accuracy of radionuclide liver/spleen imaging compared to computed tomography. Clin Nucl Med 12:268–273

Hamrick-Turner JE, Chiechi MV, Abbitt PL, Ros PR (1992) Neoplastic and inflammatory processes of the peritoneum, omentum and mesentery: diagnosis with CT. Radiographics 12:1051–1068

McCarthy SM, Stark DD, Moss AA, Golberg HI (1984) Computed Tomography of malignant carcinoid disease. J Comput Assist Tomogr 8:846–850

Merine D, Fishman EK, Jones B (1989) CT of the small bowel and mesentery. Radiol Clin North Am 27:707–715

Picus D, Glazer HS, Levitt RG, Husband JE (1984) Computed tomography of abdominal carcinoid tumors. AJR Am J Roentgenol 143:581–584

Sako M, Lunderquist A, Owman T, Martensson H, Nobin A (1982) Angiographic and computed tomographic appearance of secondary carcinoid of the liver. Cardiovasc Intervent Radiol 5:90–96

Seigel RS, Kuhns LR, Borlaza GS, McCormick TL, Simmons JL (1980) Computed tomography and angiography in ileal carcinoid tumor and retractile mesenteritis. Radiology 134:437–440

Smevik B, Kolmannskog F, Aakhus T (1983) Computed tomography and angiography in carcinoid liver metastases. Acta Radiol [Diagn] 24:189–193

Tamura Y, Katoh N, Taniguchi Y, Tanaka T, Sugawara K, Sekiya C, Naniki M (1990) A case of ileal carcinoid tumor with mesenteric retraction. Nippon Shokakibyo Gakkai Zasshi 87:2404–2409

Woodard PK, Feldman JM, Paine SS, Baker ME (1995) Midgut carcinoid tumors: CT findings and biochemical profiles. J Comput Assist Tomogr 19:400–405

13 Diffusion of Malignant Tumors of Intraperitoneal Organs to the Peritoneum, Ligaments, Mesenteries, Omentum and Lymph Nodes

CONTENTS

13.1 General Considerations

The spread of tumors arising from intraperitoneal organs occurs by permeation of tissues occupying the interstices of mesenteries and ligaments, through the lymphatic visceral network and derivative collectors, by direct or indirect invasion of the peritoneum and subsequent intraperitoneal dissemination or by the hematic route (Table 13.1).

Table 13.1. Ways of tumoral diffusion

a) Through tissue interstices of mesenteries and ligaments
b) Through the peritoneum and its cavity
c) By lymphatic route
d) By venous route

From the periphery of the tumor, the malignant cells function as plugs penetrating the tissues of all the subperitoneal interstices along the less resistant planes. They grow more slowly or stop growing only in the proximity of structures made of compact fibrous tissue, such as visceral (hepatic, splenic, renal) capsules and fasciae.

In addition, the neoplastic plugs penetrate the lymphatic collectors and are passively transported by the lymphatic flux as emboli constituted by a single cell or by groups of cells, or they grow significantly, occupying the total lumen. Once invaded, the lymphatic vessels constitute a neoplastic network called carcinomatous lymphangitis. Along their lymphatic migration, the cells cross one or more lymph node stations before reaching the intestinal and thoracic ducts and, thus, the venous circulation. In the lymph node marginal sinus, some cells are stopped and phagocytized, whereas other cells adhere to the wall of the sinus and invade the medullary or continue their trip through the efferent collectors or the venous circulation, where they arrive through numerous lymphatic-venous communications.

When a lymphatic block is caused by total invasion of one or more lymph nodes and/or obstruction of the lymphatic collectors, the neoplastic diffusion occurs in the anterograde or retrograde direction through collateral pathways, which may be close to or even far from the primary tumor. Therefore, when possible secondary lymph node localizations are searched, it is necessary not only to follow the normal lymphatic flux, but also to examine the stations that may have been reached by the neoplastic embolus through collateral or retrograde paths.

Analogously, when a suggestive lymph node is found, the primary tumor may sometimes be discovered by following the lymphatic flux in a retrograde direction.

The venous diffusion of the neoplastic cells coming from an intraperitoneal viscus follows two pathways: a direct one from the veins located in the peripheral part of the tumor, and an indirect path through the lymph nodal lymphatic-venous anastomoses or by invasion of the intra- or peri-lymph node venulae.

Most neoplastic cells reach the liver through the portal circulation whether they come directly from the primary tumor or have crossed the lymph nodal lymphatic-venous communications.

These cells stop and proliferate at the level of the sinusoids. By following the thoracic duct, only a low number of cells reach the left jugular vein and, through the systemic circulation, the lung, where they are stopped at the capillary level.

The pattern of venous diffusion of the intraperitoneal tumors explains why hepatic metastases are often observed, whereas secondary pulmonary localizations are less frequent.

The tumoral plugs invade the peritoneum by contiguous diffusion in sites where the serosa takes close contacts with the infiltrated visceral wall, by penetrating the subperitoneal interstices or by following the lymphatic collectors of the fatty tissue located between the viscus and the serosa and thus spreading to the whole serosa through the peritoneal lymphatic network. Once they are in the cavity, the tumoral cells quickly spread into all recesses and settle in the peritoneal walls. Their settlement and diffusion are favored by the flux of the peritoneal fluid and by variations in intracavitary pressure during respiration and movements, which push the cells toward the superior compartments, and by gravity, which attracts the cells toward the lowest parts. The disposition and communication between the supra- and submesocolic compartments only influence the primary and preferential localization, without stopping the neoplastic progression and spread: to the right subphrenic and subhepatic (Morrison's pouch) recesses for the supramesocolic tumors, to the pouch of Douglas for the submesocolic tumors. This distinction does not exclude the possibility that metastases originating from supramesocolic organs will first become evident in the submesocolic cavities and that pelvic tumors may initially metastasize in the supramesocolic compartments, after following the paracolic gutters, especially on the right side. A significant example of this phenomenon is provided by the peritoneal spread of ovarian tumors, which frequently metastasize into the right subphrenic recess between the diaphragm and the hepatic dome in 61% of cases (Meyers 1973, 1988).

The peritoneal invasion and spread are more frequent and rapid in the case of tumors that originate from organs with a serosa that is more closely and widely adherent (such as the stomach and the transverse colon) or constitutes part of the structure of the organ itself, such as the ovaries, because they are favored by the direct involvement of the peritoneum.

In the CT examination of the spread of an intraperitoneal tumor, the evaluation of the tumoral expansion, the involvement of the perivisceral fatty tissue, the ligaments and the mesenteries, the infiltration of the peritoneum, the extension to the peritoneal cavity, the lymphatic permeation, the lymph node enlargements and the metastases in distant parenchymatous organs must always be evaluated. The last phenomenon will not be discussed, because it is not relevant to the purpose of this text.

When the tumor has not exceeded the limits, the visceral profile is sharp and the adjacent adipose cellular is transparent, as in the other zones (Figs. 13.23–13.25, 13.46, 13.51). In contrast, in the case of tumors that have passed beyond the wall (Table 13.2) the contours are shaded or thinly dentate with linear and sinuous shoots, which sink to variable depths into the adipose tissue of the ligaments and mesenteries; these latter appear shaded or denser (Figs. 13. 26–13.37, 13.44, 13.45, 13.52–13.54).

Table 13.2. CT signs of tumoral extension outside the bowel wall

Dentate profile of the wall
Strands of soft tissue extending from the outer intestinal wall into the peritoneal fat
Higher density or loss of the fat in the perivisceral planes

The tumors that reach the peritoneum increase its thickness and density in a linear or multimicronodular fashion (Figs. 13.38–13.42, 13.48, 13.55, 13.56).

Infiltrations of the mesenteric peritoneum, especially those occurring in the diffusion of ovarian tumors, may widely involve the serosa, showing sinuous "railtrack-like" striations on both sides of the secondary branches of the mesenteric vessels. These striae are in a transverse or "fan-like" arrangement without intersections (Fig. 13.41).

When the peritoneal wall is overtaken and intraperitoneal spreading (carcinosis) occurs, various isolated or associated characteristic signs become evident. The most common, and the earliest of these signs is by ascites (Table 13.3).

Table 13.3. CT signs of peritoneal and omental spread of tumors

Peritoneal thickening with increased postcontrast density
Ascites
Peritoneal nodules, masses or plaques
Peritoneal nodular calcifications
Pseudomyxoma
Omental permeation
Omental nodules or masses with increased postcontrast density
Wide omental plaque (omental cake)

Ascites may widely occupy and swell the peritoneal cavity, pushing the lower abdominal organs away from the abdominal wall and the iliac and colic loops medially and backward; on the other hand, it may be confined in one or more spaces, preferentially in the right subphrenic and subhepatic recesses, in the pouch of Douglas and in the right paracolic gutter.

The presence of an ascitic collection clearly shows the peritoneal profile (Figs. 4.16, 4.17, 4.20, 13.1–13.3), either in normal conditions, when it

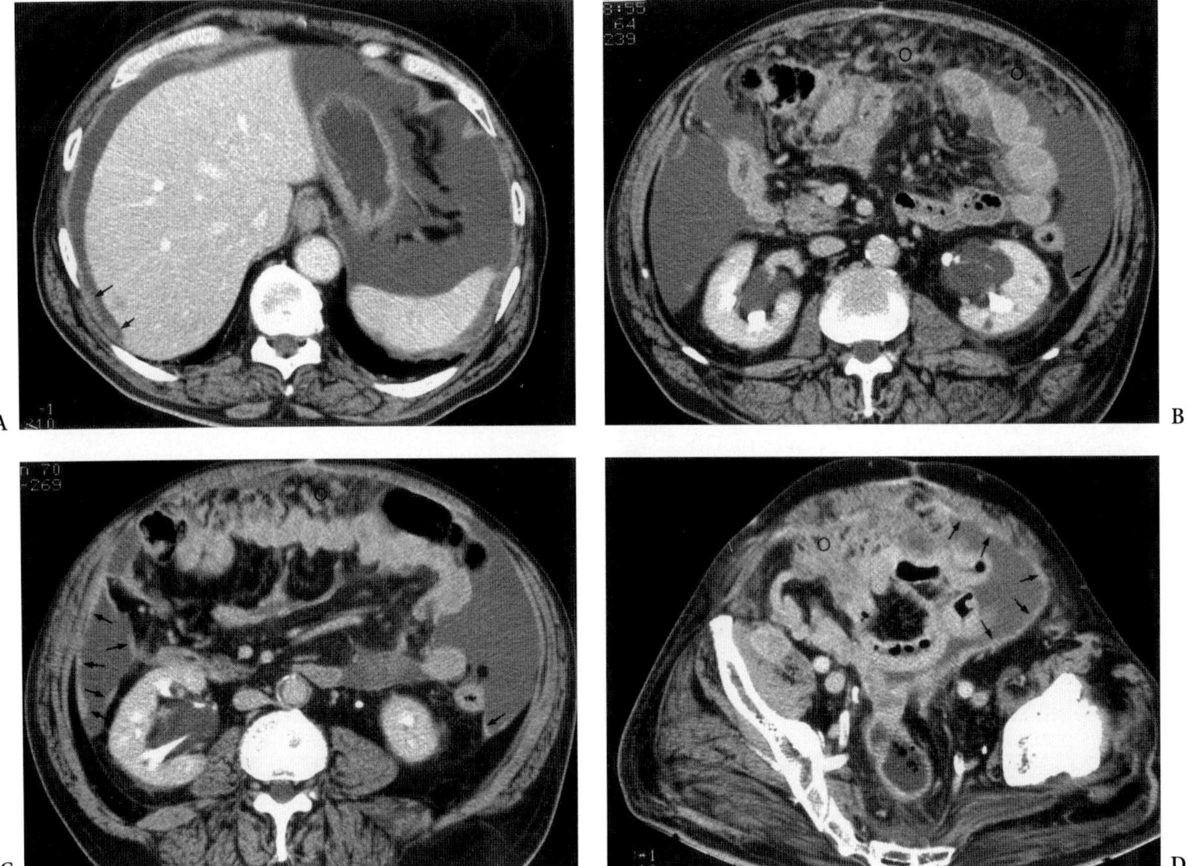

Fig. 13.1A–D. Peritoneal carcinosis and omental metastases from a tumor of the ascending colon. Ascites swelling the supra- and submesocolic peritoneal and the pelvic cavities. The parietal peritoneum is denser and thickening (*arrows*) with nodules and plaques at the abdominal level (**A–C**) and a thick pigskin-like mass in the pelvis (**D**). Dense and nonhomogeneous omental plaque including areas of adipose tissue (**B–D**)

appears as a very thin line with a smooth profile, or in the case of metastatic carcinomatosis, when the peritoneum is thickening with small nodules and plaques protruding from its surface into the cavity, and giving a fine granular appearance to its internal profile (Figs. 13.1, 13.2). Generally, these micronodules become evident in the case of ascites and more visible after contrast medium injection, because of their increased density. They may affect just a short tract of the serosa.

The extension of the tumor to the peritoneal cavity may also be shown by the presence of nodules, masses or plaques with a nonhomogeneous structure on the internal surface of the parietal peritoneum. These formations become more evident after contrast medium (Figs. 13.4, 13.6, 13.8, 13.16).

Nodules and plaques may be located everywhere in the peritoneum, but they are preferentially observed in the subphrenic recesses and in the pouch of Douglas; sometimes they are calcified (Figs. 13.2, 13.10, 13.11).These calcifications are mostly psammomatous in nature within metastases of ovarian cystadenocarcinoma, but they may also be represented by metastases of mucinous colonic carcinoma, gastric carcinoma, renal tumor or peritoneal mesothelioma; calcifications can also occur within metastatic nodules of various origins after chemotherapy.

Pseudomyxoma peritonei is characterized by the spread over the peritoneal cavity of myxomatous or gelatinous material following the rupture of a mucinous ovarian or pancreatic cystadenocarcinoma or of an appendiceal mucocele. Less frequently, it is due to a tumor of the urachus, uterus, or omphalomesenteric duct and Sertoli-Leydig's ovarian cells; it is preferentially located in the lowest parts of the cavity and tends to be made up of several pseudocysts of variable number and width.

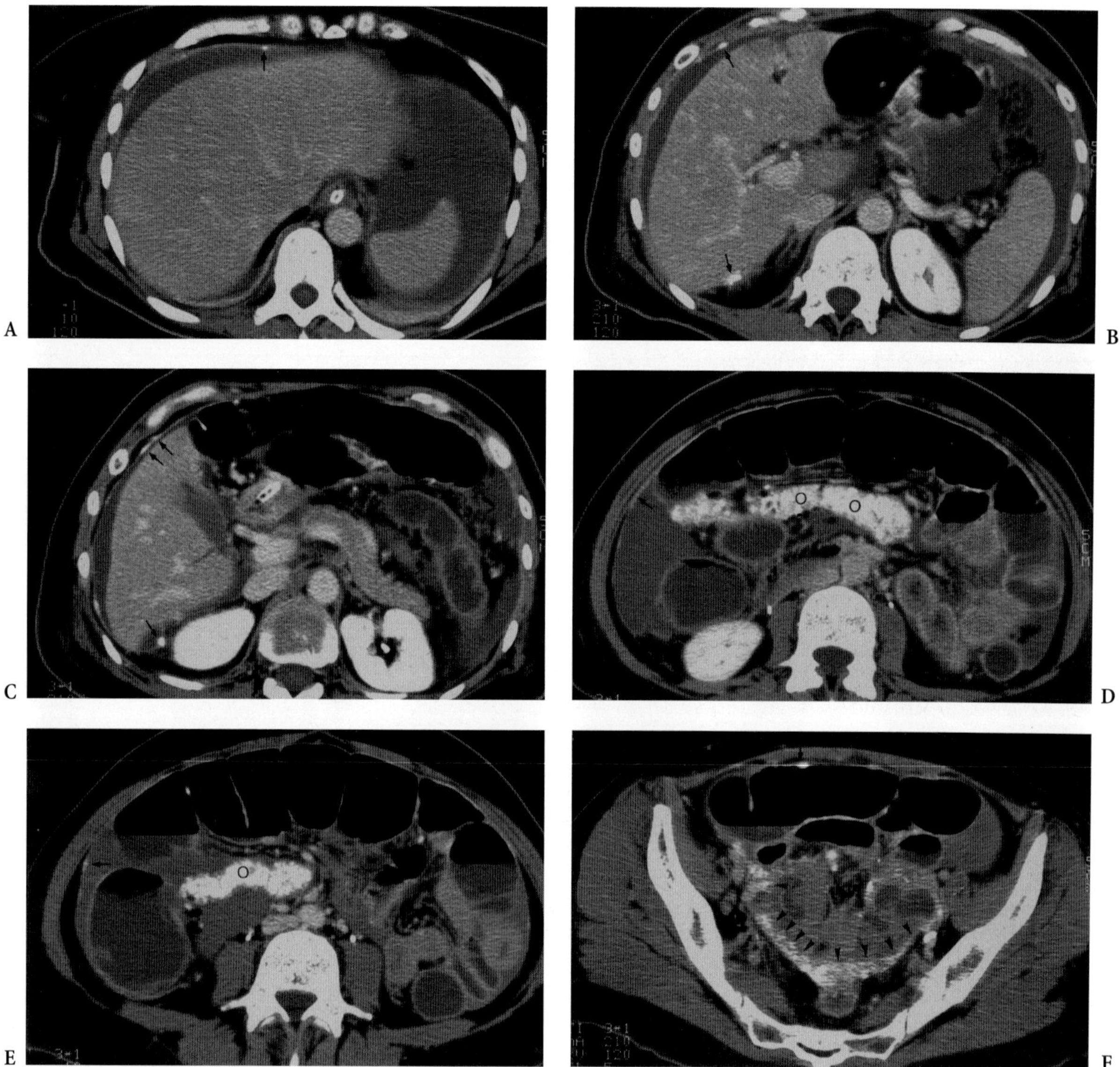

Fig. 13.2A–F. Carcinosis from ovarian cystadenocarcinoma. Ascites in the supramesocolic and pelvic cavities. Calcified nodules and plaques on the internal face of the parietal peritoneum (*small arrows*). Thick metastatic calcified plaque involving the whole omentum (*O*), which has slid under and behind the transverse mesocolon. In the pelvis, the calcified peritoneum (*arrowhead*) around the ovarian mass extends in a semicircular shape above the broad ligaments and the fundus uteri (**F**)

The pseudomyxoma is asymptomatic for a long time; it becomes evident only after abundant intraperitoneal accumulation of myxomatous material with abdominal swelling; nausea and vomiting may be present, or complications such as an obstructive acute abdominal syndrome may develop.

On CT examination, the pseudomyxoma is characterized by cyst-like round structures, which are uni- or multilocular with a low and nonhomogeneous density and a thin border becoming hyperdense after contrast medium. These masses develop in the peritoneal cavity; they displace the loops of the small intestine toward the center and push liver, spleen and intestinal loops away from the abdominal wall (Figs. 13.17–13.21, 13.71).

A characteristic scalloping of the liver and spleen edges is due to the arcuate marks impressed by the pseudomyxomatous pseudocysts on the walls (Figs. 13.17, 13.18, 13.71).

The disposition and the low density of the pseudomyxoma may sometimes simulate an ascites; however, the characteristic cyst-like images and the

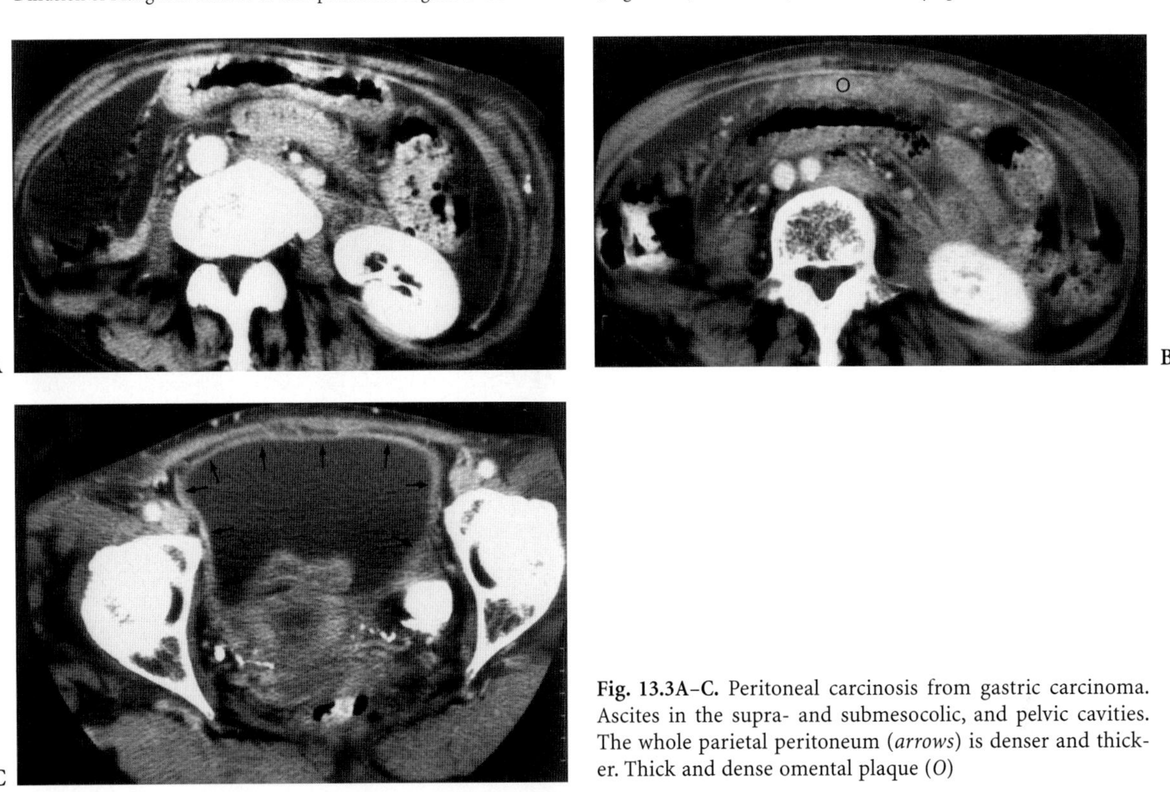

Fig. 13.3A–C. Peritoneal carcinosis from gastric carcinoma. Ascites in the supra- and submesocolic, and pelvic cavities. The whole parietal peritoneum (*arrows*) is denser and thicker. Thick and dense omental plaque (*O*)

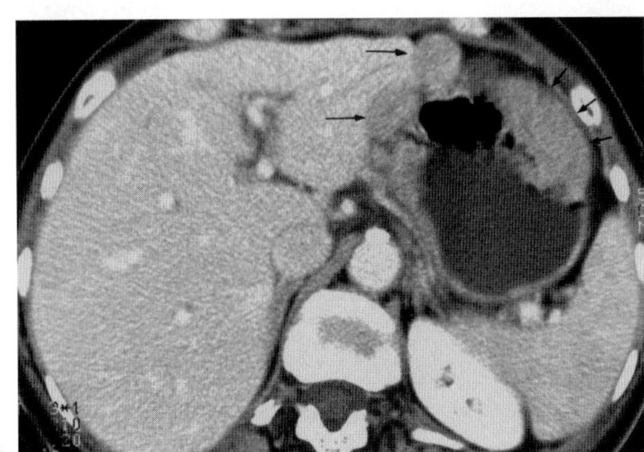

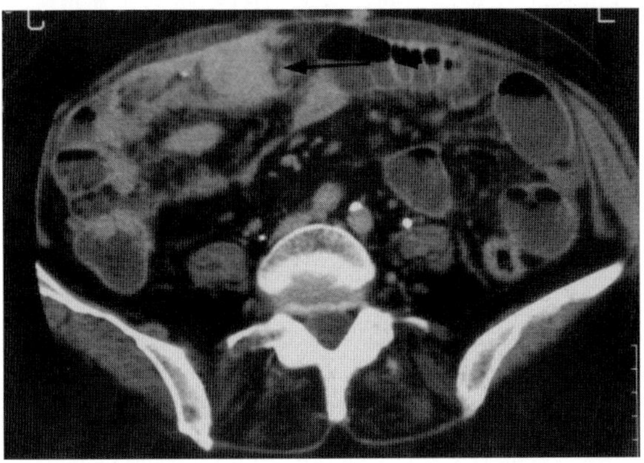

Fig. 13.4A, B. Peritoneal and omental metastasis from ovarian adenocarcinoma. Solid masses in the peritoneum constituting the gastrohepatic (*arrows*) and gastrocolic (*small arrows*) ligaments (**A**) and in the omentum (**B** *long arrow*)

incisures of the hepatic and splenic profile distinguish a pseudomyxoma from ascites.

Pseudomyxomatous pseudocysts may calcify after chemotherapy (Miller et al. 1985).

A particular form of metastatic peritoneal diffusion is that adopted by leiomyosarcomatous metastases, which develop in the peritoneal cavity as masses with a smooth surface and a necrotic-hemorrhagic center; on CT examination, they appear as structures with a well-defined profile and a solid structure containing wide central areas of low attenuation. Contrast medium strikingly increases the opacity of the solid component (Figs. 13.13, 13.14). These metastases displace the intestinal loops without infiltrations and may reach a conspicuous volume; however, they never cause ascites or lymphadenomegalies, but rather are frequently associated with hepatic metastases showing the same characteristics as the primary tumor (Figs. 13.14).

Other peritoneal metastatic masses or nodules often reproduce the characteristics of the primary tumors: for example, areas of adipose density are

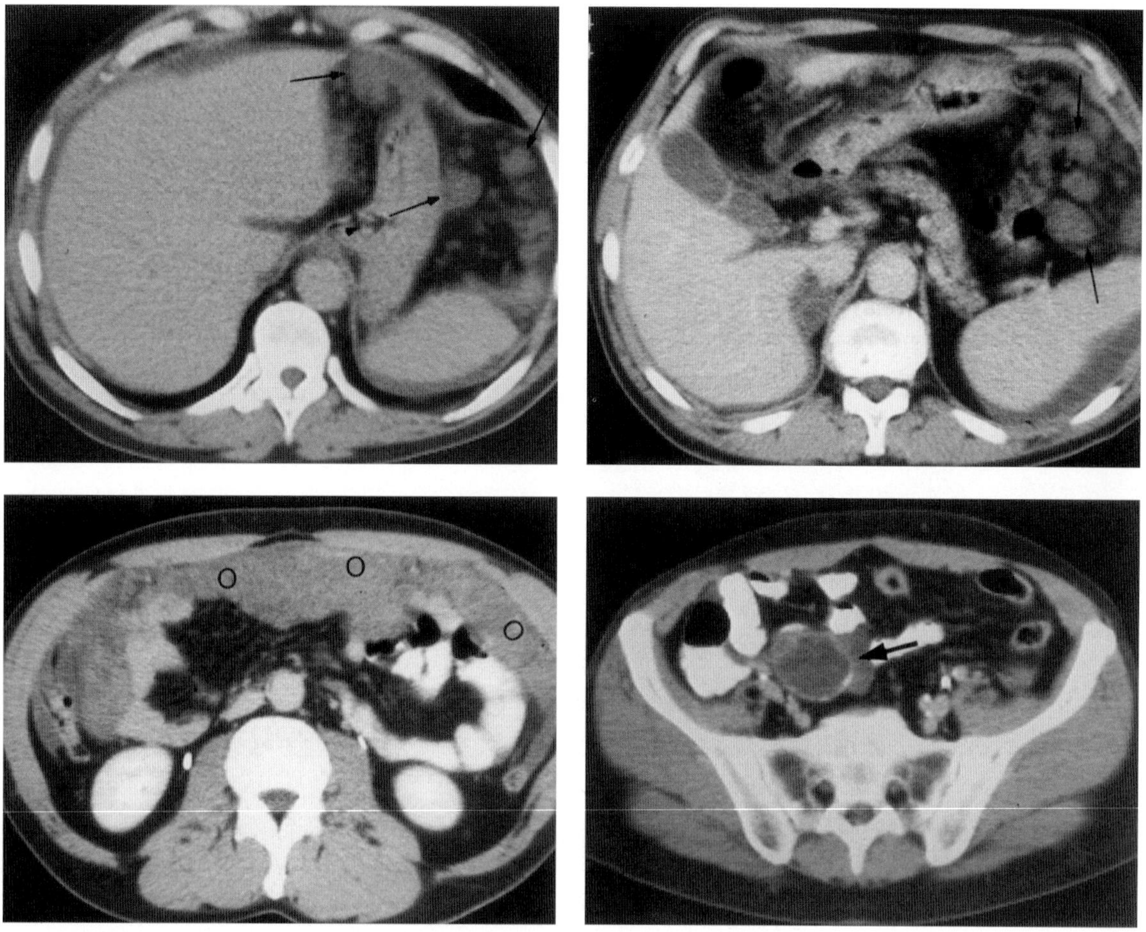

Fig. 13.5A–D. Multiple metastases from a mucoid appendiceal adenocarcinoma. **A, B** Ascitic fluid in the supramesocolic recesses and multiple subperitoneal solid nodules (*thin arrows*) in the gastrocolic and gastrosplenic ligaments. **C** Thick omental cake (*O*) extending in a semicircular shape in front of the ileal loops and the mesentery. **D** Primary tumor of the appendix with mucoid cyst-like aspect (*thick arrow*)

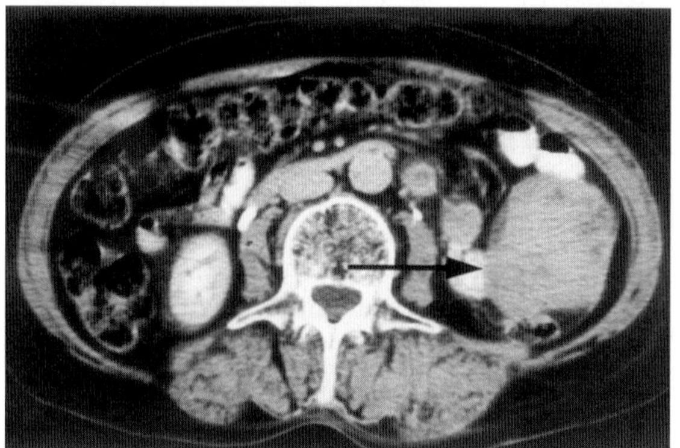

Fig. 13.6. Intraperitoneal nodular metastasis from rhabdomyosarcoma of the left quadratus lumborum muscle. Bosselated mass with a sharp profile and hypodense necrotic spots inside, located in the left paracolic peritoneal gutter in front of the ascending colon and the lateroconal compartment

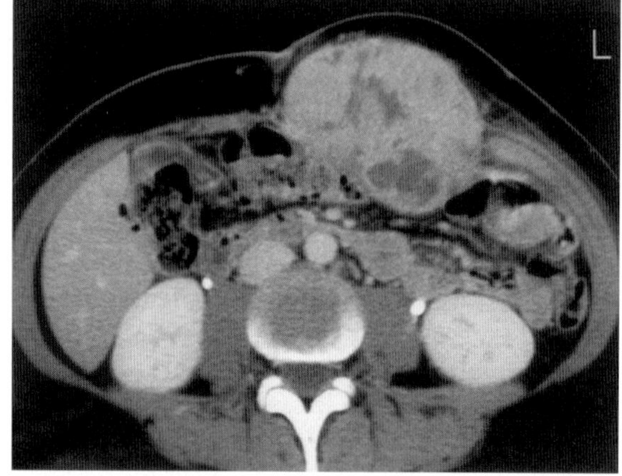

Fig. 13.7. Nodular metastasis from a hepatoma. Solid necrotic mass extending from the omentum to the skin

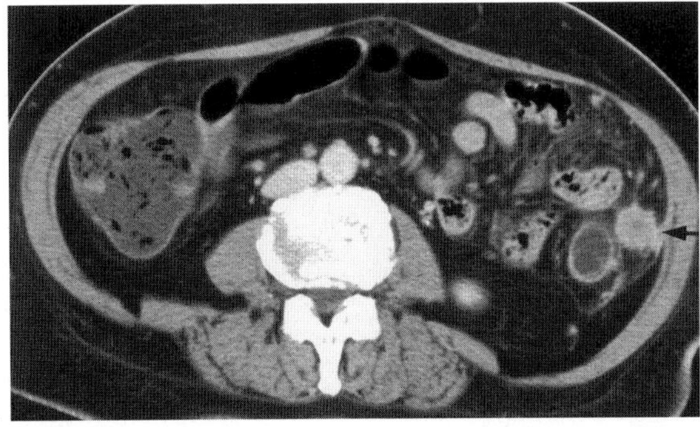
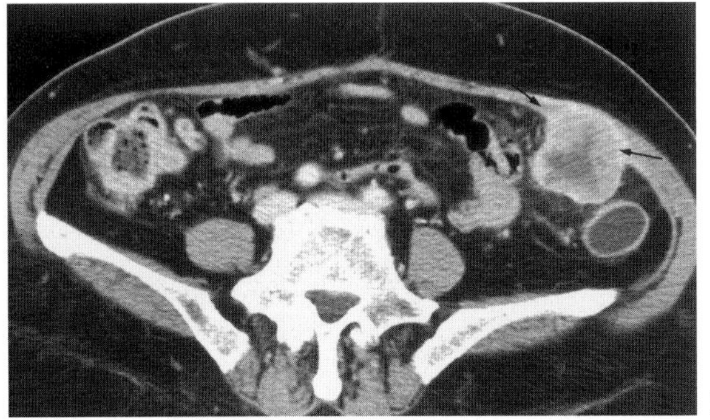

Fig. 13.8A, B. Nodular metastases from ovarian cystadenocarcinoma. Presence of two colliquative masses: **A** in the paracolic gutter, in front of the descending colon and the left lateroconal compartment (*arrowhead*); **B** the other is in the left paramedian part of the omentum and has passed the transversalis fascia, invading the obliqui abdominis muscles (*small arrows*)

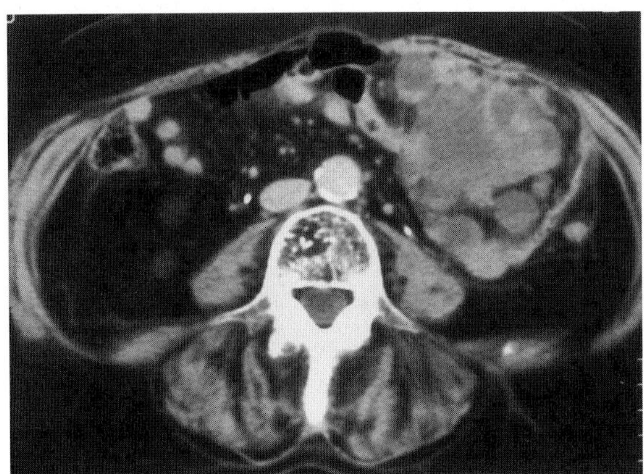
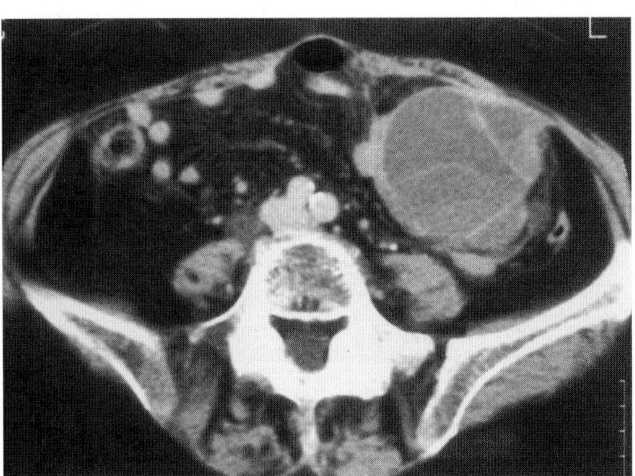

Fig. 13.9A, B. Omental metastases from ovarian cystadenocarcinoma. Multiple cyst-like nodular masses

found in metastases from liposarcomas (Fig. 13.16) and cyst-like appearances in metastases from ovarian cystadenocarcinoma (Fig. 13.9).

Round nodular images with a center of low attenuation and contours that become hyperdense after contrast medium may be due to ileal loops stretched by liquid and can sometimes simulate intraperitoneal metastatic nodules, especially when concomitant secondary lesions are present in other sites (Fig. 13.15); however, a careful examination can easily provide a differential diagnosis.

A secondary invasion of the omentum is prevalently consequent on ovarian tumors and on relapses of carcinomas of the colon and the stomach. CT shows several different aspects of omental involvement; sometimes, localizations are easily visible, whereas in other situations they are only recognizable within the transparency between the internal profile of the abdominal wall, the ileal loops and the colon. In these cases, the transparency may be more or less reduced, uniformly or irregularly distributed in spots; it is crossed by linear or serpiginous striations, which tend to constitute a very thin or rough network among the omental vessels (Fig. 13.45).

In most cases, solid nodular omental metastases become nonhomogeneously opaque after contrast medium. Furthermore, the largest masses usually show hypodense colliquative areas inside (Figs. 13.4, 13.7–13.9, 13.12, 13.16).

Like those located in the peritoneum, omental nodules may calcify, constituting psammomatous masses (Figs. 13.2, 13.10) that are typical of the secondary localizations of ovarian cystadenocarcinoma, but sometimes also of colonic mucinous carcinoma, gastric carcinoma, peritoneal mesothelioma, or they may be a consequence of chemotherapy. A massive invasion of the omentum is characterized by a thick and dense cake-like plaque, which extends transversely either uniformly or as multiple converging nodules and is sometimes calcified

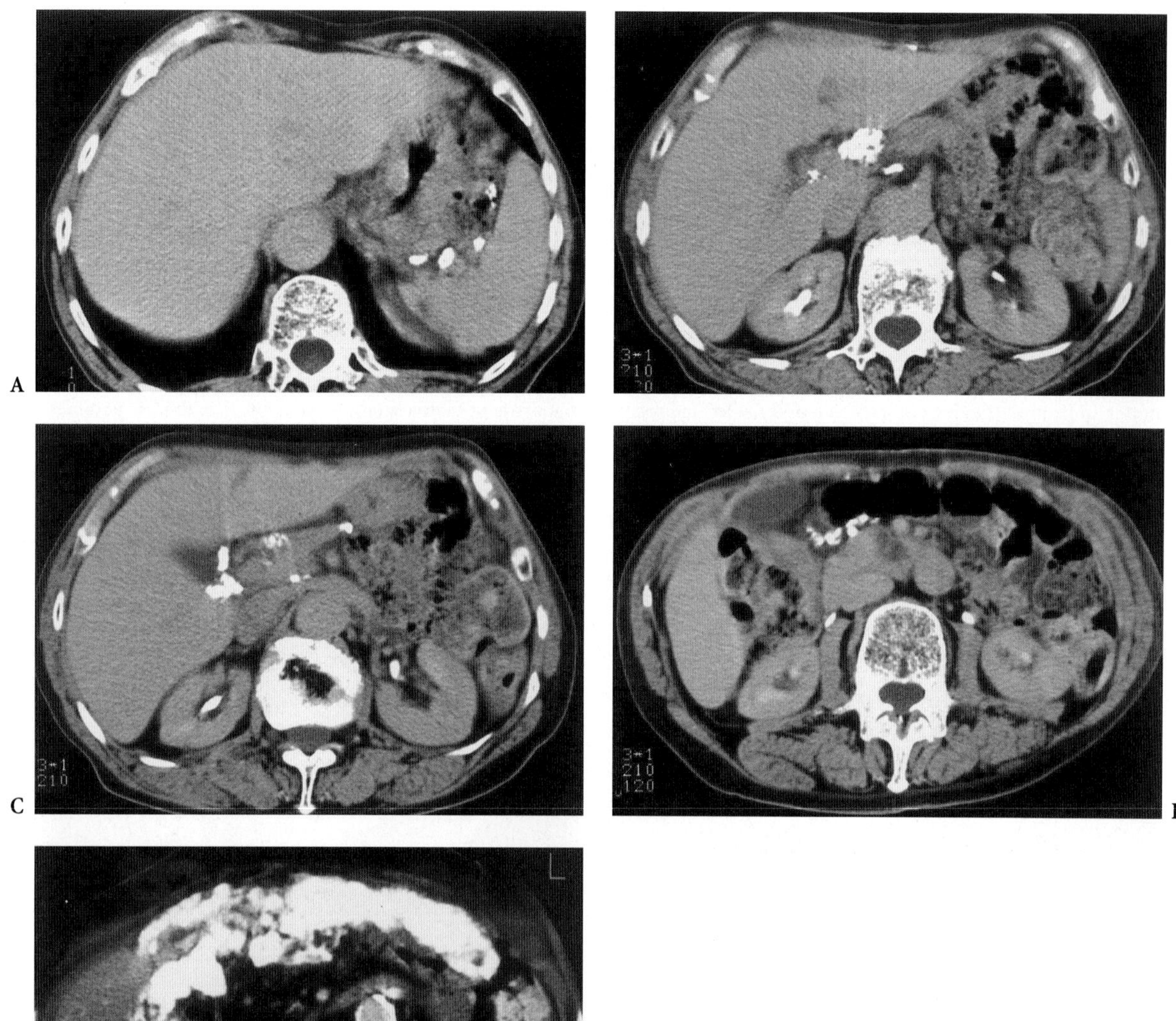

Fig. 13.10A–E. Calcified metastases from ovarian adenocarcinoma. Calcified nodules in the **A** perisplenic and **B**, **C** perihepatic peritoneum, and in the **C** gastrohepatic and **D**, **E** gastrocolic ligaments; calcified omental cake (**E**)

(Fig. 13.10). It pushes the transverse colon and the loops of the small intestine away from the anterior abdominal wall (Figs. 13.1–13.3, 13.5, 13.10). Even though this appearance is typical of this kind of secondary infiltration, it can also be observed in peritoneal mesotheliomas, tuberculous omental localizations and acute pancreatitis. This last pathology must always be considered in the differential diagnosis when abdominal tumors have not been already diagnosed (Cooper et al. 1986).

The intraperitoneal tumors spread by lymphatic pathway through collectors which drain the lymph flowing from the visceral network to lymph nodes near the tumor, then to secondary or intermediary stations located within the subperitoneal spaces of ligaments and mesenteries and finally to distal or central lymph nodes in the retroperitoneum, next to the celiac trunk and the mesenteric arteries.

In order to define a metastatic adenopathy, we consider the following parameters: dimensions, structure, density before and after contrast medium, configuration, number and position of the lymph nodes according to the tumoral location (Table 13.4).

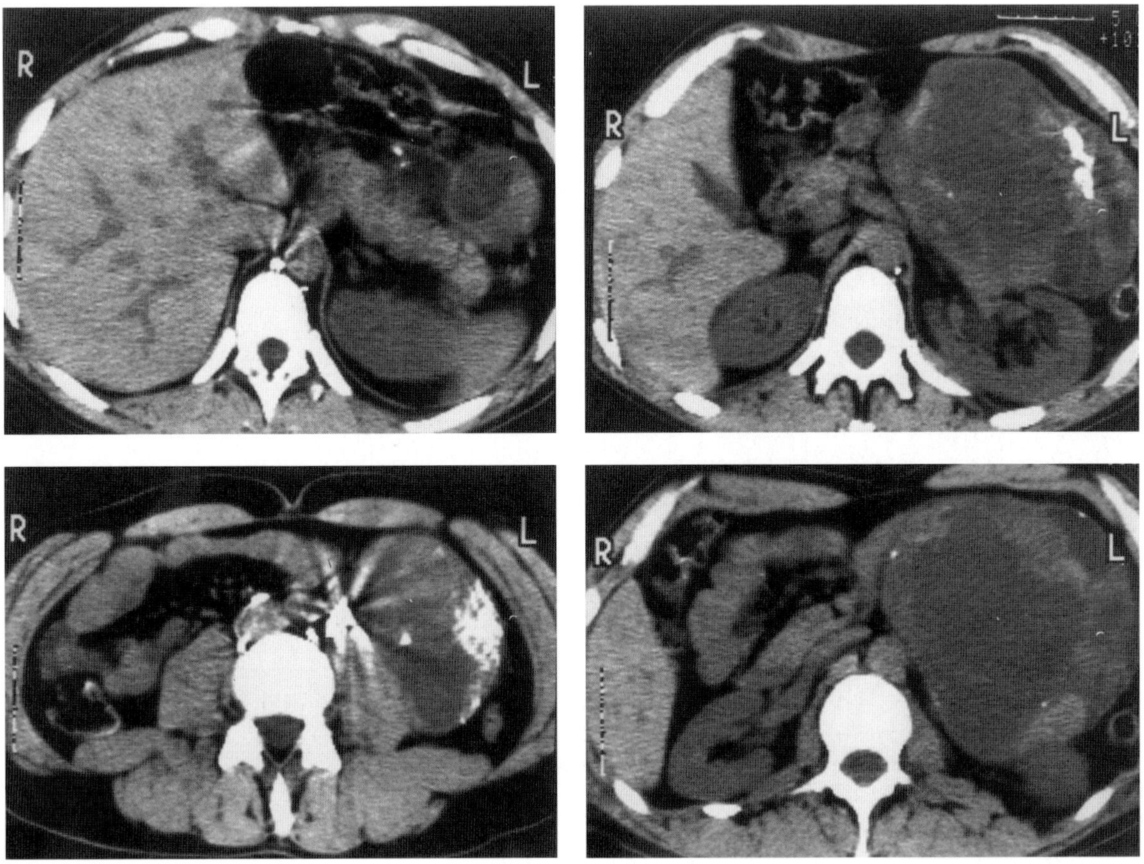

Fig. 13.11A–D. Peritoneal metastases in the left hypochondrium from ovarian dysgerminoma. Well-limited mass with a mixed structure and amorphous calcifications inside; it is separated from the pancreas, the ascending colon, and the left kidney by a transparent interstice of adipose tissue

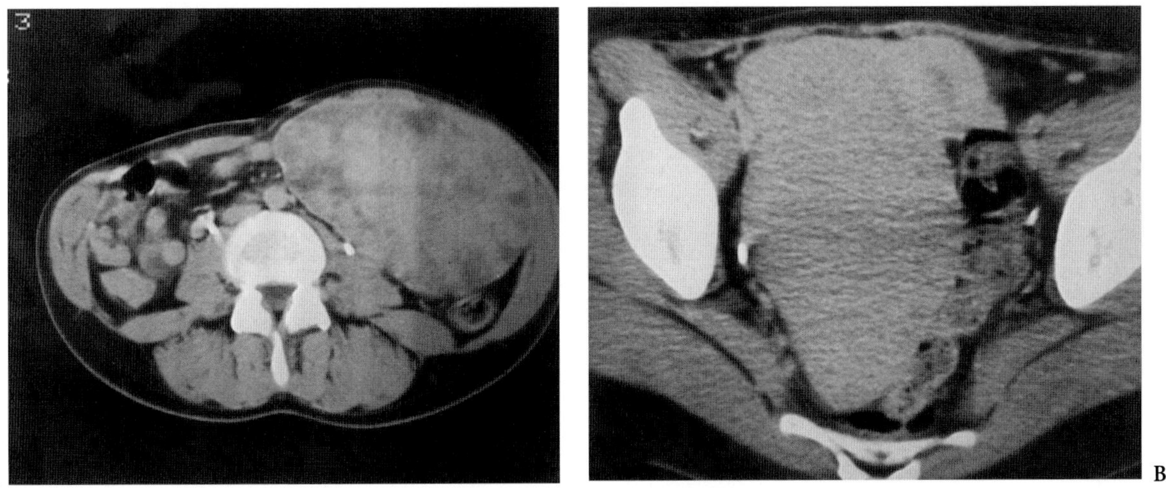

Fig. 13.12A, B. Krukenberg-type spread. Solid **A** omental and **B** ovarian metastases from gastric carcinoma

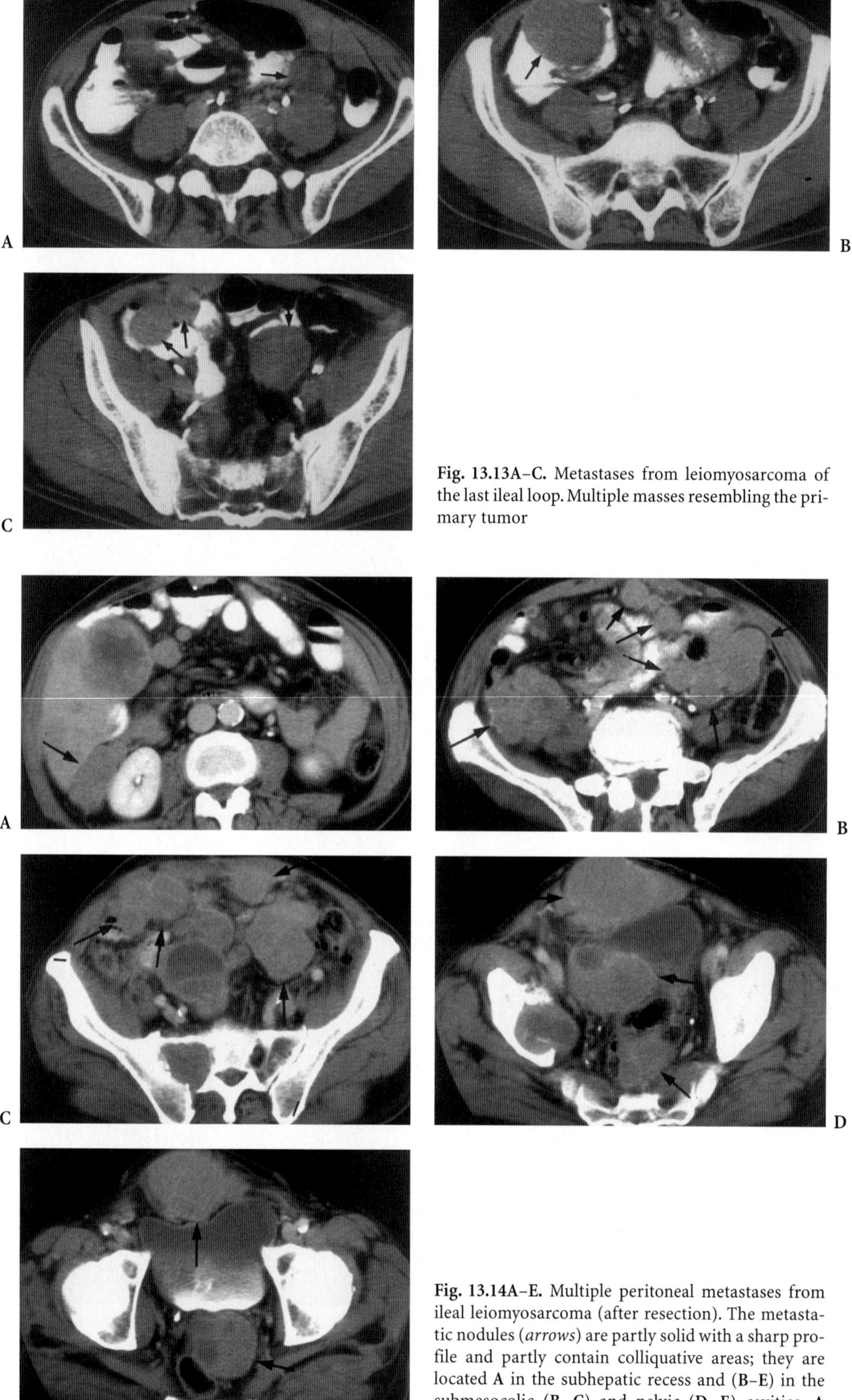

Fig. 13.13A–C. Metastases from leiomyosarcoma of the last ileal loop. Multiple masses resembling the primary tumor

Fig. 13.14A–E. Multiple peritoneal metastases from ileal leiomyosarcoma (after resection). The metastatic nodules (*arrows*) are partly solid with a sharp profile and partly contain colliquative areas; they are located **A** in the subhepatic recess and (**B–E**) in the submesocolic (**B, C**) and pelvic (**D, E**) cavities. **A** Hepatic and **C, D** osseous metastases

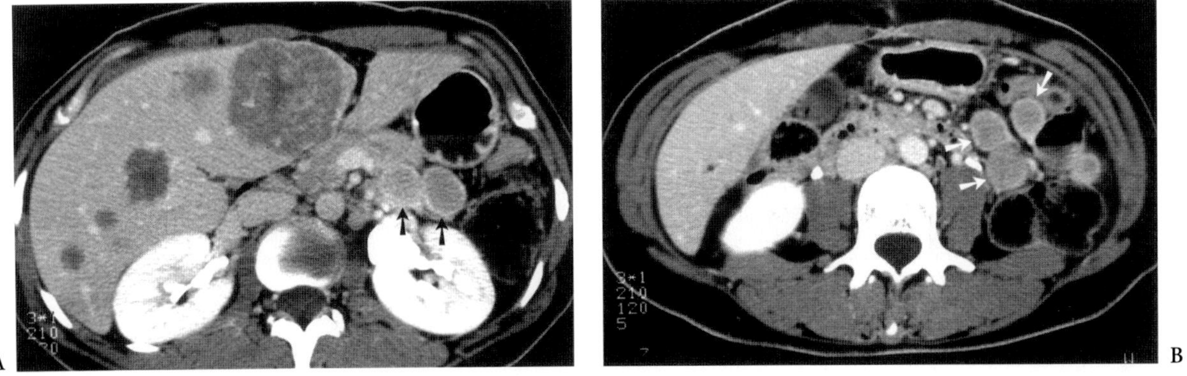

Fig. 13.15A, B. Metastatic-like aspects. Jejunal loops swelled by liquid (*arrows*) simulating nodular metastases in a patient affected by a tumor of the descending colon with hepatic metastases

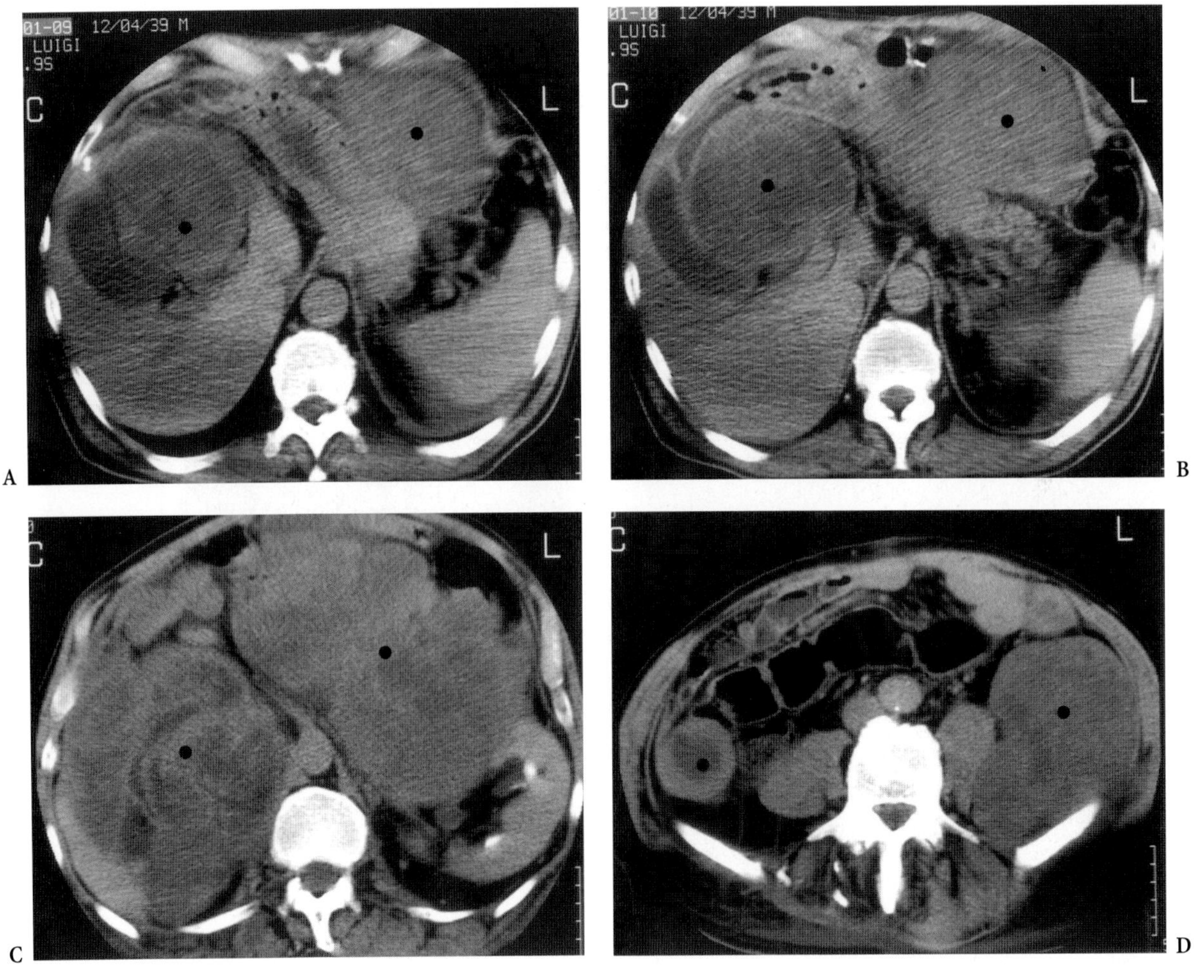

Fig. 13.16A–D. Peritoneal, omental and retroperitoneal metastases from pleiomorphous liposarcoma. Huge masses with a mixed structure and adipose component (*circles*); they show the densitometric and structural characteristics of the primary tumor

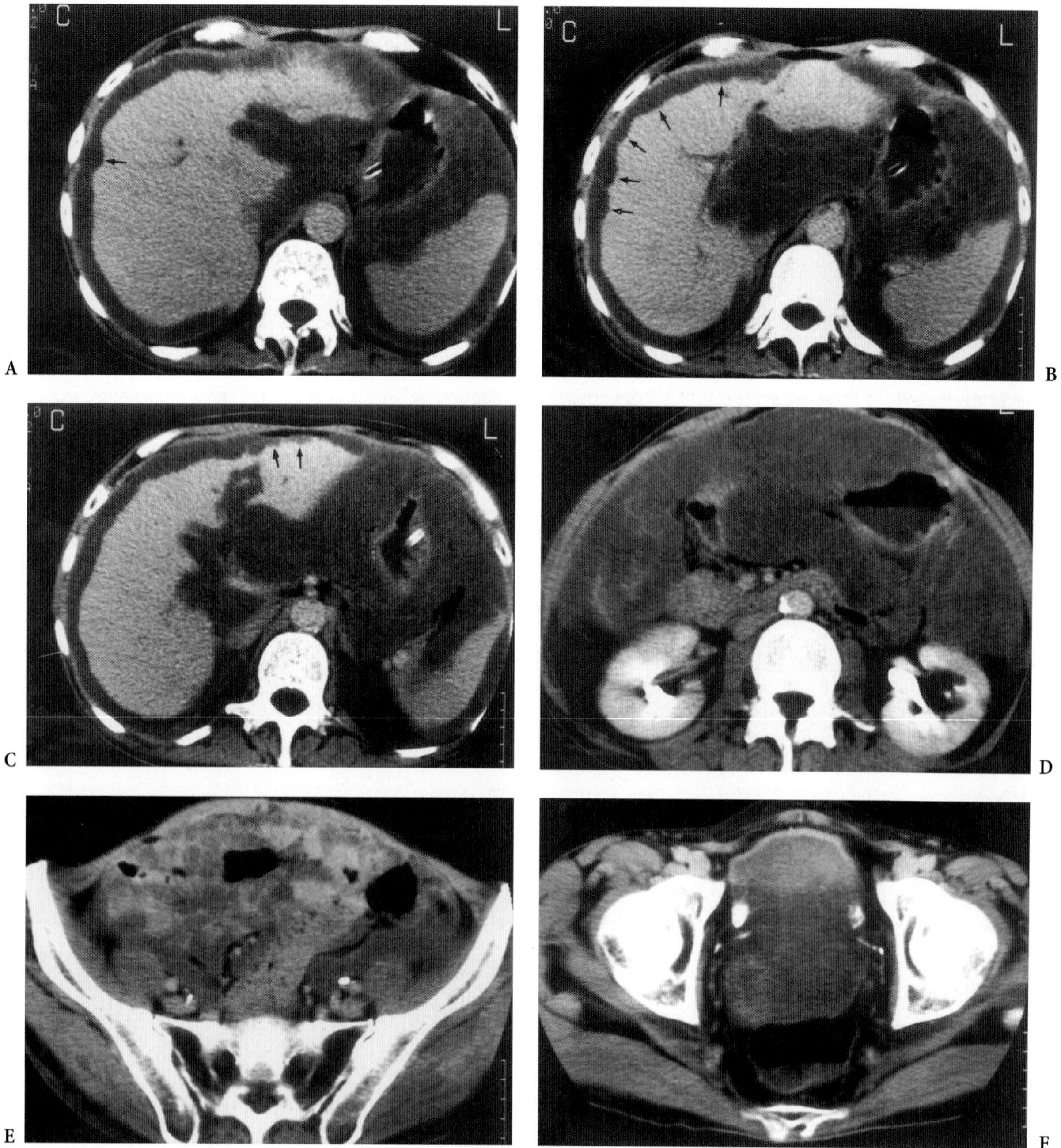

Fig. 13.17A–F. Pseudomyxoma peritonei. Peritoneal cavity occupied and swelled by multiple homogeneous cysts of low-medium attenuation (20–30 HU) mucoid material. **A–C** Scalloping of the liver edge (*small arrows*)

Fig. 13.19A–D. Pseudomyxoma peritonei due to the rupture of an appendiceal mucocele. Dense cyst-like formations overlapping each other and widely occupying the peritoneal cavity ▷

A B C D

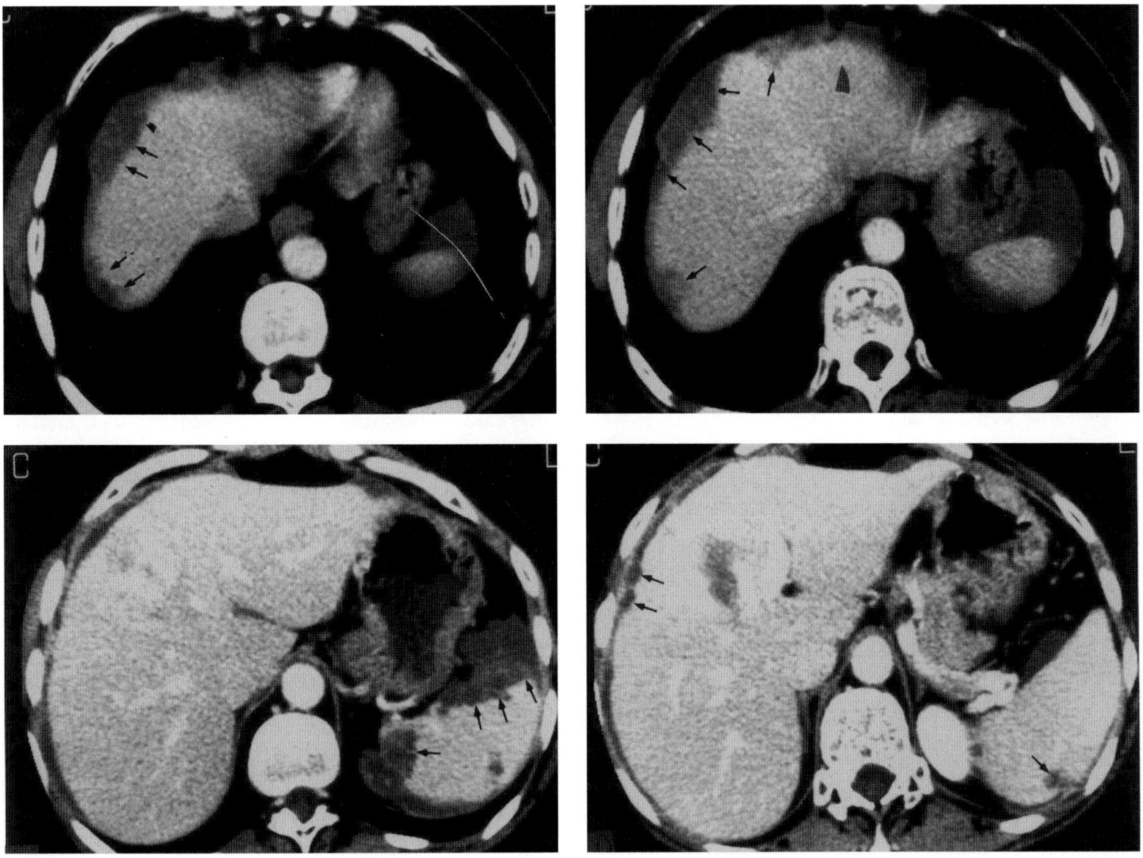

Fig. 13.18A–D. Pseudomyxoma peritonei from mucinous ovarian carcinoma. Accumulation of mucoid material with near-water density in the supramesocolic peritoneal cavities; it shows small cyst-like masses making impressions in the hepatic and splenic surface

A B C D

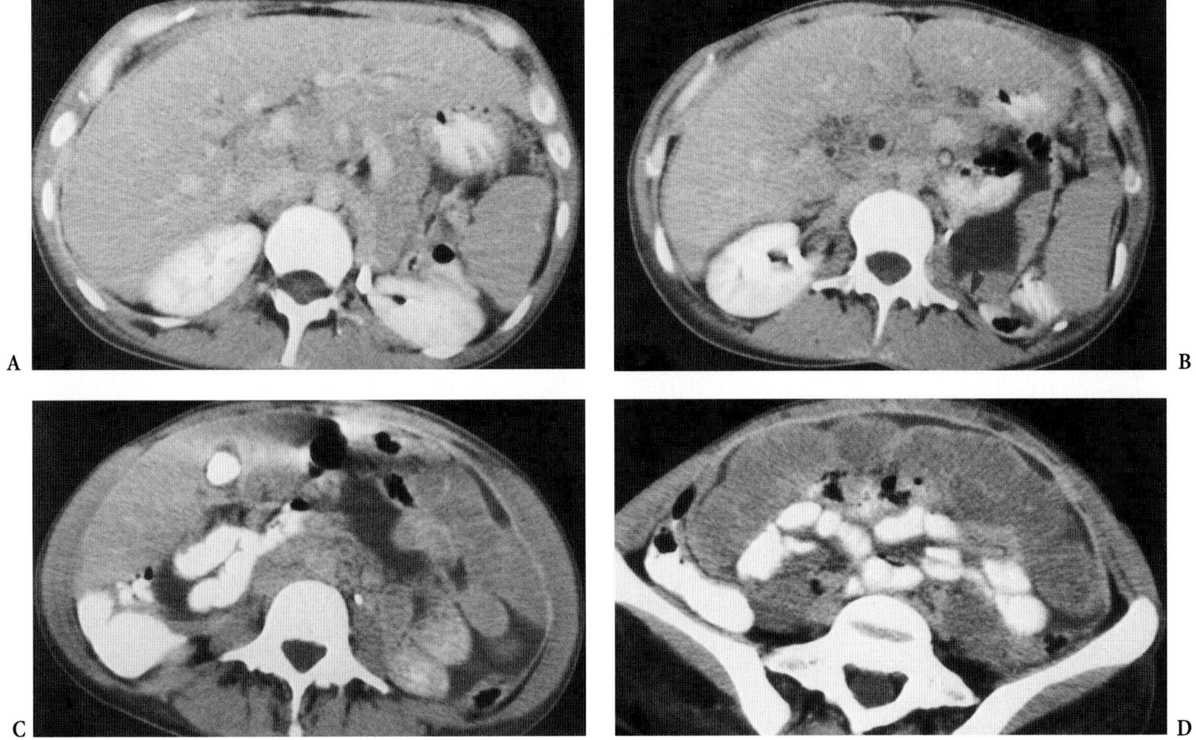

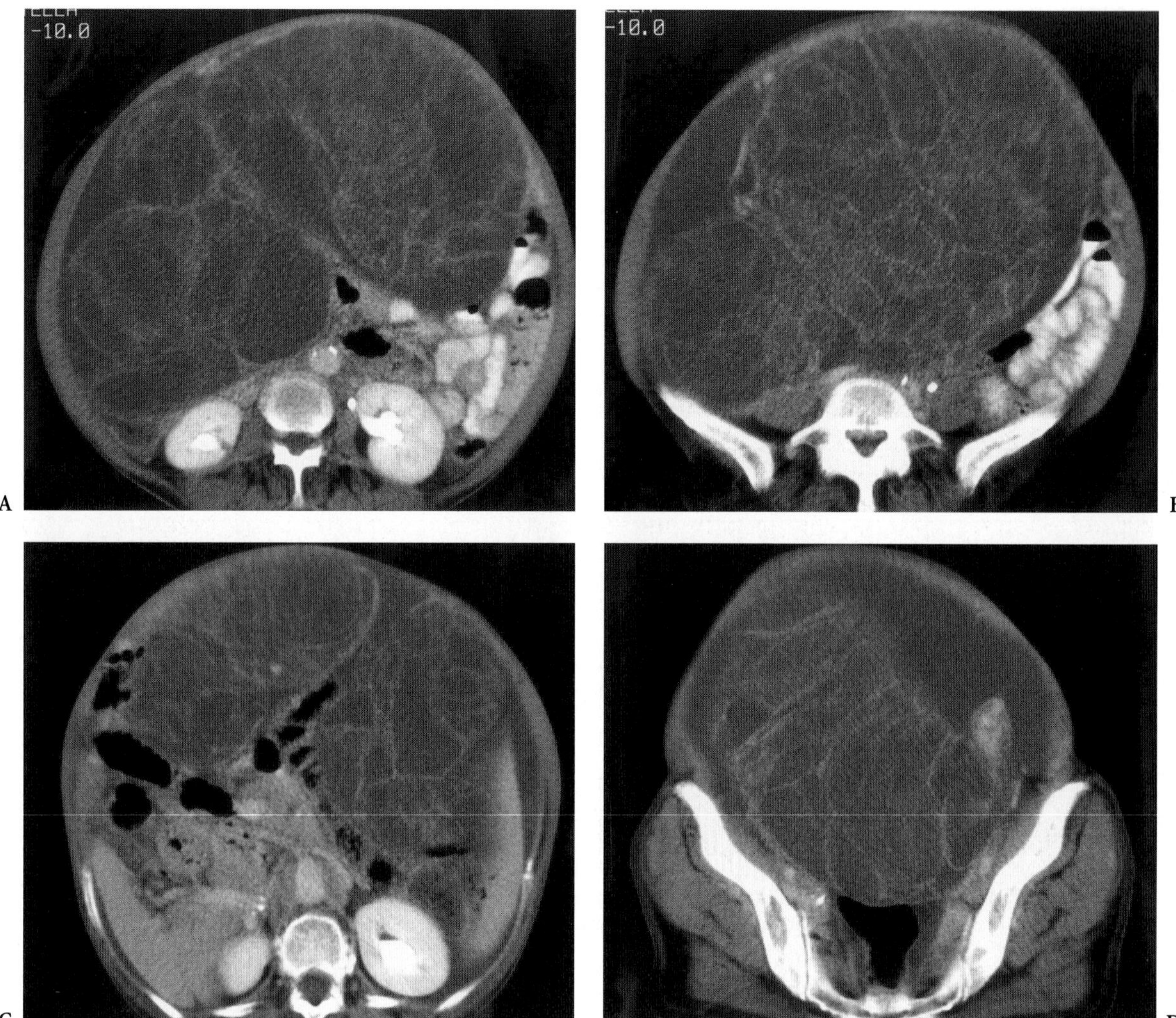

Fig. 13.20A–D. Pseudomyxoma peritonei caused by rupture of an appendiceal mucocele. The mucoid material swells the peritoneal cavity, forming a mass with a very sharp profile. The mass is constituted by multiple thick-walled cyst-like formations of near-water attenuation (0–25 HU); the walls of the mass are thin. The contrast medium only slightly enhances the opacity of the peritoneum that limits the mass

Table 13.4. CT parameters of lymph nodal metastases[a]

Diameter of the minor axis	>1 cm
Structure	Hypodense central area
Postcontrast density	>100 H.U.
Long/short diameter ratio	>0.7
Number	>3
Site	Along the lymphatic flow from the tumor

[a]When two parameters are positive the possibility of a secondary localization is high, whereas when three parameters are positive at the same time this is a definite indication of metastasis

13.1.1 Lymph Node Dimensions

One, and certainly the most significant, of the basic criteria for the diagnosis of lymph nodal metastasis is the lymph nodal dimensions The parameter that is least conditioned by the spatial disposition of the lymph node is the minor diameter, and thus, it must be utilized for lymph node measurement.

Since normal lymph nodes are not usually visible on CT, the presence of a nodular image near a tumor must always raise suspicion of a secondary lymph nodal localization, and must therefore always be reported.

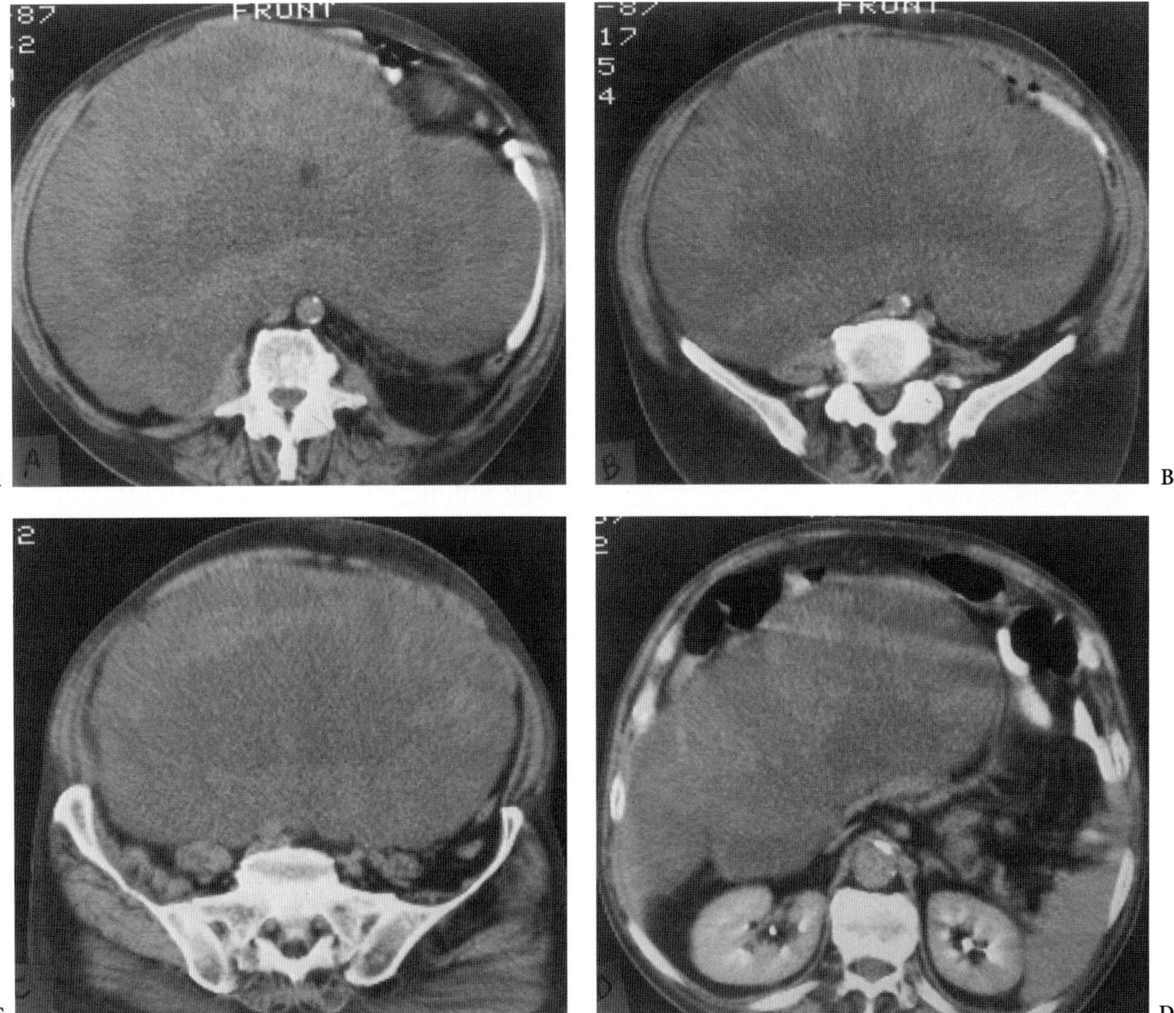

Fig. 13.21. Pseudomyxoma peritonei from ovarian mucinous cystadenocarcinoma. The peritoneal cavity is occupied by a low-density (15–35 HU) mass, which is subdivided by thin trabeculae. The intestinal loops are pushed upward and toward the left side

The probability that an enlarged lymph node is a metastatic site is directly related to its dimensions, even though a threshold value for a definite diagnosis of lymph node invasion does not exist.

Statistical reports in the literature about lymph nodal diffusion of gastric or colic tumors generally agree that lymph nodes more than 1 cm in diameter must be considered metastatic (Balthazar et al. 1988; Thoeni 1991; Angelelli and Macarini 1992; Thoeni and Rogalla 1995); this is not an absolutely valid criterion, because false-positive observations may be due to previous or present hyperplastic inflammatory processes.

However, lymph nodes with a diameter greater than 14 mm are almost always positive for metastases, whereas those with a diameter lower than 4 mm are generally negative.

13.1.2 Lymph Node Structure

The most frequent aspect of a lymph node metastasis, that is, a homogeneous nodule with an intermediate density, is not diagnostically significant per se.

In contrast, when enlarged lymph nodes are clearly hypodense with a thin dense marginal border (Figs. 13.26, 13.29–13.31, 13.37, 13.65), the presence of a metastasis is very probable, especially if the lymph nodes are located along the lymphatic pathway coming from a tumor.

However, similar aspects may be observed during antineoplastic treatment because of necroticocolliquative phenomena and in the tuberculous form (Figs. 7.8, 7.9).

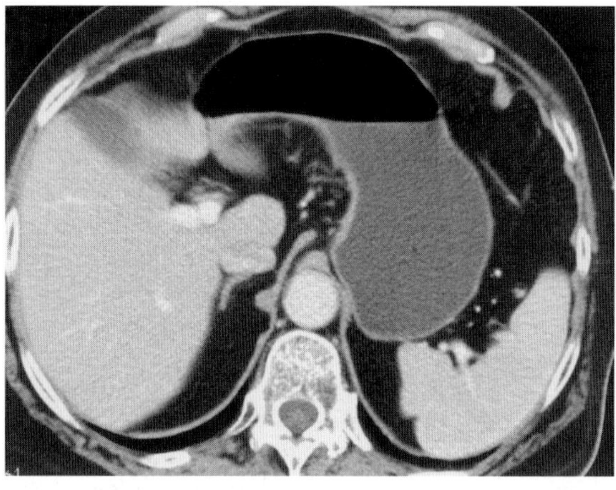

A

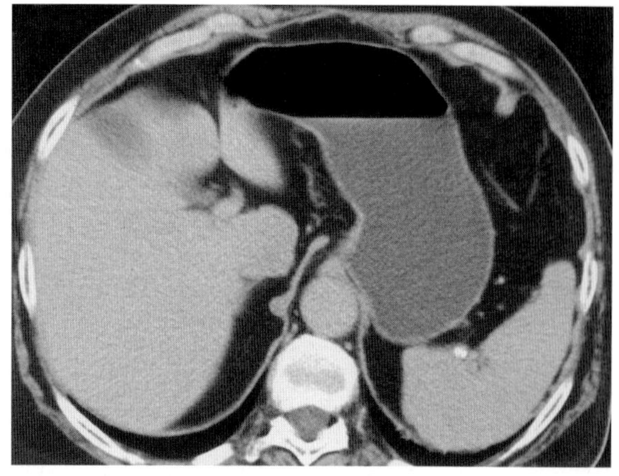

B

Fig. 13.22A, B. Normal fundus and corpus ventriculi. Sections **A** at the level of the inferior part of the esophageal hiatus and **B** 1 cm below the previous section

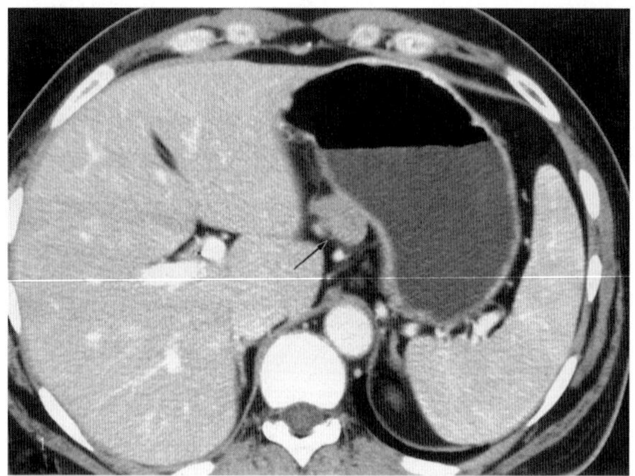

A

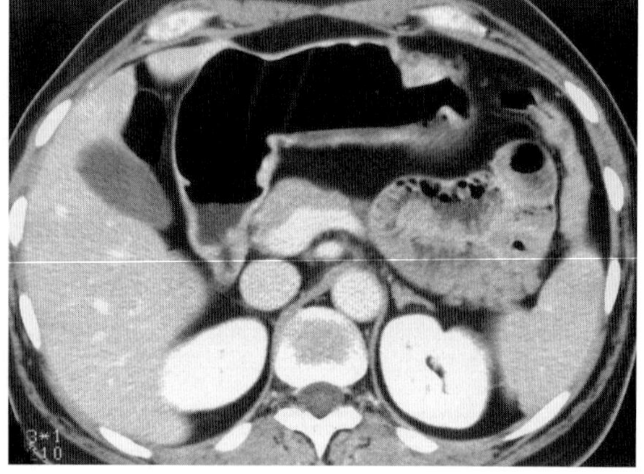

B

Fig. 13.23A, B. Gastric tumor. Preantral carcinoma infiltrating, but not passing beyond the wall of, the lesser curvature of the stomach (**B**). Left gastric lymph nodal metastases (**A** *arrow*)

In contrast, calcified lymph nodes usually represent residua of inflammatory and specific processes, but may sometimes be observed in metastases from ovarian cystadenocarcinomas (Fig. 13.10) or other tumors that are usually associated with calcifications of the primary tumor or of the peritoneal metastases.

13.1.3 Contrast Enhancement

Injection of i.v. contrast medium as a bolus by the dynamic technique induces an increase in the density, which shows values higher than 100 HU in the metastatic lymph nodes during the early arterial phase (Fukuja et al. 1995), whereas during the equilibrium phase the lymph node density becomes lower than that of a normal lymph node (Komaki 1986).

13.1.4 Lymph Node Configuration

From a statistical point of view, a ratio higher than 0.7 between greater and lesser lymph node diameters argues in favor of a metastatic localization.

13.1.5 Lymph Node Number

The probability that lymph nodes are the site of metastases increases with the increasing number of

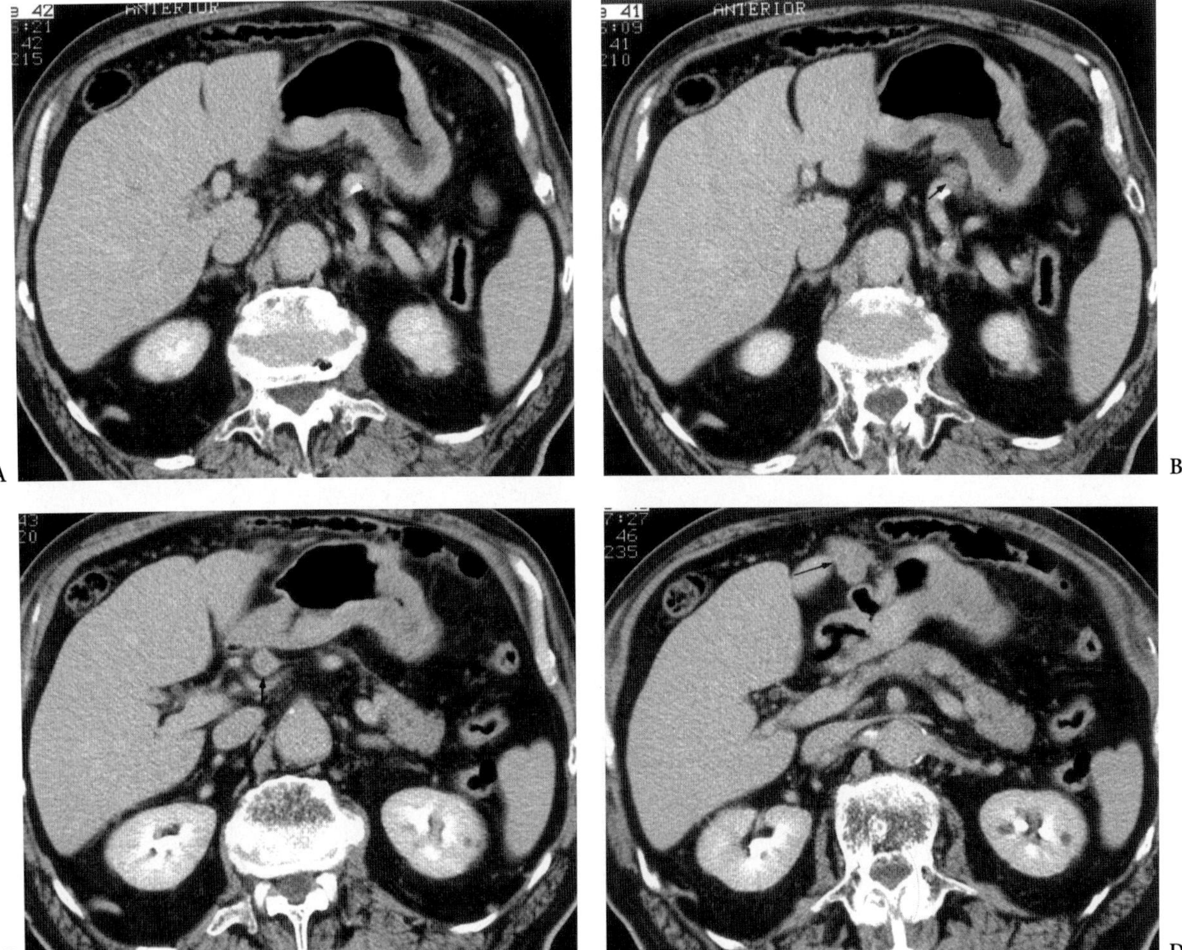

Fig. 13.24A–D. Gastric tumor. Tumor widely infiltrating the corpus and antrum ventriculi without passing beyond the wall. **B**, **C** Left gastric and **D** right gastroepiploic lymph node metastases

enlarged lymph nodes in the proximity of a tumor. We are in agreement with BALTHAZAR et al. (1988), who consider metastasis certain in the case of three or more lymph nodes with a diameter more than 1 cm along the lymphatic pathway coming from a tumor.

13.1.6 Lymph Node Position

Enlarged lymph nodes along the lymphatic pathway coming from a tumor must always raise suspicion, whereas enlarged lymph nodes located outside the paths of natural lymphatic drainage from the tumors must be carefully evaluated, because they may be just an occasional and nonrepetitive finding or a secondary localization of tumor cells coming through collateral pathways. This phenomenon may be due to the block of the main route because of massive invasion of a primary lymph node or of its afferent and efferent collectors.

13.2 Gastric Carcinoma

The CT is extremely useful to evaluate the parietal extension of the gastric carcinoma, the tumoral diffusion to perivisceral adipose cellular, ligaments and adjacent structures (liver, pancreas, transverse colon), the secondary lymph nodal and hepatic localizations and the peritoneal spread.

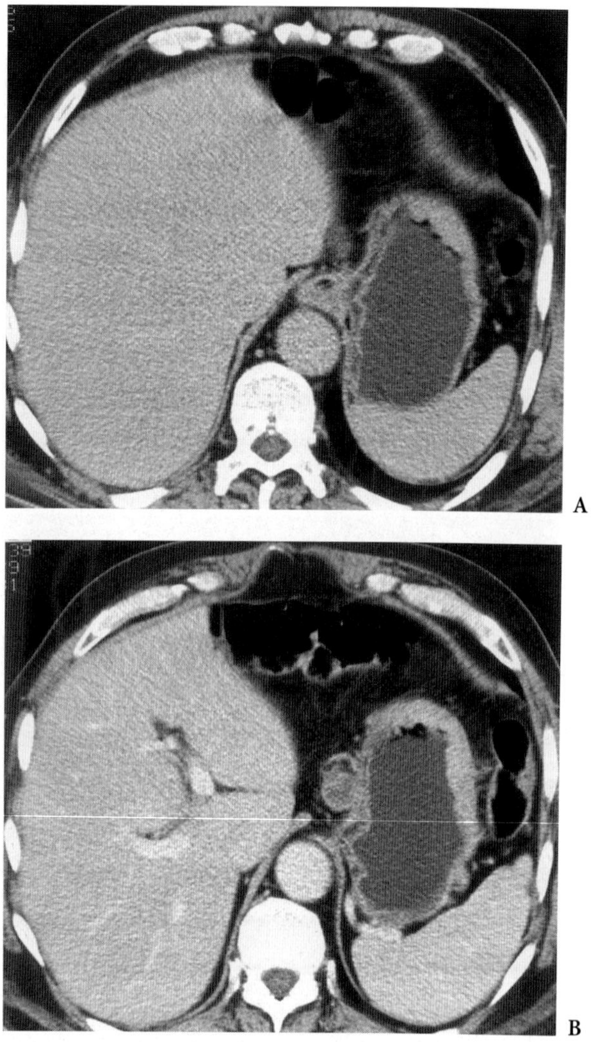

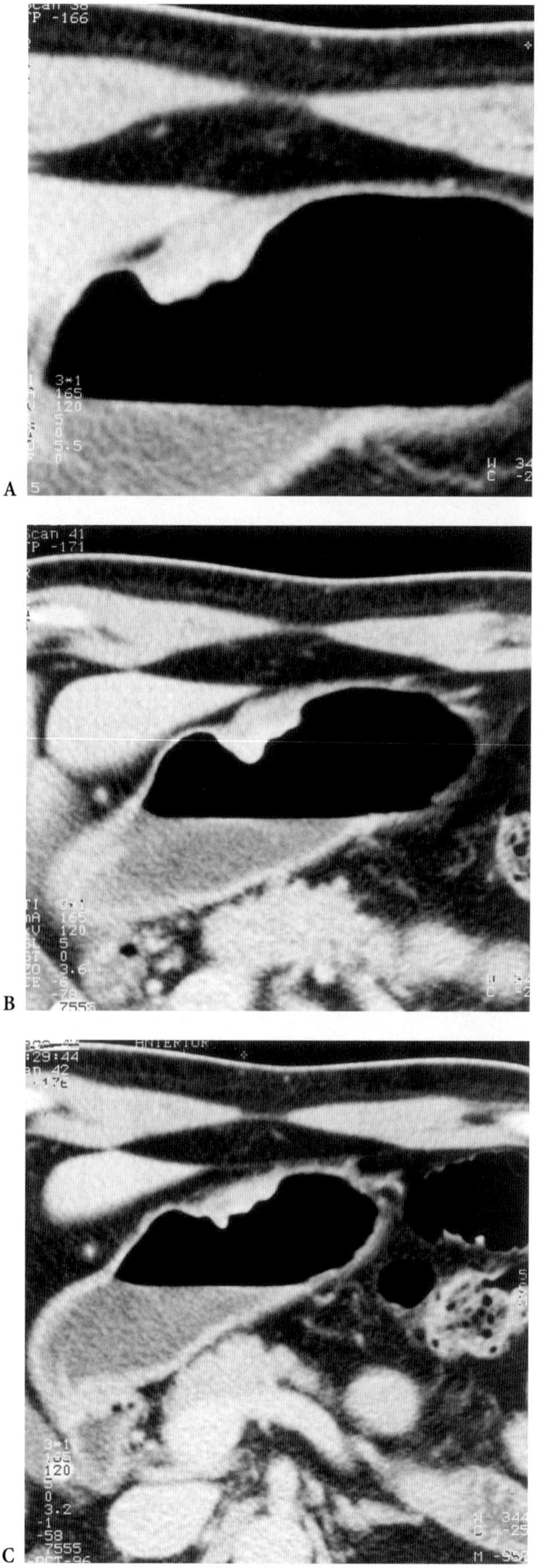

A

B

Fig. 13.26A, B. Gastric tumor. Carcinoma of the greater curvature of the corpus ventriculi with initial invasion of the gastrocolic ligament (B). Enlarged and centrally hypodense metastatic left gastric lymph node

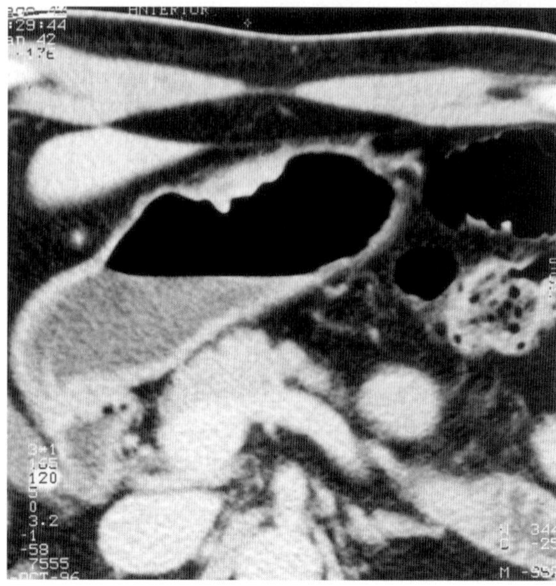

C

◁

Fig. 13.25A–C. Gastric tumor. Carcinoma infiltrating the greater curvature without passing beyond the wall

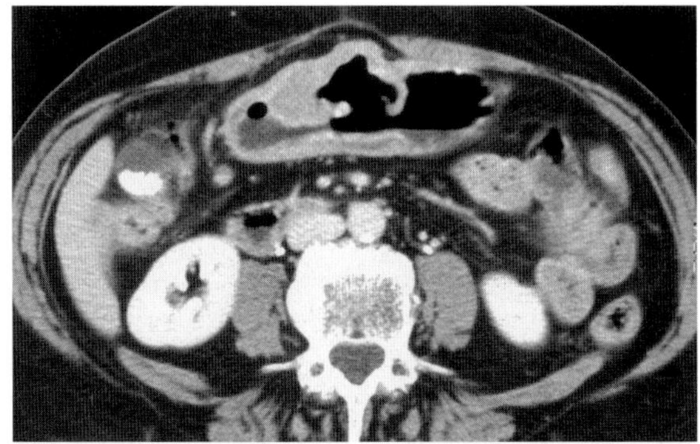
A

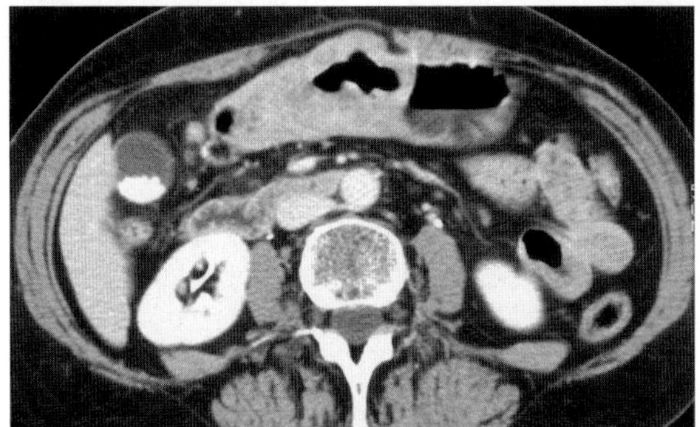
B

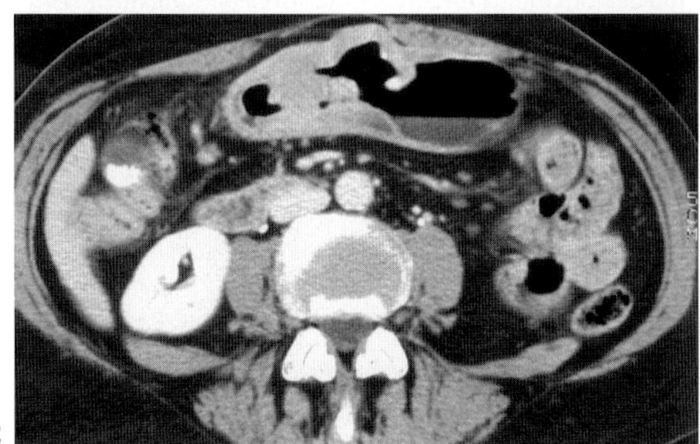
C

Fig. 13.27A–C. Gastric tumor. Circumferentially infiltrating carcinoma of the corpus and antrum: the external profile of the antrum is dentate and the adipose cellular of the hepato-duodenal ligament is shaded because of an initial invasion. **A**, **B** Gastroduodenal and **C** superior mesenteric lymph nodes found to be enlarged, but not harboring metastases on histologic examination

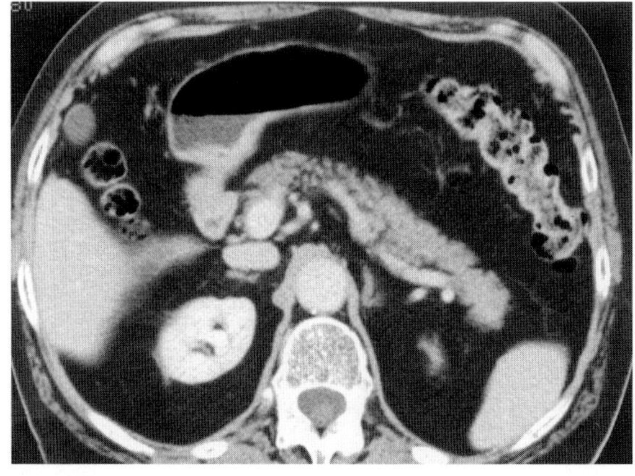

Fig. 13.28. Gastric tumor. Circumferential infiltration of the gastric antrum in a cuff-like shape. Jagged external profile of the prepyloric region because of incipient invasion

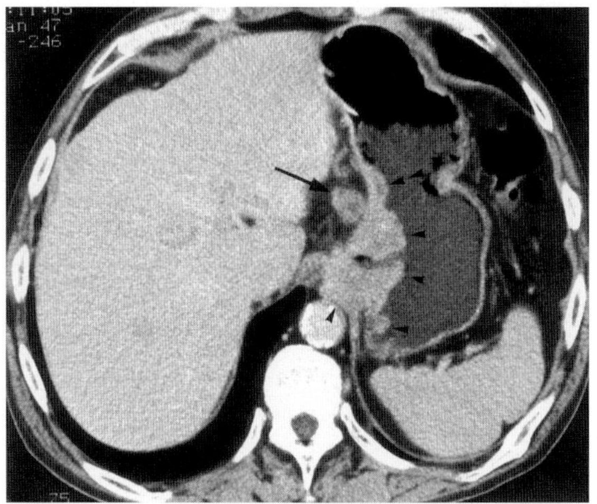
A

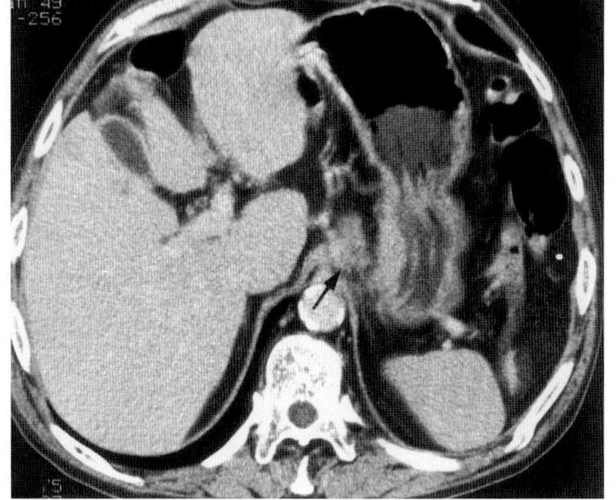
B

Fig. 13.29A, B. Gastric tumor. Cardial vegetation and infiltration by a carcinoma extending to the esophagus beyond the diaphragm and infiltrating the diaphragmatic crus (**A**). The tumor has metastasized to the subcardial coronarostomachic lymph nodes and along the lesser curvature (**A**, **B** *arrow*)

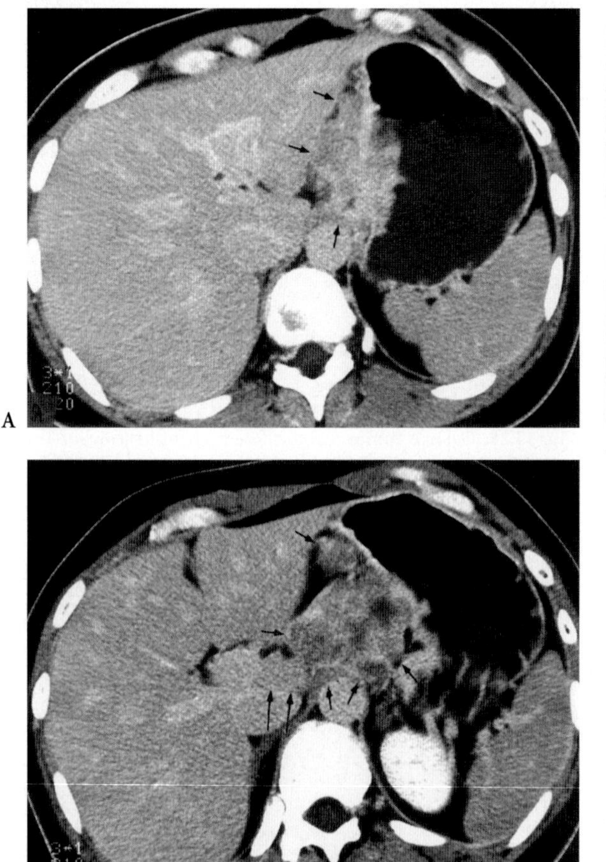
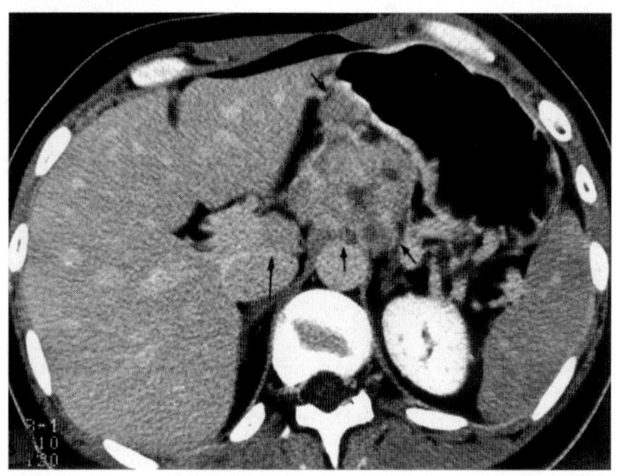

Fig. 13.30A–C. Gastric tumor. Supra- and subcardial vegetation of a carcinoma invading the gastrohepatic ligament. Large left gastric lymph nodal metastases, which constitute a unique mass together with the primary tumor and adhere to the posterior abdominal wall around the aorta (*small arrows*). Further lymph node metastases are visible in the transverse fissure of the liver (**B**, **C** *long thin arrows*)

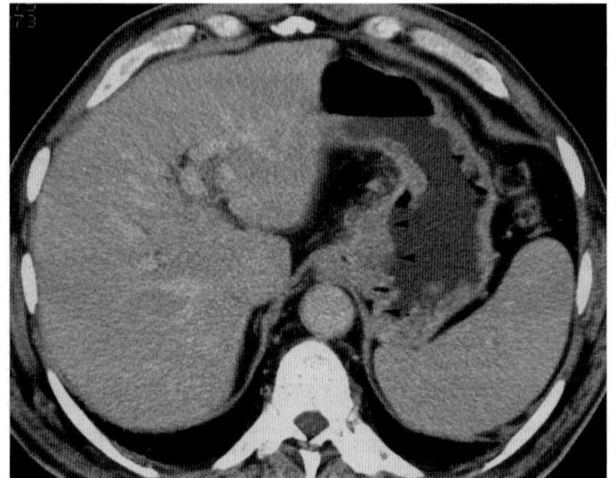
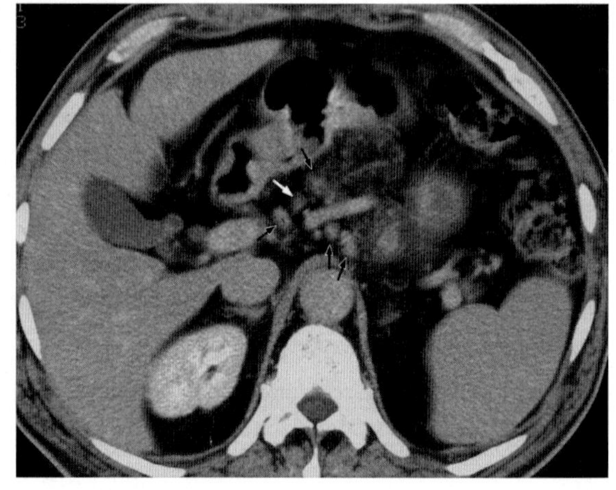

Fig. 13.31A, B. Gastric tumor. Adenocarcinoma infiltrating the lesser curvature of the fundus and corpus ventriculi and invading the gastrohepatic ligament (*arrowheads*). Metastases in **A** the subcardial lymph nodes (included in the tumoral mass), the suprapancreatic lymph nodes, and **B** those located near the celiac trunk (*small arrows*)

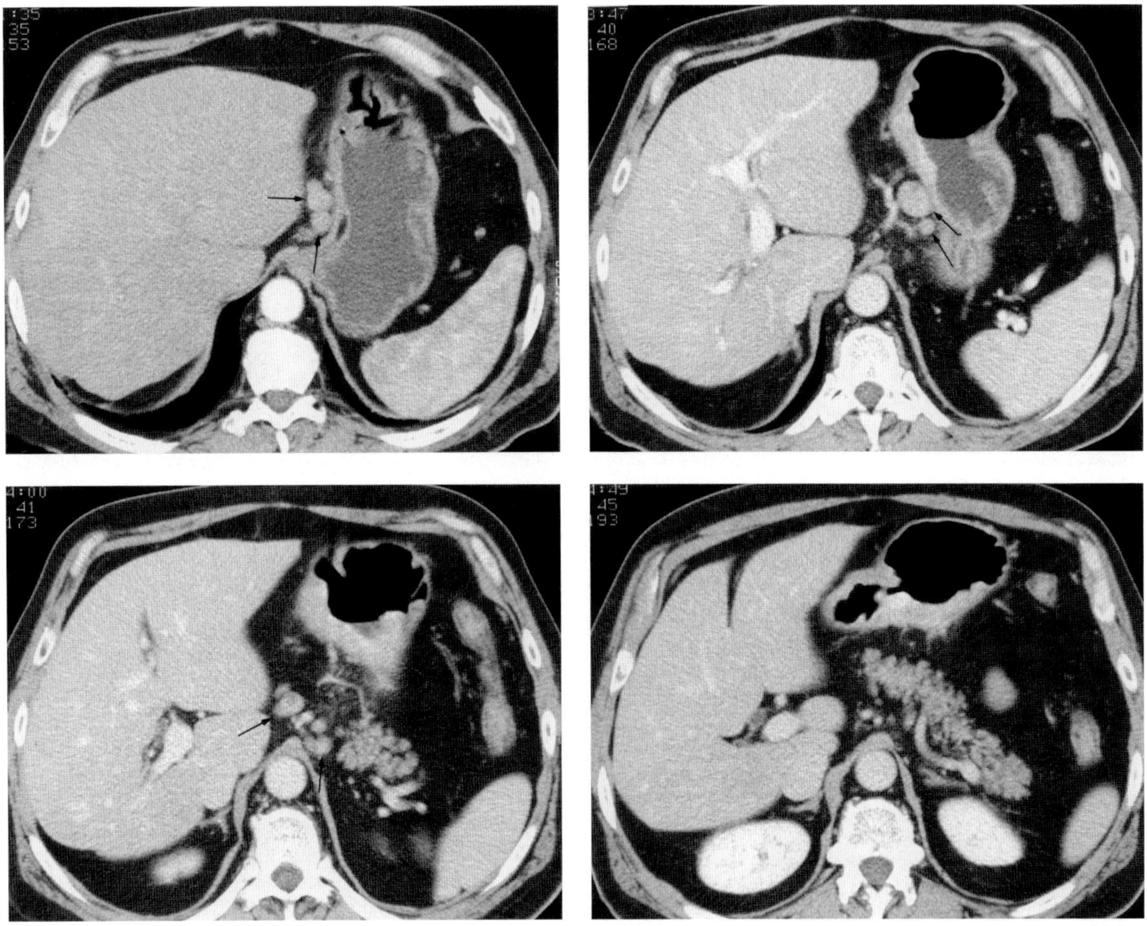

Fig. 13.32A–D. Gastric tumor. Carcinoma infiltrating the corpus and antrum ventriculi and invading the gastrohepatic ligament (**D**). Left gastric subcardial lymph nodal metastases (*arrows*) along the lesser curvature (**A**, **B**) and the ascending extension of the artery (**C**)

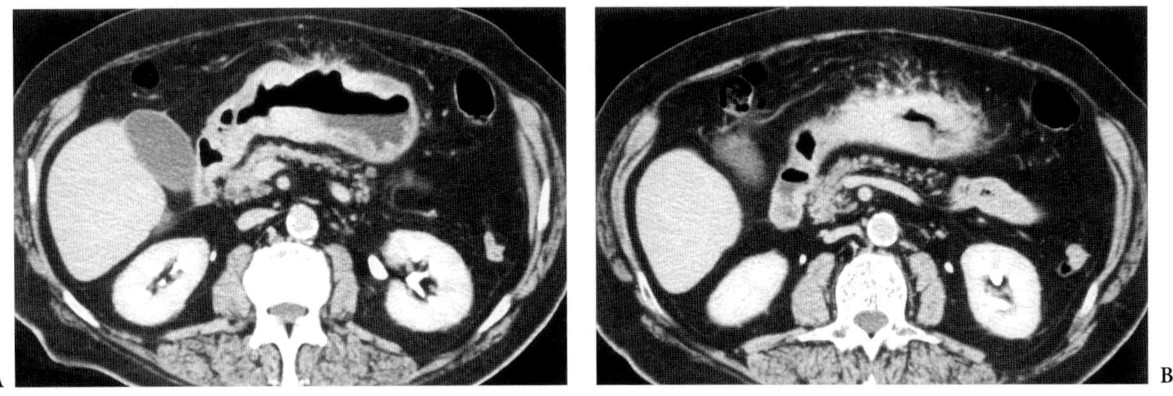

Fig. 13.33A, B. Gastric tumor. Circumferential carcinoma of the corpus and antrum ventriculi invading the gastrocolic ligament

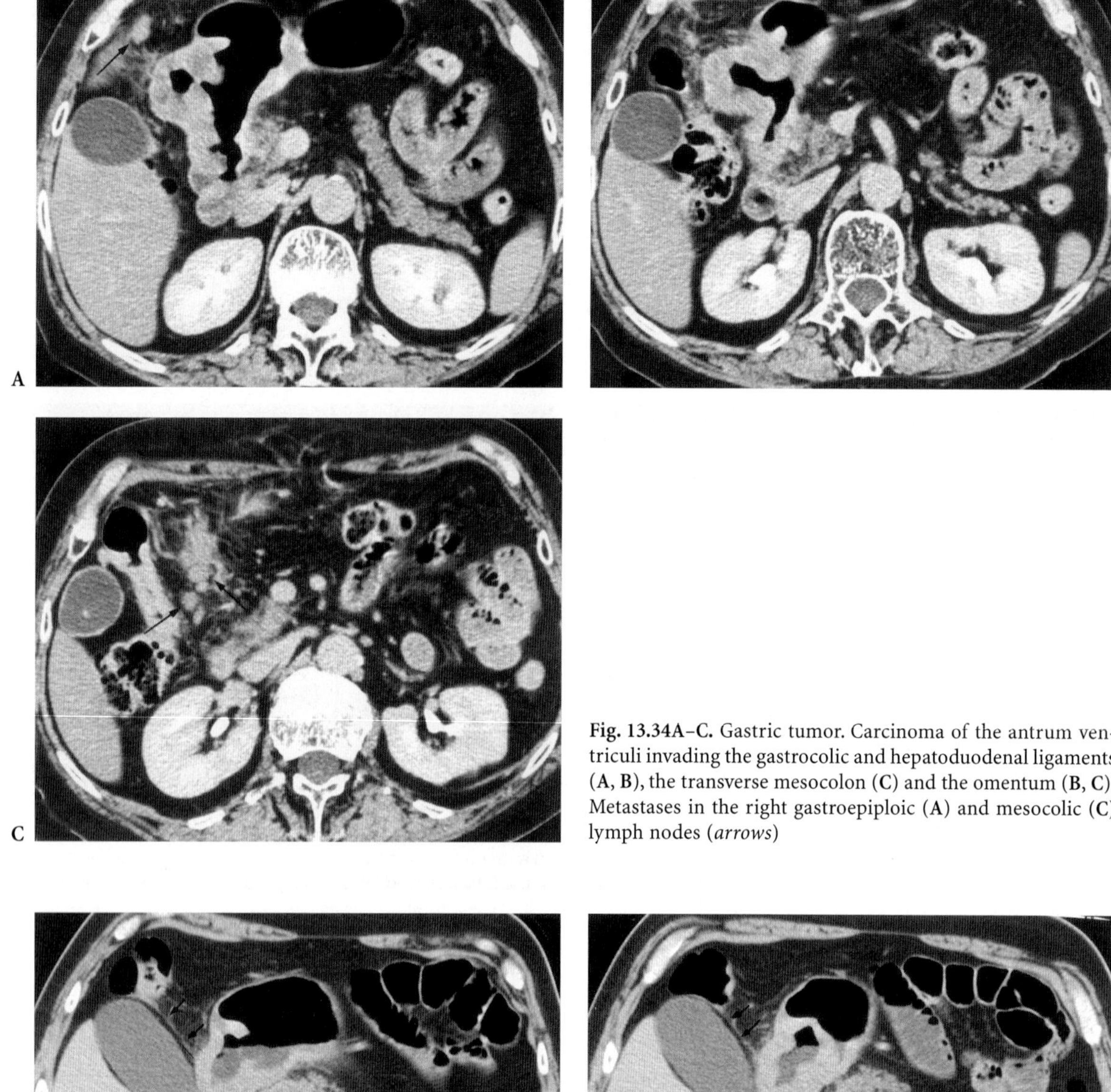

Fig. 13.34A–C. Gastric tumor. Carcinoma of the antrum ventriculi invading the gastrocolic and hepatoduodenal ligaments (**A**, **B**), the transverse mesocolon (**C**) and the omentum (**B**, **C**). Metastases in the right gastroepiploic (**A**) and mesocolic (**C**) lymph nodes (*arrows*)

Fig. 13.35A, B. Gastric tumor. Circumferential carcinoma infiltrating the antrum ventriculi, invading the gastrohepatic and hepatoduodenal ligaments and infiltrating the peritoneum that medially covers the gallbladder (*small arrows*). Metastases in the right left gastric lymph nodes (*arrow*)

Fig. 13.37A–F. Gastric tumor. Vegetation extending from the cardia to the pylorus along the lesser curvature (**A** *small arrows*) of a carcinoma with a cuff-like aspect at the level of the antrum (**B**, **C**). The tumor invades the gastrohepatic ligament, where it forms a single mass with the left gastric lymph nodes (**A**) and the gastrocolic ligament, blending with the numerous metastatic gastroepiploic lymph nodes (**B–D**). Metastases in the deep (**B**, **C**) and superficial (**C**, **D**) hepatic lymph nodes (*long thin arrows*), the pancreatoduodenal lymph nodes, the omentum (**F**), and the liver (**A–C**, **E**)

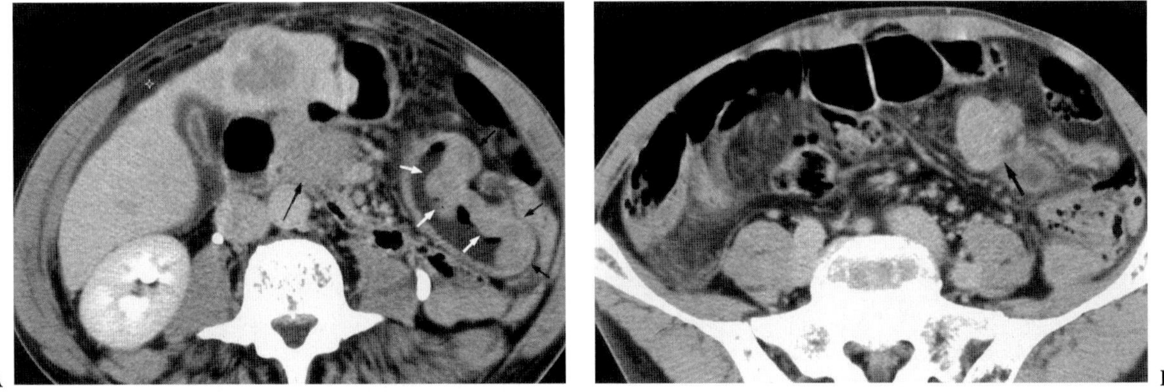

Fig. 13.36A, B. Gastric tumor. Adenocarcinoma infiltrating the greater curvature of the corpus ventriculi and invading up to the peritoneum and the omentum (**A** *small arrow*). Metastases in the left gastroepiploic (**B** *thick arrow*) and parapancreatic (**A** *long thin arrow*) lymph nodes. **A** Hepatic metastasis

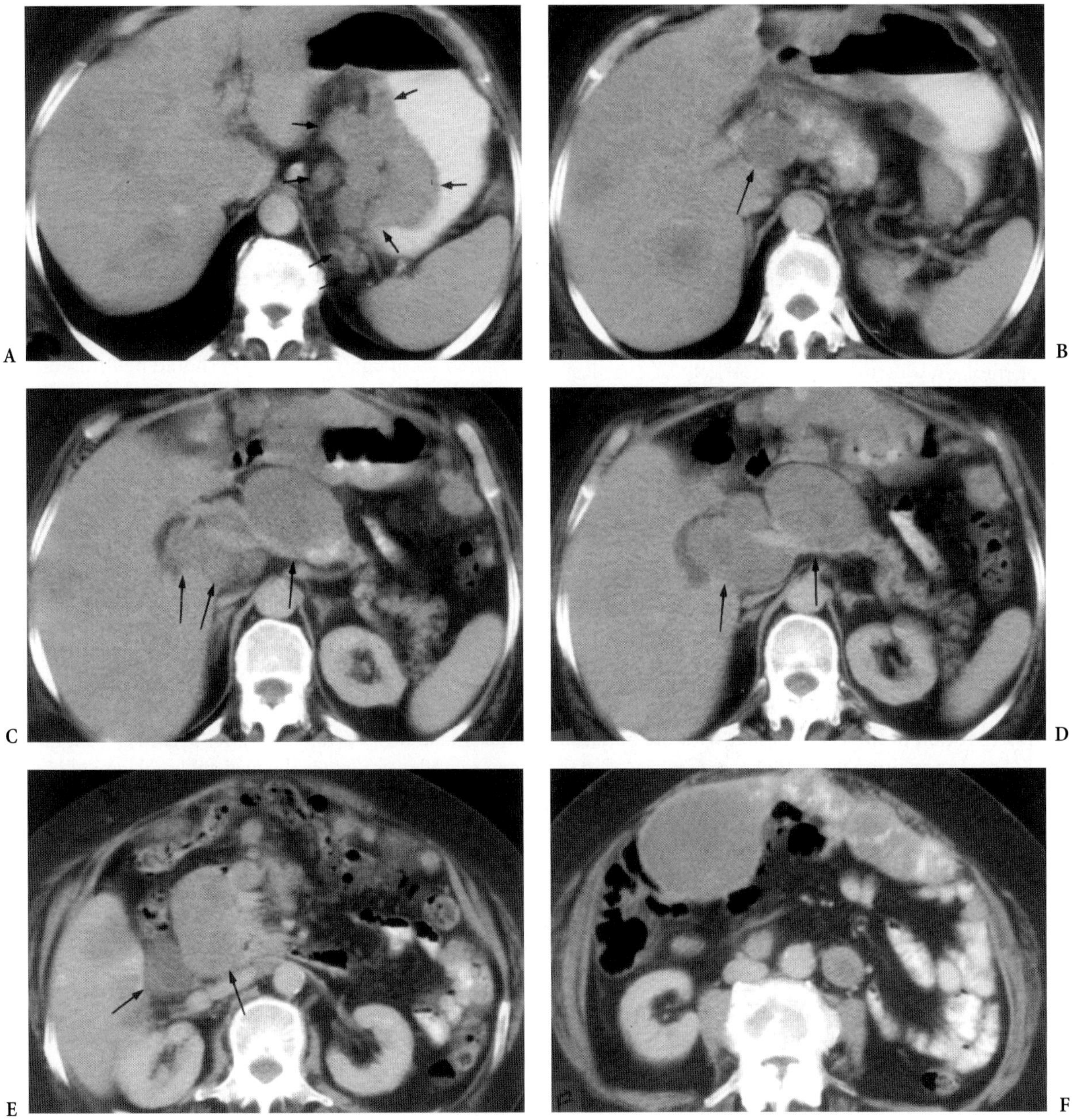

A B

C D

E F

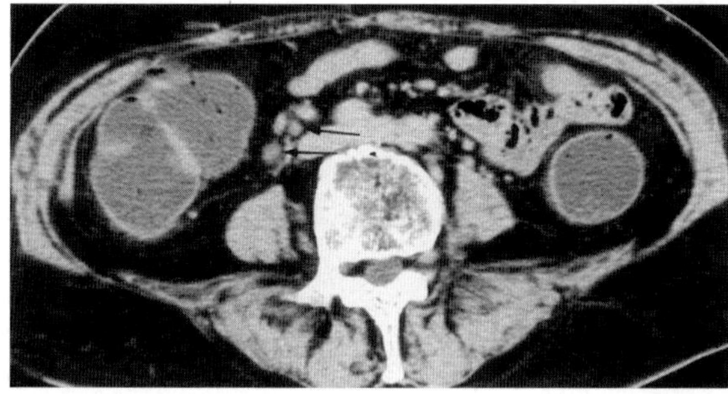

A

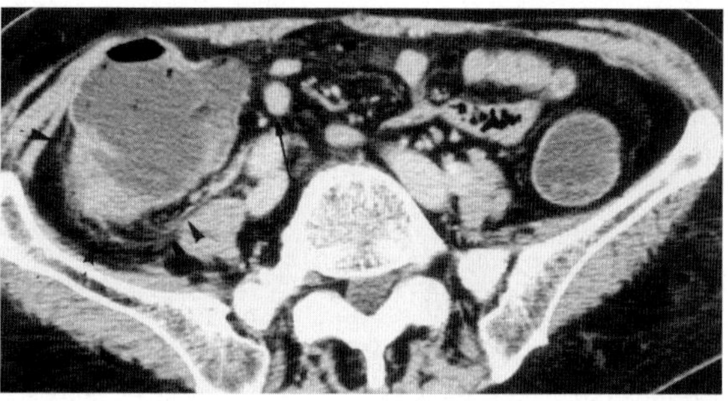

B

Fig. 13.38A, B. Colon carcinoma ascending cecum. Duke's stage C2 (T3,N2,M0). Semicircumferential thickening of the intestinal wall with strands in the pericecal fat extending to thickened peritoneum (*arrowheads*) (**B**). Enlarged metastatic ileocolic (**A**) and right colic (**B**) lymph nodes (*arrows*)

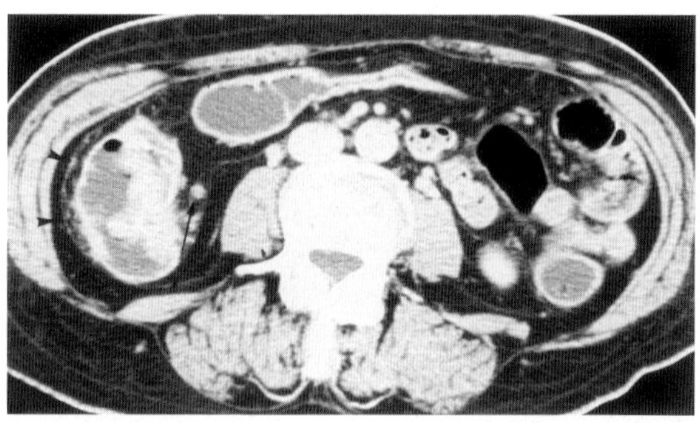

Fig. 13.39. Adenocarcinoma of ascending colon. Duke's stage C2 (T3,N1,M0). Asymmetric circumferential thickening of the intestinal wall with stranding in the pericolic fat, extending to the peritoneum and the lateroconal fascia (*arrowheads*). Metastatic paracolic lymph nodes (*arrow*)

However, high-quality instruments and a correct technique for the study of the stomach are indispensable if useful results are to be obtained in clinical practice.

In particular, we recommend:

a) Performance of a preliminary examination without contrast medium in every case.
b) Repetition of the examination with the patient in a supine position when the tumor is located in the fundus and in the corpus ventriculi or in a prone, oblique or right lateral position when it is sited in the antrum. The test should start after the stomach has been distended by oral administration of 500–800 ml of water at room temperature or i.v. infusion of 100–120 ml of 30% nonionic water-soluble contrast medium at a speed of 2 ml/s; contiguous 5-mm-thick scans should be taken, starting 45 s after the beginning of the injection.
c) Repeating the examination in the same way, except beginning the scans between 70 s 90 s after the start of the injection.
d) Perhaps, completing the study with contiguous 3-mm-thick targeted scans at the site of the invasion that had raised suspicion; an additional amount of 80 ml of contrast medium should be infused at 3 ml/s, with the scans starting 30 s.

To study the parietal and extraparietal extension of the tumor, Hori et al. (1984) and Cho et al. (1994) suggest injection of the contrast medium as an i.v. bolus followed by an immediate scan in the arterial phase and then by a second scan 2 min after the beginning of the injection during the equilibrium phase. This technique shows the gastric wall as a pluristratified structure with an internal hyperdense mucous layer, an intermediate submucous layer, which does not become opaque, and an external musculoserous layer, which becomes slightly opaque. However, since the parietal involvement is of only limited importance from a practical point of view, we believe that attention must be focused on the extraparietal diffusion, which is very important in determination of a therapeutic program.

Fig. 13.41A, B. Adenocarcinoma of ascending colon. Dukes stage D (T3,N2,M0). Adenocarcinoma infiltrating the pericolic cellular, the mesocolic peritoneum and the anterior renal and right lateroconal fasciae: thickening of the intestinal wall with pericolic reticular aspect and shading of the adipose tissue around the colon, with thickening of the peritoneum and of the fasciae (*long arrows*). Metastatic lymph nodes along the extension of the right colic artery (**B** arrows) ▷

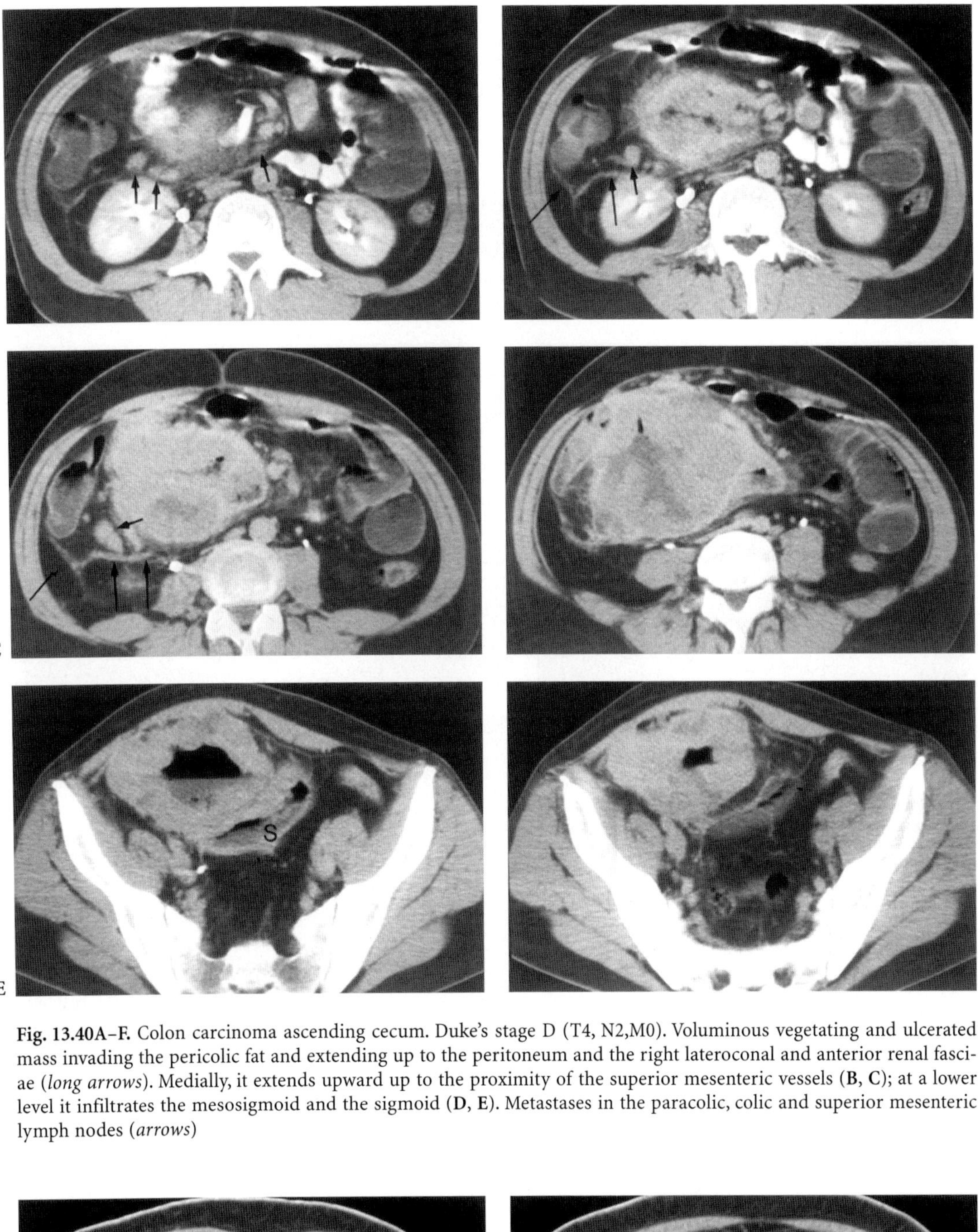

Fig. 13.40A–F. Colon carcinoma ascending cecum. Duke's stage D (T4, N2,M0). Voluminous vegetating and ulcerated mass invading the pericolic fat and extending up to the peritoneum and the right lateroconal and anterior renal fasciae (*long arrows*). Medially, it extends upward up to the proximity of the superior mesenteric vessels (**B, C**); at a lower level it infiltrates the mesosigmoid and the sigmoid (**D, E**). Metastases in the paracolic, colic and superior mesenteric lymph nodes (*arrows*)

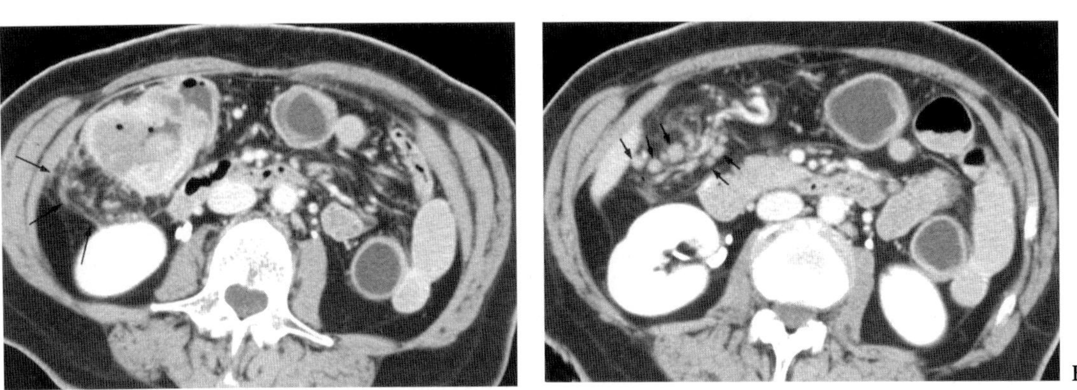

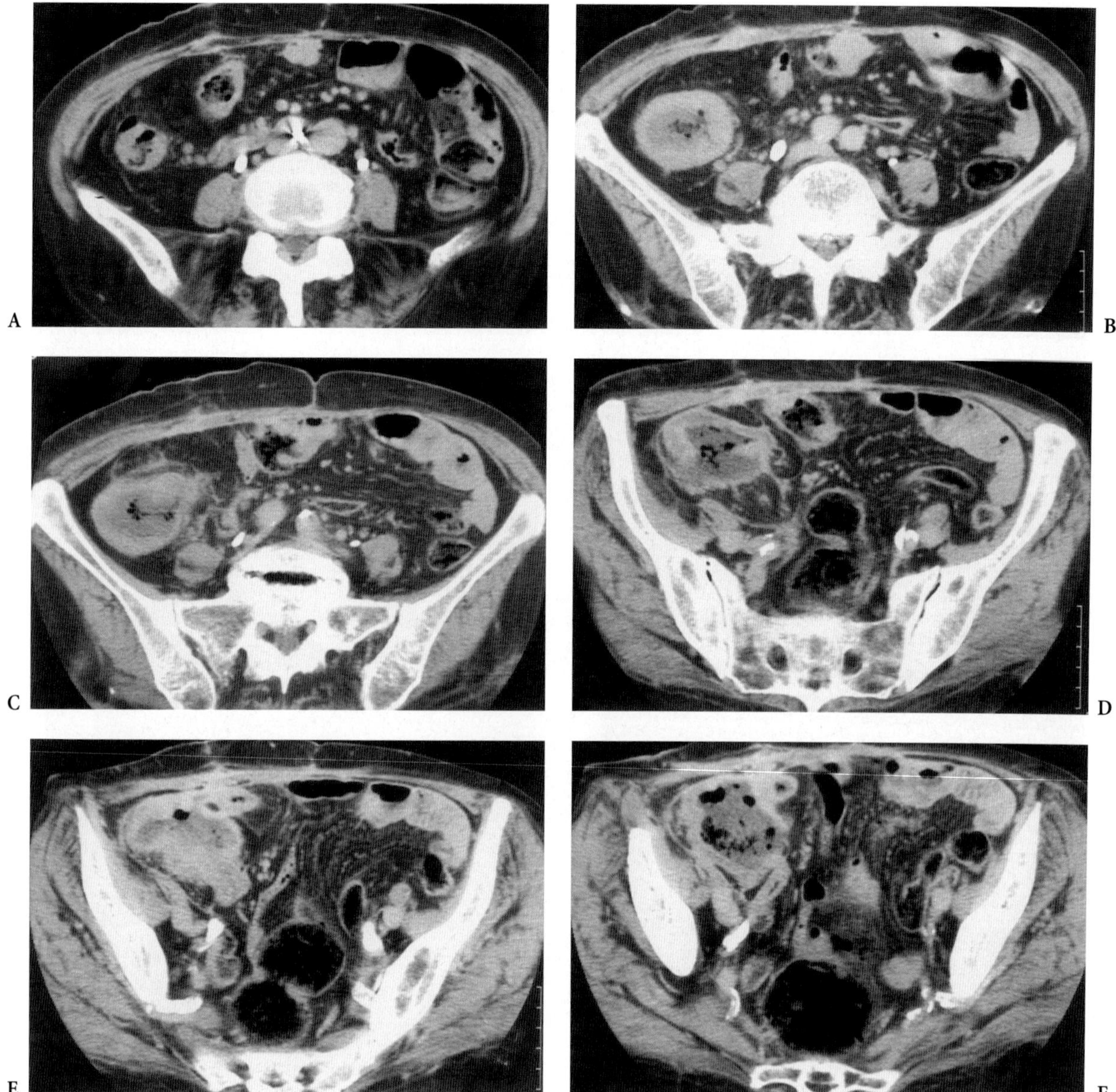

Fig. 13.42A–F. Colon carcinoma ascending cecum. Dukes stage D (T3,N2,M0). Carcinoma widely infiltrating the peritoneum and the mesentery up to the lateroconal and anterior renal fasciae. Thickening of the abdominal and pelvic parietal peritoneum around the tumor and of the mesentery around the vascular branches (**C–F**), with aspects resembling "railway track," a "fan," and a "constellation.". Metastases in paracecal, paracolic and ileocolic lymph nodes

In fact, it is particularly important to remember that the direct diffusion is closely related to the original site of the tumor:

- Tumors originating from the lesser curvature tend to invade the gastrohepatic ligament first, subsequently extending upward through this ligament to the left lobe of the liver and downward through the hepatoduodenal ligament.
- Tumors of the greater curvature of the fundus extend backward in the gastrosplenic ligament, whereas those originating from the corpus ventriculi extend forward and downward to the gastrocolic ligament and then to the greater omentum and the transverse colon.
- Tumors of the posterior wall invade the lesser sac and then the diaphragmatic crura upward and the pancreas downward.

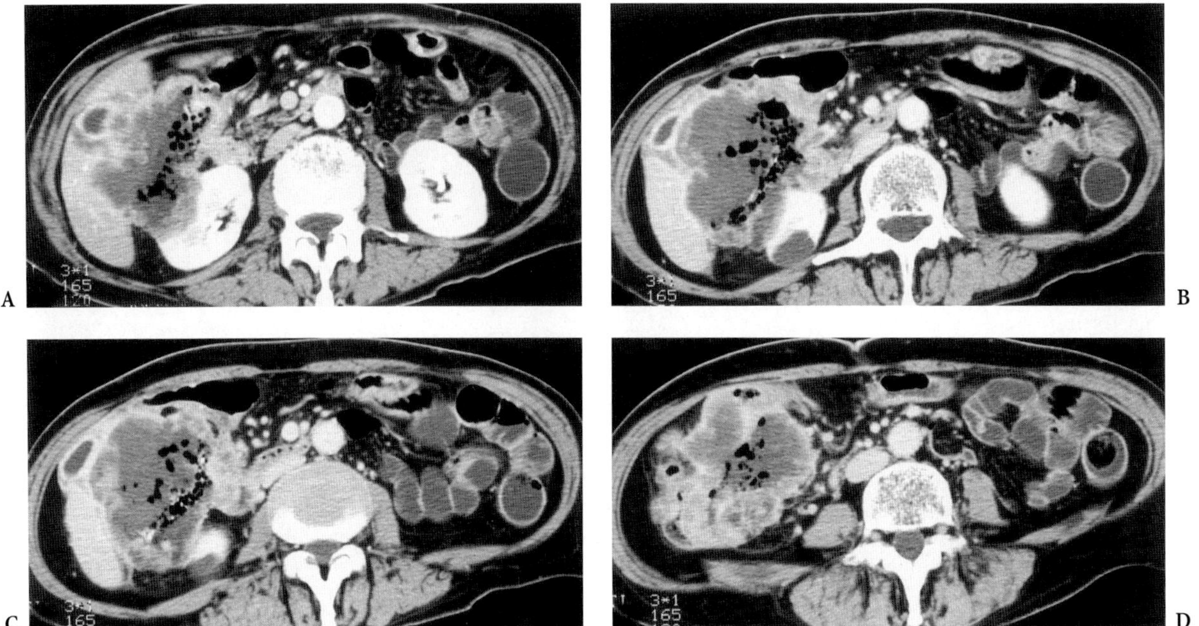

Fig. 13.43A–D. Adenocarcinoma of ascending colon. Dukes stage D (T4,N2,M1). Large, vegetating, necrotic and colliquative tumor located next to the hepatic flexure and extending beyond the mesentery and the peritoneum to the inferior pole of the liver and the gallbladder and into the renal compartment. The paracolic lymph node metastases are included in the tumoral mass

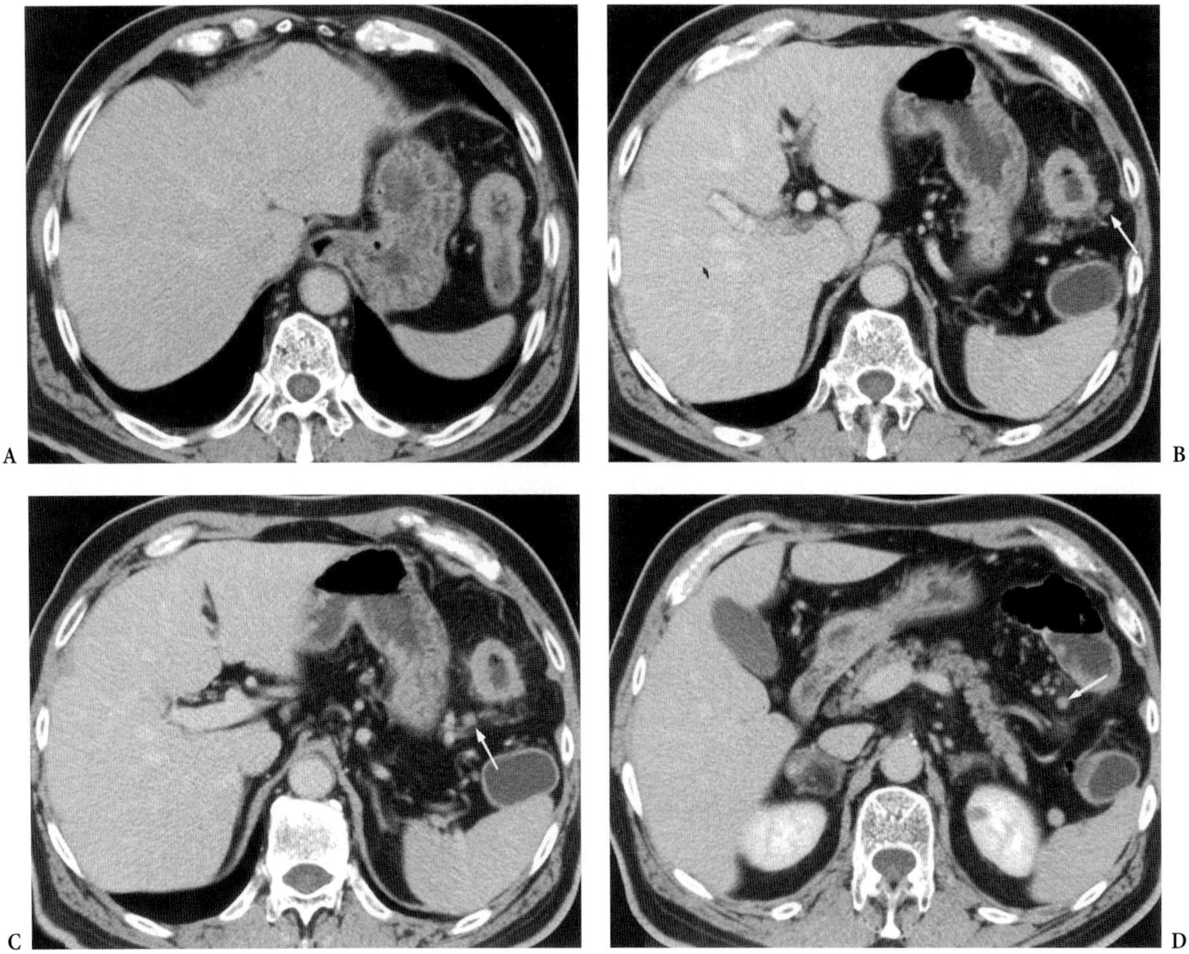

A B C D

Fig. 13.44A–D. Adenocarcinoma of colic splenic flexure. Dukes stage C2 (T3,N2,M0). Tumor infiltrating the cellular of the mesocolon. Enlarged paracolic (**B**) and left colic lymph nodes (**C, D** *arrows*)

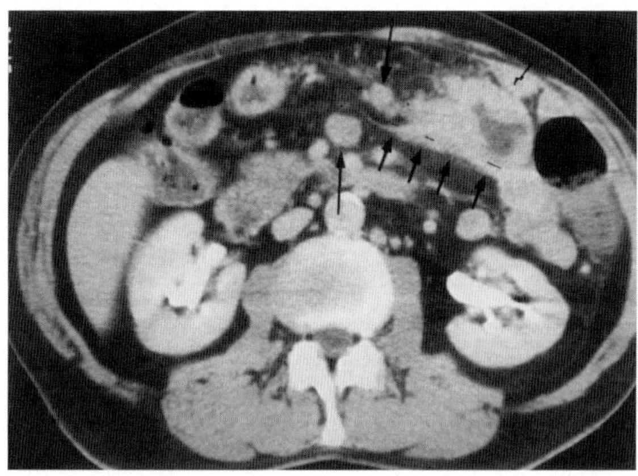

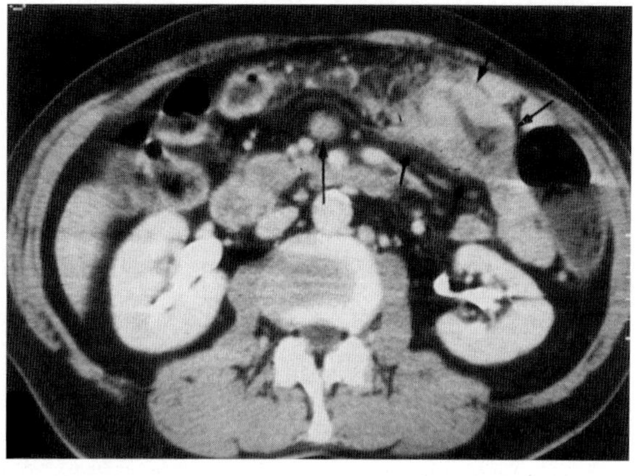

Fig. 13.45A, B. Transverse colon adenocarcinoma. Dukes stage D (T3,N2 M0). Large tumor of the transverse colon extending to the mesocolon and the omentum (*small arrows*). Metastatic paracolic and mesenteric lymph nodes (*long arrows*)

Invasion of the gastrohepatic ligament (Figs. 13.30–13.32, 13.35, 13.37) along the medial border of the lesser curvature of the stomach, either limited to the perigastric adipose tissue or extended up to the liver, can easily be recognized because it is almost constantly visible. Except in the presence of other conditions (which are common to other zones), such as lacking or insufficiently visualized adipose tissue or no cooperation from the patient, the involvement and the extension of the infiltration of this ligament is almost consistently demonstrable on CT examination.

Tumoral invasion of the gastrocolic ligament (Figs. 13.26, 13.33, 13.34, 13.37) can be recognized in front of, at the sides of and below the greater curvature in the space between the greater curvature itself and the transverse colon. Such extension is not always easily and clearly detectable in the case of small invasions below the stomach. Generally, it is not difficult to evaluate the gastrosplenic ligament, because both the subperitoneal adipose tissue of the ligament and the spleen are clearly visible on CT examination.

Evaluation of the extension of the gastric tumor to the lesser sac and to the pancreas is based on detection of the transversal transparency between stomach and pancreas; its presence generally excludes a posterior invasion. In contrast, when this transparency disappears, either a neoplastic invasion or a concomitant reactive inflammatory process can be suspected; however, it is sometimes absent just because of the absence of adipose tissue in lean or cachectic patients. Nevertheless, the extension to the pancreas is correctly recognizable in a high proportion of cases (Dehn et al. 1984; Komaki 1986; Komaki and Toyoshima 1983; Minami et al. 1992).

- To recognize a tumoral invasion of the posterior wall of the fundus ventriculi, the adipose cellular and the left diaphragmatic crus (Fig. 13.29) may be difficult because of the absence or the thinness of the adipose cellular itself. As for the retrogastric invasion toward the pancreas, in this case too, only the presence of interposed adipose tissue definitely excludes a neoplastic invasion. A thickening of the diaphragmatic crus behind the tumor is always a certain sign of neoplastic invasion if it is associated with the disappearance of the adjacent fat.

The extension of tumors to the transverse mesocolon and the greater omentum (Figs. 13.3, 13.34, 13.36, 13.37) occurs by contiguity after invasion of the gastrocolic ligament or by peritoneal spread. In the former case, the involvement of the gastrocolic ligament and the prevalently infiltrating character of the neoplastic diffusion favor a correct evaluation of the tumoral extension, whereas in the latter situation, the frequent micronodular spread raises the possibility of false-negative interpretations.

Peritoneal Diffusion. After passing the gastric wall and the serosa, the tumors may spread into the whole peritoneal cavity (carcinosis), showing the CT aspects described in the general consideration section, which are analogous to those of other intraperitoneal tumors (Fig. 13.3).

In women, a peculiar form of peritoneal spread of gastric carcinoma is seen as a secondary ovarian localization, also known as Krukenberg tumor.

On CT examination, this metastatic localization shows a prevalently bilateral character, extremely variable dimensions (3–15 cm), and different morphostructural aspects, classified into three forms:

a) Prevalently cystic, characterized by hypodense masses (5–25 HU) with a serous mucinous constitution and scarce solid protruding elements or internal septa.
b) Mixed, characterized by neoformations constituted by equal percentage amounts of solid tissue and liquid component.
c) Solid (Fig. 13.12), the most commonly observed form, prevalently made up of masses of tissue with middle-high density; sometimes, it contains areas with a nonhomogeneous structure due to extended necrosis.

Lymph Node Diffusion. The tumoral cells may spread from the parietal and perigastric lymphatic network to the primary lymph nodal stations located along the extension of the gastric arteries, the right and left gastroepiploic arteries and the short gastric arteries within the gastrohepatic, gastrocolic and gastrosplenic ligaments.

Initially, the tumors of the fundus ventriculi involve the supra- and subcardial lymph nodes medially (Figs. 13.29, 13.31) and the short gastric lymph nodes posterolaterally; on the other hand, those located along the lesser curvature initially involve the left gastric lymph nodes (Figs. 13.23, 13.29, 13.30, 13.35, 13.37) and those of the greater curvature electively affect the gastroepiploic lymph nodes (Figs. 13.34, 13.36, 13.37).

From the paracardial lymph nodes, the metastatic diffusion subsequently affects the paraesophageal lymph nodes at a high level and the lymph nodes of the proximal tract of the left gastric artery (Fig. 13.32) at a low level; on the other hand, metastases from the short gastric and gastroepiploic lymph nodes reach the splenopancreatic chain (Fig. 13.36). From the right and left gastric and gastroepiploic lymph nodes, metastases may progressively spread to pyloric, superior pancreatoduodenal (Figs. 13.31, 13.37) and superficial hepatic (Fig. 13.37) lymph nodes; the distant celiacomesenteric (Figs. 13.31, 13.37) and lumboaortic (Fig. 13.31) stations may also be reached.

The same problems as a common to all regions (scarce adipose tissue, no cooperation from the patient, etc.) may impede the CT examination of lymph node metastases; in addition, in the case of exophytic tumors it is frequently impossible to distinguish between primary tumors and adjacent metastatic lymph nodes (Fig. 13.30, 13.31, 13.37).

By analogy, when ligaments are infiltrated, the CT evaluation of metastatic lymph nodes is closely related to their site (it is easier for left gastric, right gastroepiploic, common hepatic, celiac, retropancreatic and lumboaortic lymph nodes), according to the possibility of recognizing ligaments and vessels, and thus, not only of detecting the lymph nodes, but also establishing the chain to which they belong.

To recognize the lymph nodal metastases, the site of the primary tumor, the efferent lymphatic pathways, and the lymph nodal stations (Table 13.5) must always be considered.

The proximal stations are always the primary site of the neoplastic spread; things are not the same in the case of secondary localizations, because the lymphatic flux may be partially or totally diverted because of a partial or total block of the primary lymph nodes. In this case, lymph nodes located outside the normal flux of the lymphatic stream may be involved in the metastatic diffusion.

In contrast, from a surgical point of view, the local [coronarostomachic, gastroepiploic, right gastric and supra- and subpyloric in the gastrohepatic and gastrocolic ligaments (stage N1)] adenopathies that are resected en bloc with the stomach have no negative prognostic significance.

The adenopathies affecting the secondary stations (superior and inferior pancreatoduodenal, hepatoduodenal, splenopancreatic) that are contained in the hepatoduodenal ligament or are located in the retroperitoneum (stage N2) are of critical impor-

Table 13.5. Lymph node metastatic diffusion according to the site of the gastric tumor

Site of tumor	Primary LN (N1)	Secondary LN (N2)	Distant LN (N3)
Fundus	Paracardial	Paraesophageal	
	Short gastric	Splenopancreatic	Celiaco-mesenteric; lumboaortic
	Left gastro-epiploic	Splenopancreatic	Celiaco-mesenteric; lumboaortic
Lesser curvature up to the angulus	Coronaro-stomachic		Celiaco-mesenteric; lumboaortic
Greater curvature (left part) (without the antrum)	Gastro-epiploic	Splenopancreatic	Celiaco-mesenteric; lumboaortic
Antrum	Supra-/subpyloric	Pyloric	Celiaco-mesenteric; lumboaortic
	Right gastric	Hepatoduodenal	
	Right gastro-epiploic	Pancreato-duodenal	

tance, because they may not be found during surgical exploration; if these adenopathies are not recognized and excised, they become responsible for the failure of the surgical operation.

Finally, the distant metastases [at the celiac and mesenteric level (stage N3)] require wide operations; in these cases, radical treatments are usually excluded.

At the present time, with all its limitations, CT is the best imaging method to help the surgeon in the choice of treatment.

Particularly, according to our personal experience, we believe that:

a) A tumor limited to the wall, with transparent perigastric cellular, without signs of peritoneal infiltrations, lymph node enlargements and distant secondary localizations can certainly be treated surgically.
b) Involvement of lymph nodes located around the stomach and the gastric or gastroepiploic vessels does not exclude a surgical operation, because these lymph nodes are always dissected en bloc with the stomach.
c) The neoplasms that must be considered inoperable or not suitable for radical surgery are:
   - Tumors extending to posterior structures (pancreas, splenic vessels, diaphragmatic crura, abdominal wall).
   - Tumors involving the gastrohepatic ligament and the diaphragm.
   - Tumors infiltrating the colon and the mesocolon.
   - Tumors with hepatic metastases or directly infiltrating the liver.
   - Tumors spreading over the peritoneum.
   - Tumors associated with celiac and lumboaortic lymph node enlargement.

At the present time, the accuracy of spiral CT with water-induced distension ranges around 82% in the case of gastric tumors passing the wall (Stell et al 1996), around 100% (Fukuya et al. 1997; Richter et al. 1996) for the T factor and from 65% to 82% for the N factor (Rossi et al. 1997).

13.3 Colonic Carcinoma

The pathways followed by local and lymph nodal diffusions of colonic tumors depend on the site of the wall from which they take origin, the orientation of the surrounding peritoneum, whether they are partially or totally surrounded by the peritoneum, the orientation of the mesocolic subperitoneal spaces and their continuity in the retroperitoneum, the extension of the lymphatic pathway and the position of the corresponding lymph nodes, and finally, the contiguity with organs or structures located outside the peritoneum and fasciae limiting the lateroconal compartments. The preferential pathways in the diffusion by contiguity of the colonic tumors can be classified as follows:

1) The tumors of the transverse colon tend to infiltrate the gastrocolic ligament above, the transverse mesocolon behind, and the greater omentum in the front and below (Figs. 13.44, 13.45).
2) Tumors of the ascending and descending colon develop within the fatty tissue of the mesocolon and the retroperitoneum of the corresponding lateroconal compartments, extending up to the anterior renal fascia posteriorly and the lateroconal fasciae at the sides, and infiltrating the peritoneum anteriorly (Figs. 13.38–13.43, 13.47, 13.48).
3) Tumors of the sigmoid grow within the sigmoid mesocolon (Figs. 13.52–13.55), which they pass to spread throughout the retroperitoneum. They involve the ureters and the iliac vessels (Fig. 13.57), the bladder wall (Fig. 13.58), the internal genital organs (Fig. 13.56) and the ileum.
4) Tumors of the rectum grow within the perirectal fatty tissue: in the upper third part, they may expand forward, infiltrating the posterior peritoneum by which they are covered. In the remaining two inferior parts, these tumors infiltrate the perirectal fat up to the limiting fascia; beyond the fascia they may involve the ureters, the internal genital organs and the levator ani muscles.

Lymph node metastases are located along the pathways of lymphatic flux coming from the various tracts of the colon:

- In tumors of the cecum, the first lymph nodes to be affected are those located on the internal side of the viscus (Fig. 13.42). Afterwards, the ileocolic lymph node stations located in the transparency of the mesentery, next to the homonymous vessels (Figs. 13.38, 13.40, 13.42) may be involved; finally, the lymph node stations surrounding the trunks of the superior mesenteric vessels may be invaded (Fig. 13.40).
- In tumors of the ascending colon, the primary lymph nodes are visible on the medial side of the viscus, next to the punctiform images of the right paracolic vessels (Figs. 13.34–13.43), whereas the secondary stations are located along the right colic branches (Figs. 13.38, 13.40, 13.41), which cross

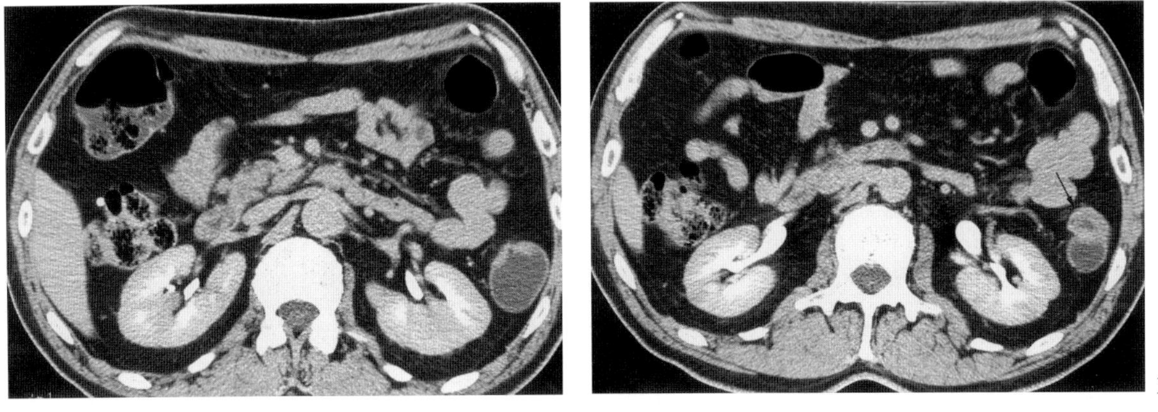

Fig. 13.46A, B. Descending colon carcinoma. Dukes stage A (T1,N0,M0). Thickened circumscribed colonic wall (*arrow*) with sharp outer margins. The paracolic fat is normal: no infiltration is present

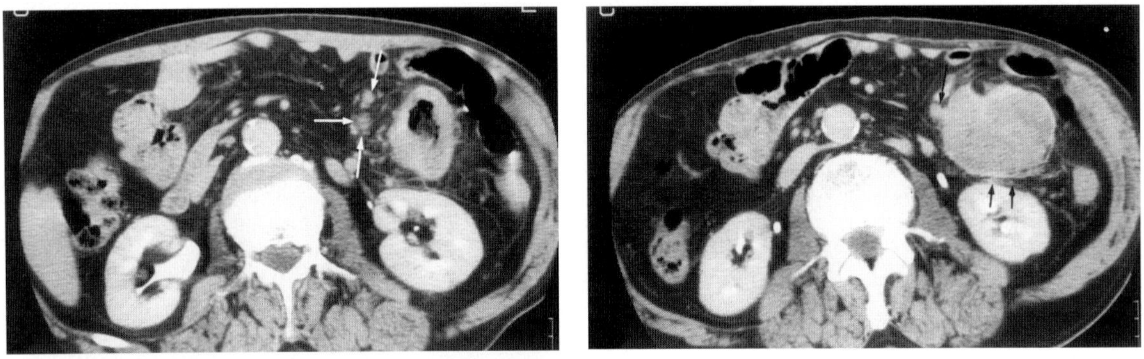

Fig. 13.47A–C. Descending colon adenocarcinoma. Dukes stage C2 (T3,N2,M0). Colonic neoplasm invading the pericolic and lateroconal spaces (higher density of the adipose tissue) up to the end of the anterior renal fascia, which appears to be slightly thicker (*small arrows*). Metastatic paracolic (**A, B**) and left colic (**C**) lymph nodes (*long arrows*)

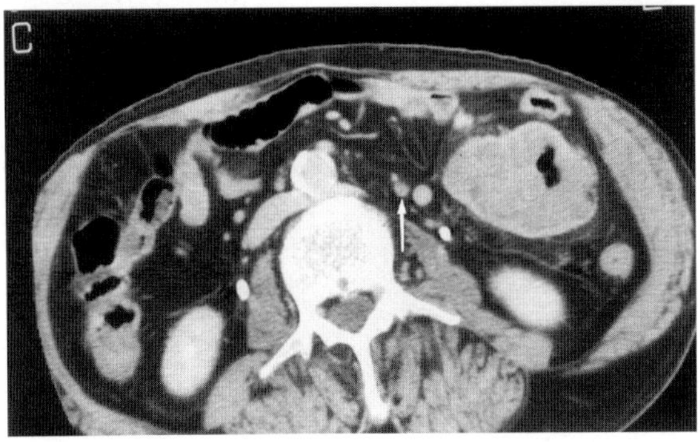

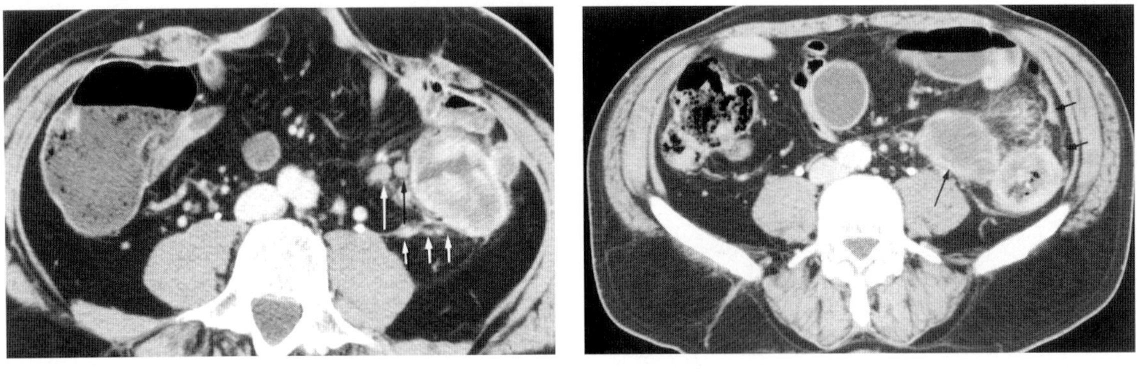

Fig. 13.48A, B. Descending colon adenocarcinoma. Dukes stage D (T3,N2,M0). Adenocarcinoma extending up to the lateroconal and the anterior renal fasciae and the posterior peritoneum (*small arrows*). Metastases in the paracolic, colic and inferior mesenteric lymph nodes (*long arrows*)

A 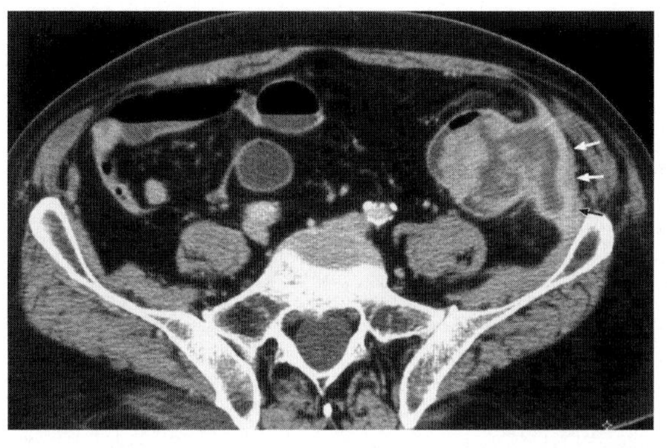 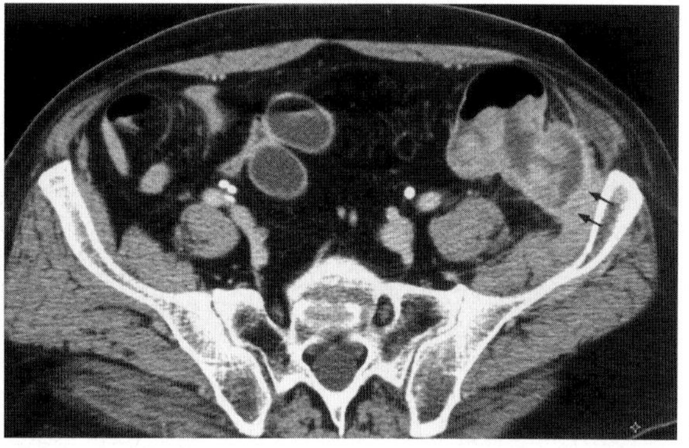 B

Fig. 13.49A, B. Descending colon carcinoma. Dukes stage D (T4,N0,M0). Extension of the tumor to the transversalis fascia and the aponeurosis of the left iliac muscle (*small arrows*)

A 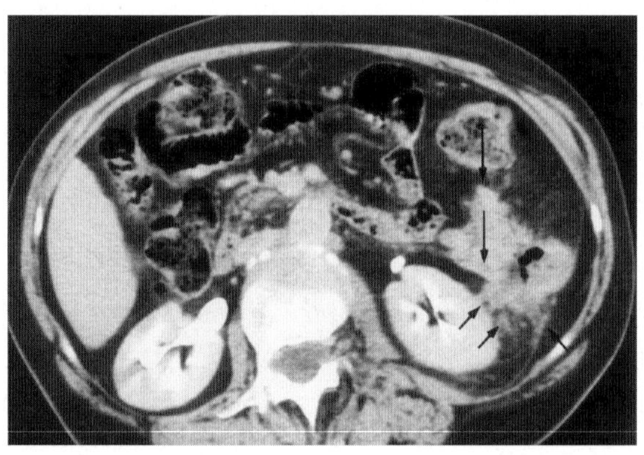 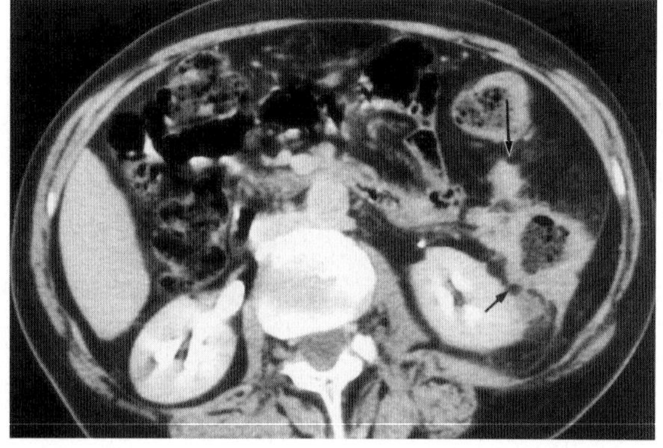 B

Fig. 13.50A, B. Descending colon carcinoma. Dukes stage D (T4,N1,MO). Wide invasion by neoplasm of the mesentery (*long arrows*), extending into the anterior pararenal and perirenal spaces (*small arrows*)

A 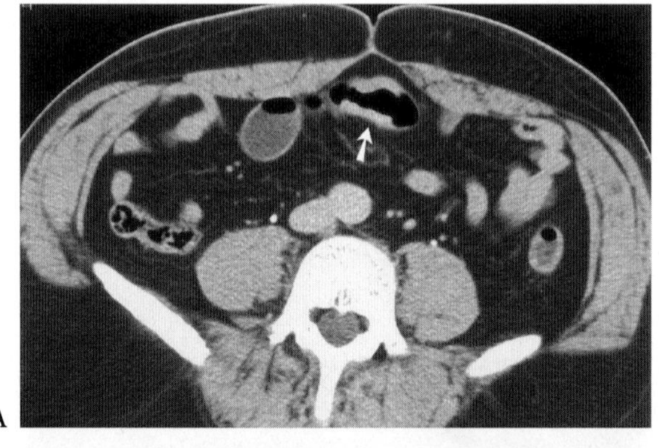 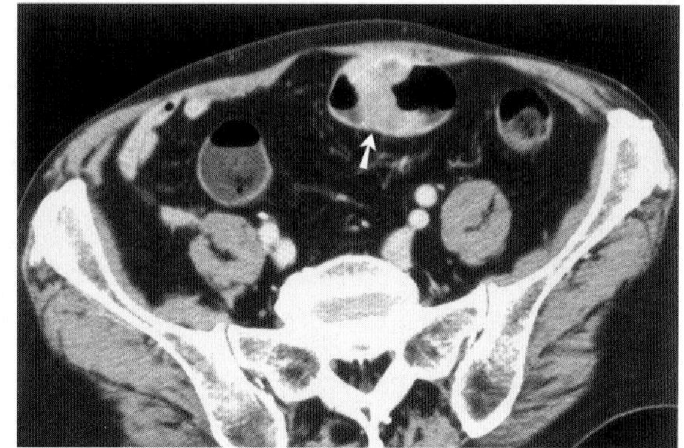 B

C 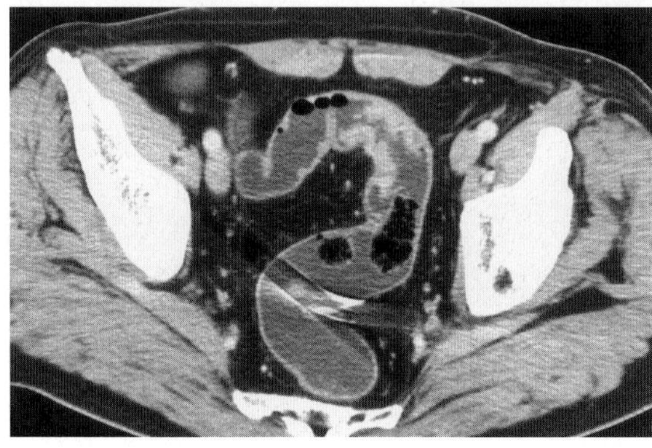

Fig. 13.51A–C. Sigmoidal adenocarcinomas (three cases). Dukes stage A (T2,N0,M0). Tumors limited to the wall: sharp outer profile of the intestinal wall also at the level of the tumor and transparency of the adjacent adipose tissue

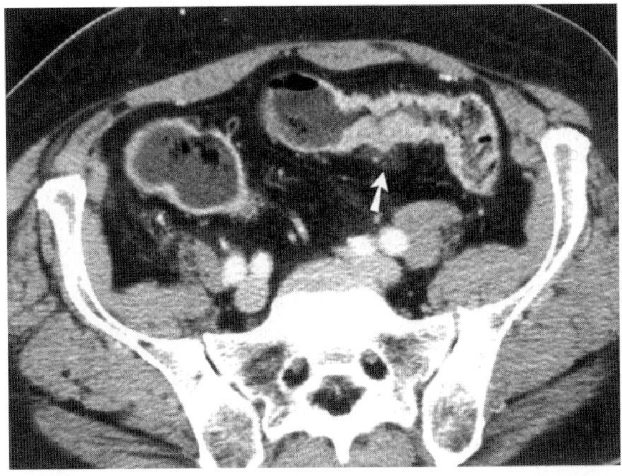

Fig. 13.52. Sigmoidal adenocarcinoma. Dukes stage B (T3, N0, M0). Initially invasive adenocarcinoma: dentate profile of the infiltrated wall and light shading of the perisigmoidal fat

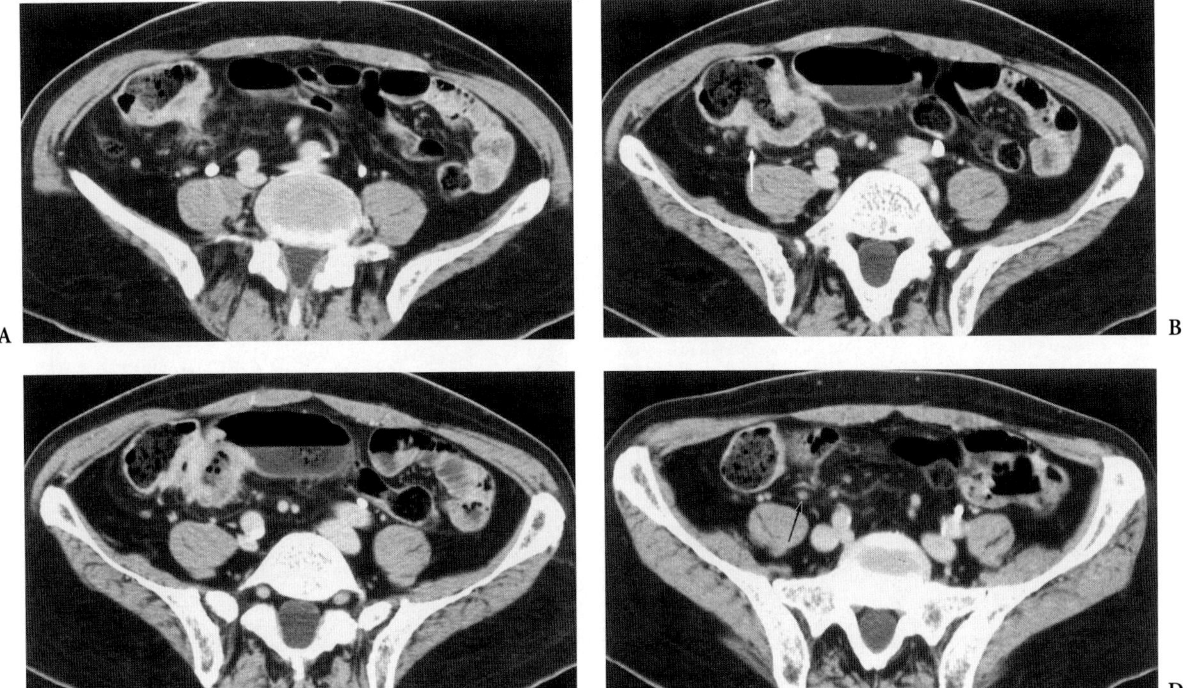

Fig. 13.53A–D. Sigmoidal adenocarcinoma. Duke stage C2 (T3,N2,M0). Tumor invading the sigmoid mesocolon with multiple lymph nodal metastases. It shows characteristic "frayed" contours. **A–C** Stranding and increased density of the perisigmoidal fat .Enlarged metastatic **B** parasigmoidal and **D** sigmoidal lymph nodes (*long arrows*)

the abdomen obliquely to reach the superior mesenteric vessels (Fig. 13.40).

- In tumors of the transverse colon, the marginal lymph nodes are usually visible behind the viscus (Fig. 13.45), but may also be located above or below, according to its position. The secondary lymph nodes are visible in the thickness of the transverse mesocolon near the middle colic vessels, which usually extend transversely (Fig. 13.45); hence, the lymphatic flux reaches the superior mesenteric lymph nodes (Fig. 13.15).
- In tumors of the splenic flexure, the primary lymph nodes are located below and on the medial side of the intestinal arcade, and the secondary lymph nodes are placed next to the ascending branches of the left colic vessels, outside and just above Treitz's duodenojejunal flexure (Fig. 13.44).
- In tumors of the descending colon, the primary lymph nodes must be sought on the medial side of the viscus, near the paracolic vascular branches (Figs. 13.47, 13.48), while the secondary lymph nodes are in a more internal position along the

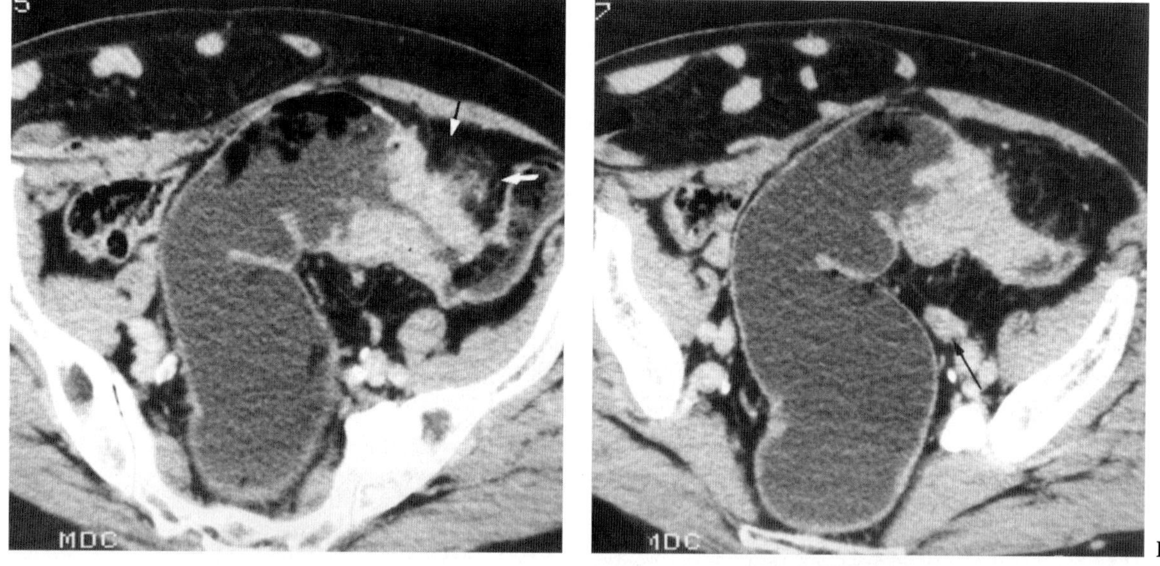

Fig. 13.54A, B. Proximal sigmoidal tract carcinoma. Dukes stage C2 (T3,N1,M0). Circumferential infiltrating neoplasm extending with dense strands in the sigmoid mesocolon (*small arrows*). Metastasis in a sigmoidal lymph node (*long arrow*)

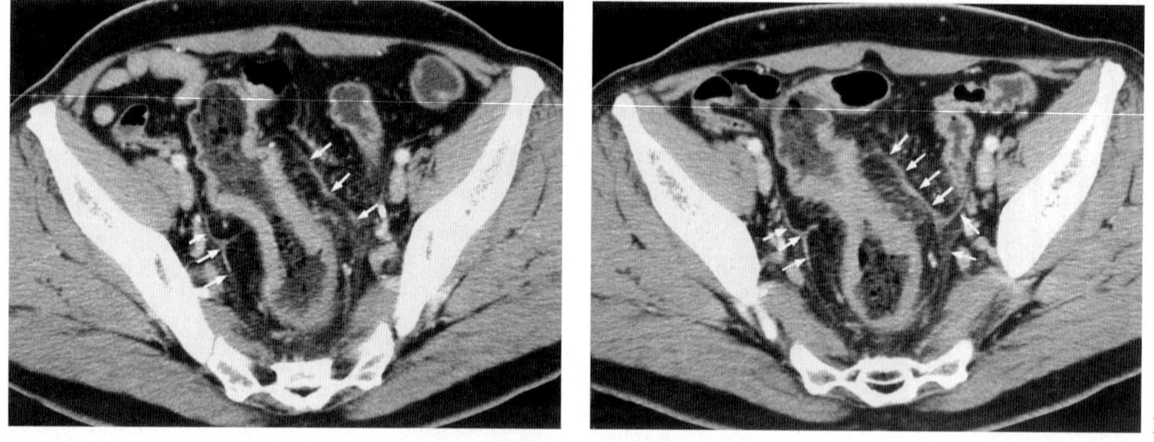

Fig. 13.55A, B. Sigmoid carcinoma. Duke's stage C1 (T3,N0,M0). Circumferential thickening of the walls of the sigmoid, with radiating soft-density stranding in the sigmoid mesocolon extending to the thickened peritoneum

path of the left colic vessels (Figs. 13.47, 13.48), which extend up to joining the inferior mesenteric vessels (Fig. 13.48).

The inferior mesenteric lymph nodal stations are located both along the homonymous artery up to the paraaortic lymph nodes and along the vein up to its junction with the superior mesenteric vein.

- In the tumors of the sigmoid, the primary lymph nodes are visible above and behind the sigmoid (Figs. 13.53, 13.54, 13.57, 13.59), while the intermediate lymph nodes are located near the sigmoidal vessels (Figs. 13.53, 13.57, 13.59). The secondary lymph nodal stations follow the inferior mesenteric vessels and are preferentially located along the extension of the artery (Figs. 13.57, 13.59).
- In tumors of the rectum, the primary lymph nodes must be sought around the viscus and the secondary lymph nodes near the two right and left branches of the superior hemorrhoidal arteries (which extend along the rectum up to their convergence with the sigmoidal artery into the inferior mesenteric artery) and then near the inferior mesenteric vessels.

The staging of colonic tumors is defined by Dukes modified classification (Turnbull 1967) based on

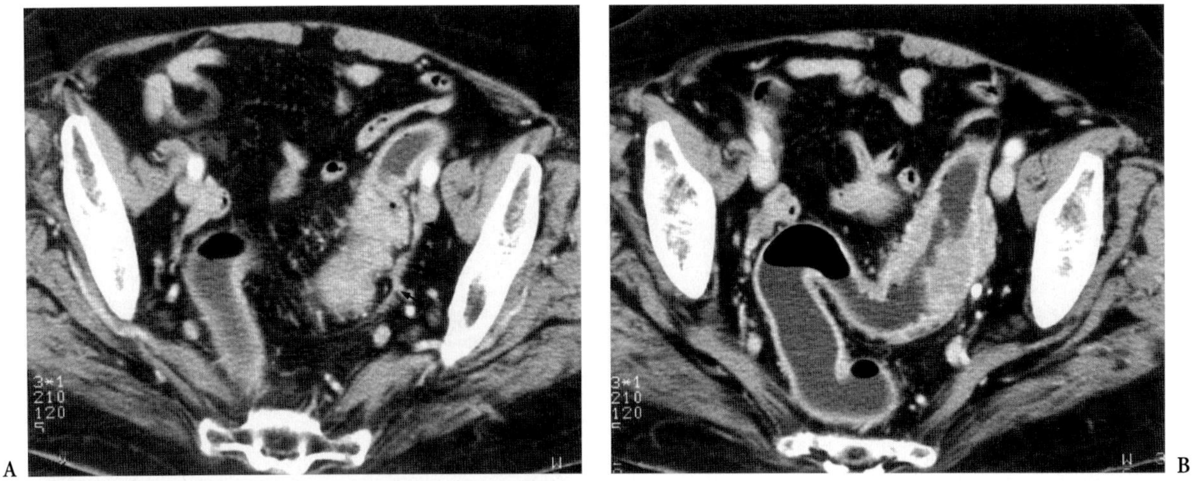

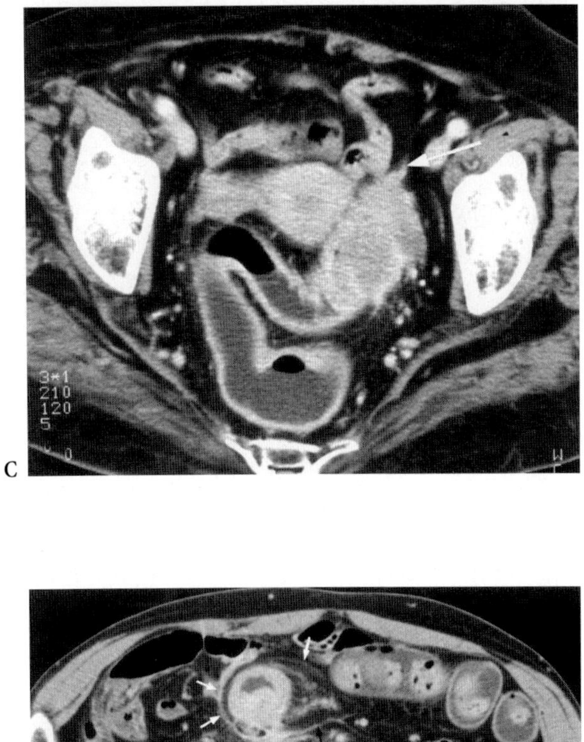

Fig. 13.56A–C. Proximal sigmoidal tract carcinoma. Duke's stage C1 (T3,N0,M0). Sigmoid neoplasm with invasion of mesosigmoidal fat extending up to the peritoneum and the left broad ligament (*long thick arrow*)

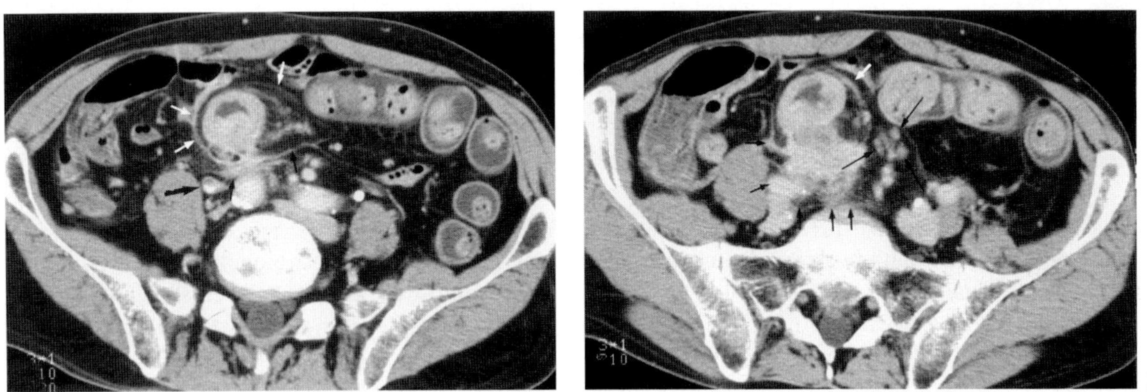

Fig. 13.57A, B. Sigmoid carcinoma. Dukes stage D (T4,N2,M1). Soft tissue sigmoidal mass extending to the sigmoid mesocolon, to the thickened peritoneum and to the retroperitoneal fat and encasing **A** the ureter (*long thick arrow*) and **B** the right iliac vessels. Enlarged metastatic sigmoidal and inferior mesenteric lymph nodes (**B** *long thin arrows*)

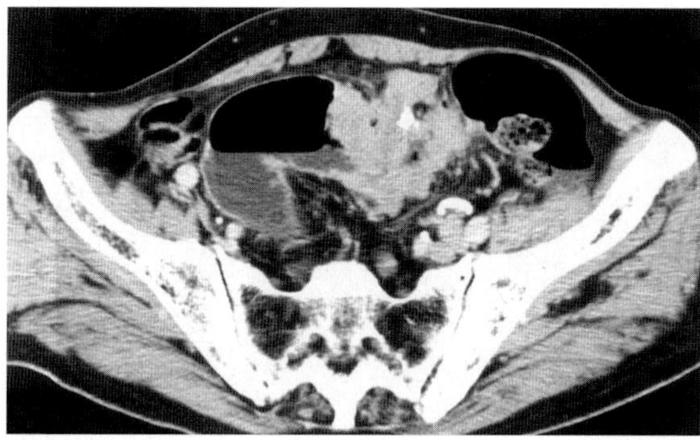
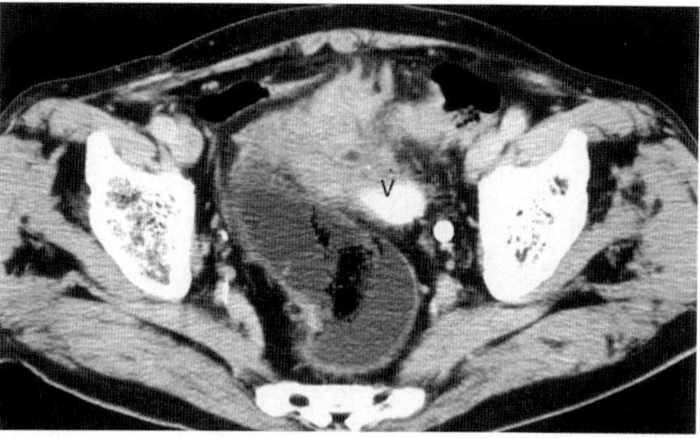

Fig. 13.58A, B. Sigmoid adenocarcinoma. Dukes stage D (T4,N0,M1). Large soft tissue mass causing a sigmoidal substenosis and invading the sigmoid mesocolon and the urinary bladder (**B**)

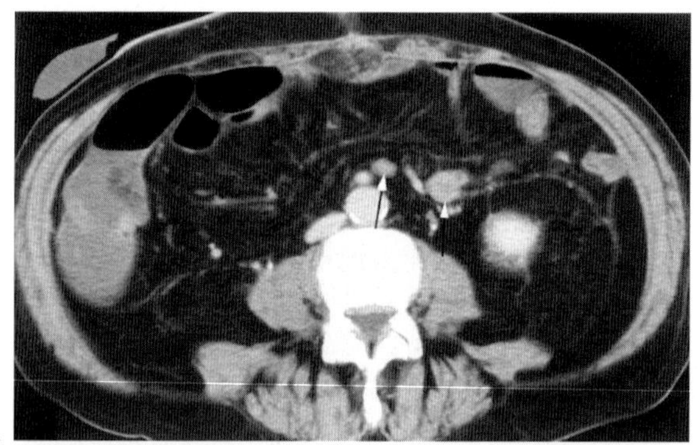
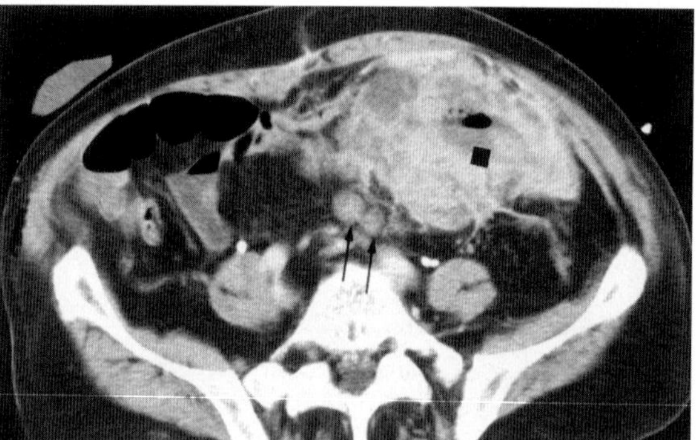
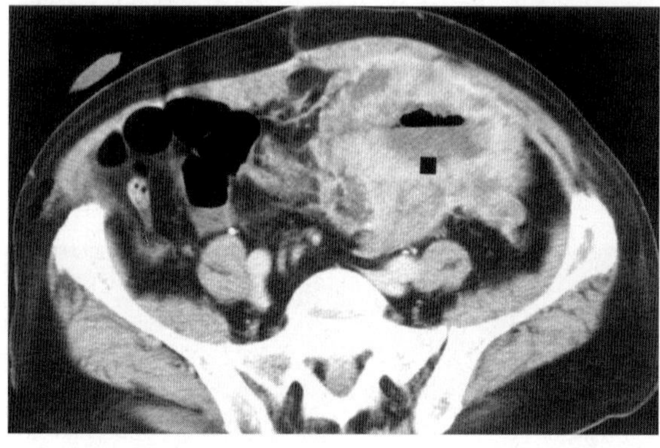

Fig. 13.59A–C. Proximal sigmoidal tract carcinoma. Dukes stage D (T3,N2,M0). Large abscessed mass with air-fluid level (*square*) owing to a neoplasm that has perforated in the sigmoid mesocolon. Enlarged metastatic sigmoidal and inferior mesenteric lymph nodes (*long thin arrows*)

the depth of invasion, the spread to adjacent organs or structures, the lymph node involvement and the presence of distal metastases (see Table 13.6).

Table 13.6. Dukes classification of colonic tumors[a]

Stage	Pathologic features
A	Limited to colonic wall
B	Extending into the pericolic fat
C1	Limited to colonic wall, positive regional nodes
C2	Extending into the pericolic fat, positive regional lymph nodes
D	Involving adjacent organs, peritoneal carcinosis, distant metastasis

[a]Modified by Tumbell

CT with spiral technique and water-induced expansion of the colon has been shown to be very reliable for a presurgical evaluation of these tumors and the selection of patients with Dukes stages A, B, and C of disease, who may be treated with a radical surgical op-eration, in contrast to those with stage D, whose tu-mors are inoperable; the latter group of patients must be treated by an oncologist and/or a radiotherapist, or may be referred for palliative surgery, such as a derivative operation (Balthazar et al. 1988; Acunas et al. 1990, 1991; Gazelle et al. 1995; Zerhouni et al. 1996).

Even though the evaluation of the local tumoral extension is not highly reliable, especially as far as the lymph nodal metastatic diffusion is concerned (48–73% reliability) (Acunas et al. 1990; Zerhouni et al. 1996) because of the frequent false-negative observations owing to micrometastases and the false-positive observations owing to reactive-inflammatory hyperplasia, at the present time the CT is the best radiological diagnostic technique for staging colonic tumors.

13.4 Carcinoma of the Gallbladder

In most cases, gallbladder carcinoma is already inoperable when it is diagnosed, because it has already invaded the liver and the adjacent structures and metastasized to the liver or lymph nodes. However, in a small number of patients a surgical operation may be successful. Ohtani et al. (1993, 1996) reported a survival rate at 5 years after operation of 45% of patients selected by means of CT and treated with radical surgery who were affected by noninfiltrating tumors with metastases only in the cystic and choledochal lymph nodes. The operation consisted in cholecystectomy, wedge resection of the hepatic gallbladder bed, resection of the suprapancreatic segment of the extrahepatic bile duct and en bloc dissection of the regional lymph nodes. An additional cephalopancreato-duodenectomy is performed when the lymph nodes located around the head of the pancreas are also involved.

During its evolution, the gallbladder carcinoma passes the wall of the viscus and spreads by contiguity over the pericholecystic and perihepatic peritoneum, to the inferior face of the liver, the hepatoduodenal ligament and the structures located inside (bile ducts and vessels), the duodenum and the pancreas. It then expands along the gastrohepatic and gastrocolic ligaments to the transverse mesocolon and the omentum, and spreads distantly into the peritoneal cavity, causing carcinosis. The involvement of the liver is favored by the communication between the venous network of the hepatic wall and that of the gallbladder.

Through the lymphatic flux, the tumor may progressively metastasize to the local and regional (cystic and pericholedochal), secondary (hepatic, gastroduodenal, superior and inferior pancreatoduodenal) and distal (celiac, paraaortic and paracaval) lymph nodes. Furthermore, the tumor may penetrate the main biliary tract through the lumen.

CT is unable to detect the pericholecystic peritoneal involvement, because the peritoneum cannot be distinguished from the cholecystic wall. In contrast, the invasion by contiguity of the inferior face of the liver appears as a hypodense area inside the hepatic parenchyma, which cannot be distinguished from the image of the primary cholecystic tumor (Figs. 13.60, 13.61, 13.63–13.65).

The involvement of the hepatoduodenal, gastrohepatic, gastrocolic ligaments and the mesocolon is characterized by the thickening of the peritoneum, by which these structures are constituted and by the presence of striations, with shading and dimming of the fat located inside (Figs. 13.61, 13.62, 13.64, 13.65).

Involvement of the choledochus makes the fat of the hepatoduodenal ligament (where the duct is placed) denser and causes swelling of the biliary structures that are located above (Fig. 13.65).

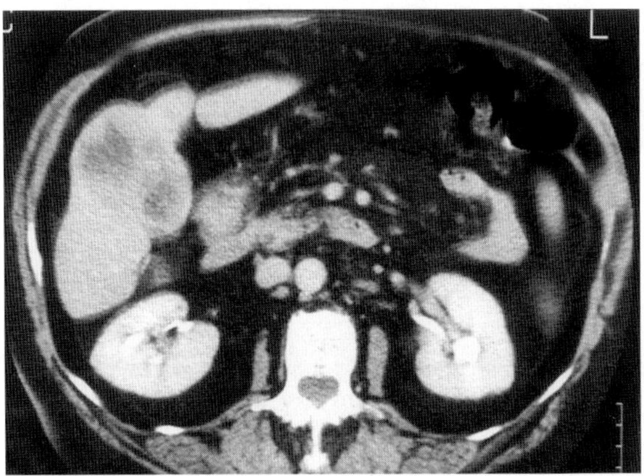

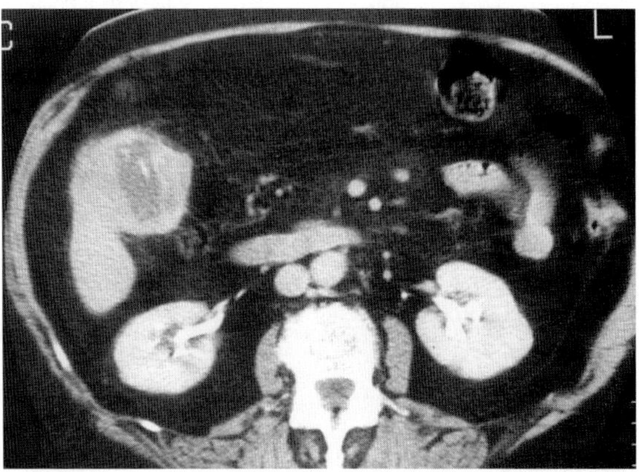

Fig. 13.60AA, B. Gallbladder carcinoma. The tumor invades the inferior face of the fifth hepatic segment, without extending beyond the pericholecystic peritoneum or producing lymph node metastases

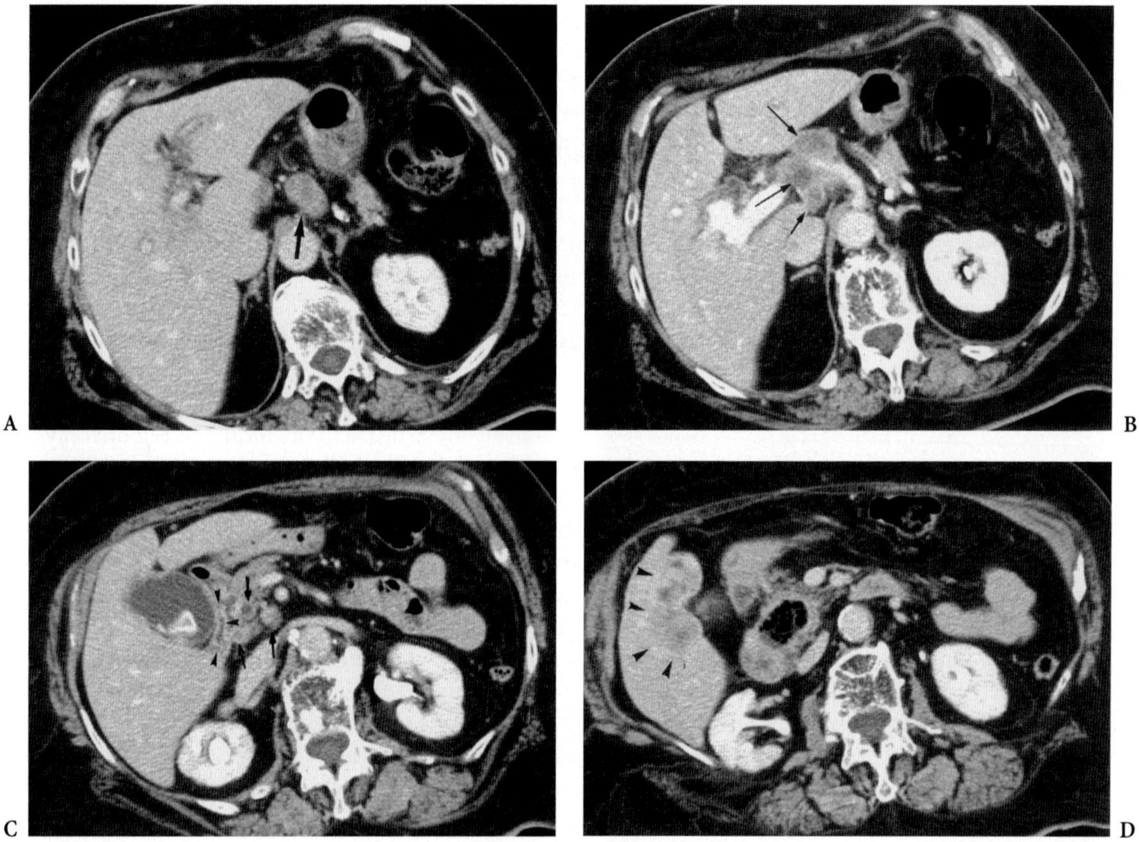

Fig. 13.61A–D. Carcinoma of the fundus of the gallbladder. Tumoral invasion by contiguity of the fifth hepatic segment (D *arrowheads*) and of the hepatoduodenal ligament (C *small arrowheads*). Metastatic involvement of the right celiac (A *thick arrow*), superficial hepatic (B *long thin arrows*), and gastroduodenal and posterior pancreatoduodenal (C *small arrows*) lymph nodes

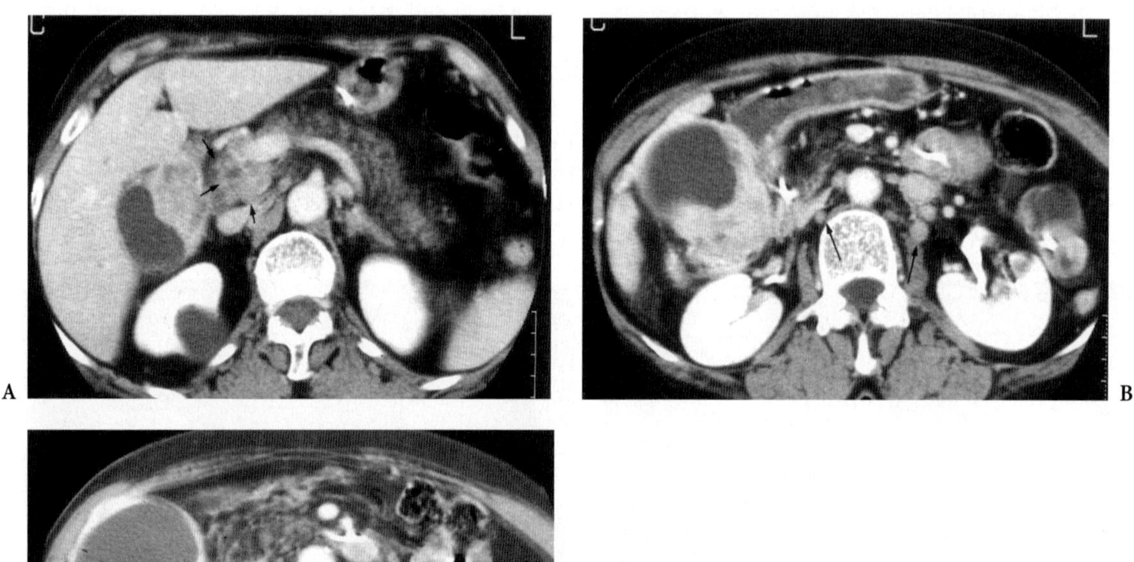

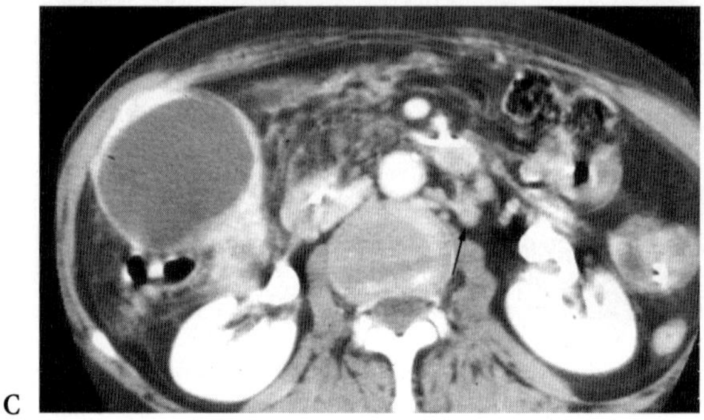

Fig. 13.62A–C. Carcinoma of the infundibular region of the gallbladder. The tumor has invaded the hepatoduodenal and gastrocolic ligaments (B, C). Metastases in the superficial hepatic lymph nodes (A small arrows), located in the hepatoduodenal ligament between the portal vein and the vena cava, and in the right and left lumboaortic lymph nodes (B, C long arrows)

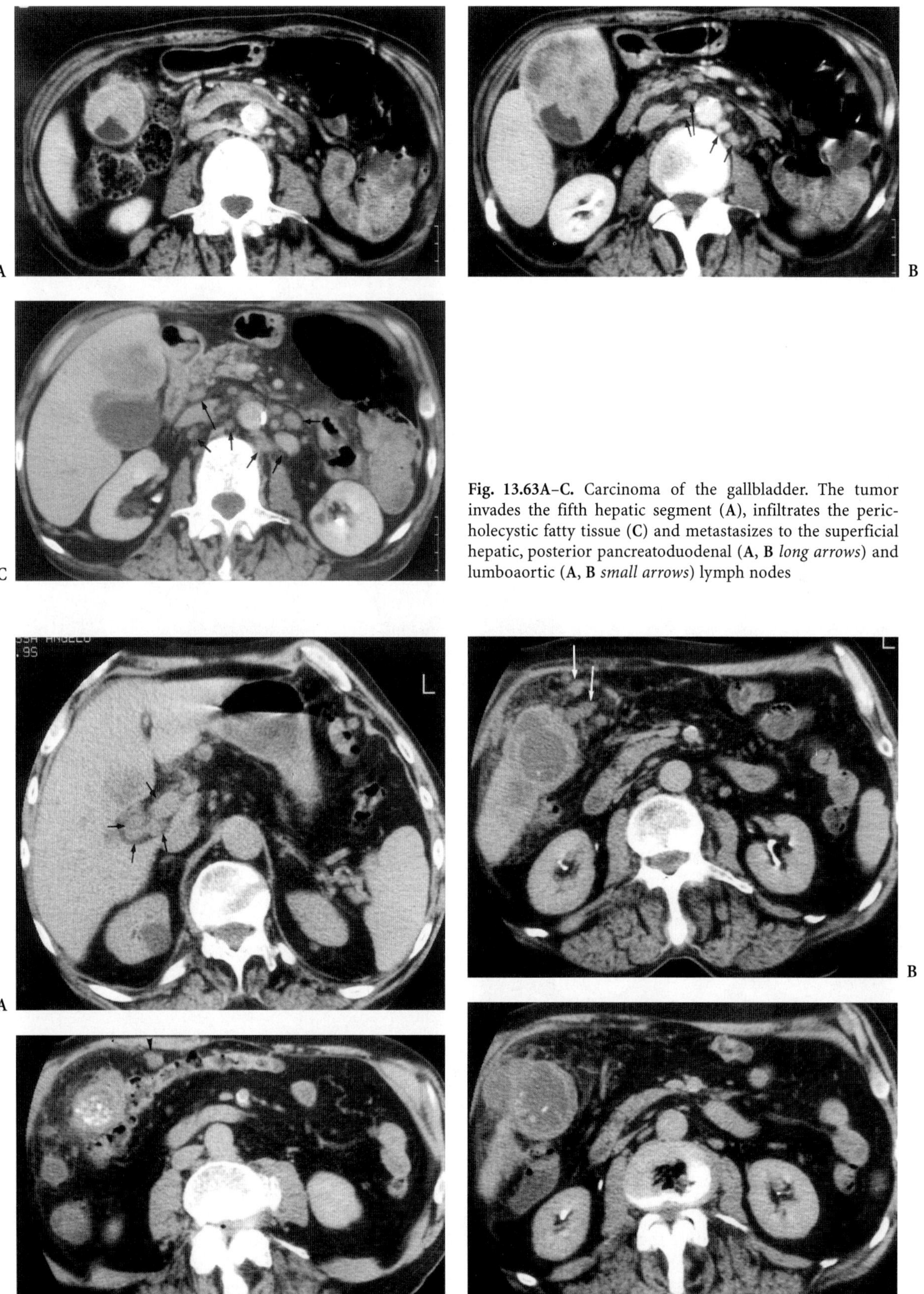

Fig. 13.63A–C. Carcinoma of the gallbladder. The tumor invades the fifth hepatic segment (**A**), infiltrates the pericholecystic fatty tissue (**C**) and metastasizes to the superficial hepatic, posterior pancreatoduodenal (**A**, **B** *long arrows*) and lumboaortic (**A**, **B** *small arrows*) lymph nodes

Fig. 13.64A–D. Abscessed carcinoma of the gallbladder, widely infiltrating the liver, the peritoneum, the hepatoduodenal (**B**) and gastrocolic (**B**, **C**) ligaments and the transverse mesocolon (**D**). Metastases in the deep hepatic (**A** *small arrows*) and right gastroepiploic (**B** *long thin arrows*) lymph nodes, and in the omentum (**C** *arrowhead*)

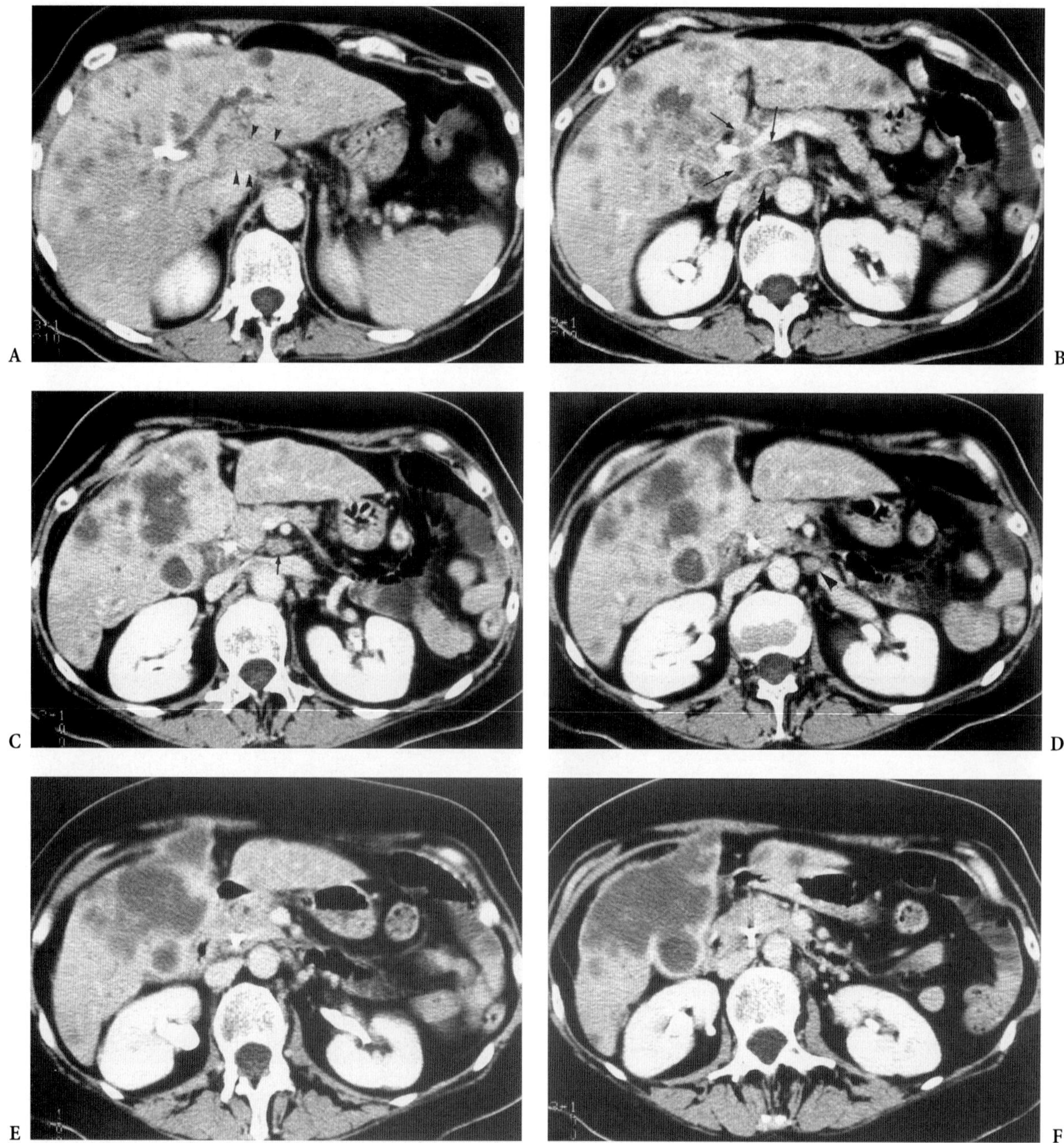

Fig. 13.65A–F. Carcinoma of the gallbladder, widely invading the inferior segments of the right lobe of the liver (**B–D**, **F**) and infiltrating the gastroduodenal ligament, the duodenum and the pancreas (**D**, **E**). The duodenum is narrowed and has thick walls (**E**). The choledochus is infiltrated and stenotic; the intrahepatic ducts are widely swelled, in spite of the intracholedochal stent (**A**). Metastases in the deep hepatic (**A** *arrowheads*), gastroduodenal (**A** *long thin arrows*), superior (**B** *long thin arrows*) and posteroinferior (**C** *small arrow*) pancreatoduodenal, retrocaval (**B** *thick arrow*) and lumboaortic (**C**) lymph nodes. Multiple hepatic metastases. Thin perihepatic ascitic layer (**B**)

In the case of spread into the peritoneal cavity, the development of ascites is observed; it is initially limited to the right perihepatic recesses (Fig. 13.65) and then expands into the whole cavity, forming nodules varying in number and width, which protrude from the wall toward the peritoneal cavity.

The first lymph nodal structures to be involved by the tumor cells are the cystic and pericholedochal stations that are located in front of the angle constituted by the cystic duct and the hepatocholedochus, and posterolaterally to the choledochus, respectively. These lymph nodes can easily be involved by the primary tumor, forming a single mass with the neoplasm. Subsequent localizations may concern the posterosuperior pancreatoduodenal lymph nodes (Figs. 13.61, 13.63, 13.65) located between the superior genu of the duodenum and the head of the pancreas, the lymph nodes of the retroportal (or Winslow's) space (Fig. 13.62) located between the portal trunk and the inferior vena cava and the right celiac lymph nodes (Fig. 13.61), behind the common hepatic artery on the right side of the celiac trunk. These last communicate with the left interaortocaval and lumboaortic lymph nodes behind the renal fascia, next to the left renal vein (Figs. 13.62, 13.63, 13.65). Frequently, the superficial and deep hepatic and the gastroduodenal lymph nodes (Figs. 13.61–13.65) located along the extension of the proprius and common hepatic artery are involved, both because they drain the lymph coming from the hepatic gallbladder bed, which is usually invaded by the tumor, and because of possible direct communications due to retrograde flux caused by pancreatoduodenal lymphatic block.

13.5 Ovarian Carcinoma

Ovarian carcinomas are characterized by the peculiarity of remaining asymptomatic for a long time; in most cases they do not become clinically evident until after local, but especially distal, spread has taken place. They expand by contiguity, through intraperitoneal invasion, and by the lymphatic and hematic routes.

The local and regional diffusion by contiguity tends to involve the urinary bladder, the sigmoid and the pelvic structures up to the lateral wall.

The intraperitoneal path is the main route of diffusion. The tumoral cells falling from the tumor into the peritoneal cavity are moved upward by the flux of the peritoneal liquid and settle over the whole serosa, the omentum and the peritoneal surface of the diaphragm.

Through the lymphatic pathway, tumoral emboli follow the ovarian collectors and can thus reach the retroperitoneal lymph nodes of the homolateral renal hilum; from here, they flow directly into the lumbar lymphatic duct and the thoracic duct, reaching the left (occasionally the right) subclavian vein and penetrating the bloodstream; finally, they stop at the level of the pulmonary capillary filter. More frequently, the lung is involved because of direct intravenous spread from either the ovarian vein or the pelvic venous

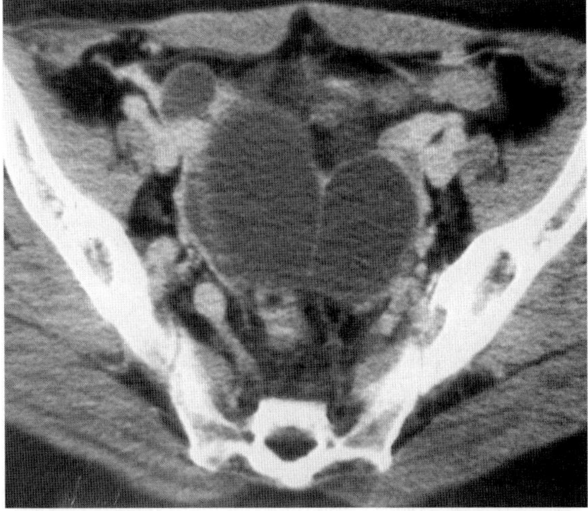
A

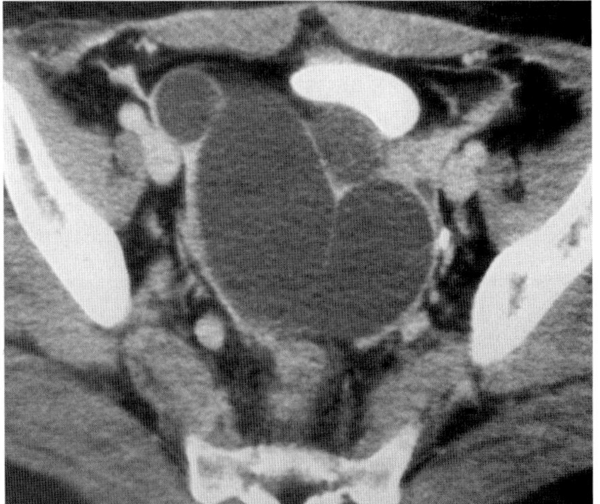
B

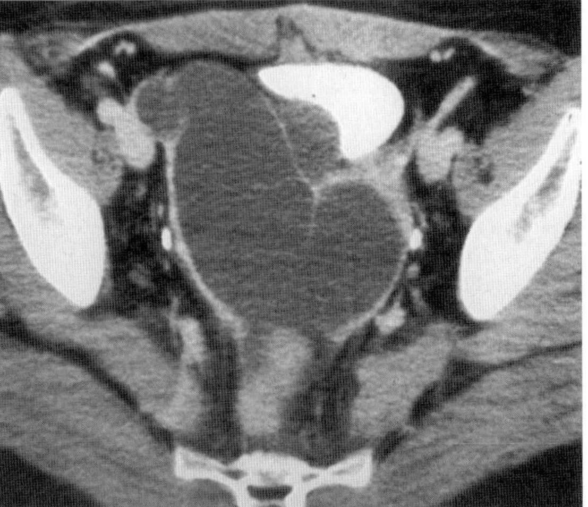
C

Fig. 13.66A–C. Ovarian cystadenocarcinoma. The tumor infiltrates the round ligaments on both sides. Evident contrast enhancement of the tumoral solid component, of the thick wall of the multicystic mass, and of the invaded round ligaments

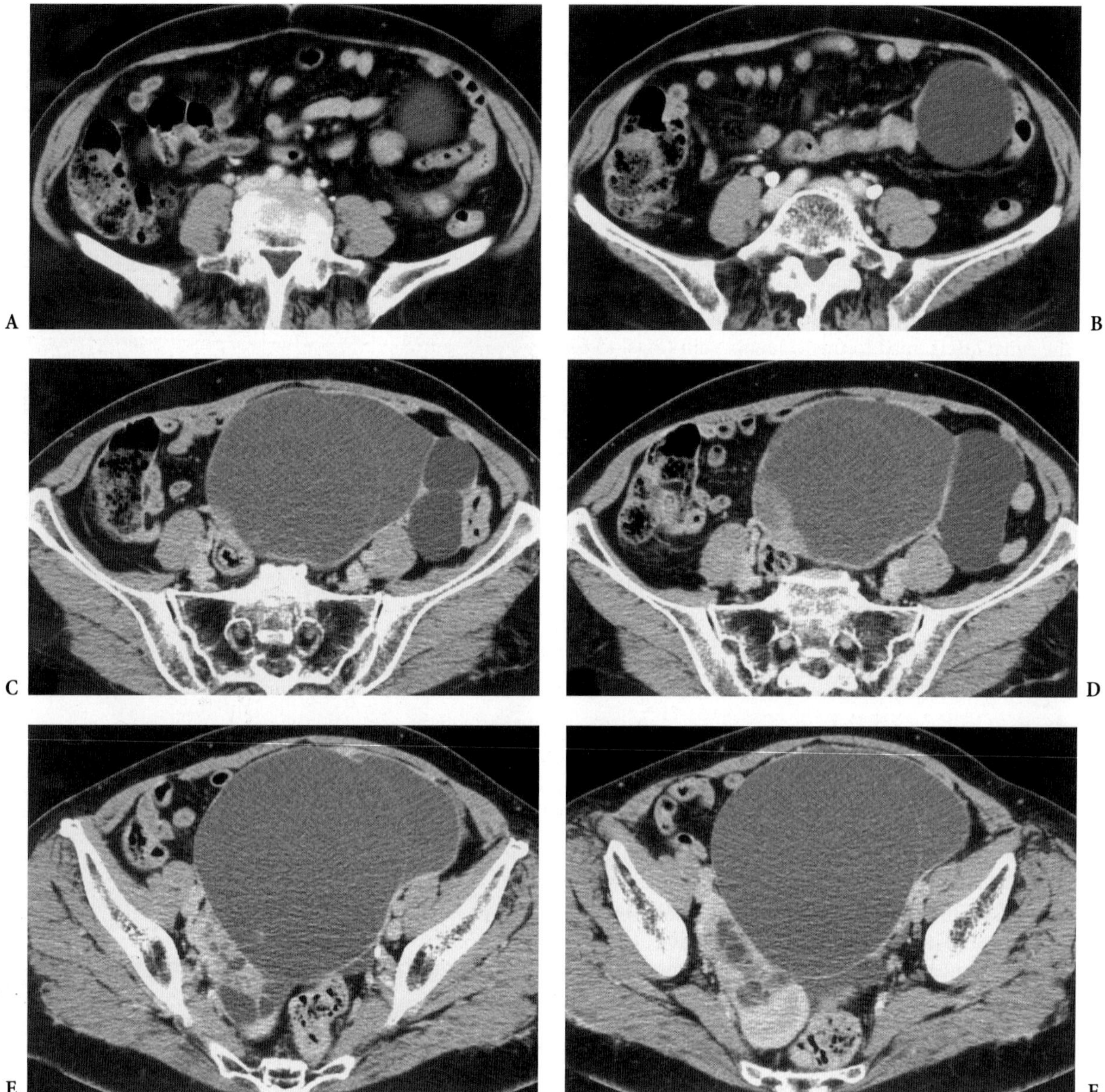

Fig. 13.67.A–F Cystadenocarcinoma of the right ovary. Mass with a prevalently cystic structure and peripheral solid component; the walls and the protrusions are made deeply opaque by the contrast medium. The sigmoid is pushed toward the left and backward; the ileal loops are raised and displaced in a semicircular shape above and on the right side of the mass, without signs of infiltration

plexus. Thus, this double route of spread explains the frequent presence of pulmonary metastases.

Secondary hepatic metastases are less frequent, because they can only be caused by portal hematic spread that has taken place since the tumor first involved the sigmoidal and superior hemorrhoidal veins.

On CT examination, ovarian tumors are variable in appearance: solid homogeneous masses, solid structures with colliquative areas (Fig. 13.68), cystic or cyst-like masses limited by a thick wall and intracystic proliferations and/or internal septa, which become more visible after contrast medium (Figs. 13.66, 13.67, 13.69).

CT signs of local and regional extension of the tumor are: the indefinite profile of the mass and the disappearance of the cleavage planes between the tumor and the various pelvic structures (sigmoid, urinary bladder, uterus, broad and round ligaments) that may

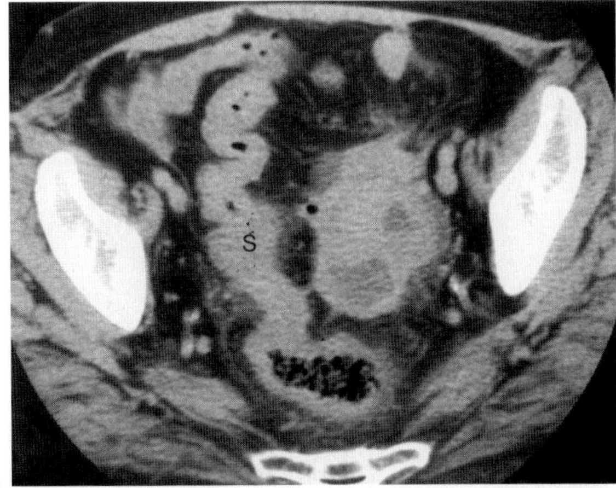

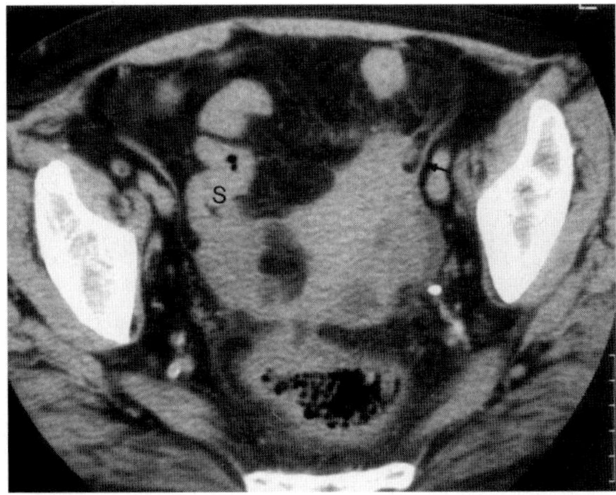

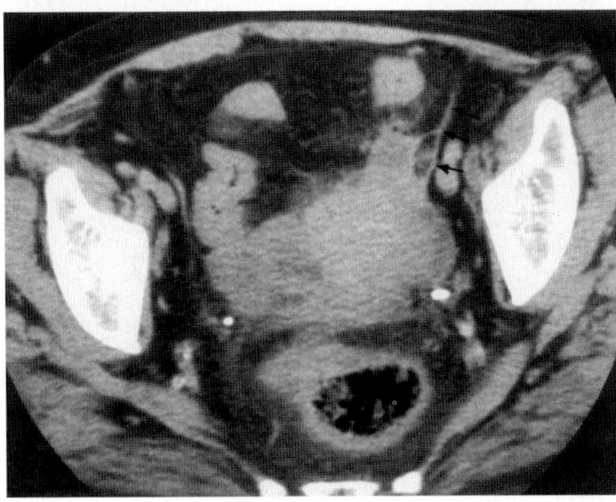

Fig. 13.68A–C. Ovarian carcinoma. Tumor made up of a solid, but partially fluid, mass infiltrating the sigmoid mesocolon and the left broad ligament (**B**, **C** *small arrows*)

be included by the tumoral mass (Figs. 13.66–13.69).

Invasion of the pelvic wall is reflected in shading of the lateral extraperitoneal fatty tissue around the iliac vessels.

Tumor spread over the peritoneum is characterized by peritoneal thickening. At the mesenteric level it produces striations or curved lines reminiscent of a "railway track" or "fan" in shape on the sides of the vessels (Fig. 13.70). At the parietal level, it shows nodules or plaques, which are sometimes very small and punctiform; these images become visible only when ascites (as frequently occurs) is present (Figs. 4.17, 5.1, 13.2, 13.70).

Omental involvement is indicated by an increased density with striations or nodules, or by the constitution of a thick transverse plaque (omental cake) within the transparency of its adipose cellular located behind the anterior abdominal wall.

Both peritoneal and omental nodules and plaques can calcify forming the psammoma bodies (Figs. 13.2, 13.10, 13.11, 13.70), which are typical of ovarian cystadenocarcinoma but are also observed in secondary localizations of mucinous colonic carcinomas or gastric carcinomas (MEGIBOW et al. 1985; PANDOLFO et al. 1986; FERROZZI and ROSSI 1991; MURPHY et al. 1992).

Furthermore, the rupture of mucinous cystadenocarcinomas in the peritoneum may cause the constitution of a pseudomyxoma (Figs. 13.21, 13.71).

It is a matter of discussion whether CT is useful for evaluation of the stage and operability of tumors and their secondary localizations; no unanimous agreement has been reached, because of the low reliability (63–67%) of the CT observations (MEGIBOW et al. 1985; KRESTIN et al. 1985; BUY et al. 1988; GIUNTA et al. 1990; SAITO 1991) owing to a high proportion of false-negative results caused by underestimation of miliary peritoneal spread and small mesenteric and omental nodules. However, the improvement in diagnostic information that can be obtained with opaque peritoneography in patients without ascites or metastases provides an increase in the sensitivity [from 67% to 84% according to GIUNTA et al. (1990) and from 64% to100% according to HALVORSEN et al. (1991)].

When peritoneal nodules with a diameter greater than 2 cm are observed at the root of the mesentery,

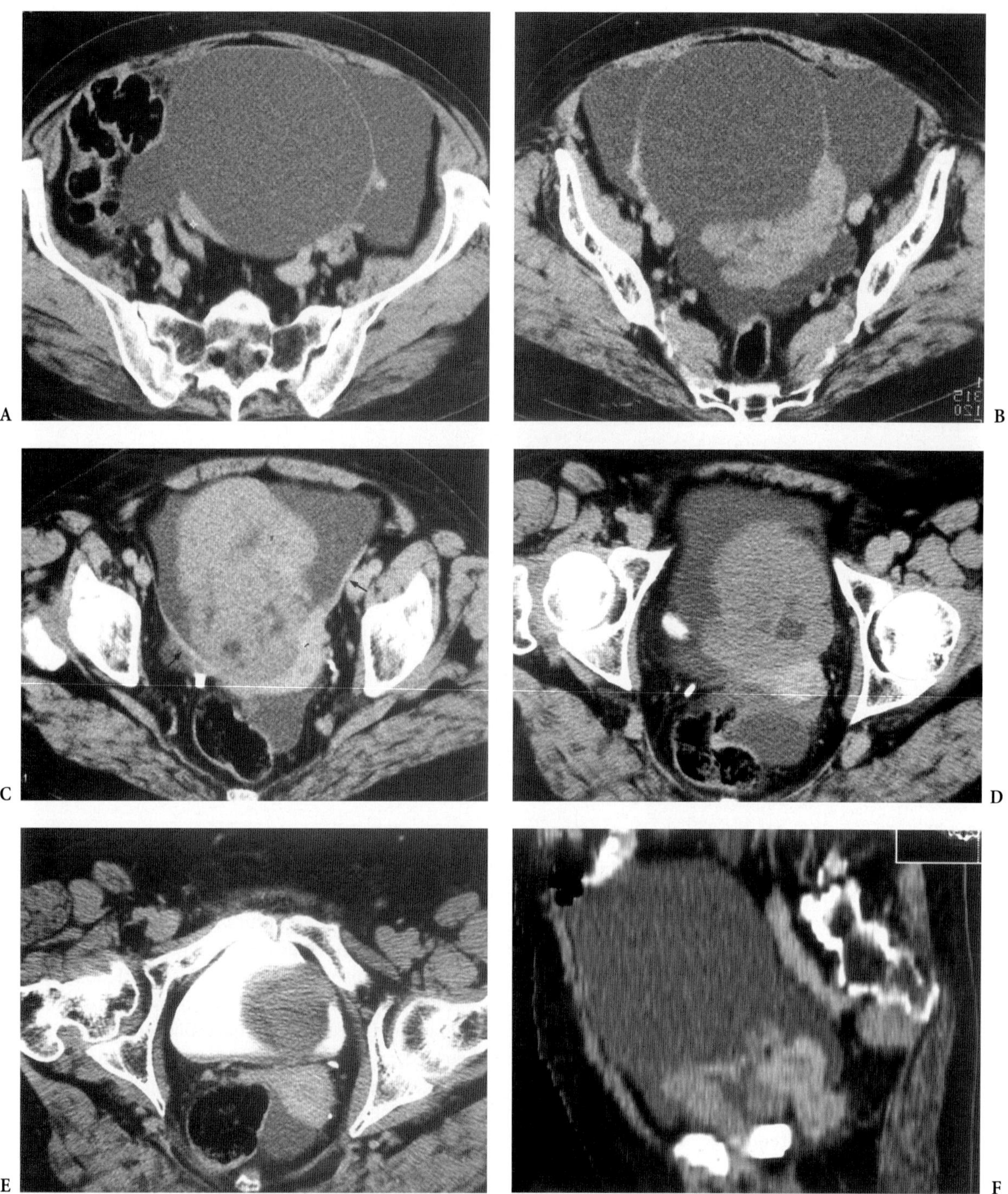

Fig. 13.69A–F. Bilateral ovarian endometrioid carcinoma. Tumor with a mixed structure, made up of a solid colliquative mass, multiple nodules and a large cyst. The tumor infiltrates the broad ligaments (**C** *small arrows*) and the fundus uteri. Carcinomatous ascites

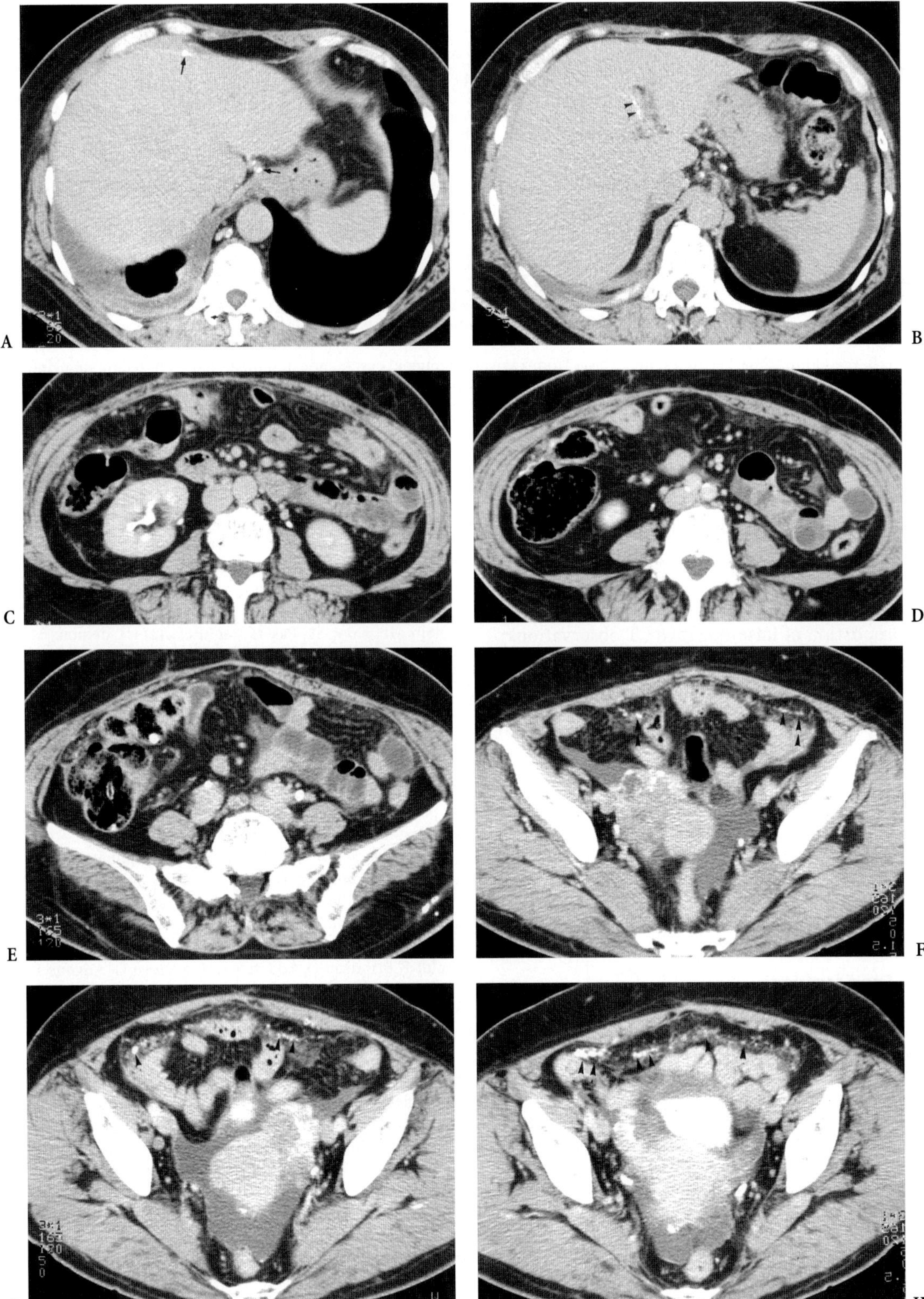

Fig. 13.70A–H. Ovarian adenocarcinoma. The tumor spreads over the perihepatic peritoneum with calcified micrometastases (**A** *small arrow*), into the falciform ligament (**B** *small arrowheads*) and the omentum (*large arrowheads*) (**F–H**). Direct diffusion to the pelvic peritoneum with ascites and linear thickening of the serosa (**F–H**), to the mesenteric peritoneum and to the omentum (**C–H**)

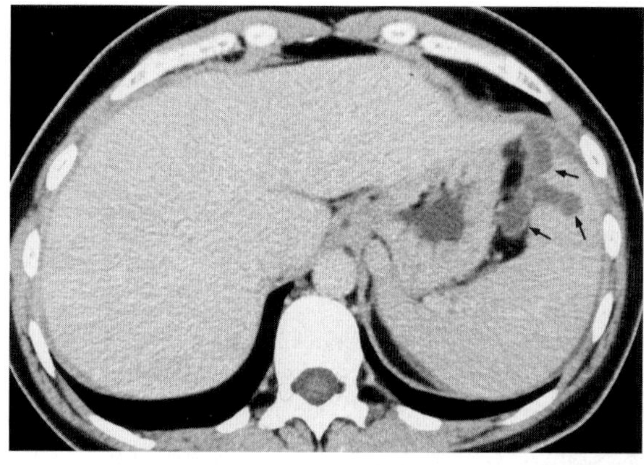
A

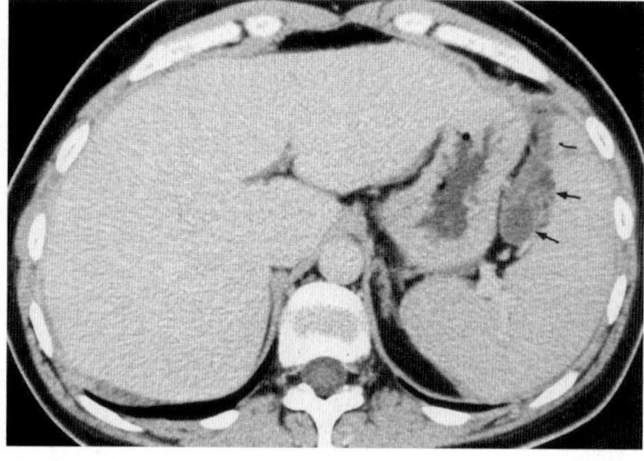
B

Fig. 13.71A, B. Pseudomyxoma. Peritoneal metastases from an ovarian mucoid cystadenocarcinoma, characterized by small low-density masses in the perisplenic recess, which make deep impressions in the spleen

in the porta hepatis, in the lesser sac, in the intersegmental fissure of the liver, on the diaphragm and on the dome of the liver or when a retroperitoneal presacral mass is detected, surgical operations cannot be recommended.

The proportion of false-negative CT observations is also high (about 50%) in check-ups after surgery or chemotherapy. However, when the CT findings are positive, chemotherapy can be started or continued, while when they are negative an exploratory operation or celioscopy can be performed (Pectasides et al. 1991).

Bibliography

General Considerations

Angelelli G, Macarini L (1992) La TC del tratto gastroenterico. Minerva Medica, Turin

Barth RA, Jeffrey RB Jr, Moss AA, Liberman MS (1981) A comparison study of computed tomography and laparoscopy in the staging of abdominal neoplasms. Dig Dis Sci 26:253

Brooke J Jr (1980) CT Demonstration of peritoneal implants. AJR Am J Roentgenol 135:323–326

Charnsangavej C, Dubrow RA, Varma DGK, Herron DH, Robinson TJ, Whitley NO (1993) CT of the mesocolon. 2. Pathologic considerations. Radiographics 13:1309

Choi BI, Lee WJ, Chi JG, et al (1990) CT manifestations of peritoneal leiomyosarcomatosis. AJR Am J Roentgenol 155:799–801

Cooper C, Jeffrey RB, Silverman PM, Federle MP, Chun GH (1986) Computed tomography of omental pathology. J Comput Assist Tomogr 10:62–66

Deutch SJ, Sandler MA, Alpern MB (1987) Abdominal lymphadenopathy in benign diseases: CT detection. Radiology 163:335–338

Dorfman RE, Alpern MB, Gross BH, Sandler MA (1991)Upper abdominal lymph nodes: criteria for normal size determined with CT. Radiology 180:319–322

Einstein DM, Singer AA, Chilcote WA, Desai RK (1991) Abdominal lymphadenopathy: spectrum of CT findings. Radiographics 11:457–472

Esenstein ML, Shaw SL, Pak HY, et al (1983) CT demonstration of multiple intraperitoneal teratomatous implants. J Comput Assist Tomogr 7:1117–1118

Fukuja T, Honda H, Hayashi T, Kaneko K, Tateshi Y, Ro T, Maehara Y, Tanaka M, Tsuneyoshi M, Majuda K (1995) Lymph-node metastases: efficacy of detection with helical CT in patients with gastric cancer. Radiology 197: 705–711

Giunta S, Tipaldi L, Diotellevi F et al (1990) CT demonstration of peritoneal metastases after intraperitoneal injection of contrast media. Clin Imaging 14:31–34

Goerg C, Schwerk WB (1991) Peritoneal carcinomatosis with ascites. AJR Am J Roentgenol 156:1185

Gore RM, Callen PW, Filly RA (1982) Lesser sac fluid in predicting the etiology of ascites: CT findings. AJR Am J Roentgenol 139:71–74

Grimaldi F, Brindicci D, Ettorre GC, Francioso G, Angone G, Monteduro M (1991) Carcinosi peritoneale. Radiol Med 81:660–665

Halvorsen RA, Panushka C, Oakley GJ, Letourneau JG, Adcock LL (1991) Intraperitoneal contrast material improves the CT detection of peritoneal metastases. AJR Am J Roentgenol 157:37–40

Hamrick Turner JE, Chiechi MV, Abbitt PL, Ros PR (1992) Neoplastic and inflammatory processes of the peritoneum, omentum, and mesentery: diagnosis with CT. Radiographics 12:1051

Jeffrey RB (1980) CT demonstration of peritoneal implants. AJR Am J Roentgenol 135:323–326

Jeffrey RB (1983) Computed tomography of the peritoneal cavity and mesentery. In: Moss AA, Gamsu GG, Genant HK (eds) Computed tomography of the body. Saunders, Philadelphia, pp 986–995

Jolles H, Coulam CM (1980) CT of ascites: differential diagnosis. AJR Am J Roentgenol 135:315–322

Lee KT, Stanley RJ, Sagel SS, et al (1978) Accuracy of CT in detecting intra-abdominal and pelvic lymph node metastases from pelvic cancers. AJR Am J Roentgenol 131:675–679

Levitt RG, Sagel SS, Stanley RJ (1978) Detection of neoplastic involvement of the mesentery and omentum by computed tomography. AJR Am J Roentgenol 131:835–838
Levitt RG, Koehler RE, Sagel SS, Lee JKT (1982) Metastatic disease of the mesentery and omentum. Radiol Clin North Am 20:501–510
Magnusson A, Anderson T, Larsson B, Hagberg H, Sundstrom CH (1989) Contrast enhancement of pathologic lymph nodes demonstrated by computed tomography. Acta Radiol 30:307–310
Matsuoka Y, Itai Y, Ohtomo K, et al (1991) Calcification of peritoneal carcinomatosis from gastric carcinoma: a CT demonstration. Eur J Radiol 13:207
Megibow AJ, Balthazar EJ (1986) Computed tomography of the gastointestinal tract. Mosby, St Louis
Megibow AJ, Hulnick DH, Bosniak MA, et al (1985) Ovarian metastases. Computed tomographic appearances. Radiology 156:161–164
Meyers MA (1973) Distribution of intra-abdominal malignant seeding: dependency on dynamics of flow of ascitic fluid. AJR Am J Roentgenol 119:198–206
Meyers MA (1975) Metastatic seeding along the small bowel mesentery. AJR Am J Roentgenol 123:67–73
Meyers MA (1988) Intraperitoneal spread of malignancies. In: Mayers (ed) Dynamic radiology of the abdomen: normal and pathologic anatomy, 3rd edn. Springer, New York, pp 91–178
Meyers MA (1992) Radiologia dinamica dell'addome. Verduci, Rome
Meyers MA, Oliphant M, Berne AS, et al (1987) The peritoneal ligaments and mesenteries: pathways of intraabdominal spread of disease. Radiology 163:593–604
Mödder U, Fiedler V, Lorenz R (1981) Computertomographische Zeichen der Peritonealkarzinose. Fortschr Rontgenstr 136:60–63
Nelson RC, Chezmar JL, Hoel MJ, Buck DR, Sugarbaker PH (1992) Peritoneal carcinomatosis: preoperative CT with intraperitoneal contrast material. Radiology 182:133
Oliphant M, Berne AS (1982) Computed tomography of the subperitoneal space: demonstration of direct spread of intraabdominal disease. J Comput Assist Tomogr 6:1127–1137
Oliphant M, Berne A, Meyers MA (1986) Subperitoneal spread of intraabdominal disease. In: Mayers MA (ed) Computed tomography of the gastrointestinal tract including the peritoneal cavity and mesentery. Springer, New York Berlin Heidelberg
Oliphant M, Berne AS, Meyers MA (1988) Imaging the direct bidirectional spread of disease between the abdomen and the female pelvis via the subperitoneal space. Gastrointest Radiol 13:285–298
Pandolfo I, Blandino A, Gaeta M, et al (1986) Calcified peritoneal metastases from papillary cystadenocarcinoma of the ovary: CT features. J Comput Assist Tomogr 10:545–546
Posniak HV, Tempany C, Demos TC, et al (1988) Computed tomography of posterior pararenal and properitoneal metastases. Urol Radiol 10:75
Rubesin SE, Levin MS (1985) Omental cakes: colonic involvement by omental metastases. Radiology 154:593–596
Solomon A, Rubinstein Z (1984) Importance of the falciform ligament, ligamentum teres, and splenic hilus in the spread of malignancy as demonstrated by computed tomography. Gastrointest Radiol 9:53–56
Thoeni RF, Rogalla P (1996) CT for evaluation of carcinomas in the colon and rectum. Semin Ultrasound CT MR 16:112–128
Walkey MM, Friedman AC, Sohotra P, Radecki PD (1988) CT manifestations of peritoneal carcinomatosis. AJR Am J Roentgenol 150:1035–1041
Walkey MM, Friedman AC, Radecki PD (1989) Computed tomography of peritoneal carcinomatosis. Radiol Report 1:152–170
Wechsler RJ, Miller CL, Kurtz AB, Needleman L, Schneck CD (1990) Anterior protrusion of retroperitoneal processes. A mimic of lesser sac or gastrohepatic masses. Clin Imaging 14:146–151
Whitley NO, Bohlman ME, Baker LP (1982) CT patterns of mesenteric disease. J Comput Assist Tomogr 6:490–496

Pseudomyxoma Peritonei

American Joint Committee on Cancer (1992) Manual for staging of cancer. 4th edn. Lippincott, Philadelphia
Dachman AH, Lichtenstein JE, Friedman AC (1985) Mucocele of the appendix and pseudomyxoma peritonei. AJR Am J Roentgenol 144:923–929
Fishman EK, Jones B, Magid D, Siegelman SS (1983) Intraabdominal abscesses in pseudomyxoma peritonei: the value of computed tomography. J Comput Assist Tomogr 7:449–453
Kevin D, Gustafson KD, Karnase GC, Hattery RR, Scheithauer BW (1984) Pseudomyxoma peritonei associated with mucinous adenocarcinoma of the pancreas: CT findings and CT guided biopsy. J Comput Assist Tomogr 8:335–338
Masaryk TJ, Chilcote WA (1984) CT of pseudomyxoma peritonei: case report. Comput Radiol 8:43–47
Matsuoka Y, Ohtomo K, Itai Y, Nishikawa J, Yoshikawa K, Sasaki Y (1992) Pseudomyxoma peritonei with progressive calcifications: CT findings. Gastrointest Radiol 17:16–18
Mayes GB, Chuang VP, Fischer RG (1981) CT of pseudomyxoma peritonei. AJR Am J Roentgenol 136:807–808
Miller DL, Udelsman R, Sugarbaker PH (1985) Calcification of pseudomyxoma peritonei following intraperitoneal chemotherapy. J Comput Assist Tomogr 9:1123–1124
Novotsky GJ, Berlin L, Epstein AJ, Lobo N, Miller SH (1982) pseudomyxoma peritonei. J Comput Assist Tomogr 6:398–399
Rieux D, Laufenburger A, Souler A, Caron-Poitreau C (1985) Aspects tomodensitometriques de la maladie gélatineuse du péritoine. J Radiol 55:297–302
Seshul MB, Coulam CM (1981) Pseudomyxoma peritonei: computed tomography and sonography. AJR Am J Roentgenol 136:803–806
Yeh HC, Shafir MK, Slater G, Meyer RJ, Cohen BA, Geller SA (1984) Ultrasonography and computed tomography in pseudomyxoma peritonei. Radiology 153:507–510

Gastric Tumors

Andaker L, Morales O, Hojer H, et al (1991) Evaluation of preoperative Computed tomography in gastric malignancy. Surgery 109:132–135
Angelelli G, Macarini L (1989) Evaluation de la paroi gastrique par tomodensitométrie. J Radiol 70:289–293
Angelelli G, Macarini L (1992) TC del tratto gastroenterico. Minerva Medica, Turin
Angelelli G, Macarini L, Favia G (1990) Aspetti TC e correlazioni patologiche nell'adenocarcinoma e nel linfoma gastrico. Radiol Med 79:191–196

Angelelli G, Brindicci D, Macarini L (1991) La TC nello studio delle lesioni di parete dell'apparato digerente. Radiol Med 81: 83–89

Arablinskii VM, Sedykh SA, Mamontov AS, Vashakmadze LA, Bakhmutskii AN, Aleinikova EI (1991) The role of computerized tomography in the diagnosis of regional metastases of cancer of the esophagus and the proximal part of the stomach. Sov Med 6:26–29

Baert AL, Roex L, Marchal G, Hermans P, Dewilde D, Wilms G (1989) Computed tomography of the stomach with water as an oral contrast agent: technique and preliminary results. J Comput Assist Tomogr 13:633–636

Baker ME, Silverman PM, Halvorsen RA, Cohan RH (1987) Computed tomography of masses in periportal/hepatoduodenal ligament. J Comput Assist Tomogr 11:258–263

Balfe DM, Koehler RE, Karstaedt N, Stanley RJ, Sagel SS (1981) Computed tomography of gastric neoplasm. Radiology 140:431–436

Botet JF, Lightdate CJ, Zauber AG, Gerdes H, Winawer SJ, Urmacher C, Brennan MF (1991) Preoperative staging of gastric cancer: comparison of endoscopic US and dynamic CT. Radiology 181:426–432

Brown BM, Federle MP, Jeffrey RB (1982) Gastric wall thickening and extragastric inflammatory processes, a retrospective CT study. J Comput Assist Tomogr 6:762–765

Chin SY, Lee BH, Kim KH, et al (1994) Radiological prediction of the depth of invasion and histological type in early gastric cancer. Abdom Imaging 19:521–526

Cho JS, Kim JK, Rho SM, Lee HY, Jeong HY, Lee CS (1994) Preoperative assessment of gastric carcinoma: value of two-phase dynamic CT with mechanical IV injection of contrast material. AJR Am J Roentgenol 163:69–75

Cho JS, Kim JK, Rho SM, Lee HY, Jeong HY, Lee CS (1994) Preoperative assessment of gastric carcinoma: value of two-phase dynamic CT with mechanical IV injection of contrast material. AJR Am J Roentgenol 163:69–75

Choi BI, Ok ID, Im J, et al (1985) Exogastric cystic gastric leiomyosarcoma with unusual CT appearance. Gastrointest Radiol 13:109–111

Cook AO, Levine BA, Sirinek KR, et al (1986) Evaluation of gastric adenocarcinoma: abdominal computed tomography does not replace celiotomy. Arch Surg 121:603–606

Dehn TCB, Reznek RH, Nocler IB, et al (1984) The preoperative assessment of advanced gastric cancer by computed tomography. Br J Surg 71:413–417

Dorfman RE, Alpern MB, Gross BH, Sandler MA (1991) Upper abdominal lymph nodes: criteria for normal size determined with CT. Radiology 180:319–322

Favagrossa GM, Aletto C (1988) La TC dell'addome nella diagnosi e follow-up delle neoplasie dello stomaco. Proceedings of the 33rd Congress of SIRM, Rome, pp 1225–1229

Forzini F, Cappelli B, Ferrari F, Terrosi Vagnoli P (1982) La TC nella valutazione della diffusione del carcinoma gastrico all'addome superiore. Radiol Med 68:561–563

Fukuya T, Honda H, Hayashi T, Kaneku K, Tateshi Y, Ro T, Maeharay, Tanaka M, Tsuneyoshi M, Masuda K (1995) Lymph-node metastases: efficacy of detection with helical CT in patients with gastric cancer. Radiology 197:705–711

Fukuya T, Honda H, Kaneko K, Kuroiwat T, Yoshimitsu K, Irie H, Maehara Y, Masuda K (1997) Efficacy of helical CT in T-staging of gastric cancer. J Comput Assist Tomogr 21:73–81

Gossios K, Tsianos EV, et al (1996) CT evaluation of the resectability of gastric cancer post-chemotherapy. Abdom Imaging 21:293–298

Grosser G, Wimmer B, Ruf G (1985) The diagnostic value of computed tomography in carcinoma of the stomach. Fortschr Rontgenstr 142:514–519

Hada M, Hihara T, Kakishita M (1984) Computed tomography in gastric carcinoma: thickness of gastric wall and infiltration to serosa surface. Radiat Med 2:27–30

Halvorsen RA Jr, Thompson WM (1987) Computed tomographic staging of gastrointestinal malignancies. Esophagus and stomach. Invest Radiol 22:2–16

Halvorsen RA Jr, Thompson WM (1989) Gastrointestinal cancer: diagnosis, staging, and the follow-up role of imaging. Semin Ultrasound CT MR 10:467–480

Halvorsen RA Jr, Thompson WM (1991) Primary neoplasms of the hollow organs of the gastrointestinal tract. Straging and follow-up. Cancer 67 [Suppl 4]:1181–1188

Hori M, Watanabe S, Matsubara T, et al (1984) Detection of lymph nodes of the stomach cancer with computed tomography. Rinshogeka 39:543–546

Hori S, Tsuda K, Murayama S, Matsushita M, Yukawa K, Kozuka T (1992) CT of gastric carcinoma: preliminary results with a new scanning technique. Radiographics 12:257–268

Inzerillo M, De Maria M, Bianco BP, Calabrese A, Calistre V, Di Gesù C, Feo M (1988) Studio TC degli spazi sub-peritoneali perigastrici nei pazienti affetti da neoplasie dello stomaco. Proceedings of the 33rd National Congress on Radiology, Rome, pp 1721–1724

Kleinhaus U, Militianu D (1988) Computed tomography in the preoperative evaluation of gastric carcinoma. Gastrointest Radiol 13:97–101

Koehler RE, Balfe DM, Stanley RJ (1989) Gastrointestinal tract. In: Lee JKT (ed) Computed body tomography with MRI correlation. Raven Press, New York

Komaki S (1986) Gastric carcinoma. In: Meyers MA (ed) Computed tomography of the gastrointestinal tract. Springer, New York Berlin Heidelberg, pp 23–54

Komaki S, Toyoshima S (1983) CT's capability in detecting advanced gastric cancer. Gastrointest Radiol 8:397–413

Lee KR, Levine E, Moffat RE, Bignongiari LR, Hermreck AS (1979) Computed tomographic staging of malignant gastric neoplasm. Radiology 133:151–155

Lee KS, Choi YT, Lee JH, Park YH, Park KS, Ko YT, Lim JH, Auh YH (1994) Exophytic adenocarcinoma of the stomach: CT findings. AJR Am J Roentgenol 163:77–80

Lee WB (1988) Left gastric and coeliac lymph nodes: a problem area for CT staging of carcinoma of the gastro-oesophageal junction. Australas Radiol 32:230

Levine MS, Megibow AJ (1994) Stomach and duodenum: carcinoma. In: Gore RM, Levine MS, Laufer I (eds) Textbook of gastrointestinal radiology. Saunders, Philadelphia, pp 660–683

Matsuoka Y, Itai Y, Ohtomo K, et al (1991) Calcification of peritoneal carcinomatosis from gastric carcinoma: a CT demonstration. Eur J Radiol 13:207

Matsushita M, Oi H, Murakami T, et al (1994) Extraserosal invasation in advanced gastric cancer: evaluation with MR imaging. Radiology 192:87–91

Minami M, Kawauchi N, Itai Y, Niki T, Sasaki Y (1992) Gastric tumors: radiologic-pathologic correlation and accuracy of T staging with dynamic CT. Radiology 185:173–178

Miyake H, Maeda M, Kurauki S, Watanabe H, Kawaguchi M, Tsuji K (1989) Thickened gastric walls showing diffuse low attenuation on CT. J Comput Assist Tomogr 13:253–255

Moss AA (1982) Computed tomography in the staging of gastrointestinal carcinoma. Radiol Clin North Am 20:761–780

Moss AA, Schnyder P, Marks WM, Margulis AR (1981) Gastric adenocarcinoma: a comparison of the accuracy and economics of staging by computed tomography and surgery. Gastroenterology 80:45–50

Ohkuma K, Hisashi N, Hiramatsu K (1984) Computed tomography for staging of gastric cancer. I to Cho 19:1313–1318

Oliphant M, Berne AS (1982) Computed tomography of the subperitoneal space: demonstration of direct spread of intraabdominal disease. J Comput Assist Tomogr 6:1127–1137

Ozaki M (1984) Preoperative diagnosis of lymph node metastasis of gastric cancer using CT scan. Nisho Gekaishi 17:1507–1516

Ozaki M, Byu T, Watanabe Y, et al (1984) Diagnosis of metastatic lymph node of gastric cancer. Igakunoayumi 128:115–118

Potente G, Osti MF, Torriero F, Scattoni Padovan F, Maurizi Enrici R (1994) La tomografia computerizzata nella stadiazione preoperatoria del cancro gastrico. Radiol Med 87:76–81

Richter GM, Dux M, Roeren T, et al (1996) Gastrointestinale Diagnostik mit Hydrosonographie und Hydro-CT. 1. Magen-Karzinom. Rofo Fortschr Geb Rontgenstr Neuen Bildgeb Verfahr 164:281–289

Rossi M, Broglia L, Arata FM, Di Girolamo M, Petrone A, Coniglio M, Rossi P (1997) Accuratezza e riproducibilità diagnostica della tomografia computerizzata con distensione idrica e ipotonia indotta nella stadiazione pre-operatoria dei tumori gastrici. Radiol Med 94:486–491

Rubesin SE, Levine MS, Glick SN (1986) Gastric involvement by omental cakes: radiographic findings. Gastrointest Radiol 11:223–228

Scatarige JC, Di Santis DJ (1989) CT of the stomach and duodenum. Radiol Clin North Am 27:687–706

Stell DA, Carter CR, Stewart I, Anderson JR (1996) Prospective comparison of laparoscopy, ultrasonography and computed tomography in the staging of gastric cancer. J Surg 83:1260–1262

Sussman SK, Halvorsen RA Jr, Illescas FF, et al (1988) Gastric adenocarcinoma: CT versus surgical staging. Radiology 167:335–340

Takao M, Fakuda T, Iwanaga S, Hayashi K, Kusano K, Okudaira S (1998) Gastric cancer: evaluation of triphasic spiral CT and radiologic. Pathologic correlation. J Comput Assist Tomogr 22:288–294

Terrier F, Schapira C, Fichs WA (1984) CT assessment of operability in carcinoma of the oesophagogastric junction. Gastroint Radiol 8:307–313

Thompson WM, Halvorsen RA, Foster WL, et al (1983) Computed tomography for staging esophageal and gastroesophageal cancer. AJR Am J Roentgenol 141:951–958

Triller J, Roder R, Stafford A, Schröder R (1986) CT in advanced gastric carcinoma: is exploratory laparotomy avoidable? Eur J Radiol 6:181–186

Ziegler K, Sanft C, Weitz M, et al (1993) Comparison of computed tomography, endosonography, and intraoperative assessment in TN staging of gastric carcinoma. Gut 34:604–610

Colonic Tumors

Acunas B, Rozanes I, Acunas G, Celik L, Sayi I, Gokmen E (1990) Preoperative CT staging of colon carcinoma (excluding the rectosigmoid region). Eur J Radiol 11:150–153

Angelelli G, Macarini L, Lupo L, Caputi-Jambenghi O, Pannarale O, Mereo V (1990) Rectal carcinoma: CT staging with water as contrast medium. Radiology 177:511–514

Angelelli G, Brindicci D, Macarini L (1991) la TC nello studio delle lesioni di parete dell'apparato digerente. Radiol Med 81:83–89

Balthazar EJ (1991) CT of gastrointestinal tract: principles and interpretation. AJR Am J Roentgenol 156:23–32

Balthazar EJ, Megibow AJ, Hulnick D, Naidich DP (1988) Carcinoma of the colon: detection and preoperative staging by CT. AJR Am J Roentgenol 150:301–306

Balthazar EJ, Siegel SE, Megibow AJ, Scholes J, Gordon R (1995) CT in patients with scirrhous carcinoma of the GI tract: imaging findings and value for tumor detection and staging. AJR Am J Roentgenol 165:839–845

Becker CD, Fucs WA (1986) Colorectal carcinoma. In: Meyers MA (ed) Computed tomography of the gastrointestinal tract. Springer, New York Berlin Heidelberg, pp 253–272

Charnley RM (1990) Imaging of colorectal carcinoma. Radiology 174:283

Charnsangavej C, Whitley NO (1993) Metastases to the pancreas and peripancreatic lymph nodes from carcinoma of the right side of the colon: CT findings in 12 patients. AJR Am J Roentgenol 160:49–52

Chen YM, Ott DJ, Wolfman NT et al (1987) Recurrent colorectal carcinoma: evaluation with barium enema examination and CT. Radiology 163:307–310

Diamond RT, Greenberg HM, Boult IF (1981) Direct metastatic spread of right colonic adenocarcinoma to duodenum: barium and computed tomographic findings. Gastroint Radiol 6:339–341

Ellert J, Kreel L (1980) The value of CT in malignant colonic tumors CT. 4:225–240

Freeny PC, Marks WM, Ryan JA, Bolen JW (1986) Colorectal carcinoma evaluation with CT: preoperative staging and detection of postoperative recurrence. Radiology 158:347–353

Freeny PC, Marks WM, Ryan JA, et al (1987) Computed tomography of colorectal carcinoma: preoperative staging and detection of recurrence. Semin Ultrasound CT MR 8:432–445

Gazelle GS, Gaa J, Saini S, Shellito P (1995) Staging of the colon carcinoma using water enema CT. J Comput Assist Tomogr 19:87–91

Gossios KJ, Tsianos EV, Kontogiannis DS, et al (1992) Water as contrast medium for computed tomography study of colonic wall lesions. Gastrointest Radiol 17:125–128

Granfield CAJ, Charnsangavej C, Dubrow RA, et al (1992) Regional lymph node metastases in carcinoma of the left side of the colon and rectum: CT demonstration. AJR Am J Roentgenol 159:757–761

Hara AK, Johnson CD, Reed JE, et al (1996) Colorectal polyp detection with CT colography: two- versus three- dimensional techniques. Work in progress. Radiology 200:49–54

Hulnick DH, Megibow AJ, Balthazar EJ, et al (1987) Perforated colorectal neoplasms: correlation of clinical, contrast enema and CT examinations. Radiology 164:611–615

Keeney G, Jafri SZH, Mezwa DG (1989) Computed tomographic evaluation and staging. Gastrointest Radiol 14:65

Kelvin FM, Maglinte DT (1987) Colorectal carcinoma. A radiologic and clinical rewiew. Radiology 164:1–8

Krestin GP, Beyer D, Lorenz R (1985) Secondary involvement of the transverse colon by tumors of the pelvis: spread of malignancies along the greater omentum. Gastroint Radiol 10:283–288

Mayes GB, Zornoza J (1980) Computed tomography of colon carcinoma. AJR Am J Roentgenol 135:43–46

McDaniel K, Charnsangavej C, Dubrow RA, Varma DGK, Granfield CAJ, Curley S (1993) Pathway of nodal metastasis in carcinomas of the cecum, ascending colon and transverse colon: CT demonstration. AJR Am J Roentgenol 161:61–64

Moss AA (1989) Imaging of colorectal carcinoma. Radiology 170:308

Okizuka H, Sugimura K, Shinozaki N, Watanabe K (1995) Colorectal carcinoma: evaluation with ultrafast CT. Clin Imaging 19:247–251

Rubesin SE, Levin MS (1985) Omental cakes: colonic involvement by omental metastases. Radiology 154:593–596

Scharling ES, Wolfman NT, Bechtold RE (1996) Computed tomography evaluation of colorectal carcinoma. Semin Roentgenol 31:142–153

Solomon A, Bar-Ziv J, Stern D (1988) Staging cecal and ascending colon carcinoma with computed tomography. Gastrointest Radiol 13:152

Thoeni RF (1989) CT evaluations of carcinomas of the colon and rectum. Radiol Clin North Am 27:731–741

Thoeni RF (1991) Colorectal cancer: cross-sectional imaging for staging of primary tumor and detection of local recurrence. AJR Am J Roentgenol 156:909–915

Thoeni RF, Laufer I (1994) Polyps and cancer. In: Gore RM, Levine MS, Laufer I (eds) Textbook of gastrointestinal radiology. Saunders, Philadelphia

Thoeni RF, Moss AA, Schnyder P, et al (1981) Detection and staging of primary rectal and rectosigmoid cancer by computed tomography. Radiology 141:135–138

Thompson WM, Halvorsen RA, Foster WL Jr, et al (1986) Preoperative and postoperative CT staging of rectosigmoid carcinoma. AJR Am J Roentgenol 146:703–710

Turnbull RB, Kyle K (1967) Cancer of colon: the influence of the no touch isolation technique on survival rates. Ann Surg 160:420-425

Zerhouni ER, Rutter C, Hamilton SR, Balfe DM, Megibow AT, Francis IR, Moss AA, Heiken JP, Tempany CMC, Aisen AM, Weinreb JC, Gatsonis C, Neil BJ (1996) CT and MR imaging in the staging of colorectal carcinoma: report of the Radiology Diagnostic Oncology Group II. Radiology 200:443–451

Gallbladder Tumors

Araki T, Hihara T, Karikomi M, et al (1988a) Hepatocellular carcinoma: metastatic abdominal lymph nodes identified by computed tomography. Gastrointest Radiol 13:247

Araki T, Hihara T, Karikomi M, Kachi K, Uchiyama G (1988b) Intraluminal papillary carcinoma of the gallbladder: prognostic value of computed tomography. Gastrointest Radiol 13:261–265

Baker ME, Silverman PM, Halvorsen RA Jr, Cohan RH (1987) Computed tomography of masses in periportal/hepatoduodenal ligament. J Comput Assist Tomogr 11:258–263

Collier NA, Carr D, Hemingway A, Blumgart LH (1984) Preoperative diagnosis and its effect on the treatment of carcinoma of the gallbladder. Surg Gynecol Obstet 159:465–470

Engels JT, Balfe DM, Lee JKT (1989) Biliary carcinoma: CT evaluation of extrahepatic spread. Radiology 172:35–40

Fahim RB, McDonald JR, Richard JC, Ferris DO (1962) Carcinoma of the galbladder: a study of its modes of spread. Ann Surg 156:114–124

Fraquet T, Monets M, Ruize AY, Jimenez FJ, Cozcolluela R (1991) Primary gallbladder carcinoma: imaging findings in 50 patients with pathologic correlation. Gastrointest Radiol 16:143–148

Fultz PJ, Skucas J, Weiss SL (1988) Comparative imaging of gallbladder cancer. J Clin Gastroenterol 6:683–692

Harris RD (1979) Computed tomography of retroperitoneal lymphadenopathy: benign or malignant? Comput Tomogr 3:73–80

Itai Y, Araki T, Yoshikawa K, Furui S, Yashiro N, Tasaka A (1980) Computed tomography of gallbladder carcinoma. Radiology 137:713–718

Lane J, Buck JL, Zeman RK (1989) Primary carcinoma of the gallbladder: a pictorial essay. Radiographics 9:209–227

Magnano San Lio V, Milone P, Coppola G, Dall'Aira S, Magnano M, Patanè D, Petrillo G (1990) La TC nello staging delle neoplasie della colecisti. Radiol Med 80:451–454

Mori H, Aikawa H, Hirao K, et al (1989) Exophytic spread of hepatobiliary disease via perihepatic ligaments: demonstration with CT and US. Radiology 172:41–46

Nesbit GM, Johnson CD, James EM, et al (1988) Cholangiocarcinoma: diagnosis and evaluation of resectability by CT and sonography as procedures complementary to cholangiography. AJR Am J Roentgenol 151:933–938

Ohtani T, Shirai Y, Tsukada K, Hatakeyama K, Muto T (1993) Carcinoma of the gallbladder: CT evaluation of lymphatic spread. Radiology 189:875–880

Ohtani T, Shirai Y, Tsukada K, et al (1996) Spread of gallbladder carcinoma: CT evaluation with pathologic correlation. Abdom Imaging 21:195–201

Scribano E, Saccà F, Pandolfo I, et al (1986) Rilievi diagnostici TC del cancro della colecisti. Ital Curr Radiol 5:217–220

Shirai Y, Yoshida K, Tsukada K, Ohtani T, Muto T (1992) Identification of the regional lymphatic system of the gallbladder by vital staining. Br J Surg 79:659–662

Winstein JB, Heiken JP, Lee JK, et al (1986) High resolution CT of the porta hepatis and hepatoduodenal ligament. Radiographics 6:55–74

Zeman RK, Schieber M, Clark LR, et al (1985) The clinical and imaging spectrum of pancreatoduodenal lymph node enlargement. AJR Am J Roentgenol 144:1223–1227

Zirinsky K, Auh YH, Rubenstein WA, Kneeland JB, Whalen JP, Kazam E (1985) The portacaval space: CT with MR correlation. Radiology 156:453–460

Ovarian Tumors

Amendola MA (1985) The role of CT in the evaluation of ovarian malignancy. Crit Rev Diagn Imaging 24:329–368

Amendola MA, Walsh JW, Amendola BE, Tisnado J, Hall DJ, Goplerud DR (1981) Computed tomography in the evaluation of carcinoma of the ovary. J Comput Assist Tomogr 5:179–186

Brenner DE, Shaff MI, Jones HW, Grosh WW, Greco FA, Burnett CS (1985) Abdominopelvic computed tomography: evaluation in patients undergoing second-look laparotomy for ovarian carcinoma. Obstet Gynecol 65:715–719

Buist MR, Golding RP, Burger CW, et al (1994)Comparative evaluation of diagnostic methods in ovarian carcinoma with emphasis on CT and MRI. Gynecol Oncol 52:191–198

Buy JN, Moss AA, Ghossain MA, Sciot C, Malbec L, Vadrot D, Taniel BJ, Pecroix Y (1988) Peritoneal implants from ovarian tumors: CT findings. Radiology 169:691–694

Feldman GB, Knapp RC (1974) Lymphatic drainage of the peritoneal cavity and its significance in ovarian cancer. Am J Obstet Gynecol 119:991–994

Ferrozzi F, Rossi A (1991) Aspects tomodensitométriques des metastases à forme calcifiante. A propos de 40 cas. J Radiol 72:305-312

Forstner R, Hrirack H, Occhipinti KA, Powell CB, Francel SD, Stern JL (1995) Ovarian cancer: staging with CT and MR imaging. Radiology 197:619–626

Fukuda T, Ikeuchi M, Hashimoto H, et al (1986) Computed tomography of ovarian masses. J Comput Assist Tomogr 10:990–996

Ghossian MA, Buy JN, Ligneres C, et al (1991) Epithelial tumors of the ovary: comparison of MR and CT findings. Radiology 181:863–878

Giunta S, Tipaldi L, Diotallevi F, et al (1990) Demonstration of peritoneal metastases after intraperitoneal injection of contrast media. Clin Imaging 14:31–34

Giwerc M, Masselot J, George M, Rochard F, Haie C (1986) Intérêt de l'examen tomodensitométrique dans la surveillance des cancers de l'ovaire. A propos de 69 observations. J Radiol 67:769–774

Jaquet P, Jelinek JS, Steves MA, Sugarbaker PH (1993) Evaluation of computed tomography in patients with peritoneal carcinomatosis. Cancer 72:1631–1636

Johnson RJ, Blackledge G, Eddleston B, Crowther D (1983) Abdomino-pelvic computed tomography in the management of ovarian carcinoma. Radiology 146:447–452

Krestin GP, Beyer D, Lorenz R (1985) Secondary involvement of the transverse colon by tumors of the pelvis: spread of malignancies along the greater omentum. Gastrointest Radiol 10:283–288

Kalovidouris A, Gouliamos A, Pontifex GR, Gennatas K, Dardoufas K, Papavasiliou C (1984) Computed tomography of ovarian carcinoma. Acta Radiol 25:203–208

Kerr-Wilson RHJ, Shingleton HM, Orr JW, Hatch KD (1984) The use of ultrasound and computed tomography scanning in the management of gynecologic cancer patients. Gynecol Oncol 18:54–61

Lee KT, Stanley RJ, Sagel SS, McClennan BL (1978) Accuracy of CT in detecting intra-abdominal and pelvic lymph node metastases from pelvic cancers. AJR Am J Roentgenol 131:675–679

Low RN, Carter WD, Saleh F, Sigeti JS (1995) Ovarian cancer: comparison of findings with perfluorocarbon-enhanced MR imaging, In-111-CYT-103 immunoscintigraphy, and CT. Radiology 195:391–400

Lundstedt C, Holmin T, Thorvinger B (1992) Peritoneal ovarian metastases simulating liver parenchymal metastases. Gastroint Radiol 17:250–252

Maxwell AJ, Boggis CRM, Sambrook P (1990) Computed tomographic peritoneography in the investigation of abdominal wall and genital swelling in patients on continuous ambulatory peritoneal dialysis. Clin Radiol 41:100–104

Megibow AJ, Hulnick DH, Bosniak MA, et al (1985)Ovarian metastases. Computed tomographic appearances. Radiology 156:161-164

Megibow AJ, Bosniak MA, Ho AG, Beller U, Hulnick DH, Beckman EM (1988) Accuracy of CT in detection of persistent or recurrent ovarian carcinoma: correlation with second-look laparotomy. Radiology 166:341–345

Mitchell DG, Hill MC, Hill S, Zaloudek C (1986) Serous carcinoma of the ovary: CT identification of metastatic calcified implants. Radiology 158:649–652

Miller DS, Spirtos NM, Ballon SC, et al (1992) Critical reassessment of second look laparotomy for epithelial ovarian cancer. Cancer 69:502–510

Moncada R, Cooper RA, Garces M, Badrinath K (1974) Calcified metastases from malignant ovarian carcinoma. Radiology 113:31–35

Murphy D, Hughes PM, Zammit-Maempel I (1992) Computed tomographic assessment of intraperitoneal fluid distribution prior to intraperitoneal chemotherapy for ovarian cancer. Br J Radiol 65:295

Nelson BE, Rosenfield AT, Schwartz PE (1993) Preoperative abdominopelvic computed tomographic prediction of optimal cytoreduction in epithelial ovarian carcinoma. J Clin Oncol 11:166–172

Pandolfo I, Blandino A, Gaeta M, et al (1986) Calcified peritoneal metastases from papillary cystadenocarcinoma of the ovary: CT features. J Comput Assist Tomogr 10:545–546

Pectasides D, Kayianni H, Facou A, Bobotas N, Barbounis V, Zis J, Athanassiou A (1991) Correlation of abdominal tomography scanning and second-look operation findings in ovarian cancer patients. Am J Clin Oncol 14:457–462

Rieber A, Brambs HJ (1990) A calcified tumor in the mesenterium. Ovarian carcinoma with a calcified metastasis in the abdominal wall ("omental cake"), histologically cystadenocarcinoma. Radiologe 30:145–6

Saito T (1991) Role of X-ray CT in the evaluation of extension of ovarian cancer. Nippon Sanka Fujinka Gakkai Zasshi 43:93–100

Sanders RC, McNeil BJ, Finberg HJ, et al (1983) A prospective study of computed tomography and ultrasound in the detection and staging of pelvic masses. Radiology 146:439–442

Semelka RC, Lawrence PH, Shoenut JP, et al (1993) Primary ovarian cancer: prospective comparison of contrast-enhanced CT and pre- and postcontrast fat-suppressed MR imaging, with histologic correlation. JMRI 3:99–106

Shiels RA, Peel KR, MacDonald HM, Thorogood J, Robinson PJ (1985) A prospective trial of computed tomography in the staging of ovarian malignancy. Br J Obstet Gynaecol 92:407–412

Silverman PM, Osborne M, Dunnick NR, Bandy LC (1988) CT prior to second look operation in ovarian cancer. AJR Am J Roentgenol 150:829–832

Soloman A, Brenner HJ, Rubinstein Z, Chaitchik S, Morag B (1983) Computerized tomography in ovarian cancer. Gynecol Oncol 15:48–55

Teplik JG, Haskin ML, Alavi A (1976) Calcified intraperitoneal metastases from ovarian carcinoma. AJR Am J Roentgenol 127:1003–1006

Walkey MM, Friedman AC, Sohotra P, Radecki PD (1988) CT manifestations of peritoneal carcinomatosis. AJR Am J Roentgenol 150:1035–1041

Whitley NO, Brenner DE, Francis A, Kwon T, Villa Santa U, Aisner J, Wiernik P, Whitley J (1981) Use of the computed tomographic whole body scanner to stage and follow patients with advanced ovarian carcinoma. Invest Radiol 16:479–486

Subject Index

Medical Radiology
Diagnostic Imaging and Radiation Oncology

Titles in the series already published

Diagnostic Imaging

Innovations in Diagnostic Imaging
Edited by J. H. Anderson

Radiology of the Upper Urinary Tract
Edited by E. K. Lang

The Thymus – Diagnostic Imaging, Functions, and Pathologic Anatomy
Edited by E. Walter, E. Willich, and W. R. Webb

Interventional Neuroradiology
Edited by A. Valavanis

Radiology of the Pancreas
Edited by A. L. Baert, co-edited by G. Delorme

Radiology of the Lower Urinary Tract
Edited by E. K. Lang

Magnetic Resonance Angiography
Edited by I. P. Arlart, G. M. Bongartz, and G. Marchal

Contrast-Enhanced MRI of the Breast
S. Heywang-Köbrunner and R. Beck

Spiral CT of the Chest
Edited by M. Rémy-Jardin and J. Rémy

Radiological Diagnosis of Breast Diseases
Edited by M. Friedrich and E.A. Sickles

Radiology of the Trauma
Edited by M. Heller and A. Fink

Biliary Tract Radiology
Edited by P. Rossi

Radiological Imaging of Sports Injuries
Edited by C. Masciocchi

Modern Imaging of the Alimentary Tube
Edited by A. R. Margulis

Diagnosis and Therapy of Spinal Tumors
Edited by P. R. Algra, J. Valk, and J. J. Heimans

Interventional Magnetic Resonance Imaging
Edited by J. F. Debatin and G. Adam

Abdominal and Pelvic MRI
Edited by A. Heuck and M. Reiser

Orthopedic Imaging
Techniques and Applications
Edited by A.M. Davies and H. Pettersson

Radiology of the Female Pelvic Organs
Edited by E. K. Lang

Magnetic Resonance of the Heart and Great Vessels
Clinical Applications
Edited by J. Bogaert, A. J. Duerinckx, and F. E. Rademakers

Modern Head and Neck Imaging
Edited by S. K. Mukherji and J. A. Castelijns

Radiological Imaging of Endocrine Diseases
Edited by J. N. Bruneton in collaboration with B. Padovani and M.-Y. Mourou

Trends in Contrast Media
Edited by H. S. Thomsen, R. N. Muller, and R. F. Mattrey

Functional MRI
Edited by C. T. W. Moonen and P. A. Bandettini

Radiology of the Pancreas
2nd Revised Edition
Edited by A. L. Baert
Co-edited by G. Delorme and L. Van Hoe

Radiology of Peripheral Vascular Diseases
Edited by E. Zeitler

Emergency Pediatric Radiology
Edited by H. Carty

Spiral CT of the Abdomen
Edited by F. Terrier, M. Grossholz, and C. D. Becker

Liver Malignancies
Diagnostic and Interventional Radiology
Edited by C. Bartolozzi and R. Lencioni

Medical Imaging of the Spleen
Edited by A. M. De Schepper and F. Vanhoenacker

Diagnostic Nuclear Medicine
Edited by C. Schiepers

Radiology of Blunt Trauma of the Chest
P. Schnyder and M. Wintermark

Portal Hypertension
Diagnostic Imaging-Guided Therapy
Edited by P. Rossi
Co-edited by P. Ricci and L. Broglia

Recent Advances in Diagnostic Neuroradiology
Edited by Ph. Demaerel

Virtual Endoscopy and Related 3D Techniques
Edited by P. Rogalla, J. Terwisscha Van Scheltinga, and B. Hamm

Multislice CT
Edited by M. F. Reiser, M. Takahashi, M. Modic, and R. Bruening

Pediatric Uroradiology
Edited by R. Fotter

Radiology of AIDS
A Practical Approach
Edited by J.W.A.J. Reeders and P. C. Goodman

CT of the Peritoneum
Armando Rossi and Giorgio Rossi

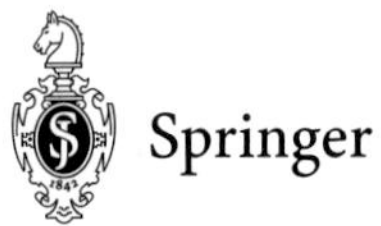

Medical Radiology
Diagnostic Imaging and Radiation Oncology

Titles in the series already published

Radiation Oncology

Lung Cancer
Edited by C. W. Scarantino

Innovations in Radiation Oncology
Edited by H. R. Withers
and L. J. Peters

Radiation Therapy of Head and Neck Cancer
Edited by G. E. Laramore

Gastrointestinal Cancer – Radiation Therapy
Edited by R. R. Dobelbower, Jr.

Radiation Exposure and Occupational Risks
Edited by E. Scherer, C. Streffer,
and K.-R. Trott

Radiation Therapy of Benign Diseases - A Clinical Guide
S.E. Order and S.S. Donaldson

Interventional Radiation Therapy Techniques - Brachytherapy
Edited by R. Sauer

Radiopathology of Organs and Tissues
Edited by E. Scherer,
C. Streffer, and K.-R. Trott

Concomitant Continuous Infusion Chemotherapy and Radiation
Edited by M. Rotman
and C. J. Rosenthal

Intraoperative Radiotherapy – Clinical Experiences and Results
Edited by F. A. Calvo,
M. Santos, and L. W. Brady

Radiotherapy of Intraocular and Orbital Tumors
Edited by W. E. Alberti
and R. H. Sagerman

Interstitial and Intracavitary Thermoradiotherapy
Edited by M. H. Seegenschmiedt
and R. Sauer

Non-Disseminated Breast Cancer
Controversial Issues in Management
Edited by G. H. Fletcher
and S. H. Levitt

Current Topics in Clinical Radiobiology of Tumors
Edited by H.-P. Beck-Bornholdt

Practical Approaches to Cancer Invasion and Metastases
A Compendium of Radiation Oncologists' Responses to 40 Histories
Edited by A. R. Kagan with the
Assistance of R. J. Steckel

Radiation Therapy in Pediatric Oncology
Edited by J. R. Cassady

Radiation Therapy Physics
Edited by A. R. Smith

Late Sequelae in Oncology
Edited by J. Dunst and R. Sauer

Mediastinal Tumors. Update 1995
Edited by D.E. Wood
and C.R. Thomas, Jr.

Thermoradiotherapy and Thermochemotherapy

Volume 1:
Biology, Physiology, and Physics

Volume 2:
Clinical Applications
Edited by M. H. Seegenschmiedt,
P. Fessenden, and C. C. Vernon

Carcinoma of the Prostate
Innovations in Management
Edited by Z. Petrovich,
L. Baert, and L.W. Brady

Radiation Oncology of Gynecological Cancers
Edited by H. W. Vahrson

Carcinoma of the Bladder
Innovations in Management
Edited by Z. Petrovich,
L. Baert, and L. W. Brady

Blood Perfusion and Microenvironment of Human Tumors
Implications for Clinical Radiooncology
Edited by M. Molls and P. Vaupel

Radiation Therapy of Benign Diseases. A Clinical Guide
2nd Revised Edition
S. E. Order and S. S. Donaldson

Carcinoma of the Kidney and Testis, and Rare Urologic Malignancies
Innovations in Management
Edited by Z. Petrovich,
L. Baert, and L. W. Brady

Progress and Perspectives in the Treatment of Lung Cancer
Edited by P. Van Houtte, J. Klastersky,
and P. Rocmans

Combined Modality Therapy of Central Nervous System Tumors
Edited by Z. Petrovich, L. W. Brady,
M. L. Apuzzo, and M. Bamberg

Age-Related Macular Degeneration
Current Treatment Concepts
Edited by W. A. Alberti, G. Richards,
and R. H. Sagerman

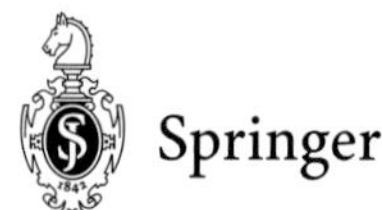

Printing and Binding: Stürtz AG, Würzburg